RECENT ADVANCES IN THEORIES AND PRACTICE OF CHINESE MEDICINE

Edited by **Haixue Kuang**

Recent Advances in Theories and Practice of Chinese Medicine
Edited by Haixue Kuang

Published by InTech
Janeza Trdine 9, 51000 Rijeka, Croatia

Publishing Process Manager Ivona Lovric

Technical Editor Teodora Smiljanic

Cover Designer InTech Design Team

Additional hard copies can be obtained from orders@intechopen.com

Recent Advances in Theories and Practice of Chinese Medicine, Edited by Haixue Kuang
p. cm.
ISBN 978-953-307-903-5

Meet the editor

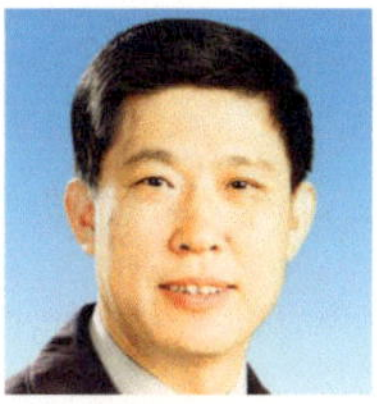

Prof. Kuang Haixue is the Director of the laboratory Chinese Materia Medica (Heilongjiang University of Chinese Medicine, Ministry of Education). He graduated from the Meiji Pharmaceutical University, obtaining his PhD in the field of pharmaceutical chemistry. So far he has been awarded a number of honorary titles for his contributions to Traditional Chinese Medicine (TCM) development in China, including: state-level teaching; winner of the State Council Special Allowance; supervisor of National Excellent Doctoral Dissertation; member of the China Pharmacopoeia Committee; China Food and Drug Administration's Commissioner's special citation, and China new drug appraisal expert. Prof. Kuang is always engaged in Chinese Medicine research and has acquired a significant number of achievements in natural product research, theory of TCM property, and creative drugs. He has led many multidisciplinary research programs and published over 50 scientific papers in international journals in the TCM filed. His current research interests are focused on the theory of TCM property, notably the discovery approach for new drug research and development based on the theory of TCM property. He is also an editorial member on many journals such as Chinese Medicine, Chinese Journal of Natural Medicine, Chinese Herbal Medicine, Chinese Traditional Patent Medicine, Drug Standards of China, Chinese Journal of Experimental Traditional Medical Formulae, and so on.

Contents

Preface

During recent years, traditional Chinese medicine (TCM) has attracted the attention of researchers all over the world. With rich history in China, it is looked upon not only as a bright pearl, but also a treasure house of ancient Chinese culture. TCM has made a great contribution to the health of Chinese people for thousands of years, and it became an independent medical system within world medicine as a result of its special clinical effects, a rational theoretical system and rich practical experience. TCM is holistic medicine guided by a systematic theoretical background, based on the harmony between human and nature, emphasizing equilibrium and balance, and focusing on the state of a functioning system and the normal function of the human organism, which is viewed as the integral entity.

Although TCM at present is based on phytochemistry and pharmacology research, this study provides an example for TCM modernization with certain research ideas. In fact, it has followed the research methods common to that of western medicine. From the TCM theory of the system, the unique character of TCM has not been fully and correctly explained. It is extremely essential to clarify the role of TCM theory, principles of TCM and material basis. In a manner of speaking, this is an effective way to develop TCM industry in the direction of TCM theory using the idea of modern science. This leads us to conclude that Chinese medicine is a subject area with high potential and the possibility for original innovation. So, it is necessary to discuss practical application, promotion and worldwide spreading of TCM knowledge. Moreover, it presents a new chance and challenge for the TCM industry. Keeping all that in mind, we wrote the book Recent Advances in Theories and Practice of Chinese Medicine. It is divided into four sections: the basic theories of TCM, clinical practice, pharmacological experimental research and pharmacodynamic material base research.

In order to ensure a better understanding of the contents of this Chinese medicine book, we have recognized that different readers have different needs and desires. The authors of this book comprise an international group of recognized researchers who possess abundant clinical knowledge and research background due to their years of practicing TCM. During the process of compiling this book, we have consulted with a variety of specialists to collect advice and suggestions and also to summarize their experience by presenting a collection of effective treatments. We have also referenced a large number of national and international documents that analyze and explore the subject based on current research results. I recommend the book to either those who have recently embarked on TCM research work or to those who are considering it. The book may also be valuable to those who are just starting out as academics and are new to research practice. It discusses many often neglected important issues, such as the theory of TCM property, and how to carry out TCM research in the direction of TCM property theory using modern scientific technology.

Hopefully, this book will help our readers gain a deeper understanding of the unique characteristics of Chinese medicine, its application, diagnosis and treatment in all fields. We also aim to bridge the gap between the methods of Chinese medicine and modern biomedicine through the discussion of integrative treatment approaches. We believe that it will provide authoritative and cutting-edge information about TCM research. Recent Advance in Theories and Practice of Chinese Medicine has the objective of providing a platform for all who concentrate their efforts on the modernization of TCM.

Prof. Kuang Haixue
Key Laboratory of Chinese Materia Medica,
Heilongjiang University of Chinese Medicine,
Ministry of Education,
Harbin,
China

Introductory Chapter

Haixue Kuang
Key Laboratory of Chinese Materia Medica (Heilongjiang University of Chinese Medicine), Ministry of Education, Harbin
China

1. Introduction

The long-term clinical practice of traditional Chinese medicine (TCM) confirms its importance and essential role in the health care system in China, especially in the prevention and treatment of chronic diseases [1]. TCM is not only looked upon as a bright pearl, but also a treasure house in Chinese ancient culture. TCM has made great contribution to the health of Chinese people for thousands of years, and it became an independent medical system in world medical field with its special clinical effect, rational theory system and rich practice experience [2]. TCM is the holistic medicine under the guidance of system theory, emphasizing harmony between human and nature, focusing on equilibrium and balance, and focusing on state of functional system and normal function of the human organism viewing it as the integral entity. TCM is based on the Chinese philosophy of Yin-Yang and Five Elements. The oldest classic of TCM is *Huangdi Neijing* (Inner Canon of Huangdi or the Yellow Emperor's Medicine Classic), which was written around 2300 years ago. The basic theory of TCM includes five-zang organs and six-fu organs, qi (vital energy), blood, and meridians. TCM is based on the holistic principles and emphasizes harmony with the universe. It categorizes the causes of diseases into two groups: external causes and internal causes. It differentiates syndromes according to the eight principles (yin, yang, exterior, interior, cold, heat, deficiency (*xu*) and excess (*shi*)). Besides, the theory of TCM property is also one of the basic theories of the science of TCM. It is the connection between the TCM theory and the clinic. The interpreting of the scientific meaning of TCM property is one of the critical problems for the modernization process of TCM. It mainly includes four properties, five flavors, toxicity, and raising, lowering, floating, and sinking.

Although, TCM at present is based on the phytochemistry and the pharmacology research, this study provides an example for the modernization of TCM with certain research ideas. In fact, it has followed the study of Western medicine research method [3]. Nowadays, though a large number of young researchers are engaged in the study of TCM, some are deviating from unique characteristics of Chinese medicine. With the developing of their research work, people come to realize the importance of TCM characteristics, and begin to lay more emphasis on its special clinical effect, rational theory system and rich practice experience. Otherwise, the essential character of the role of TCM cannot be fully and correctly explained. It is essential to clarify the role of TCM theory, principles of TCM and material basis. In a manner of speaking, this is an effective way to develop TCM industry in the direction of TCM theory with the idea of modern scientific technology. This leads us to conclude that Chinese medicine is the subject area with the most potentiality and the possibility for original innovation. So, it is necessary for discussing practical application, promotion and worldwide spreading of TCM knowledge. Moreover, there is a new chance and challenge for the TCM industry.

2. Discussion

Chinese medicines have been attracting interest and acceptance in many countries. An estimated 1.5 billion people now use these preparations worldwide. This may be primarily because of the general belief that herbal drugs are without any side effect besides being cheap and locally available [4]. The abundant philosophical connotation of TCM, its profound cultural foundation, and its integration with great wisdom of the world are still amazing the world. TCM theories are originated from the profound experiences and understanding of ancient Chinese medicine practitioners. As far as I am concerned, digging TCM theories is able to effectively break through the bottleneck of the development of Chinese medicine. In order to make sufficient use of the advantages of TCM, it is essential to clarify the role of TCM theory, principles of TCM and material basis. In that case, we wrote this book *Recent Advances in Theories and Practice of Chinese Medicine* with 26 chapters. It is divided into four sections, namely, basic theories of TCM, clinical practice, pharmacological experimental research and pharmacodynamic material base research, respectively. Next, we make a briefly introduction of these four sections by several representative chapters, respectively.

2.1 Studies on basic theories of TCM

2.1.1 Metabonomics research of the four properties in TCM based on UPLC-QTOF-MS

The theory of TCM property is an important part of theories of TCM. It is one of the basic theories of the science of TCM, which is composed of multiple contents. It mainly includes four properties(Si Xing), five flavors(Wu Wei), channel tropism (Guijing), toxicity, and raising, lowering, floating and sinking (Sheng Jiang Fu Chen). It is the connection between the TCM theory and the clinic. The interpreting of the scientific meaning of TCM property is one of the critical problems for the modernization process of TCM. In TCM, diagnosis and medication are based on "Syndrome" ("ZHENG" in Chinese Mandarin), which can be regarded as a profile of symptom combination, or clinical phenotypes, such as Cold or Hot Syndrome, and "Hot medication curing Cold Syndrome and Cold medication curing Hot Syndrome" is a standard therapeutic guide line. This classical systems medicine at the macro level has been validated and developed by its repeated clinical practice for thousands of years. Hot and Cold medication are the four properties of Chinese medicinal herbs, precisely including cold, hot, warm and cool, which are also called the four natures or "four xing" in TCM. Cold-cool and warm-hot are two completely opposite categories of natures, whereas cold and cool or hot and warm differ in the degree. Chinese medicinal herbs with cold and cool nature can clear away heat, purge fire and eliminate toxic materials, which are mainly used for heat-syndrome; while with hot and warm nature have the actions of expelling cold, which are mainly used for cold syndrome. The four natures are summarized mainly from the body's response. On the base of syndrome differentiation theory, only distinguish heat or cold nature of disease, and have a good understanding of the cold or hot property of TCM, so selectively apply corresponding medicinal herbs that you could achieve the desired effect.

The theories of TCM are so broad and profound, and considered the civilization treasure of China. The four properties, the essence and important component of TCM theories, the high generalization on the basic property and typical characteristics of TCM, are a significant theoretical foundation for the clinical use of Chinese medicine. In recent 30 years more and more reports on the four natures of TCM have appeared in the literature. To date several aspects of research such as the characteristics of thermodynamics, the changes of nervous system and the endocrine glands, energy metabolism, the systems biology analysis include genome, transcriptome, proteome, and metabolome are all supposed to explored the macro and micro framework on the four properties, among which metabonomics is the most novel tool. It is a rapidly growing area of scientific research, which has been widely used in disease diagnosis, biomarker discovery, and research into the disease mechanisms.

Metabonomics is an emerging subject of the post-genome era, which, together with genomics, transcriptomics and proteomics, jointly constitutes the 'Systems Biology'. Metabonomics is the branch of science concerned with the quantitative understandings of the metabolite component of integrated living systems and its dynamic responses to the changes of both endogenous factors (such as physiology and development) and exogenous factors (such as environmental factors and xenobiotics). Recently, as a novel systemic approach to study metabolic profile and accelerate the course of drug development, metabonomics has achieved great growth, which is attracting more and more concerns from the academic community [5]. Metabolite or metabolic profiling, the compositional analysis of low molecular-weight (MW) species in biological samples (urine, plasma and serum), has been in existence for at least 35 years and has traditionally used mass spectrometry (MS) coupled to some modern separation technique such as ultra-performance liquid chromatography (UPLC) and gas chromatography (GC) for resolution and detection [6]. Integrity of metabonomic processes includes sample collection and pretreatment, data collection and analysis, and metabolic variation interpretation.

In this study, UPLC-QTOF-MS techniques coupled to metabonomics methods were used to prove the existence of the four properties in TCM, to illustrate its multi-component, multi-target, multi-channel and the complex mechanism. Metabonomics aims to assess metabolic changes in a comprehensive and global manner in order to infer biological functions and provide the detailed biochemical responses of cellular systems. We successfully established predict models based on cold and hot medicines as references. To estimate the predictive ability of our model, we used herb-Flos Datura to cross-validation, and excellent separation among the TCM varieties obtained by OPLS-DA, which a hot medication belonging to the hot medication group, are presented in terms of recognition and prediction abilities. It represented the percentage of the samples correctly classified during model training and cross-validation, respectively, while the prediction ability was only qualitative rather than quantitative.

This chapter is aimed at guiding researchers to understand a new way of drug discovery based on the theory of TCM property. More commonly, some researchers focused on traditional chemical constituents and ignore many other effective ones in TCM so that the characteristics of TCM were seriously lost. Also, it could be applied to explore Western medicine properties to effectively guide the clinical application. Considering the encouraging results obtained in this study, it seems to be very promising approach to apply metabonomics for further study on theory of TCM property.

2.1.2 An approach to the nature of Qi in TCM-Qi and bioenergy

TCM has been practiced for more than five thousand years, is a complete ancient medical system that takes a deep understanding of the laws and patterns of nature and applies them to the human body. TCM believes that the human body is a microcosm of the Universal macrocosm. Therefore, humans must follow the laws of the Universe to achieve harmony and total health. Even today TCM practitioners use these essential theories to understand, diagnose and treat health problems. In TCM, "harmony" is the ultimate goal. So, when nature's Qi undergoes change as it does seasonally, a person's internal Qi will respond automatically. If, for any reason, it can't make a smooth transition to the energy of the next season, TCM understands that illness will result. Often Western Complementary and Alternative Medicine (CAM) practitioners and their patients or clients derive their understanding of TCM from acupuncture. However, acupuncture is only one of the major treatment modalities of this comprehensive medical system based on the understanding of Qi or vital energy. These major treatment modalities are Qigong, herbal therapy, acupuncture, foods for healing and Chinese psychology.

Meridians, or channels, are invisible pathways through which Qi flows that form an energy network that connects all parts of the body, and the body to the universe. The ancient medical text 'The Yellow Emperor's Inner Canon (Nei Jing)' states: "The function of the channel (meridian) is to transport the Qi and blood, and circulate yin and yang to nourish the body". The energy practice of Qigong, with its postures and movements, also affects the flow of Qi. The energy pathways and the Organ Systems they link provide TCM with a framework for identifying the root cause of health problems and the diagnoses to heal them. Meridians work by regulating the energy functions of the body and keeping it in harmony. If Qi stagnates for too long in any meridian, it can become blocked and eventually turn into matter, setting the stage for conditions that can create a physical mass. TCM Meridian Theory states: "As long as Qi flows freely through the meridians and the Organs work in harmony, the body can avoid disease".

The study of Qi phenomena in this Chapter may help bridge some of the apparent difference between Western and Eastern culture. This chapter covered the nature of Qi as well as its philosophical aspects and the significance in the modern civilization because the true foundation of TCM is Qi.

2.1.3 A geomedical approach to Chinese medicine: The origin of the yin-yang symbol

This chapter shows how to compute Yin and Yang for different latitudes so traditional Chinese herbalists can quantify the efficacy of herbal drugs. Based on daylight hours, the chapter provides a simple formula that allows computation of Yin and Yang for each day of the year. Moreover, using daily Yin and Yang values, the chapter shows how to render the Yin-Yang symbol properly in accordance with its original meaning. Considering the importance of Yin and Yang in TCM, the rendering method presented in this chapter provides evidence that TCM, in its origin, is a geomedical science.

Herbal medicines collected from different geographic locations can significantly differ in their therapeutic efficacy. The concentration of bioactive substances varies depending on many local factors, such as sunshine hours or chemical and physical properties of the soil. To guarantee the optimal composition of herbal drugs, Chinese herbalists use "geo-authentic" herbs from recognized locations. However, it is often difficult to confirm geographical authenticity. The lack of formal models for Yin and Yang, and herbal efficacy in general, complicates objective comparisons and evaluations. Herbalists and practitioners of TCM need a better formal understanding of the Yin-Yang composition of each herb. This chapter contributes to the solution to this problem by providing a formal description of Yin and Yang. It shows in a mathematical way how Yin and Yang vary depending on latitude. The latitude of a herb's location determines the number of daylight hours and sunshine the herb is exposed to during the year. The number of daylight hours is one of the components affecting the concentration and composition of bioactive substances and therefore the efficacy of the herb. To standardize herbal preparation and administration, rigorous mathematical methods are essential to measure the Yin-Yang composition of herbs quantitatively. The work presented in this chapter is a first step towards such standardization.

2.2 Clinical practice of TCM

2.2.1 A comparison study on arterial blood pressure and pulse data of condenser microphone

As a pilot study to investigate the relationship between Chinese and modern medicines with microphone pressure sensor, we conduct a cross analysis of pulse data measured by microphone sensor and intra-arterial catheter, and Electrical CardiaoGram (ECG.). Unlike the ABP and ECG data, which are widely applied in most modern hospitals, the microphone data acquisition system is noninvasive and is easy to construct. It uses the commercial microphone, the software and hardware built in a personal or notebook computer and the data analysis of time series data. The measuring point of the microphone data should have prominent feeling of pulse when one touches his forefinger's tip to the wrist skin. Then, one just firmly presses the front head of the small microphone to the point. Since a commercial electret condenser microphone is generally very sensitive, the time series data can be successfully picked up. This measuring technique is closely related to the ancient Chinese diagnostic technique via three fingers.

As to the post processing, a fast and diffusive filter is first used to remove the trend of all the data. The remaining part is just the Fourier spectrum of the periodic part of the time series because the fast filter is carried out on the spectral domain. By imposing a Gaussian window, the band-pass- limited spectra are obtained and the corresponding results of applying the inverse Fast Fourier Transforms (FFT) is the real part of the wavelet coefficient. Then, using the Hilbert transform, the energy or amplitude of the spectral bands is evaluated. The cross correlation coefficients of the real part between the ECG, ABP, and microphone data are separately calculated with the spectral center of the Gaussian window scans over the range of 0.1 to 10 Hz which are corresponding to several organ-meridian modes. Six test cases in an intensive care unit were examined. Most numerical results show that the microphone data is related to ABP data in the real part correlation in the spectral region around the heart rate mode. The similarity between two spectrograms is considered to have the partial energy correlation. It seems that all the test cases are not in critical situations because ABP to ECG or microphone data to ECG are either correlated or partially correlated and all of them still alive. Although the sample size does not achieve a reasonable statistical level, these limited cases show that the Chinese and modern medicines are closely related to each other.

In this Chapter, the ECG signals were obtained from the three-lead ECG recording device. The ABP signals were conveyed from an invasive arterial-line system which involves an insertion of an arterial catheter connecting to a conducting tube filled with properly pressured fluid. The mechanical signals were then transformed to the electrical ones with a midway pressure transducer. Both ECG and ABP data were transferred back to the Philips MP60 module which was the physiological signal monitoring system used in our study. The analog signals were output to the data acquisition card where they would be converted to the digital signals with a sampling rate of 500Hz and then forwarded to the portable computer for further analysis.

If we can prove that the microphone arterial signal's heart rate mode can be used to provide the index, the preventive medicine would become a practical issue for the general population. Moreover, the connection between the ancient Chinese and modern medicines will become more solid in near future.

2.2.2 Hyperspectral imaging technology used in tongue diagnosis

Among the four diagnostic processes of TCM: inspection, auscultation and olfaction, inquiry, and pulse feeling and palpation, the examination of tongue is one of the most important approaches for getting significant evidences in diagnosing the patient's health conditions. However, owing to its drawbacks in quantification and standardization, the development of tongue diagnosis is stagnated. Computerized methods for TCM allow researchers to identify required information more efficiently, discover new relationships which are obscured by merely focusing on Western medicine, and bridge the gaps between Western Medicine and TCM. Therefore, getting the overall information about tongue surface is very important for computerized tongue diagnosis system. In this chapter, an an acousto-optic tunable filter (AOTF) based hyperspectral tongue imaging system (THIS) which can capture hyperspectral images of human tongue at a series of wavelengths is developed and used in tongue diagnosis. The basic principles and instrumental systems of the new system, the data pre-processing method as well as some applications are presented. Compared with the pushbroom hyperspectral tongue imager used in our previous works, this new type of hyperspectral tongue imaging system has the advantage of having no moving parts and can be scanned at very high rates. As the hyperspectral tongue images can provide more information than the traditional charge coupled device CCD based images, we can find some successful applications in computerized tongue diagnosis such as tongue body segmentation, tongue colour analysis and discrimination, tongue cracks extraction and classification, sublingual veins analysis, etc. Preliminary experiments show that the AOTF-based hyperspectral tongue imaging system is superior to the traditional CCD based methods because the hyperspectral images can provide more information about the tongue surface. In future studies, we will extract the quantitative features of the tongue surface and find some methods to model the relationship between these features and certain diseases.
The new system can capture image scenes in contiguous but narrow spectral bands under the control of the AOTF controller. The hyperspectral tongue images provided by the instrument can be visualized as a 3D cube because of its intrinsic structure, where the cube face is a function of the spatial coordinates and the depth is a function of wavelength. In this case, each spatial point on the face is characterized by its own spectrum (often called spectral signature). This spectrum is directly corresponds to the amount of energy that the tongue represented, as hyperspectral sensors commonly utilize the simple fact that a tongue can emits light in certain frequency bands. Consequently, the hyperspectral tongue image data provides a wealth of information about an image scene which is potentially very helpful to tongue diagnosis.

2.2.3 Advances in Chinese medicine diagnosis: From traditional methods to computational models

Although Chinese and Western physicians were not distinct in their conceptual framework, their respective medical practices evolved on different cultures and historical contexts. Therefore, it is expected that the advances on medical knowledge represent this cultural divergence.

Many efforts have been made to integrate the ancient, traditional knowledge of Chinese medicine into contemporary, Eastern medical practice. Diagnosis is the key element in this integration of medical systems since it links the patient's needs to the available therapeutic resources. The art of Chinese medicine diagnosis was enriched throughout history but it main traditional aspect remains unchanged: the exclusive use of information available to the naked senses. Clinical information provided by vision, hearing, smelling, and touching is interpreted in a framework of Chinese medicine theories of physiology. No equipment or instrument was developed with specific diagnostic purposes or based on Chinese medicine theories. However, advances in computation and biomedical instruments allowed more powerful analysis of clinical data and quantification of parameters otherwise assessed only in a qualitative fashion. As a consequence, computer models for diagnosis in Chinese medicine were developed and tested in the last few decades and are promising tools in the clinical environment.

This chapter introduces the traditional methods of diagnosis in Chinese medicine and introduces their evolution into computational models. Current methods for validation of computational model by the assessment of their diagnostic accuracy and possible sources of errors are also presented. Finally, perspectives on the issue of computational diagnosis are discussed.

2.3 Pharmacological experimental research

2.3.1 Effects of vasoactive Chinese herbs on the endothelial NO system

Nitric oxide (NO) produced by the endothelial NO synthase (eNOS) plays a protective role in the vasculature. It is a potent vasodilator and protects blood vessels from thrombosis by inhibiting platelet aggregation and adhesion. In addition, endothelial NO possesses multiple anti-atherosclerotic properties. Interestingly, the purported effects of "circulation-improving" herbs used in TCM show striking similarities with the vascular actions of eNOS-derived NO. Therefore, we hypothesized that part of the pharmacological effects of such TCM herbs may be mediated by NO.

This Chapter studied the effects of 17 Chinese herbs with potential effects on the vasculature, and have identified *Salviae miltiorrhizae radix*, *Zizyphi spinosae semen* and *Prunella vulgaris* L. as potent eNOS-upregulating agents. In cultured human endothelial cells, aqueous extracts of these herbs increased eNOS promoter activity, eNOS mRNA and protein expression, as well as NO production in a concentration- and time-dependent manner. In addition, we have studied the constituents from the abovementioned Chinese herbs and have found that ursolic acid and betulinic acid are capable of enhancing eNOS gene expression. More recently, we have found that betulinic acid also stimulated NO production through post-translational mechanisms. By enhancing eNOS phosphorylation at serine 1177 and dephosphorylation at threonine 495, betulinic acid also increases eNOS enzymatic activity. In summary, we have described the pharmacological effects of Chinese herbs on endothelial NO system and have identified some active compounds from these plants. By performing modern pharmacological studies, we have provided some molecular mechanisms that may partially explain the therapeutic effects described in TCM.

2.3.2 Traditional Chinese herbal medicine – East meets West in validation and therapeutic application

The holistic views of TCM generally have no conflicts with the western medicine, perhaps they were just expressed in different terms. Western medicine is usually more concrete in diagnosis and judgment. Treatment is often quicker, particularly in acute cases, and surgery is its strength. Its weak points are that it sees disease as something to be measured and quantified and often ignores the psychological, social and behavioral factors involved in illness. Chinese medicine, on the other hand, can be too flexible and too general where diagnosis and judgment are concerned, and sometimes relies too heavily on the individual practitioner's experiences. Its strong points are its highly flexible approach, which enabling treatments to be changed as the patient improve, and its emphasis on preventive medicine. The Chinese way tends to treat the whole body rather than to try to isolate a particular infected area. And, finally, the herbs themselves, compared with chemically produced medicines, are relatively cheap and easy to use. They have minimal side-effects, and most have been tried and tested for over many thousand years. Western medicine focuses more on symptomatic management, whereas TCM focuses more on cause and effect. Western medicine is more useful for first-aid and surgical interventions, whereas TCM is more useful in treating internal and chronic illnesses. An ideal health care system should be established to concern people's physical and mental health, to deal with all personal problems, and to improve people's quality of life. A new model of health care should be composed by a different medical system to provide a holistic approach. TCM, today as an alternative and complementary medicine should be included into the conventional medicine to form the new modern medicine. This is in line with the aim of the WHO to promote recognition of traditional medicine and to support its integration into the mainstream health service. There is space of integration for TCM and modern medicine. A new paradigm for developing medicine is needed, and Chinese medicine could make a significant contribution in this field. To achieve such integration, modern science and technology had to be used to study the action, efficacy and toxicity of Chinese medicines. Although, there are many issues to concern, especially safe and effectiveness, some compromise and agreement are needed.

Thus botanicals should be defined, authenticated and documented as to their source and conditions of cultivation using modern methodology. Manufacturing and preparation processes of Chinese medicine should be carefully monitored and standardized. Claims for Chinese medicine should be verified from rigorous controlled trials. Interaction between Western and Chinese medicines should be better studied and information obtained centralized into accessible databases. This would be an enormous undertaking requiring international collaboration and participation of governments worldwide. In fact, the feasibility of herbal validation by using Western methods is well-illustrated. In particular, concerns about identity authentication, quality control, evidences of efficacy and safety of herbal remedies, are being addressed with the modern science and technology, and ultimately allow the gathering of information necessarily to support clinical trials. Along with this route, efforts being played will return with the transition of TCM into a recognized science specialty to fill up the gaps between Eastern and Western medical approaches. In this perspective, it may not be necessary to isolate the active ingredients from herbal remedies or purity them to finally become chemical drugs. To promote the effectiveness, Chinese herbal medicine can remain in formulae but standardizations are needed. Meanwhile, both Chinese and western practitioners should come together and sort out the best treatment they can offer to patients, which very often may be the combination of the modern and Chinese medicine, instead of favoring one over the other. Conventional Western medicine and Chinese medicine should be seen as complementary to each other, rather than as alternatives. Both types of medicine have their advantages and drawbacks, which is why they need to work hand in hand for optimal results. Together, Chinese and Western medicine could form the most effective disease treatment the world has ever known.

2.3.3 Targeting effect of traditional Chinese medicine

Meridian guide drug had the effect of synery and attenuation, and this effect based on concentrated drug at target-site. Meridian guide effect had an close relatiship with drug transporters and metabolism enzyme. Differnert components had different affinity to transporters or enzymes, and meridian guide effect is the combination of all components in meridian guide drug. Therefore, it is necessary to investigate the exact effect of main components of meridian guide drug on transporters and metabolism enzyme, establish the relationship between its dose and its effect as well as effects in kinds of diseases. As we known more about the relatiship among components in meridian guide drug, kinds of transporters and metabolism enzymes, activity in nomal and disease state, we could design target delivery system freely as we like.

2.4 Pharmacodynamic material base research

2.4.1 Therapeutic effects of lignans isolated from schisandra chinesis on hepatic carcinoma

The development of novel therapeutic drugs for hepatic carcinoma is a very important objective in the field of pharmacological research. Among the variety of approaches thus far pursued to develop novel drugs, identification and screening of natural compounds from medical herbs has proven a very effective one—not least, because this method saves a great deal of time and cost. Recently, many institutes and companies in advanced countries have focused on an approach to novel drugs for hepatic carcinoma via the use of various lignins isolated from *S. chinensis.* This chapter introduces three lignans and one blend which may prove valuable in efforts to combat hepatic carcinoma. Gomisin A at high concentration was found to significantly induce anti-proliferative and pro-apoptotic effects in hepatic carcinoma. Schizandrin A markedly increased vincristine-induced hepatic carcinoma apoptosis and anti-tumor activity. Additionally, tigloygomisin H induced the death of hepatic carcinoma cells and inhibited quinone reductase activity. Furthermore, KY88 was a blend composed of 10 herbal extracts and effects a dose-dependent inhibition of hepatocellular carcinoma cellular proliferation. Collectively, the results of this chapter demonstrated that these lignins and the blend from *S. chinensis* were regarded as an anti-cancer drug candidate capable of inducing apoptosis and inhibiting the cell proliferation of hepatocellular carcinoma via a variety of mechanisms.

2.4.2 Separation and quantification of component monosaccharides of polysaccharide extracts from ephedra sinica by MECC with photodiode array detector

TCM polysaccharides with multiple pharmacological activities have recently stimulated the interest of academia and the pharmaceutical industries. In fact, the roles of water-soluble polysaccharides from traditional Chinese medicines in biological processes have been studied with increasing attention over the past recent years because of their broad spectrum of therapeutic properties and relatively low toxicity. Indeed, immunomodulation, anti-tumour, antivirus, anticoagulant, hypoglycaemic, anti-complementary, anti-inflammatory and antioxidation bioactivities have been presented by many polysaccharides extracted from medicinal fungi and plants.

The *Ephedra* plant, or "Mahuang" of traditional Chinese medicine, is one of the oldest medicinal plants known to mankind. More than 45 species of *Ephedra* plants exist and are indigenous to regions of Asia, North, Central and South America and Europe. Mahuang contains ephedrine alkaloids as their principal components, which are primarily localized in

the aerial parts of the plant. In recent years, many herbs used in popular medicine have been reported to contain polysaccharides with a great variety of biological activities and the water-soluble Mahuang polysaccharides are also demonstrated to be one of the main bioactive constituents of *Ephedra* plant except for a series of ephedrine alkaloids. For these reasons, great interest arose on the reliable analytical methods of the Mahuang polysaccharides, which can be used for exploring the new functional products with polysaccharides due to its pharmacological importance and application in the pharmaceutical industry. Immunosuppressive effects of acidic polysaccharides from the stems of *E. sinica* have been demonstrated by carbon clearance test, delayed type hypersensitivity reaction and humoral immune response *in vivo*.
In this chapter, a rapid and sensitive method was optimized and validated for the separation and quantification of derivatized monosaccharides in cold water-soluble polysaccharide extract from the stems of *E. sinica* using 1-phenyl-3-methyl-5 -pyrazolone (PMP) as precolumn derivatization reagent by micellar electrokinetic capillary chromatography (MECC) with photodiode array detector. The separation was carried out on a on an unmodified fused silica capillary and UV detection at 250 nm, and the 8 PMP derivatives of mannose, rhamnose, glucuronic acid, galacturonic acid, glucose, xylose, galactose and arabinose were baseline separated within 12 min.

3. Conclusion

This book may help our readers gain a deeper understanding of unique characteristics of TCM and will bridge the gap between the methods of Chinese medicine and modern biomedicine through the discussion of TCM with advanced instrumental methods. Also, it will be providing cutting-edge information about TCM research including its basic theories, diagnostic approach, current clinical applications, latest advances, and so on. Hopefully, it could play a very important role in disseminating TCM knowledge, promoting TCM influence in the world and accelerating the modernization of TCM.

4. References

[1] Jiang, M., Zhang, C., Cao, H., Chan, K., & Lu, A. The Role of Chinese Medicine in the Treatment of Chronic Diseases in China. *Planta Medica*, 2011, 77, 873-881.

[2] David, M., Eisenberg, Eric, S. J., Harris, Bruce, A. Littlefield, et al. (2011). Developing a library of authenticated Traditional Chinese Medicinal (TCM) plants for systematic biological evaluation -Rationale, methods and preliminary results from a Sino-American collaboration. *Fitoterapia*, 82, 17–33.

[3] Dou,S.S., Liu, R.H., Jiang, P., *et al*. System biology and its application in compound recipe of traditional Chinese medicine study. *Mode Tradit Chin Med Mater Med*, 2008, 10, 116-121.

[4] Li, S.P., Zhao, J., Yang, B. Strategies for quality control of Chinese medicines. *Journal of* Pharmaceutical and Biomedical Analysis 2011, 55, 802-809.

[5] Lao, Y.M., Jiang, J.G., and Yan L. Application of metabonomic analytical techniques in the modernization and toxicology research of traditional Chinese medicine. *British Journal of Pharmacology*, 2009, 157, 1128-1141.

[6] Keun, H.C. Metabonomic modeling of drug toxicity. *Pharmacology & Therapeutics*, 2006, 109, 92-106

Part 1

Basic Theories of TCM

1

Metabonomics Research of the Four Properties in Traditional Chinese Medicine Based on UPLC-QTOF-MS System

Haixue Kuang, Yanyan Wang, Qiuhong Wang,
Bingyou Yang and Yonggang Xia
Key Laboratory of Chinese Materia Medica (Heilongjiang University of Chinese Medicine), Ministry of Education, Harbin, China

1. Introduction

TCM has long been practised as an empirical system and retrieved tens of millions of lives from historically to currently [1]. It is considered as an ancient and classical paradigm of systems biology. In TCM, diagnosis and medication are based on "Syndrome" ("ZHENG" in Chinese Mandarin), which can be regarded as a profile of symptom combination, or clinical phenotypes, such as Cold or Hot Syndrome, and "Hot medication curing Cold Syndrome and Cold medication curing Hot Syndrome" is a standard therapeutic guide line. This classical systems medicine at the macro level has been validated and developed by its repeated clinical practice for thousands of years [2]. Hot and Cold medication are the four properties of Chinese medicinal herbs, precisely including cold, hot, warm and cool, which are also called the four natures or "four xing" in TCM. Cold-cool and warm-hot are two completely opposite categories of natures, whereas cold and cool or hot and warm differ in the degree. Chinese medicinal herbs with cold and cool nature can clear away heat, purge fire and eliminate toxic materials, which are mainly used for heat-syndrome; while with hot and warm nature have the actions of expelling cold, which are mainly used for cold-syndrome. The four natures are summarized mainly from the body's response. On the base of syndrome differentiation theory, only distinguish heat or cold nature of disease, and have a good understanding of the cold or hot property of TCM, so selectively apply corresponding medicinal herbs that you could achieve the desired effect.

Herbal medicine has attracted much attention as a means of alternative therapy along with the orthodox medical system [3, 4]. In recent 30 years more and more reports on the four natures of TCM have appeared in the literature. To date several aspects of research such as the characteristics of thermodynamics, the changes of nervous system and the endocrine glands, energy metabolism, the systems biology analysis include genome, transcriptome, proteome, and metabolome are all supposed to explored the macro and micro framework on the four properties, among which metabonomics is the most novel tool [5]. It is a rapidly growing area of scientific research, which has been widely used in disease diagnosis, biomarker discovery, and research into the disease mechanisms [6-10]. Metabonomics aims at comparing the pattern of endogenous metabolites under defined temporal conditions as comprehensively as possible. In the past few years, widely used analytical techniques in metabonomics were nuclear magnetic resonance spectroscopy (NMR) [11], mass spectrometry in combination with gas chromatography (GC-MS) [12], capillary electrophoresis (CE-MS) [13] and especially liquid chromatography (LC-MS) [14]. Because of the advantages of robust operation and usability, separation with a reversed-phase column is a routine in LC-MS based metabonomic analysis. Advances in mass spectrometric techniques, particularly when linked to liquid chromatography, have resulted in the development of robust methods for low molecular mass organic molecules in biological matrices [15, 16]. Indeed in a preliminary study the potential for LC-MS to detect differences in the composition of urine from control and dosed animals in a properties study of TCM has been demonstrated. Here we describe preliminary studies on the variety of the endogenous metabolite of different herbs.

Metabonomic strategies produces complex data sets, and therefore, the uses of appropriate multivariate statistical and visualization tools are mandatory keys that include efficient and robust methods to model, analyze, and interpret the complex chemical and biological data [21]. In metabonomics studies chemometrics analysis techniques including PCA and OPLS-DA are often used to classify the samples[17]. Loading plots and Variable importance in the Project (VIP) value are commonly used for biomarker selection. Besides, the S-plot also plays an important role in screening for statistically significant compounds. It is a scatter plot which combines the covariance and correlation in loading results.

In this work, we employed a metabonomics strategy based on UPLC-QTOF-MS to discriminate the global urine profiles, and PCA was performed to detect the perturbation metabolites as many as possible. Furthermore, the potential biomarkers were screened out, which might be the target components in the future pathogenesis research, as well as predicted model was builded up using OPLS-DA. One of the intentions is to discuss whether this model is suitable for other herbs. The other purpose is to find potential criterion to evaluate the properties in TCM.

2. Experimental

2.1 Reagents and materials

Acetonitrile (HPLC grade) was purchased from Fisher Scientific (Loughborough, UK); formic acid (HPLC grade) used as mobile phase additives (each of purity ≥ 99%), were supplied by Sigma-Aldrich (MO, USA); the distilled water was purified by a Milli-Q system (Millipore, MA, USA); Pentobarbital sodium was purchased from the Shanghai Chemical Agent Company of China Medicine Clique (Shanghai, China); Leucine-enkephalin was obtained from Sigma-Aldrich (MO, USA).

The six crude drugs, Rhizoma Coptidis, Radix Scutellariae, Cortex Phellodendri, Radix Aconiti Lateralis Preparata, Rhizoma Zingiberis Pricklyash Peel and Flos Datura were purchased from the Harbin Tongrentang Drugstore and were authenticated by Professor Zhenyue Wang of the Department of Pharmacognosy, Heilongjiang University of Chinese Medicine. The crude drugs were refluxed extraction with distilled water two times for an hour each time. The extracts of the six herbs were filtered and concentrated, their concentrations were shown in Table 1, and stored in 4°C for animal experimental usage.

2.2 Animals and dosing

Male Sprague-Dawley rats (n = 8 per group), approx. 220 g in weight, were allowed to acclimatize in metabolism cages for 5 days prior to treatment. Food and water was provided ad libitum. The whole procedure of administration for each group was shown in Table 1. Urine was collected every other day (7:00 pm-7:00 am) from metabolism cages at ambient temperature throughout the whole procedure and centrifuged at 12,000 rpm at 4°C for 10 min, and then the supernatants were aliquot into eppendorf tubes with 1.5 mL urine in each stored at -20°C until analysis. In the exploratory study, in order to improve the matching rate of subjects, all groups were male. And there were no diet while drink free in the sample collection.

No.	Groups	Concentrations of crude drugs (g/ml)	Administration dosage (g/kg)
1	control	-	-
2	Rhizoma Coptidis	0.35	7.0
3	Radix Scutellariae	0.30	6.0
4	Cortex Phellodendri	0.42	8.4
5	Radix Aconiti Lateralis Preparata	0.525	10.5
6	Rhizoma Zingiberis	0.42	8.4
7	Pricklyash Peel	0.20	4.0

Table 1. The whole procedure of administration for each group, mean±SD, n = 8.

2.3 UPLC-QTOF-MS

2.3.1 Reversed-phase liquid chromatography

Urine samples were centrifuged again at 12,000 rpm for 10 min at 4°C, the supernatants were transferred to autosampler vials for analysis. The autosampler was maintained at a temperature of 4°C for the duration of the analysis. The UPLC-MS analysis was performed on a Waters ACQUITY™ UPLC system (Waters Corporation, MA, USA). Separation was achieved on an ACQUITY UPLC™ BEH C_{18} column (50 mm×2.1 mm, i.d., 1.7 μm) maintained at 40 °C. The column was eluted with a linear gradient of 2-40 % B over 0-8.0 min, 40-98 % B over 8.0-10.0 min, 98-2 % B over 10.0-12.0 min and kept at 2% B for 2 min, the composition was held at a flow rate of 600 μl/min, where mobile phase A consisted of 0.1% formic acid in demonized water and mobile phase B consisted of 0.1% formic acid in acetonitrile. The injection volume was 2 μl and the gradient duration was 14 min. A blank was analyzed between every five samples to wash the column.

2.3.2 Mass spectrometry

A Waters Xevo quadrupole time-of-flight Mass Spectrometer (Manchester, UK) equipped with an electrospray ionization (ESI) source was used to collect metabolic profiling. Mass spectrometry was operated in the positive ion mode, according to our preliminary experiments for determination of system, the optimal conditions were as follows: capillary voltage of 3.0 kV, cone voltage of 40 V, source temperature of 120°C and desolvation temperature of 400°C. Nitrogen was used as the desolvation and cone gas with the flow rate of

800 and 50 L/h, respectively. The data acquisition rate was set to 0.2 s with a 0.02 s interscan delay. The scan range was from 100 to 1000 *m/z*. All analyses were acquired by using the lock spray to ensure accuracy and reproducibility, leucine-enkephalin was used as the lock mass at a concentration of 400 pg/ml in acetonitrile (0.1% formic acid): H_2O (0.1% formic acid) for the positive ion mode ($[M+H]^+$ = 556.2771). Data were collected in pareto mode, the lock spray frequency was set at 1 s and the lock mass data were averaged over 10 scans for correction. A "purge-wash-purge" cycle was employed on the autosampler with 90% aqueous formic acid used for the wash solvent and 0.1% aqueous formic acid used as the purge solvent.
For the further identification of potential markers, a mass spectrometric data were collected in full scan auto mode from 0 to 14 min in positive ion mode. In the MS/MS experiments, the conditions were the same as above except the collision energy was set from 15 to 30 eV for each analyte.

2.4 Data processing and statistical analysis

UPLC-MS data were analyzed with the MassLynx software version V4.1 (Waters Corporation, Milford, USA). Before multivariate statistical analysis, the data of each sample was normalized to total area to correct for the MS response shift from the first injection to the last injection due to the long duration, overnight or longer, of an LC-MS analysis in metabonomics studies. The main parameters were set as follows: retention time range 1-9 min, mass range 100-1000, mass tolerance 0.05, mass window 0.05, retention time window 0.20, noise elimination level 6. the MarkerLynx Application Manager (Waters Corporation, Milford, USA) was used for the peak detection and the EZinfo software was used for PCA and OPLS-DA. Pareto scaling was used in all the models to avoid chemical noise. Potential biomarkers were selected according to Variable importance in the Project (VIP) value, the loading plot and the S-plot. For the identification of potential markers, the following databases have been used: HMDB (http://www.hmdb.ca/), METLIN (http://metlin.scripps.edu/), Massbank (http://www.massbank.jp), PubChem (http://ncbi.nim.nih.gov/) and KEGG (http://www.kegg.com/).

3. Results

3.1 UPLC-QTOF-MS method development

In this study, non-targeted analyses of Urine samples metabolic components were performed. As there was no specific group of target analyses, some generic settings had to be applied both to LC separation and MS detection during the method development, in order to obtain urine metabolic profiling containing as many compounds as possible. UPLC employs smaller stationary phase particle size column, generating high efficiency to the separation, which concurrently increases resolution and sensitivity. All urine metabolites were eluted in 14 min and full scan was set in the positive ion mode because it gave more information rich data than negative ion mode. For LC-MS-based metabonomics, the stability of analytical system is one of the most important factors to obtain the valid data. Extracted ion chromatographic peaks of seven ions (m/z 105.04, 154.02, 267.08, 271.08, 338.04, 340.03 and 675.13 in positive ion mode) were selected for method validation. Method repeatability was evaluated by five replicate analysis of a urine sample. The relative standard deviations (R.S.D.s%) of peak areas and retention times were estimated to be 1.14-3.52% and 0.445-1.36%, respectively. The stability of sample was tested by analyzing a sample left at autosampler (maintained at 4 ℃) for 4, 8, 12 and 24 h. The R.S.D.s% of peak areas were from

4.58% to 7.54%. These results demonstrated the excellent stability and reproducibility of chromatographic separation and mass measurement during the whole sequence [18].

3.2 Chemometric analysis

3.2.1 Metabolic profiling analysis

The positive ion base peak intensity (BPI) chromatograms of urine samples collected from representative rats for each of the different groups are presented in Fig. 1 Urine samples on the 30th day from each group were used for UPLC-MS analysis. Some differences could be visually noted among these chromatograms.

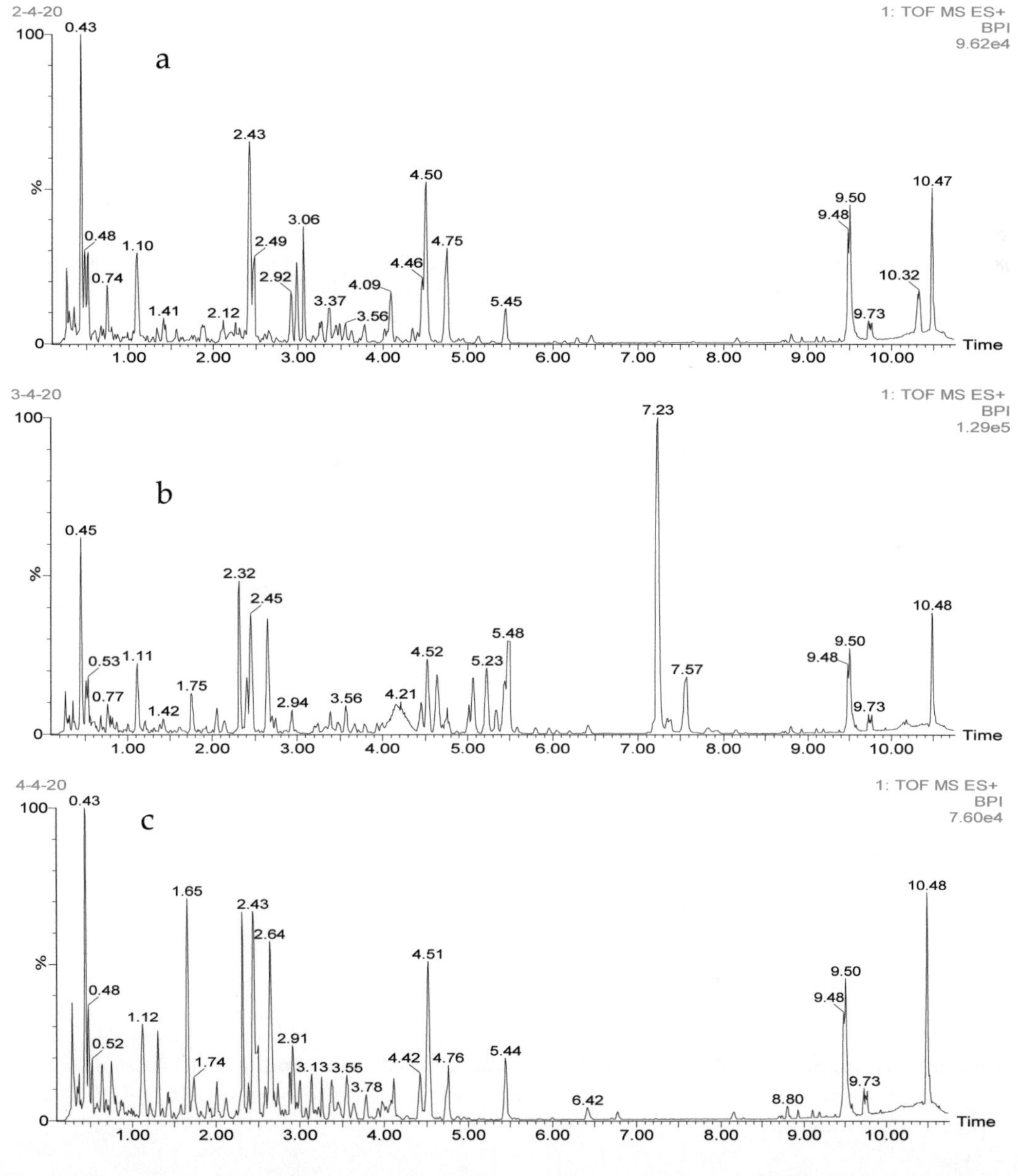

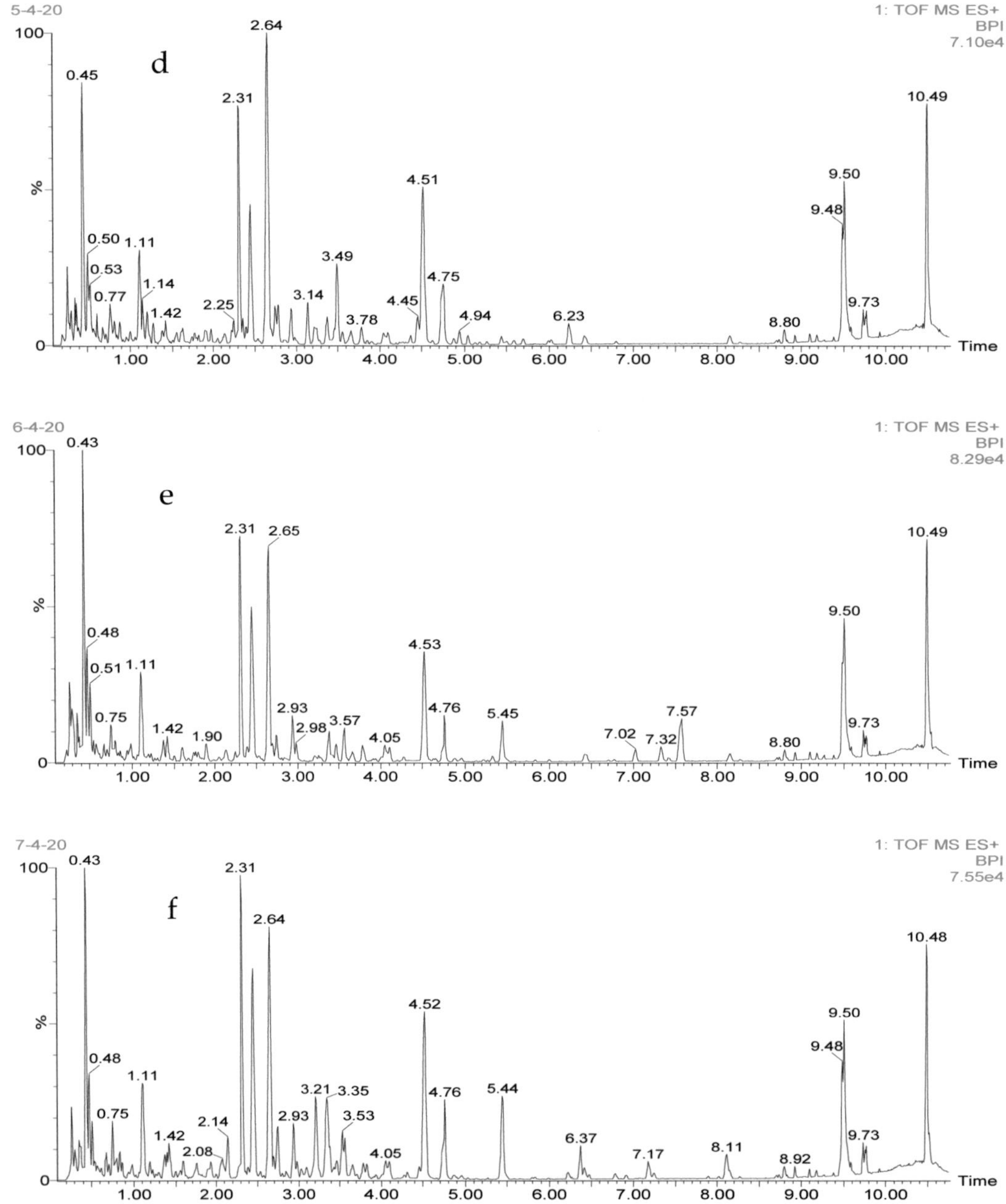

Fig. 1. BPI chromatograms of (a) Rhizoma Coptidis, (b) Radix Scutellariae, (c) Cortex Phellodendri, (d) Radix Aconiti Lateralis Preparata (e) Rhizoma Zingiberis (f) Rhizoma Zingiberis and Pricklyash Peel groups urine samples on the last day analyzed by UPLC-MS in positive ESI mode.

3.2.2 PCA analysis

In order to clearly differentiate among groups, unsupervised pattern recognition PCA was used for analyzing the chromatographic data. PCA is a bilinear decomposition method that allows original data to be reduced to a few principal components while retaining the features that contribute most to the variance. It does not require any prior knowledge of class membership and was used here to detect any inherent trends within the data and to identify potential markers. The urinary data was subjected to EZinfo software, PCA score plots separated urine samples into different blocks, and samples with the same treatment were located on the same trajectory, indicating that treatments have greatly disturbed the normal urine metabolic profiles of rats (Fig. 2). Urine from the 2-4 groups were further from control group, suggesting the metabolic profiles have significantly changed as a result of Cold-cool medication administration. Rats in 5-7 groups were administrated with warm-hot medication for 24 consecutive days, the results were separated from the control group, demonstrating that the endogenous metabolic disorders occured after stimulus from warm-hot medication, nevertheless, the perturbation of metabolic profiles are different from Cold medication group even with opposite trend. It was consistent with the clinical report that the four natures cold and hot are summarized mainly from the body's response after taking Chinese medicinal herbs are taken. Following the above data pre-treatment, PCA was employed in the first phase of chemometric analysis for positive data to evaluate urine sample clustering according to the character of the herbs variety, which is the most suitable for discrimination among the sample classes.

3.2.3 OPLS-DA analysis

In order to obtain better discrimination between different characteristic herbs and find the significant change of endogenous metabolites (i.e. potential biomarkers), an OPLS-DA model was constructed. OPLS-DA score plots separated urine samples of control group and Chinese medicinal herbs with cold nature groups as well as hot nature groups into two blocks, respectively, especially in the component P1 direction, and component P2 properly explained individual variation in each group (Fig. 3), which indicates biochemical changes happened in the urinary of male rats after the treatment of different property herbs. Loadings for component P1 indicated the content of each ion in the control and herbs groups; the Y+ axis represented the herbs group; the Y-axis represented the control group; the X-axis represented the number of detected ions. To exhibit the responsibility of each ion for these variations more intuitively, S-plots and VIP-value plots were shown (Fig. 4). In the S-plot, most of the ions were clustered around the origin point; only a few of them scattered in the margin region, and just these few ions contributed to the clustering observed in the score plot and were also the differentiating metabolites. The VIP-value plot represents the value of each ion. The farther away from the origin, the higher the VIP value of the ions was. As illustrated in Fig. 3, Urine of the six herbs-treated groups were analyzed by OPLS-DA, the result of score plots indicating Cold and hot medication could separated well from each other, Rhizoma Coptidis, Radix Scutellariae and Cortex Phellodendri-treated groups have similar metabolic profiles were located the same quadrant, Similarly to Radix Aconiti Lateralis Preparata, Rhizoma Zingiberis and Pricklyash Peel-treated groups. The analysis of the chromatographic data identified the Cold and hot medication-treated rats based on the differences in their metabolic profiles, demonstrating that the classic herbs showed significant intervened effects on the normal rats, which was consistent with the theory of clinical medicine.

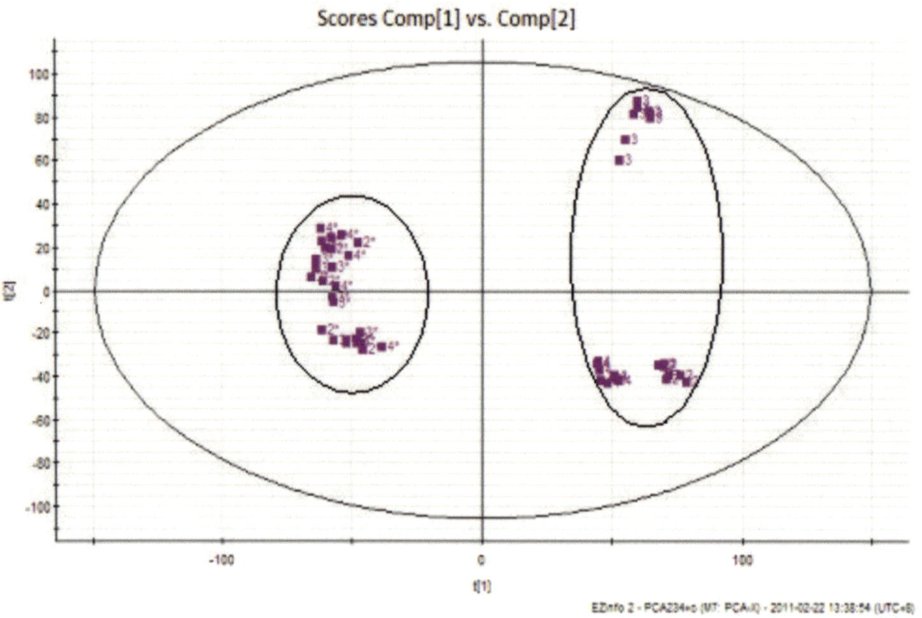

A

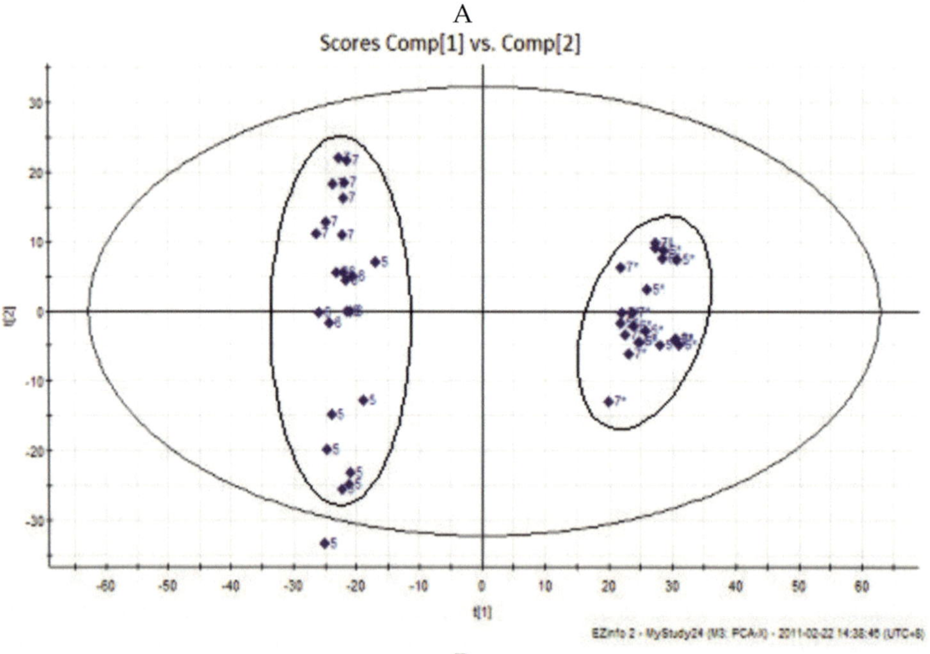

B

Fig. 2. PCA scores plots derived from the UPLC-QTOF spectra of the urine in positive mode. (A) 2-4 groups originated from Rhizoma Coptidis, Radix Scutellariae and Cortex Phellodendri, belong to cold medication 2*-4* groups originated from control groups. (B) 5-7 groups originated from Radix Aconiti Lateralis Preparata, Rhizoma Zingiberis and Rhizoma Zingiberis and Pricklyash Peel groups, belong to hot medication groups and 5*-7* groups originated from control groups.

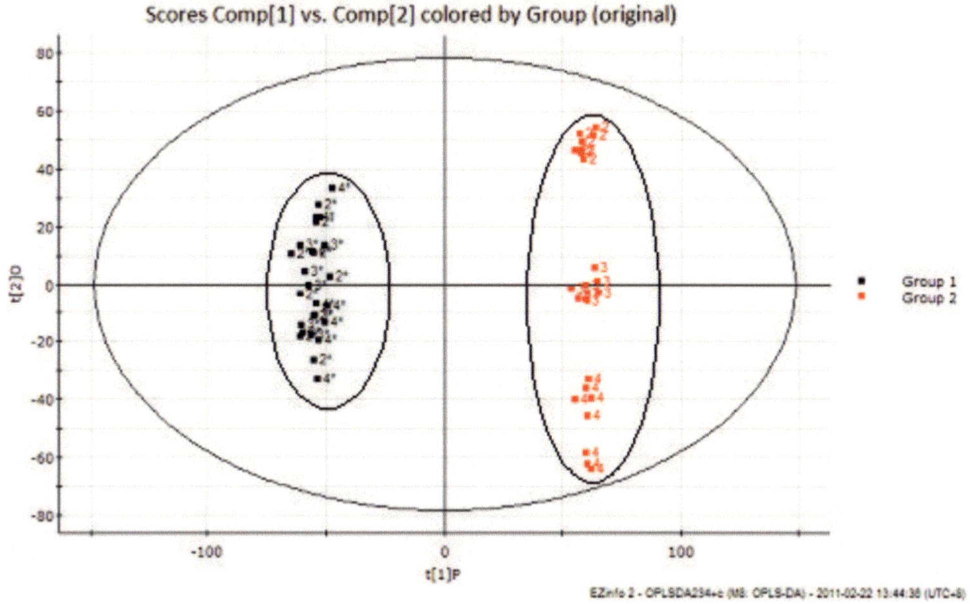
Scores Comp[1] vs. Comp[2] colored by Group (original)
t[2]O
t[1]P
Group 1
Group 2

A

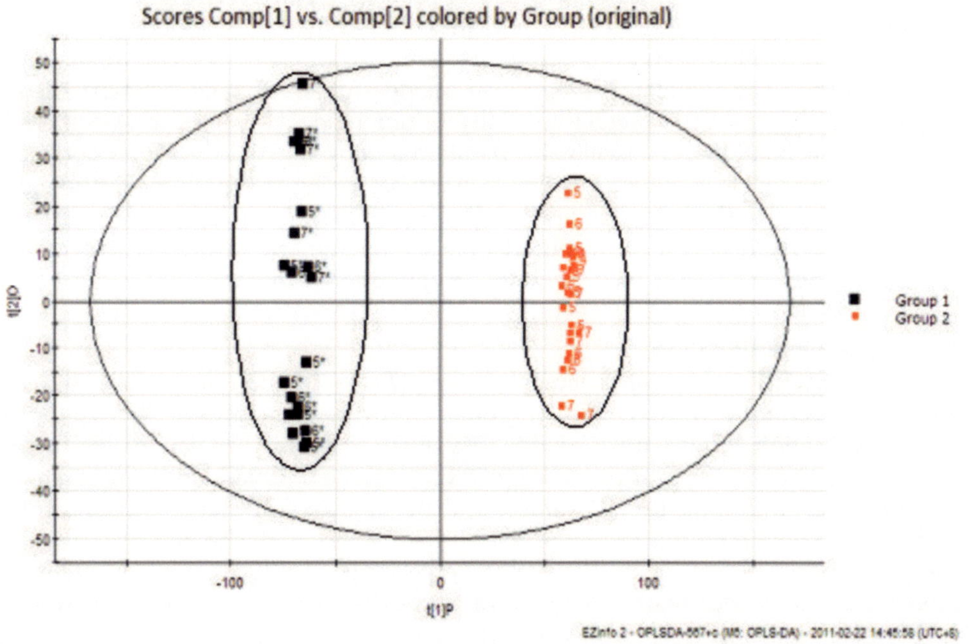
Scores Comp[1] vs. Comp[2] colored by Group (original)
t[2]O
t[1]P
Group 1
Group 2

B

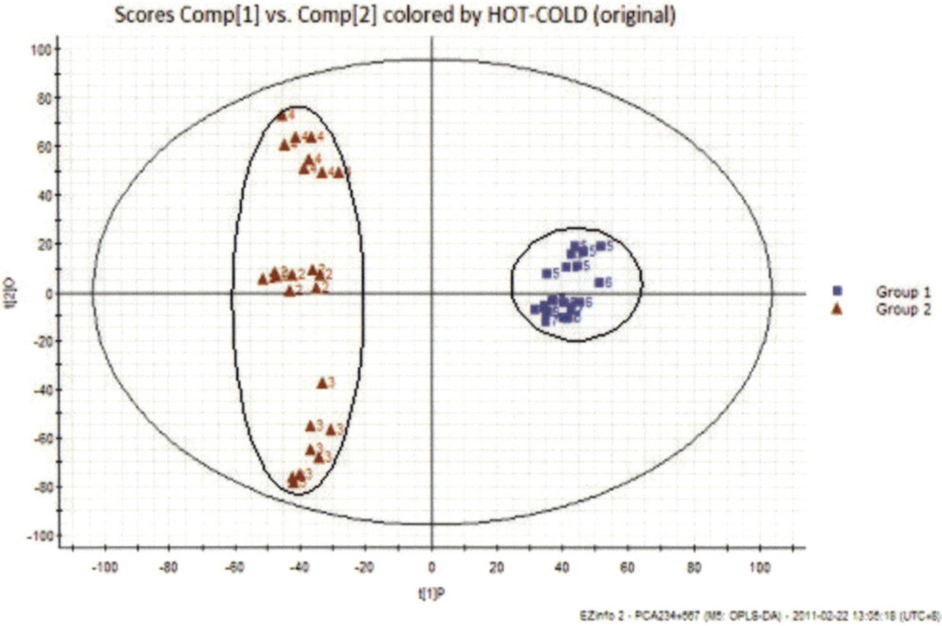

C

Fig. 3. OPLS-DA scores plots to classification the six groups of cold and hot medication. A, (■) Group 1 is cold medication group and (■) group 2 is control group. B, (■) Group 1 is hot medication group and (■)group 2 is control group. C, (■) Group 1 is hot medication group and (▲) group 2 is cold medication group.

For demonstration of the discrimination potential offered by the above data, OPLS-DA, a widely used supervised pattern recognition method capable of sample class prediction, was used to construct and validate a statistical model for traditional Chinese medicine classification. To estimate the predictive ability of our model, we used another herb-Flos Datura to cross-validation, and excellent separation among the TCM varieties obtained by OPLS-DA is shown in Fig. 5, which a hot medication belonging to the hot medication group, are presented in terms of recognition and prediction abilities. It represented the percentage of the samples correctly classified during model training and cross-validation, respectively, while the prediction ability was only qualitative rather than quantitative.

3.2.4 Biomarker identification

According to the VIP values of independent test (Table 2), these ions show significant differences between the controls and TCM groups. The same trend ions of three cold-cool or warm-hot medication groups were found, they may be biomarker candidates to reflect metabolic differences on the four properties of TCM. All the detected ions were arranged in descending order according to VIP values, and the highest VIP value was 20.75 in the positive mode. Combining the results of the OPLS analysis with the amount variation of ions in each group, 9 ions with VIP values exceeding two were selected preliminary identified in the Cold medication groups. At the same time, the highest VIP value was 12.73 in the positive mode, and 9 ions with VIP values exceeding two were selected and preliminary identified. The UPLC-MS segregation analysis platform provided the retention

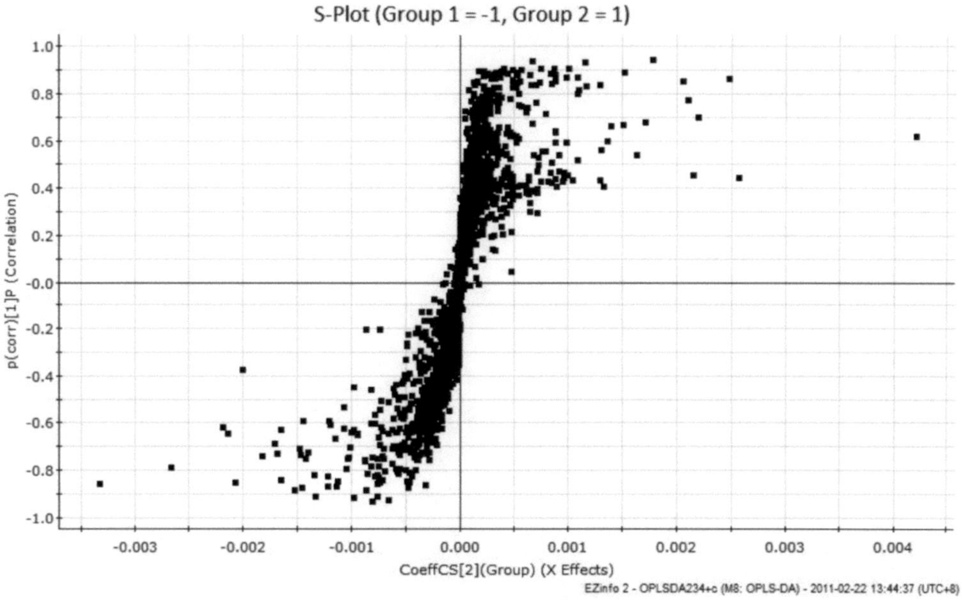

A

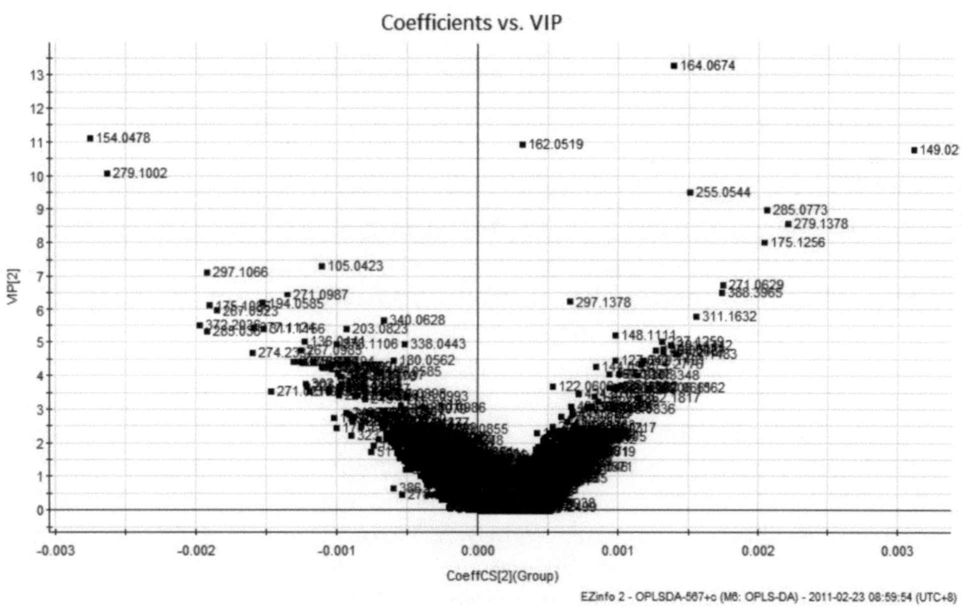

B

Fig. 4. S-plot and VIP values in positive ESI mode. A, S-plot of Cold medication group(Gruop 1 originated from cold medication, and group 2 originated from control ones). B, VIP values plot of Hot medication group.

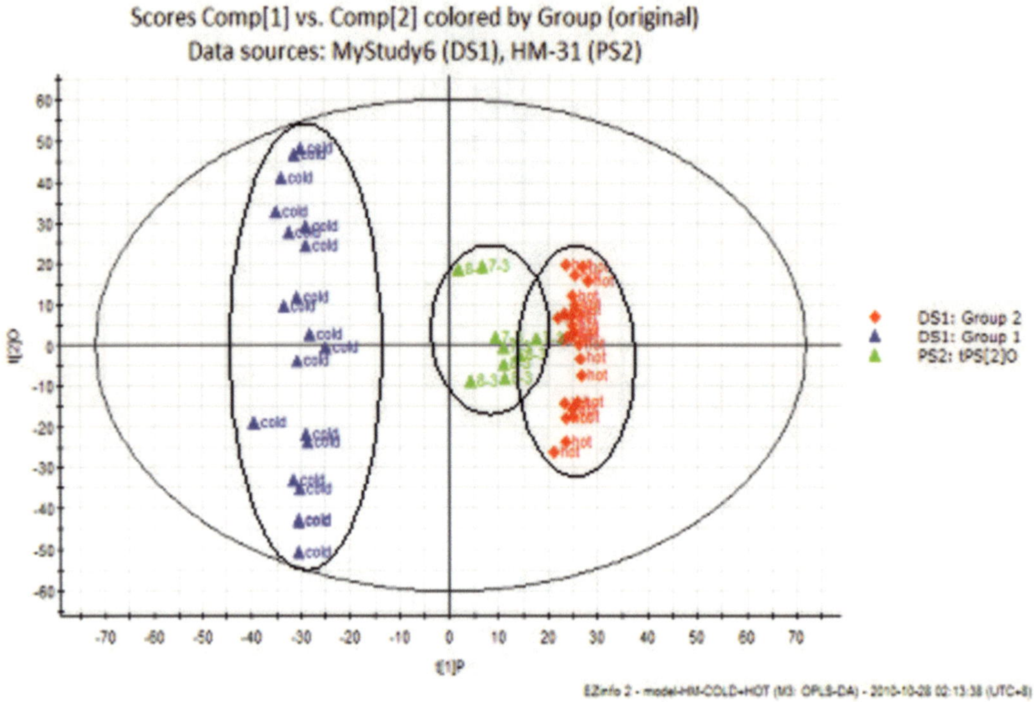

Fig. 5. Another hot medication-Flos Datura was used to verify the reliability of the forecasting model of OPLD-DA. (▲) cold medication group, (◆) hot medication group. (▲) Flos Datura.

time, precise molecular mass and MS/MS data for the structural identification of biomarkers. The precise molecular mass was determined within measurement errors (<5 ppm) by Q-TOF, and meanwhile, the potential elemental composition and fractional isotope abundance of compounds were obtained. The presumed molecular formula was searched in METLIN Database and other databases to identify the possible chemical constitutions, and MS/MS data were screened to determine the potential structures of the ions. Taking two ions as examples, the identification procedure was as follows. Taking two ions as examples, the identification procedure was as follows. In the positive mode, the ion at Rt = 5.46 and $[M+H]^+$ = 146 has a high VIP value. This ion might contain an odd number of nitrogen atoms because its precise molecular weight was 145.0739, and its molecular formula was speculated as $C_6H_{11}NO_3$ from the analysis of its elemental composition and fractional isotope abundance. The main fragment ions analyzed by MS/MS screening were m/z 128 and 101, which could be the $[M+H]^+$ of lost $-NH_4$, and $-C_2H_7N$, respectively. Finally, it was speculated as (S)-5-Amino-3-oxohexanoic acid, the ion at Rt = 4.26 and $[M+H]^+$ = 162 has a high VIP value, and the main fragment ions were m/z 145, 144 and 117, which could be the $[M+H]^+$ of lost $-NH_4$, $-NH_3$ and $-NO_2$, respectively. Finally, it was speculated as L-2-Aminoadipic acid.

NO.	VIP values	Rt-M+	Actual M	Proposed compound	Trend	MS/MS	Losses	Proposed structure
1	2.70	5.25_134.0986	133.0375	Aspartic Acid $C_4H_7NO_4$	Hot↑	118 103	O HNO	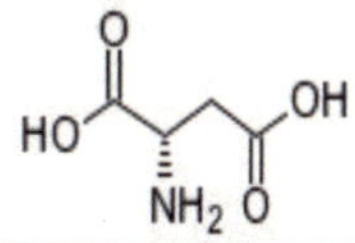
2	3.00	3.64_190.041	189.0637	N-Acetyl-L-glutamate $C_7H_{11}NO_5$	Cold↓	172 146 133	CH_6 C_2H_4O C_2H_3NO	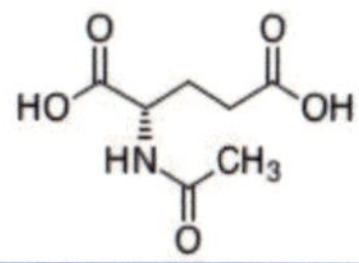
3	2.71	3.94_135.0962	134.0215	L-Apple acid $C_4H_6O_5$	Cold↓	104	NO	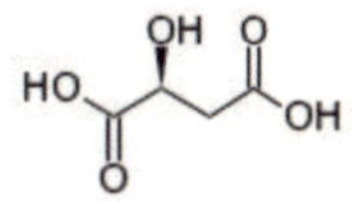
4	2.13	4.73_233.0837	232.1212	Melatonin $C_{13}H_{16}N_2O_2$	Cold↓	191 174	C_2H_2O C_2H_5NO	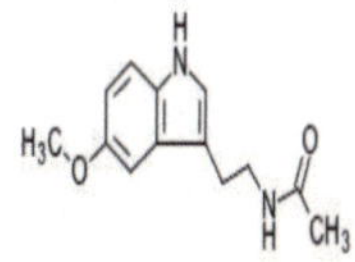
5	3.25	2.62_137.0683	136.0385	Hypoxanthine $C_5H_4N_4O$	Cold↑	120	HO	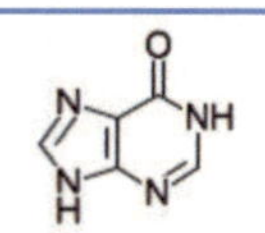
6	5.84	2.7_180.0886	179.0582	Acetylisoniazid $C_8H_9N_3O_2$	Cold↑	135	CHO_2	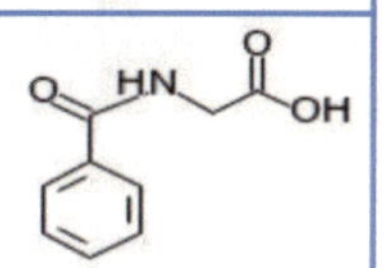
7	2.20	6.25_285.0773	284.0757	Xanthosine $C_{10}H_{12}N_4O_6$	Cold↑	267 228	H_2O CHN_2O	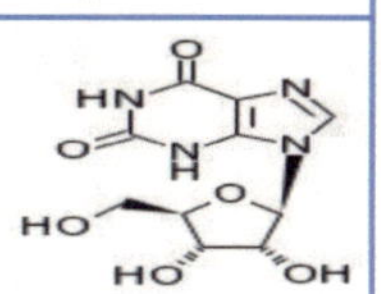
8	7.76	2.81_300.1645	299.0770	D-4'-Phosphopantothenate $C_9H_{18}NO_8P$	Cold↑	242 187 114	$C_2H_2O_2$ H_2O_5P $C_3H_9NO_6P$	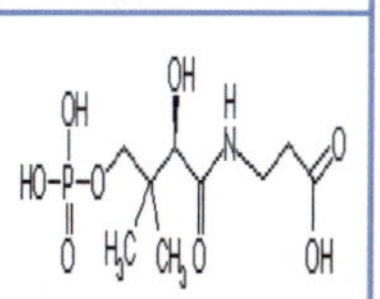
9	2.91	3.26_308.0929	307.0838	Glutathione $C_{10}H_{17}N_3O_6S$	Cold↑	262 179 147	CH_2S $C_5H_7NO_3$ $C_5H_7NO_3S$	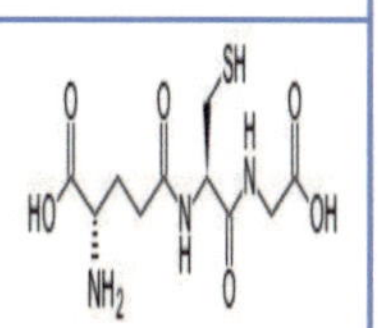
10	2.25	3.04_133.0853	132.0535	L-Asparagine $C_4H_8N_2O_3$	Hot↓	118	HN	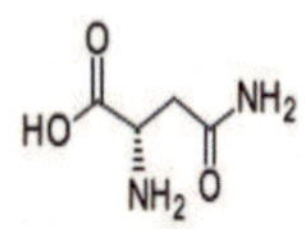

NO.	VIP values	Rt-M+	Actual M	Proposed compound	Trend	MS/MS	Losses	Proposed structure
11	5.02	4.14_146.0618	145.0739	(S)-5-Amino-3-oxohexanoic acid $C_6H_{11}NO_3$	Hot↓	128 101	H_4N C_2H_7N	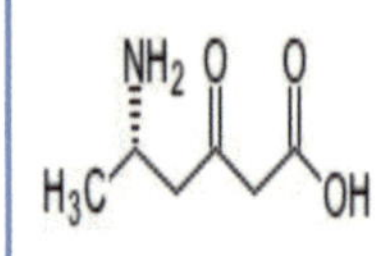
12	3.23	3.5_178.0469	177.046	N-Formyl-L-methionine $C_6H_{11}NO_3S$	Hot↓	148 132 104	CH_2O CH_2S C_2H_2OS	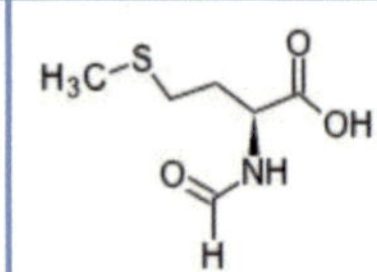
13	4.31	9.57_301.1442	300.2089	Vitamin A acid $C_{20}H_{28}O_2$	Hot↓	284 175	HO C_9H_{18}	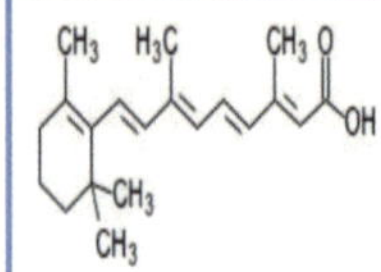
14	5.13	4.1_289.1075	288.0246	2-Dehydro-3-deoxy-D-arabino-heptonate 7-phosphate (DAHP) $C_7H_{13}O_{10}P$	Hot↑	242 158	CH_3O_2 H_4O_6P	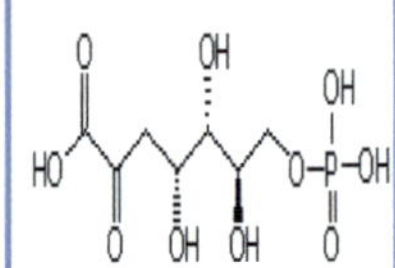
15	2.78	4.05_151.0389	150.1045	Myrtenal $C_{10}H_{14}O$	Hot↑	123 108	C_2H_4 C_3H_7	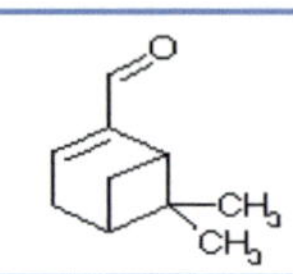
16	12.73	4.26_162.0519	161.0688	L-2-Aminoadipic acid $C_6H_{11}NO_4$	Hot↑	145 144 117	NH_3 NH_4 NO_2	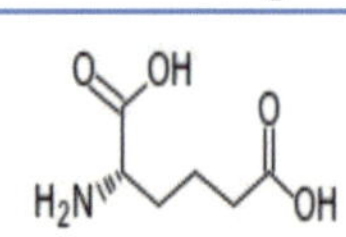
17	2.04	3.89_319.1289	318.2195	Leukotriene A4 $C_{20}H_{30}O_3$	Hot↑	273 259 162	C_3H_{10} C_4H_{12} $C_8H_{13}O_3$	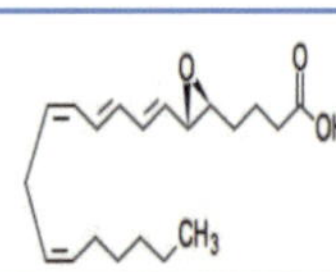
18	20.75	4.48_164.0674	163.0633	3-Methyldioxyindole $C_9H_9NO_2$	Cold↓	146 122	-H2O -CNO	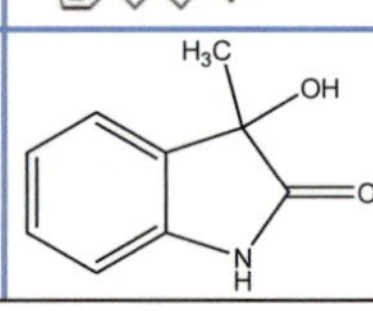

Table 2. Potential biomarkers identified in positive ESI mode.

4. Discussion

Metabonomics aims to assess metabolic changes in a comprehensive and global manner in order to infer biological functions and provide the detailed biochemical responses of cellular systems [19]. In this study the successful discrimination and classification of the four properties in TCM was made. Multivariate statistical analysis was used to find the most characteristic markers in complex records. This demonstrates the potential of UPLC-QTOF-MS combined with metabonomics to determine the four properties of TCM. It should be noted that for this particular purpose, the molecular identification of these marker compounds is not necessary, some different chemometric tools, such as PCA and OPLS-DA have been proposed as powerful tools for the four properties classification [20]. However, the benefit of obtaining MS/MS accurate mass spectra of marker compounds (metabolites) were shown to provide a high level of confidence for the identification process. Even with this data, the identification of true unknowns is a rather difficult task. Biological Interpretation of several biomarkers: L-Apple acid is a tart-tasting organic dicarboxylic acid that plays a role in many sour or tart foods. In its ionized form it is malate, an intermediate of the TCA cycle along with fumarate. It can also be formed from pyruvate as one of the anaplerotic reactions. It is a key intermediate in energy metabolism and the change indicated that energy metabolism was perturbation by Chinese herbs.

5. Conclusion

The four properties, the essence and important component of TCM theories, the high generalization on the basic property and typical characteristics of TCM, are a significant theoretical foundation for the clinical use of Chinese medicine. In this study, UPLC-QTOF-MS techniques coupled to metabonomics methods were used to prove the existence of the four properties, to illustrate its multi-component, multi-target, multi-channel and the complex mechanism. All the work are aimed at guiding researchers to carry out new drug develop work with the theory of Chinese medicine, simultaneously, eliminating too much emphasis the effective chemical composition while ignore the many other ones, result in the loss of characteristics of Chinese herbs and even highlights the toxicity and side effects. This theory also could apply to explore Western medicine properties to effectively guide the clinical application. Considering the encouraging results obtained in this study, the application of metabonomics for authentication and other purposes in TCM seems to be very promising approach [22].

6. Acknowledgements

Our work was supported by the Major State Basic Research Development Program of China (973 Program 2006CB504708) the National Natural Science Foundation of China (No. 30371736, 30672633) and Special Fund Project of National Excellent Doctoral Dissertation of China (200980).

7. References

[1] C. Auffray, Z. Chen, L. Hood, Genome Med.1 (2009) 1-2.
[2] T. Ma, C.g. Tan, H. Zhang, M.Q. Wang, W. J. Ding, S. Li, Mol. BioSyst. 6 (2010) 613-619.
[3] A.P. Lu, H.W. Jia, C. Xiao, Q.P. Lu.. World J Gastroenterol 13 (2004) 1854-1856.
[4] D. Normile. Science 299(2003) 188-190.
[5] J. Lindon, J. Nicholson, E. Holmes, Elsevier, Amsterdam, (2007) 279-287.

[6] J. Chen,W.Z.Wang, S. Lv, P. Y. Yin, X. J. Zhao, X. Lu, F. X. Zhang, G.W. Xu, Analytica Chimica Acta 650 (2009) 3-9.
[7] D.M. Drexler, J.H.M. Feyen, M. Sanders, Drug Discov. Today Technol. 1 (2004) 17-23.
[8] J.C. Lindon, E. Holmes, M.E. Bollard, E.G. Stanley, J.K. Nicholson, Biomarkers 9 (2004) 1-31.
[9] D.G. Robertson, M.D. Reily, J.D. Baker, J. Proteome Res. 6 (2007) 526-539.
[10] I.D. Wilson, R. Plumb, J. Granger, H.Major, R.Williams, E.M. Lenz, J. Chromatogr. B 817 (2005) 67-76.
[11] E. Holmes, P.J.D. Foxall, M. Spraul, R.D. Farrant, J.K. Nicholson, J.C. Lindon, J. Pharm. Biomed. Anal. 15 (1997) 1647-1659.
[12] C. Wang, H.W. Kong, Y.F. Guan, J. Yang, J.R. Gu, S.L. Yang, G.W. Xu, Anal. Chem. 77 (2005) 4108-4116.
[13] F. Benavente, R. van der Heijden, U.R. Tjaden, J. van der Greef, T. Hankemeier, Electrophoresis 27 (2006) 4570-4584.
[14] J. Zhang, L. J. Yan, W. G. Chen, L. Lin, X. Y. Song, X. M. Yan,W. Hang, B. l. Huang, Analytica Chimica Acta 650 (2009) 16-22.
[15] R.S. Plumb, J.H. Granger, C.L. Stumpf, K.A. Johnson, B.W. Smith, S. Gaulitz, I.D. Wilson, J. Castro-Perez, Analyst 130 (2005) 844-849.
[16] J.H. Granger, R. Williams, E.M. Lenz, R.S. Plumb, C.L. Stumpf, I.D. Wilson, Rapid Commun. Mass Spectrom. 21 (2007) 2039-2045.
[17] R. Madsen, T. Lundstedt, J. Trygg, Analytica Chimica Acta 659 (2010) 23-33.
[18] P. Wang, H. Sun, H.T. Lv, W. J. Sun, Y. Yuan, Y. Han, D. W. Wang, A. H. Zhang, X. J. Wang, J. Pharm. Biomed. Anal. 53 (2010) 631-645.
[19] O. Fiehn;, B. Kristal, B. van Ommen, L. W. Sumner, S. A. Sansone, C. Taylor, N. Hardy, R. Kaddurah-Daouk, OMICS, 10 (2006), 158-63.
[20]L. Rafael, U. S. Mireia, J.Olga, M.Maria, A. L. Cristina, Journal of Proteome Research, 8(2009), 5060-5068.
[21] S.Wiklund, E. Johansson, L. Sjostrom, E. J. Mellerowicz, U. Edlund, J. P. Shockcor, J. Gottfries, T. Moritz, J. Trygg, Anal. Chem., 80 (2008), 115-22.
[22] F. Y. Du, Y. Bai, Y. Bai, H.W. Liu, Anal. Chem. 82 (2010), 9374-9383.

2

A Geomedical Approach to Chinese Medicine: The Origin of the Yin-Yang Symbol

Stefan Jaeger
*National Library of Medicine**
United States

1. Introduction

This chapter shows how to compute Yin and Yang for different latitudes so traditional Chinese herbalists can quantify the efficacy of herbal drugs. Based on daylight hours, the chapter provides a simple formula that allows computation of Yin and Yang for each day of the year. Moreover, using daily Yin and Yang values, the chapter shows how to render the Yin-Yang symbol properly in accordance with its original meaning. Considering the importance of Yin and Yang in traditional Chinese medicine (TCM), the rendering method presented in this chapter provides evidence that TCM, in its origin, is a geomedical science.

Herbal medicines collected from different geographic locations can significantly differ in their therapeutic efficacy. The concentration of bioactive substances varies depending on many local factors, such as sunshine hours or chemical and physical properties of the soil. To guarantee the optimal composition of herbal drugs, Chinese herbalists use "geo-authentic" herbs from recognized locations. However, it is often difficult to confirm geographical authenticity. The lack of formal models for Yin and Yang, and herbal efficacy in general, complicates objective comparisons and evaluations. Herbalists and practitioners of TCM need a better formal understanding of the Yin-Yang composition of each herb. This chapter contributes to the solution to this problem by providing a formal description of Yin and Yang. It shows in a mathematical way how Yin and Yang vary depending on latitude. The latitude of a herb's location determines the number of daylight hours and sunshine the herb is exposed to during the year. The number of daylight hours is one of the components affecting the concentration and composition of bioactive substances and therefore the efficacy of the herb. To standardize herbal preparation and administration, rigorous mathematical methods are essential to measure the Yin-Yang composition of herbs quantitatively. The work presented in this chapter is a first step toward such standardization.

The chapter structure is as follows: Section 2 discusses the main ideas of the philosophical Yin-Yang concept. Section 3 shows today's most common Yin-Yang symbol and discusses its typical shape. Then, Section 4 presents the origin of the Yin-Yang symbol and introduces a daylight model that allows computation of Yin and Yang depending on the daylight hours for each geographic latitude. Using the computed values for Yin and Yang, the section will show how to render the Yin-Yang symbol properly, and in accordance with its original meaning. The chapter concludes with a discussion of the consequences of the results for researchers in TCM and herbal medicine. Finally, the appendix contains examples of Yin-Yang symbols computed for different latitudes in the northern and southern hemispheres.

---

*Work on this study began while the author was affiliated with the Chinese Academy of Sciences.

2. Yin and Yang

Yin-Yang has become a universal philosophical concept that many people readily embrace to their advantage. The concept of Yin and Yang is deeply rooted in Chinese philosophy (Miller, 2003; Watts, 1999). Its origin dates back at least 2500 years, probably much earlier, playing a crucial role in the formation of the Chinese ancient civilization. Chinese thinkers have attached great importance to Yin and Yang ever since. In Asia's search for a universal formula describing balance and harmony, Yin-Yang today appeals to fields as different as medicine, arts, religion, sports, or politics.

According to the Chinese philosophical concept, there are two opposing forces in the world, namely Yin and Yang, which are constantly trying to gain the upper hand over each other. However, neither one will ever succeed in doing so, though one force may temporarily dominate the other one. Both forces cannot exist without each other; it is rather the constant struggle between both forces that defines our world and produces the rhythm of life. Yin and Yang are not only believed to be the foundation of our universe, but also to flow through and affect every being. For example, typical Yin-Yang opposites are night/day, cold/hot, rest/activity.

Chinese philosophy does not confine itself to a mere description of Yin and Yang; it also provides guidelines on how to live in accordance with Yin and Yang. The central statement is that Yin and Yang need to be in harmony. Any imbalance of an economical, biological, physical, or chemical system can be directly attributed to a distorted equilibrium between Yin and Yang. For example, an illness accompanied by fever is the result of Yang being too strong and dominating Yin. On the other hand, for example, dominance of Yin could result in a body shivering with cold. The optimal state every being, or system, should strive for is therefore the state of equilibrium between Yin and Yang. It is this state of equilibrium between Yin and Yang that Chinese philosophy considers the most powerful and stable state a system can assume.

Yin and Yang already carry the seed of their opposites: A dominating Yin becomes susceptible to Yang and will eventually turn into its opposite. On the other hand, a dominating Yang gives rise to Yin and will turn into Yin over time. This defines the perennial alternating cycle of Yin or Yang dominance. Only the equilibrium between Yin and Yang is able to overcome this cycle.

3. Yin-Yang symbol

Figure 1 shows the well-known black-and-white symbol of Yin and Yang. This Yin-Yang

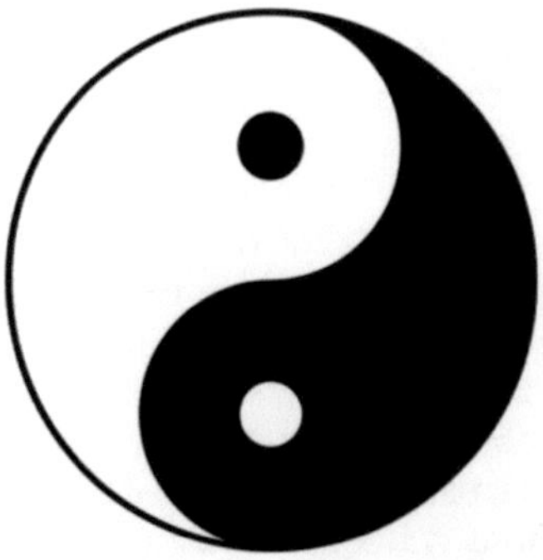

Fig. 1. A common Yin-Yang symbol.

symbol, also known under the name Tai Chi symbol, is arguably one of the most flamboyant symbols today. It stands on the same level as the Christian cross and other mainstream religious symbols. We can see the intertwining spiral-like curves in Figure 1, which are actually semicircles, separating the Yin and Yang area. The small spots of different color in each area indicate the above mentioned conception that both Yin and Yang carry the seed of their opposites; Yin cannot exist without Yang, and Yang cannot exist without Yin. These spots will play no role in this chapter. Neither will the assignment of black and white to Yin and Yang have any significance here, though Yin is typically associated with black and Yang with white.

Spiral-like curves are a common occurrence in nature. They appear in various forms in a wide range of living beings and processes; e.g., mollusk shells, hurricanes, or galaxies (Cook, 1979; Séquin, 1999). Depending on the form of these curves, the Yin-Yang symbol can take on different shapes. It is therefore necessary to define a standard rendering method before plotting the Yin-Yang symbol. For example, Figure 2 shows two versions of the South Korean Flag.

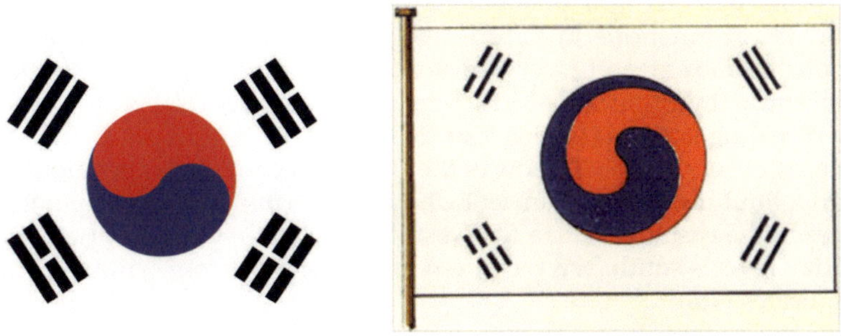

(a) Modern flag (b) Older version

Fig. 2. Flag of South Korea (Wikipedia).

The South Korean flag's modern version is on the left-hand side of Figure 2. On the right-hand side is an older version of the flag. Both versions feature the Yin-Yang symbol prominently in their center, which is again testimony of the importance of the Yin-Yang concept for Asian countries. However, the shapes of the Yin-Yang spirals are clearly different for both flags. To agree on a common flag, it is necessary to define a standard construction scheme for rendering the Yin-Yang symbol. Figure 3 shows the standard construction sheet for the modern South Korean flag. However, the next section shows that the rendering method in Figure 3 does not reflect the original meaning of the Yin-Yang symbol.

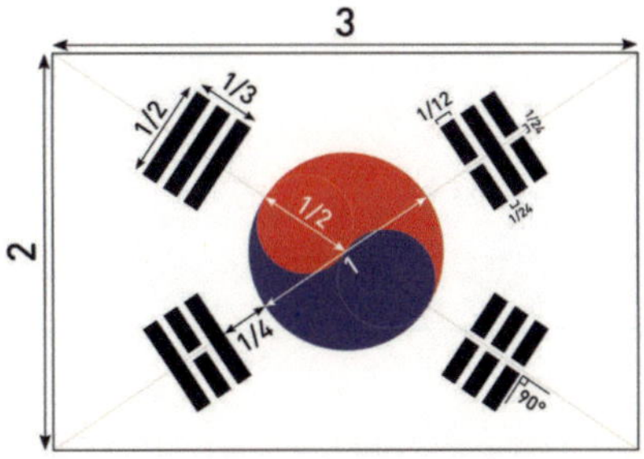

Fig. 3. Construction sheet for the South Korean flag (Wikipedia).

Contemporary literature has been mostly neglecting the plotting of the Yin-Yang symbol, paying more attention to philosophical questions. However, a mathematical formalization of the Yin-Yang symbol is desirable to open hitherto mathematically inaccessible fields, such as Chinese traditional medicine, for rigorous scientific research.

4. The origin of the Yin-Yang symbol

Despite its presence in everyday life, it is fair to say that only a few people know about the origin of the Yin-Yang symbol. Very often, even the most devoted practitioners have to pass on the question about its origin. Contrary to what one would expect, literature dealing with the origin of the Yin-Yang symbol is rare. Contemporary books and articles typically deal in detail with the philosophical facets of Yin and Yang, but do not address the origin of the Yin-Yang symbol. It turns out that the original Yin-Yang symbol is more complex than its modern representation as two semicircles suggests (Browne, 2007; Graf, 1994).

The Yin-Yang symbol has its origin in the I-Ching; one of the oldest and most fundamental books in Chinese philosophy. The I-Ching, which is typically translated as "The Book of Changes", deals with natural phenomena and their seasonal cycles. From the constant changes and transformations in nature, the I-Ching tries to derive the unchanging rules governing our cosmos and our very existence. The observation of celestial phenomena is therefore of central importance to the I-Ching (Hardaker, 2001). It is here, where one finds the roots of the Yin-Yang symbol (Tian & Tian, 2004).

For example, by observing the shadow of the sun and recording the positions of the Big Dipper at night throughout the year, the ancient Chinese determined the four points of the compass: The sun rises in the east and sets in the west. The direction of the shortest shadow measured on a given day reveals south (www.chinesefortunecalendar.com/yinyang.htm). At night, the Pole Star indicates North.

4.1 Shadow model

The Yin-Yang symbol is tightly connected with the annual cycle of the earth around the sun, and the four seasons resulting from it. To investigate this cycle, the ancient Chinese used a pole that they put up orthogonally to the ground, as shown in Figure 4. With this setup, the

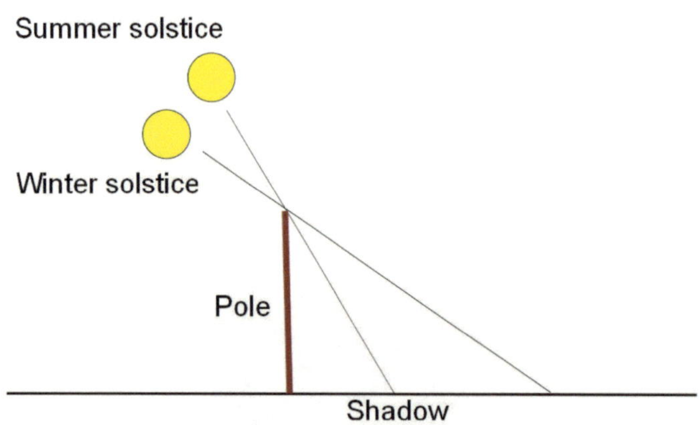

Fig. 4. Shadow model.

ancient Chinese were able to record precisely the positions of the sun's shadow and divide the year into different sections. They found the length of a year to be about 365.25 days.

Furthermore, they divided the circle of the year into segments, including the vernal equinox, autumnal equinox, summer solstice, and winter solstice. In addition, they used concentric circles around the pole, helping them to record the length of the sun's shadow every day. As a result, they measured the shortest shadow during the summer solstice, and measured the longest shadow during the winter solstice. After connecting the measured points and dimming the part that reaches from summer solstice to winter solstice (Yin), they arrived at a chart like the one in Figure 5. The resemblance between this chart and the modern Yin-Yang

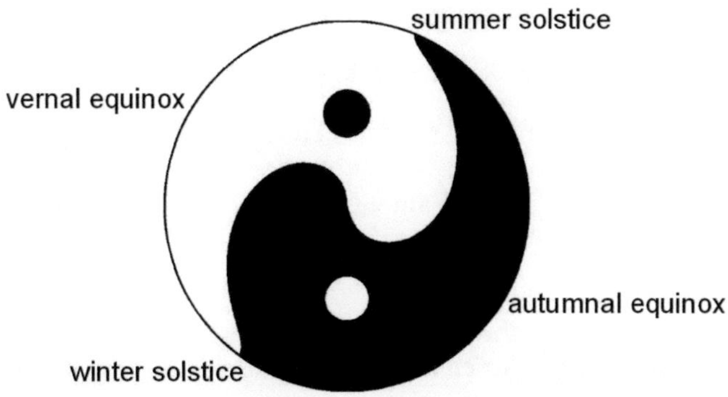

Fig. 5. Yin-Yang symbol for Latitude $L = 68°$ (near polar circle) with equinoxes and solstices.

symbol in Figure 1 is striking. Figure 5 provides visual evidence that the original Yin-Yang symbol describes the change of a pole's shadow length during a year. In fact, by rotating the chart and positioning the winter solstice at the bottom, the Yin-Yang chart of the ancient Chinese becomes very similar to the modern Yin-Yang symbol depicted in Figure 1.

The white area of the Yin-Yang symbol is typically called Yang. It begins at the winter solstice and indicates a beginning dominance of daylight over darkness, which is the reason why the ancient Chinese associated it with the sun (or male). Accordingly, the dark area of the Yin-Yang symbol represents Yin, which begins with the summer solstice. Yin indicates a beginning dominance of darkness over daylight. The ancient Chinese therefore associated it with the moon (or female).

Note that the shape of the Yin-Yang symbol also depends on the ecliptic angle of the earth. The ecliptic affects the angle between the white Yang area, or black Yin area, and the outer circle of the Yin-Yang symbol. The ecliptic is the sun's apparent path around the earth. It is tilted relative to the earth's equator. As a result, one can observe four different seasons throughout the year. In the year 2000, the obliquity of the ecliptic was about $23°26'19''$. The ecliptic's obliquity is not stable and can change during the millennia. This is due to the different forces exerted by the bodies in the solar system on the earth. The obliquity varies between about $21°55'$ and $24°18'$ within a period of $40,000$ years (Wikipedia, March 2008). For example, in the year $3,000$ BC, the ecliptic was about $24°1.6'$. Therefore, the ancient Yin-Yang symbol looks slightly different than the modern Yin-Yang symbol when rendered based on the shadow model.

4.2 Daylight model

This section presents a rendering method for the Yin-Yang symbol based on daylight hours, which are connected with shadow lengths. A long day has the sun standing high on the

horizon at noon, casting a short shadow. On the other hand, a short day is the result of the sun standing low on the horizon at noon, which in turn produces a long shadow. For computing the daylight time for a given day in the year, this section uses the formula given in (Forsythe et al., 1995). The formula takes many different factors into account, most notably the refraction of the earth's atmosphere. The daylight model presented here is therefore an accurate description of the actual daylight measurement of an observer on the ground. A detailed investigation of the formula is beyond the scope of this paper, though.
The formula requires two input parameters, namely the day of the year J and the latitude L of the observer's location. It consists of two parts. The first part computes an intermediate result P, which is the input to the second part. The equation for the first part is as follows:

$$P = \arcsin[0.39795 * \cos(0.2163108 + 2 * \arctan\{0.9671396 * \tan[0.00860(J - 186)]\})] \quad (1)$$

Given P, the second part then computes the actual day length D in terms of sunshine hours:

$$D = 24 - \left(\frac{24}{\pi}\right) * \arccos\left\{\frac{\sin\left(\frac{0.8333*\pi}{180}\right) + \sin\left(\frac{L*\pi}{180}\right) * \sin(P)}{\cos\left(\frac{L*\pi}{180}\right) * \cos(P)}\right\} \quad (2)$$

Using Equation 2, Figure 6 shows the daylight time for each day of the year and a latitude of 68°. This latitude is close to the polar circle, or Arctic Circle, in the northern hemisphere. The

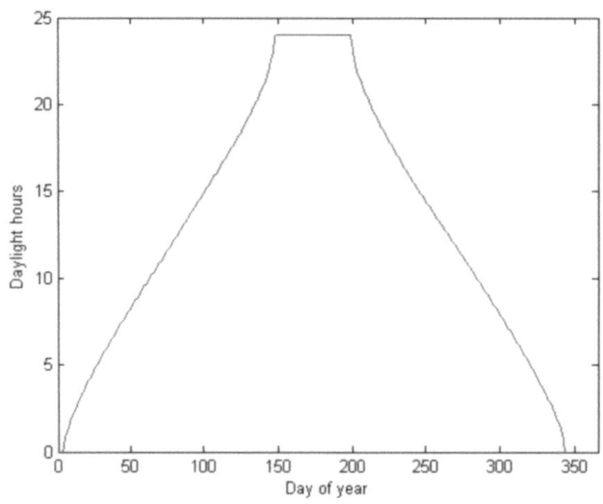

Fig. 6. Daylight hours for Latitude $L = 68°$ (near polar circle).

equivalent latitude in the southern hemisphere is the Antarctic Circle. The Arctic Circle marks the southernmost latitude in the northern hemisphere where the sun shines for 24 hours at least once per year (midnight sun) and does not shine at all at least once per year. Theoretically, the Arctic Circle marks the area where these events occur exactly once per year, namely during the summer and winter solstices. However, due to atmospheric refractions and because the sun is a disk rather than a point, the actual observation at the Arctic Circle is different. For example, the midnight sun can be seen south of the Arctic Circle during the summer solstice. According to Figure 6, the midnight sun shines for about 50 days at latitudes around 68°.
Figure 7 shows the daylight hours in Figure 6 as a polar plot. In this polar plot, the distance to the origin stands for the daily sunshine hours. One full turn of 360° corresponds to one year. There is another important difference to Figure 6, though. For the second half of the

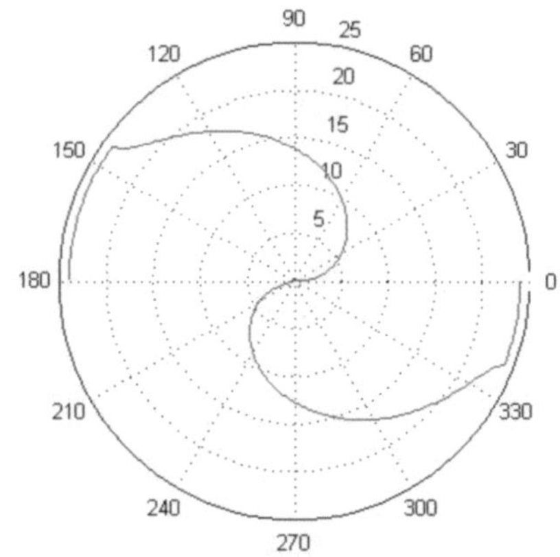

Fig. 7. Polar daylight plot for Latitude $L = 68°$ (near polar circle).

year, Figure 7 shows the hours of darkness instead of the daylight hours. The number of hours with darkness is simply the number of daylight hours subtracted from 24. Drawing the daylight hours in such a way produces the two spirals depicted in Figure 7. Coloring the areas delimited by both spirals and the outer circle in black and white then produces a rotated version of the Yin-Yang symbol in Figure 5. Note that this symbol is not quite symmetrical. This is correct because spring and fall are not completely symmetrical in terms of the solar cycle; a fact not discussed further in this chapter. For latitudes around the polar circle, the spirals in Figure 7 originate either directly in the origin of the polar plot or in a point close to it. This is because there will be at least one day with no sunshine.

Figure 8 shows the daylight hours and polar plots generated in the same way for different latitudes L, according to Equations 1 and 2. In particular, Figure 8 shows plots for $L = 40°$ (near Beijing), $L = 0°$ (Equator), and $L = 88°$ (near North Pole). For Latitude $L = 40°$, which is about the latitude of Beijing, the daylight curve is flatter compared to the daylight curve for $L = 68°$ in Figure 6. The reason for the flatter shape is that each day of the year has sunshine as well as darkness at $L = 40°$. For this latitude, the shapes of the spirals in the polar plot are approaching semicircles. Their starting points are relatively far from the center of the polar plot. This degeneration into semicircles continues with decreasing latitude. It reaches its extreme at the equator, with $L = 0°$. Here, each day has the same number of sunshine hours, namely exactly 12 hours. Consequently, the Yin and Yang spirals complement each other to form a perfect cycle for observers on the equator.

The last example in Figure 8 shows the daylight hours and polar plot when the observer's location is close to one of the earth's poles. For $L = 88°$, which is close to the North Pole, the year is split into two halves. For one half, the sun shines continuously for 24 hours on each day. For days in the other half, the sun does not shine at all. The transition from one half to the other happens very quickly. Due to this rapid transition between day and night, each of the Yin and Yang spirals in Figure 8 covers a sector in the polar plot. Both spirals together describe an almost vertical axis.

5. Conclusion

The chapter shows that the origin of the Yin-Yang symbol lies in the graphical representation of the daily change of a pole's shadow length. This length varies for each day, when measured

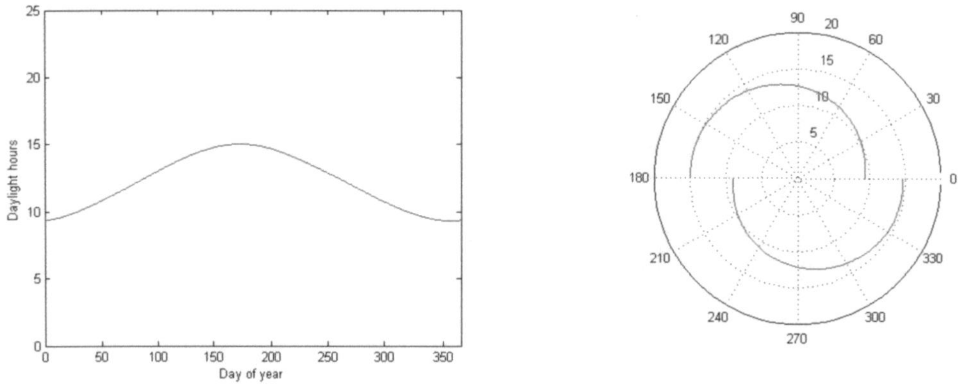

(a) Daylight hours and polar plot for Latitude $L = 40°$ (near Beijing).

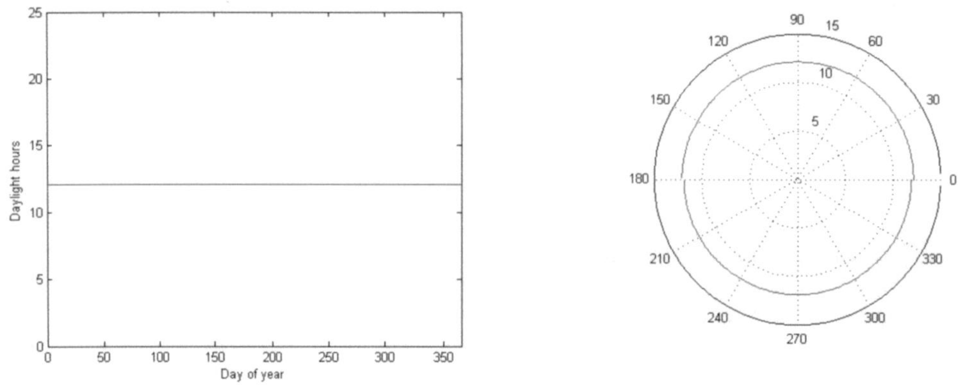

(b) Daylight hours and polar plot for Latitude $L = 0°$ (Equator).

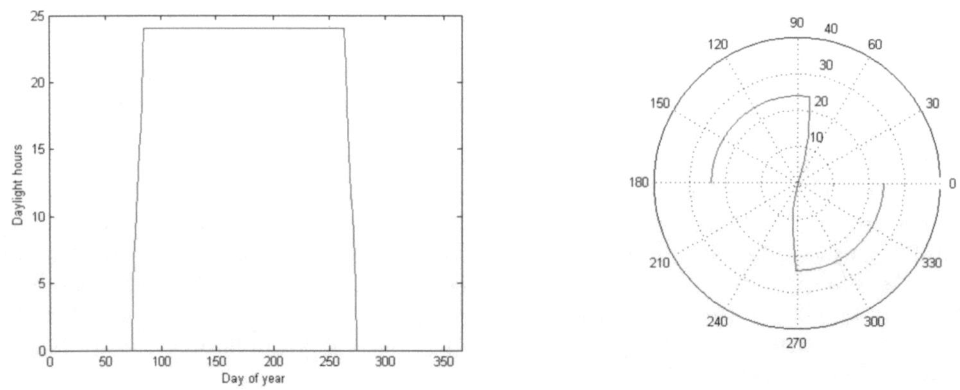

(c) Daylight hours and polar plot for Latitude $L = 88°$ (near North Pole).

Fig. 8. Daylight hours and polar plots for different latitudes.

at the same time, and depends on the geographic latitude of the observer. Given the significant role the Yin-Yang symbol plays in TCM, ancient herbalists and practitioners of TCM must have attached great importance to geographic location from the outset. It is reasonable to assume that they considered geographical aspects for both drug preparation as well as administration. To ensure an authentic TCM treatment, modern practitioners of TCM need to take geographic location into account not only when preparing drugs but also during the treatment of their patients. They must be aware of the geomedical origin of TCM. Latitude is one important factor in finding geo-authentic herbs. A mathematical formalization of this factor is a first step toward a well-defined and standardized TCM; a TCM that has the same scientific foundation as western medicine. This chapter equips herbalists with a means to compute Yin and Yang for different locations. They can now begin formalizing their daily work routine, such as herb evaluation, with the results presented here. The mathematical formalization of other factors determining the geo-authenticity of herbs, such as the physical and chemical soil properties, is a goal of future research. With a formalization of all these factors, herbalists can compute the overall Yin-Yang composition of herbs and herb combinations.

To render the Yin-Yang symbol, the chapter presents a daylight model to compute daylight hours for each day and latitude. However, the rendered Yin-Yang symbols differ from the common Yin-Yang symbol shown in Figure 1. The common symbol is an oversimplification. It represents Yin and Yang as two semicircles, which is a rough approximation at best. Therefore, the most popular Yin-Yang symbol is not in accordance with the original meaning of the Yin-Yang symbol. In fact, none of the symmetrical symbols existing today can coincide with any of the asymmetric symbols generated by the rendering method presented in Section 4. In particular, all symbols presented in the appendix of this chapter are asymmetric. This raises the question whether the common Yin-Yang symbol should be replaced by a symbol closer to the original meaning. In principle, any of the Yin-Yang symbols presented here could replace the common symbol and serve as a new standard. A particular good candidate would be the Yin-Yang symbol of the Arctic Circle, shown in Figure 5, because it looks very similar to the common symbol. Whatever the choice, there is yet another problem. Due to the cyclic change of the earth's ecliptic, any chosen Yin-Yang symbol is only a snapshot in time. It will eventually become less accurate. To avoid this problem, one could simply continue using the old Yin-Yang symbol or design a new symbol that does not feature these defects. Anyway, the choice of the standard Yin-Yang symbol depends on many factors, including personal taste. The ultimate answer to this question is therefore beyond the scope of this chapter.

6. Appendix

On the following six pages, the appendix shows examples of Yin-Yang symbols computed for different latitudes in the northern and southern hemispheres. All examples are polar plots of the output of Equations 1 and 2 for different input latitudes. All polar plots are rotated counter-clockwise by 45° so the x-axis is vertical. A closer inspection shows that none of the symbols is symmetrical. The symbols of the southern hemisphere are mirrored versions of the corresponding symbols in the northern hemisphere, apart from some numerical inaccuracies close to the polar circles and poles. Several popular variants of the Yin-Yang symbol are visible north of the Arctic Circle and south of the Antarctic Circle. Both spots in each Yin-Yang symbol lie on the vertical axis, plotted halfway between the polar plot's origin and the outer circle.

Note that for latitudes L with $|L| \leq 68°$, the Yin-Yang symbol will look similar to the symbols observed at the polar circles when plotted as a polar plot in the following way: Instead of the daylight hours, the polar plot shows the daylight hours minus the minimum day length. Furthermore, instead of the number of hours with darkness, the polar plot shows the difference between the maximum day length and the number of daylight hours.

6.1 Yin-Yang symbols for the northern hemisphere

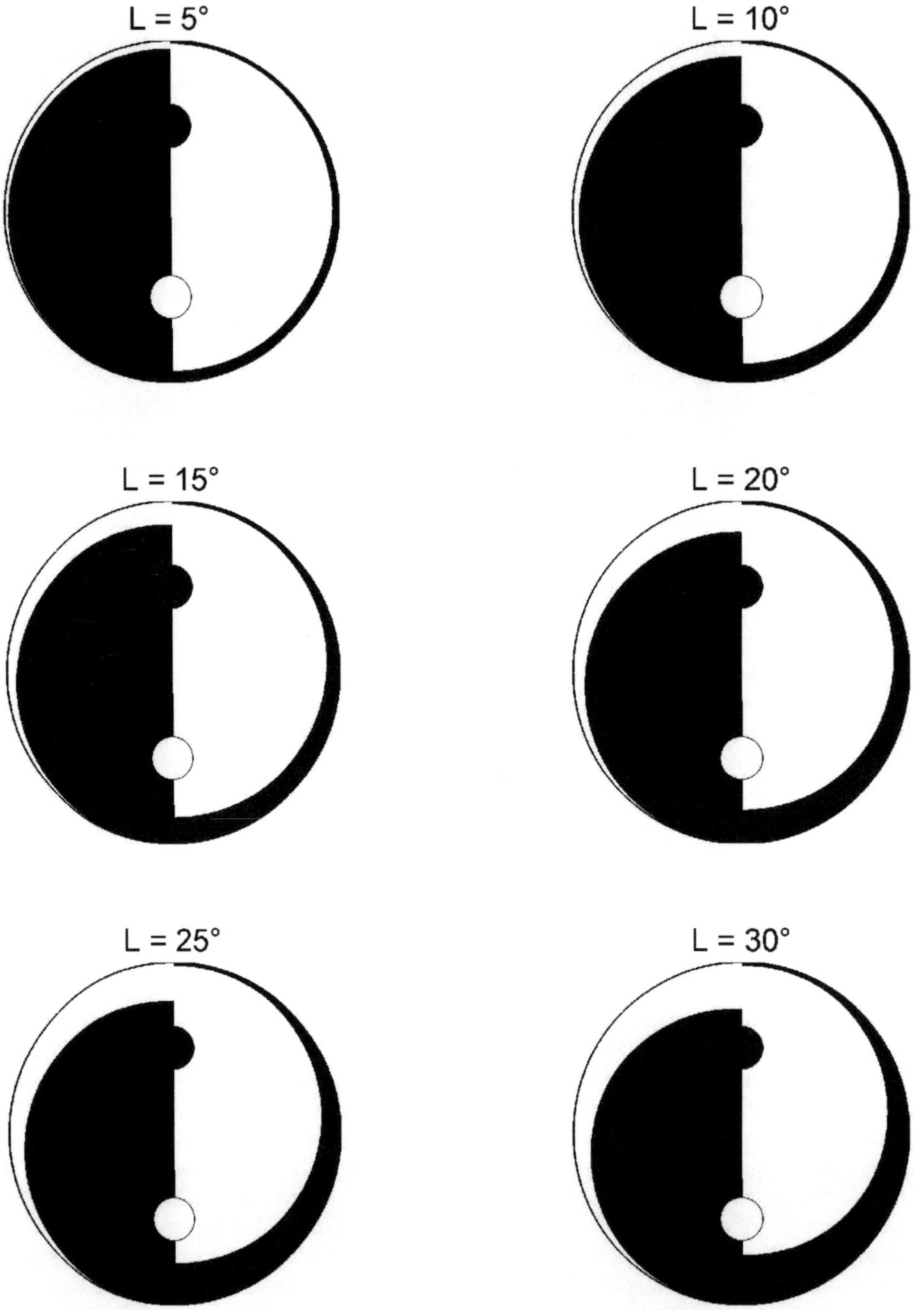

Fig. 9. Yin-Yang symbols for $L = 5°, 10°, 15°, 20°, 25°, 30°$.

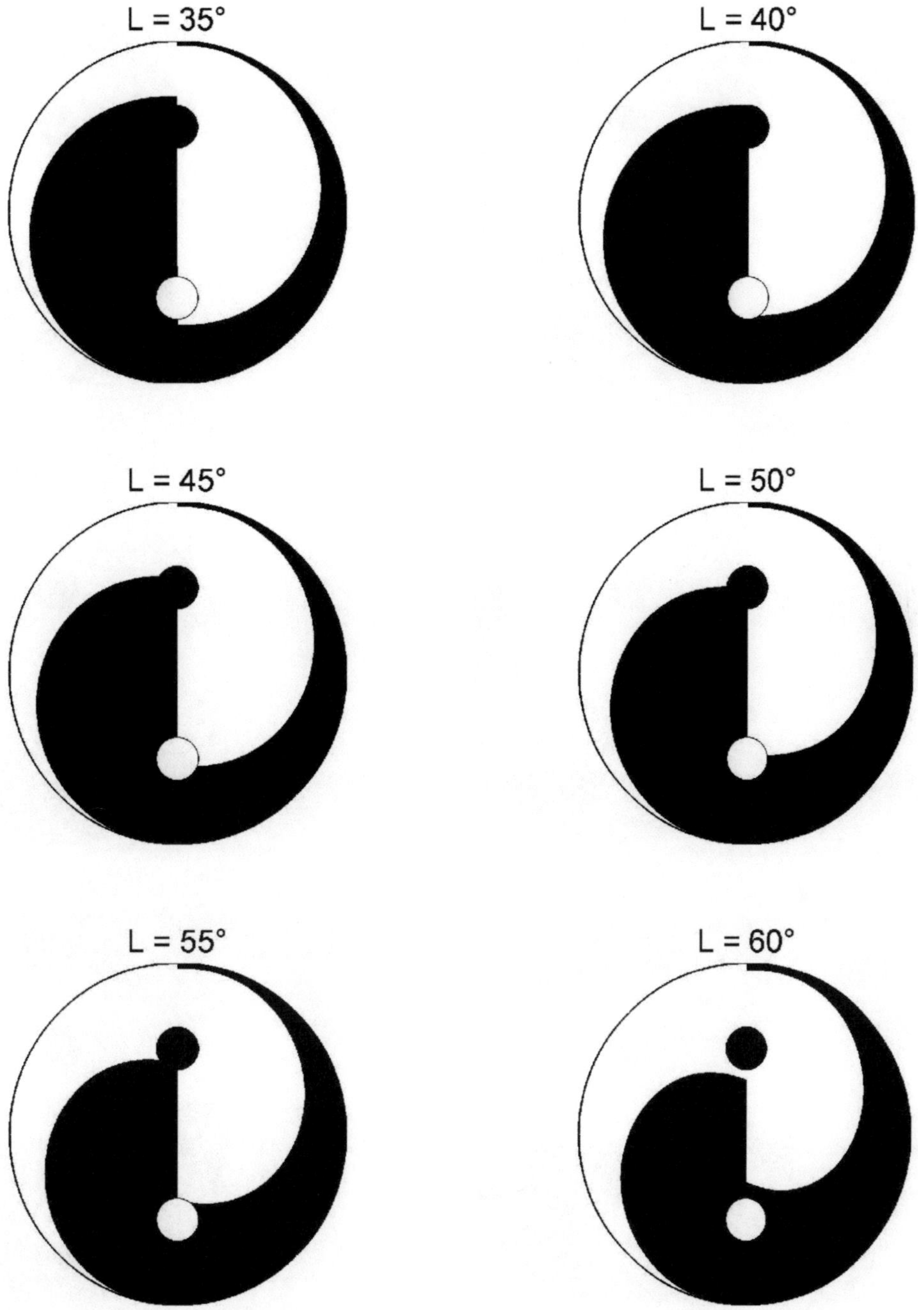

Fig. 10. Yin-Yang symbols for $L = 35°, 40°, 45°, 50°, 55°, 60°$.

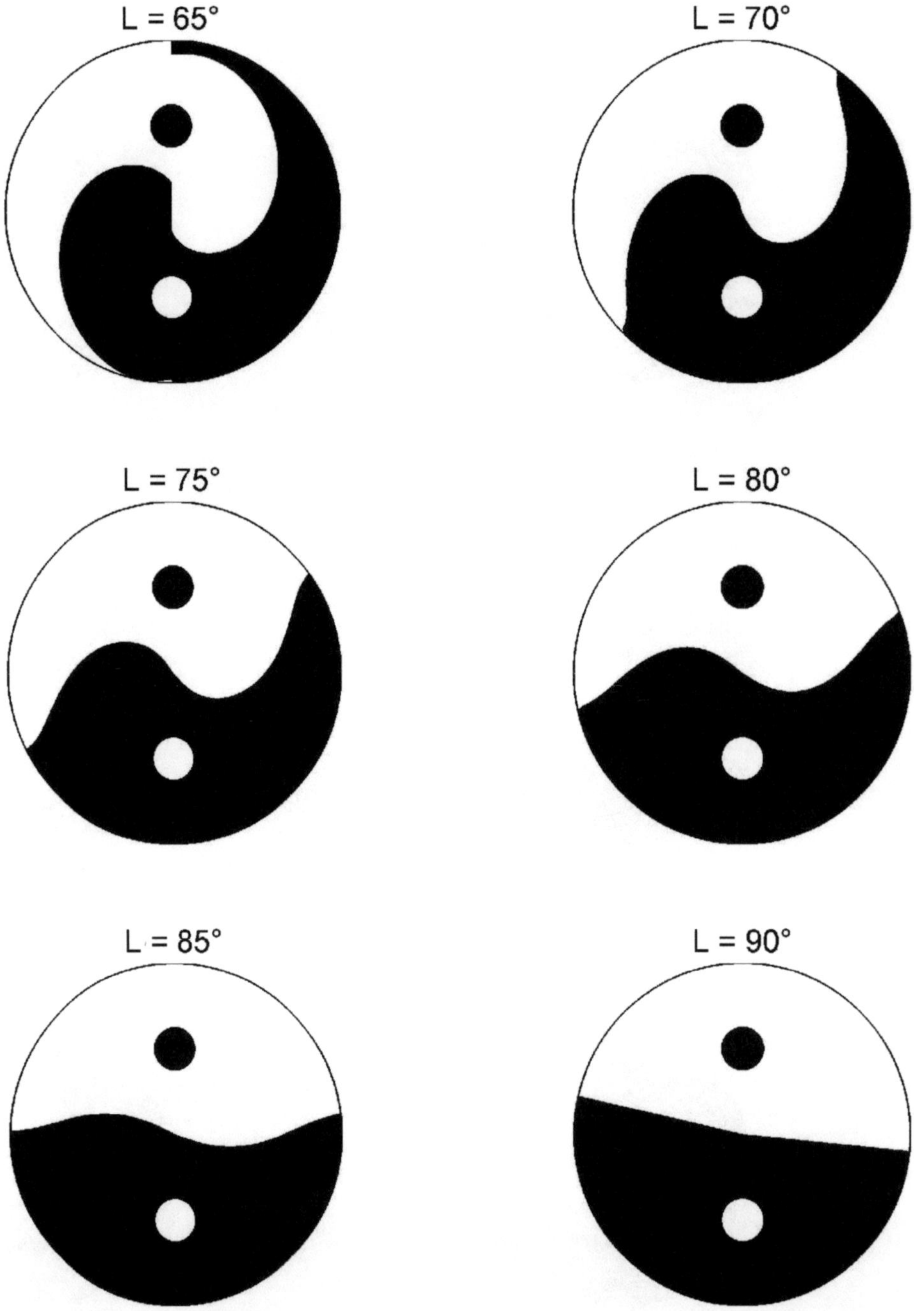

Fig. 11. Yin-Yang symbols for $L = 65°, 70°, 75°, 80°, 85°, 90°$.

6.2 Yin-Yang symbols for the southern hemisphere

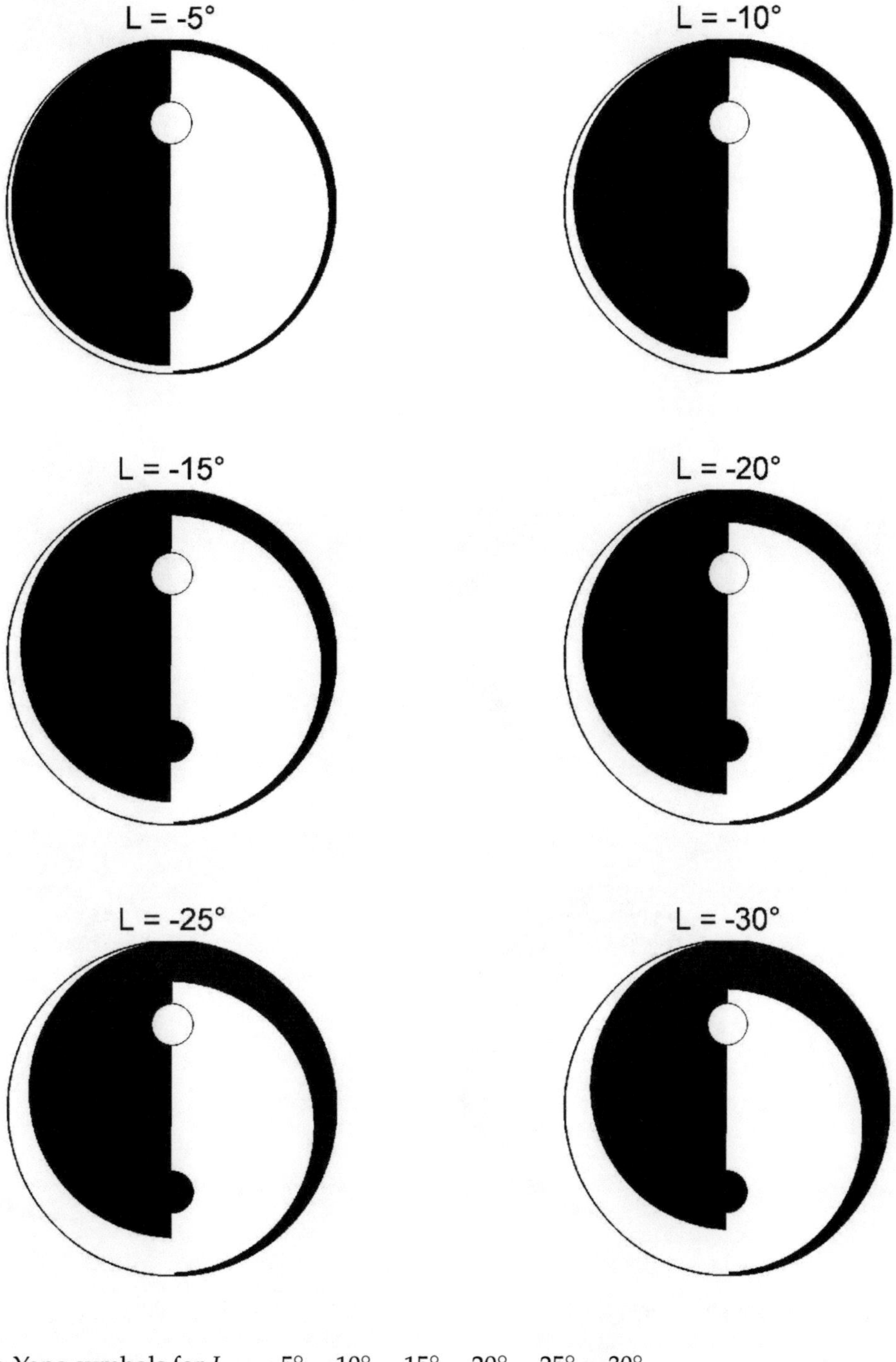

Fig. 12. Yin-Yang symbols for $L = -5°, -10°, -15°, -20°, -25°, -30°$.

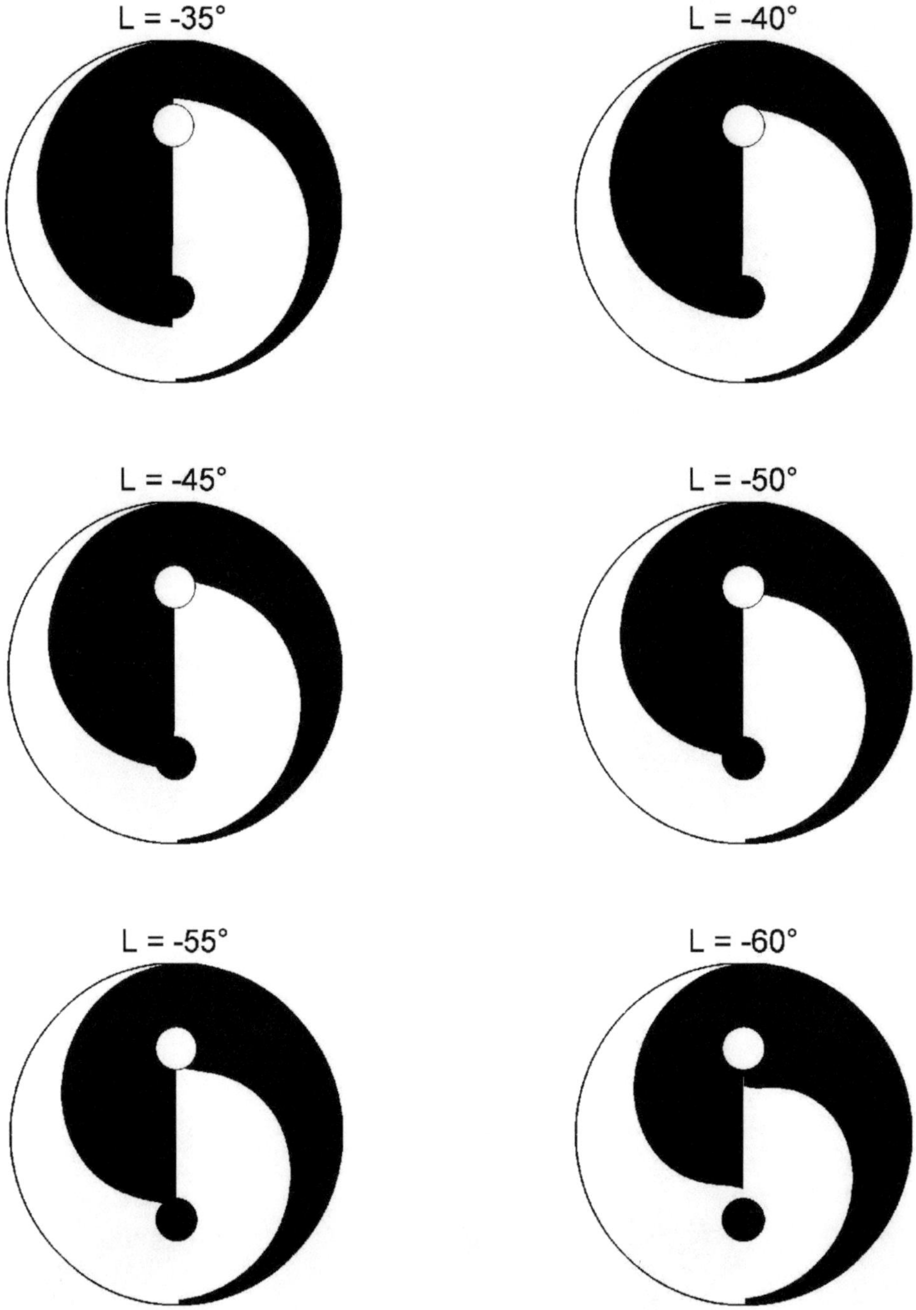

Fig. 13. Yin-Yang symbols for $L = -35°, -40°, -45°, -50°, -55°, -60°$.

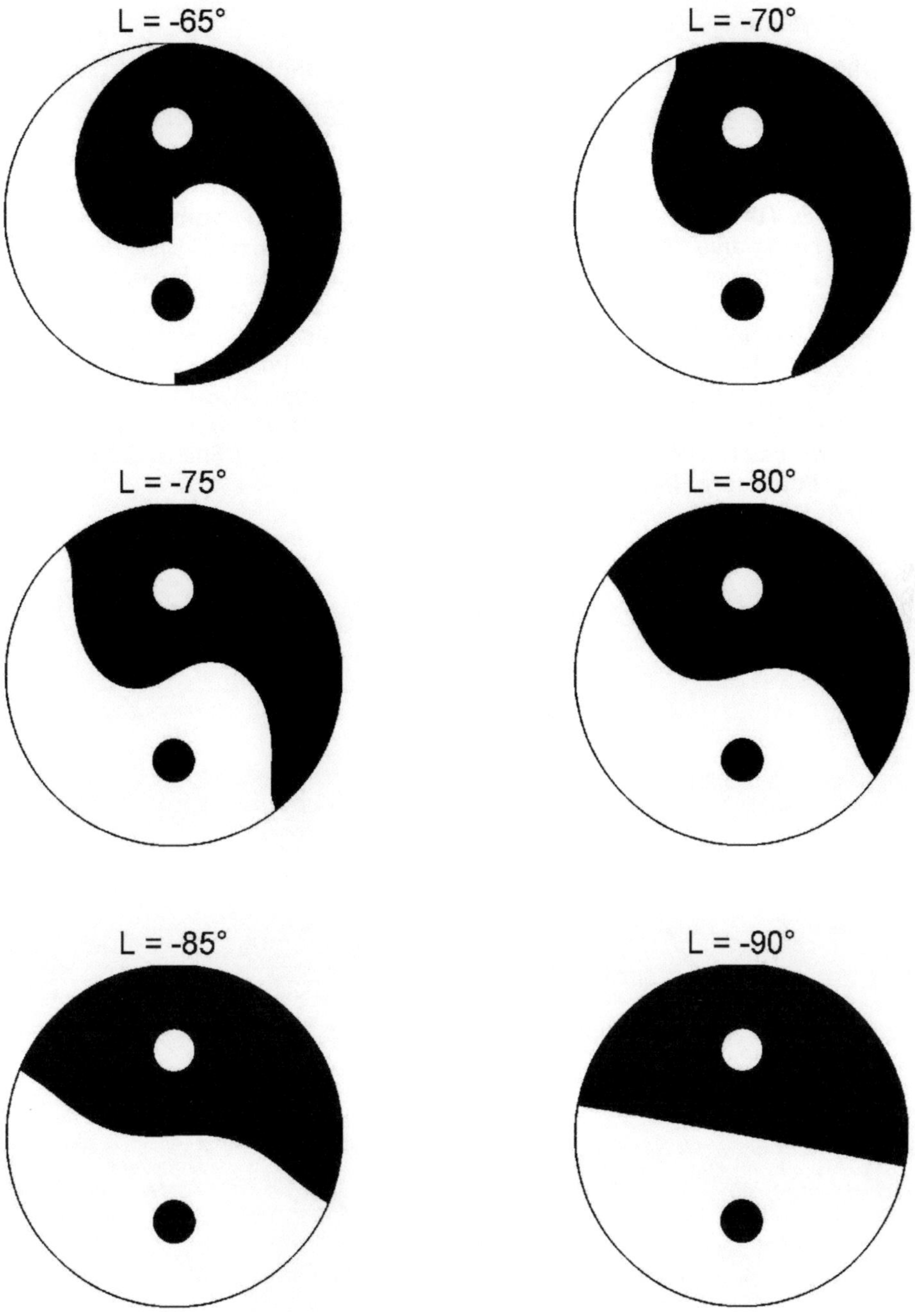

Fig. 14. Yin-Yang symbols for $L = -65°, -70°, -75°, -80°, -85°, -90°$.

7. References

Browne, C. (2007). Taiji variations: Yin and Yang in multiple dimensions, *Computers & Graphics* 31(1): 142–146.

Cook, T. (1979). *The Curves of Life*, Dover Publications.

Forsythe, W., Rykiel, E., Stahl, R., Wu, H.-I. & Schoolfield, R. (1995). A model comparison for daylength as a function of latitude and day of year, *Ecological Modelling* 80(1): 87–95.

Graf, K.-D. (1994). Mathematics and Informatics in old symbols: Tai Chi symbol and hexagrams from the I Ging, *K. Yokochi and H. Okamori (Eds): Proceedings of the Fifth Five Nations Conference on Mathematics Education*, Osaka, Japan, pp. 15–21.

Hardaker, C. (2001). The hexagon, the solstice and the kiva, *Symmetry: Culture and Science* 12(1-2): 167–183.

Miller, J. (2003). *Daoism: A Short Introduction*, Oneworld Publications.

Séquin, C. H. (1999). Analogies from 2D to 3D, exercises in disciplined creativity, *BRIDGES - Mathematical Connections in Art, Music, and Science*, Winfield KS.

Tian, H. & Tian, F. (2004). *The true origin of Zhou Yi (in Chinese)*, Shanxi Science and Technology Publishing House.

Watts, A. (1999). *The Way of Zen*, Vintage.

3

Application of "Five Elements Theory" for Treating Diseases

Yasuyo Hijikata
Toyodo Hijikata Clinic
Japan

1. Introduction

The ancients thought that there were five indispensable qualities for living. These are Wood, Fire, Earth, Metal and Water, and they are otherwise known as the five phases. They each possess different characteristics, and all phenomena and substances within the universe belong to one of these five phases.

The idea which has developed into the five-phase theory is that all phenomena and substances in the universe are the products of the movement and mutation of these five phases. The five-phase theory, as described in the Neijing, is a philosophical theory of medical practice in ancient China.

This theory has served as the guiding ideology and methodology of physiology, pathology, clinical diagnosis and treatment. The characteristics of each phase in this theory have been derived from the observations of countless generations over the millennia, and they are reflected in clinical experiences. As will be mentioned, among these phases both engendering and restraining patterns exist. In the case of the excess of one phase, engendering becomes overwhelming, and restraint becomes rebellion.

However, in five-phase theory, not every situation is well-defined because there are some contradictions and cross-overs in the signs of various physiological features. In both Yin Yang theory and five-phase theory, not all notions are necessarily clear. Nonetheless, despite such a lack of clarity, intractable diseases are sometimes cured or else ameliorated by applications of five-phase theory.

More details about five-phase theory will be described below.

2. Characteristics and categorization

Wood signifies both bending and straightening, and has the characteristics of growth, up-bearing and effusion. It refers to the state of the growing tree. All things which are characteristic of growth, development and elongation belong to Wood.

Fire flares upwards, and has the characteristic of blazing heat. Things which have the characteristics of heat and rising belong to Fire.

Earth is the source of everything, and it represents the characteristics of sowing, reaping and engendering transformation. Things which form and grow, or are sown, raised, and reaped belong to Earth.

Metal is the working of change, and it has the characteristics of purification, elimination and malleability. Things which are constantly changing or are involved in purification and elimination belong to Metal.

Water is the moistening and descending element. It has the characteristics of moistening, downward movement and coldness. Things which are cold, cool, humid and move downwards belong to Water.

3. The relation between the five phases and the five viscera

The five viscera (Liver, Heart, Spleen, Lung, and Kidney: the first capital letter means Viscus in TCM) are related to the five phases according to their own properties. The physiological characteristic of Liver is to govern free-coursing, to thrive by orderly reaching, to rise and to move. As it is likened to spring - when plants grow - and since of the five elements spring relates to Wood, Liver is attributed to Wood. As Liver controls the sinew, and the eyes express the function of Liver, these also belong to Wood.

The function of Heart is to control blood vessels and to warm the whole body by propelling qi and blood. It is likened to the summer heat. As the summer is attributed to Fire, Heart belongs to Fire. As pulse is caused by blood flow and Heart meridian leads to the tongue, they also belong to Fire.

Spleen controls the transportation and transformation of the essence of food, and it is the origin of the engendering transformation of qi and blood. It is likened to the late summer and humid weather - when all things grow - and to Earth which brings up all things. As late summer corresponds to Spleen, Spleen belongs to Earth. Since the condition of Spleen is expressed in muscle and lips, they belong to Earth as well.

Lung pertains to purification and down-sending. It is likened to the cool, crisp air of autumn - a quiet time when everything contracts. As autumn corresponds to Metal, Lung belongs to Metal. Equally, as the condition of Lung is expressed in body hair and the surface of the skin, as well as the nose, these also belong to Metal.

The function of Kidney is to store essence and fluid. It is likened to the winter, when all things are stored and the bitter cold exists. As winter corresponds to Water, Kidney belongs to Water. Kidney opens into bone, ears and two yins. Accordingly, they belong to Water. Other correspondences between the natural world and the human body are shown in Table 1.

Elements	Viscera	Bowels	Color	Flavor	Emotions	Senses	Climate	Season	Tissues	Direction
Wood	**Liver**	**Gall - bladder**	**Green**	**Sour**	**Anger**	**Eyes**	**Wind**	**Spring**	**Tendon**	**East**
Fire	**Heart**	**Small Intestine**	**Red**	**Bitter**	**Joy**	**Tong**	**Heat**	**Summer**	**Vessels**	**South**
Earth	**Spleen**	**Stomach**	**Yellow**	**Sweet**	**Pre-occupation**	**Mouth**	**Damp**	**Late summer**	**Muscle**	**Center**
Metal	**Lung**	**Large Intestine**	**White**	**Pun-gent**	**Sorrow**	**Nose**	**Dryness**	**Autumn**	**Skin & Body Hair**	**West**
Water	**Kidney**	**Urinary Bladder**	**Black**	**Salty**	**Fear**	**Ears**	**Cold**	**Winter**	**Bones**	**North**

Table 1. Categorization of objects and phenomina based on Five Phase theory.

4. Engendering and restraining in the five elements and the five viscera

The five phases of engendering and restraining are seen in Wood, Fire, Earth, Metal and Water. Engendering denotes the principle whereby each of the phases nurtures, produces and benefits another specific element or phase. Restraining denotes the principle by which each of the phases constrains another phase. Arranged in cyclic form, the engendering cycle is shown below:

Wood→Fire→Earth→Metal→Water→Wood

The restraining cycle is shown as follows:

Wood→Earth→Water→Fire→Metal→Wood

Applied to the viscera, these cycles are:

Engendering: Liver→Heart→Spleen→Lung→Kidney→Liver

Restraining: Liver→Spleen→Kidney→Heart→Lung→Liver

According to the *Lei-jing*, Nature requires both engendering and restraining forces. Without engendering nothing will arise. Without restraining, things will become powerful without limitation and will therefore become harmful. Thus, the successful functioning of the united whole is considered to be based on the existence of mutual engendering and restraining. Concerning this fact, two key maxims are advanced: "In engendering, restraint exists" and "With restraining, things work". Accordingly, within the movement and changes in nature, engendering and restraining exist. Interestingly, Si-sheng-xin-yuan instead describes the engendering and restraining work through qi transformation rather than through change of quality.

Relationships of engendering among the various viscera are well-defined by the five-phase theory. Kidney stores essence and Liver stores and controls the blood, and Kidney essence forms the liver blood (Kidney engenders Liver). The ability of Liver in blood storing and free-coursing engenders the heart to control blood vessels (Liver engenders Heart). Heat produced by Heart warms Spleen yang. Spleen controls the transportation, transformation and the origin of the engendering transformation of qi and blood, and so controls the blood. Accordingly, Heart supports the ability of Spleen to control the blood (Heart engenders Spleen). Spleen engenders transformation of food to qi and blood, and carries them to Lung and so supports Lung in working efficiently (Spleen engenders Lung). Kidney controls Water, stores essences and absorbs qi. If Lung qi works smoothly, Lung can regulate the waterway and supports Kidney in controlling Water (Lung engenders Kidney).[Ref 1]

Relations of restraining among the viscera are also well defined. The characteristic of Lung function is purification and down-sending. Accordingly, it can restrain the ascending Liver qi and the ascendant hyperactivity of Liver yang (Lung restrains Liver). As Liver has the ability of free-coursing, it can dissipate stagnated Spleen qi (Liver restrains Spleen). Spleen's function of transportation and transformation supports Kidney in controlling the water and also protects the overflow of water moisture (Spleen restrains Kidney). The moistening action of Kidney restrains the progression of Heart "Fire" (Kidney restrains Heart). The yang heat of Heart restrains the excessive purification and down-sending of Lung (Heart restrains Lung).

Engendering and restraining among the five viscera keeps the body in balance. Wherever a viscus is functionally suppressed by the restraining viscus, it is simultaneously engendered so that it doesn't become deficient or damaged. Likewise, where a viscus is supported by its engendering viscus, it is also restrained by its restraining viscus, so that it maintains a sound state, without acceleration.[Ref 2]

5. Overwhelm and rebellion amongst the five phases

When the normal restraining element gets excessive power, so-called overwhelm occurs. Overwhelm is an abnormal, excessive restraint. This happens in two cases. First, it may occur when one phase becomes excessively powerful and so overwhelms the corresponding viscera. Second, it may also arise when the restrained viscera becomes too weak and hence is overwhelmed by its restraining viscera [Ref 3].

Conversely, when the restraining viscera becomes too weak, or the restrained viscera becomes excessively powerful, the opposite of restraining occurs. This is called rebellion. For example, Metal naturally restrains Wood. However, when Wood gets too much power, Metal can't, not only restrain Wood, but it is also injured by Wood's excessive rebellion against Metal.

Similarly, and in applying this concept to the viscera, Lung normally restrains Liver. Nonetheless, when Liver becomes excessively powerful, Lung is not only unable to restrain Liver, but it is injured by Liver's reaction to Lung. Again, this is called Rebellion.

In Zhong-yi-bing-yin-bing-ji-xue,[Ref 4] engendering and restraining concern the mutual relations among human viscera. Overwhelm and rebellion relate to a pathological idea concerning the mutual influences and actions among viscera. For example, when Fire (Heart) gets excessive power, Water (Kidney) cannot ordinarily restrain Fire and so Fire overwhelms Metal to the point of damage; at this stage, inferior Water is boiled down by Fire qi (rebellion). In this way - in illness - overwhelm and rebellion always appear at the same time."

6. The physiological function and condition of the five viscera

Liver lies on the right side, beneath the diaphragm, whilst Gallbladder sticks to the under-surface of the right hepatic lobe. Liver is connected to Gallbladder with channels. Liver is an "exterior" organ and Gallbladder is an "interior" organ.

Liver controls free-coursing, blood storage and the sinews. Free-coursing relates to the regulation of qi movement, psychological and emotional activity, and bile secretion etc. Blood storage means that it controls the blood in circulation as well. Controlling the sinews implies that Liver works to maintain the normal movement of the muscles and joints of the whole body. Liver channel starts from the great toe, climbing the leg and passing through the genitals and the lower abdomen, and then goes up through the costal region to the eyes and the vertex of the head. When pathological changes appear along Liver channel, they are described as Liver diseases.

Dysfunction of the free-coursing causes change to Liver qi depression[*1], stagnated Liver qi transforming into fire, damage to Liver yin, yin deficiency, ascendant hyperactivity of Liver yang[*2], and further progresses to" Liver wind[*3]. On the contrary, dysfunction of storing blood[*4] is caused by blood deficiency as has been mentioned, "Liver yang and Liver qi exist always in excess and Liver yin and Liver blood exist always in insufficiency."[Ref 5, Ref 6]

The treatment for dysfunction of free-coursing is to smooth Liver and regulate the qi, and to apply drugs to pacify Liver and purge Fire. The treatment for dysfunction of blood storage is to tonify Blood and emolliate Liver, enrich Liver and tonify Kidney and so on.[Ref 7]

(Symptoms of *1 include depression, chest and side pain, and digestive symptoms; of *2, nervousness, surliness, headache, vertigo, tinnitus, insomnia, and lumbago; of *3, severe dizziness, headache, stiffness in the neck, tingling in the limbs, trembling lips and fingers, convulsive spasms and inhibited speech; and of *4, dizziness, insomnia, excessive dreams, flowery vision, inhibited sinew-vascular movement, lustreless nails, and reduced menstrual flow).

Heart is in the chest and is covered by the pericardium. Heart controls the blood vessels and the spirit. Heart opens at the tongue. Heart meridian is entangled with the meridian of Small Intestine, which is the corresponding interior viscus.

Pathologies based on Heart qi deficiency*1, Heart yang deficiency*2, Heart blood deficiency*3 and Heart yin deficiency*4 involve diseases of the blood vessels, including arrhythmia, some psychological diseases and ulceration and/or pain of the tip of the tongue.[Ref 8] Treatment is based on the pathology of the Heart [Ref 9].

(Each of *1,*2,*3, and *4 show symptoms of a dull pale complexion, palpitations, dyspnea and arrhythmia. Symptoms of *1 also include hyperhidrosis and a weak, fine and slow pulse; of *2, a dark grey, cyan or purple complexion, inversion frigidity of the limbs, and cold sweats; of *3, dizziness, insomnia, excessive dreams, a fine pulse, and palpitation; and of *4, vexing heat in the chest, the palms and the soles, and night sweats including the symptoms of *3).

The digestive system is composed mainly of Spleen, Stomach, Large Intestine and Small Intestine, of which Spleen and Stomach are the most important. The meridian of Spleen is external and that of Stomach is internal, and they communicate closely with each other.

Spleen controls the transportation and transformation of water and food, whilst Stomach controls the acceptance of food. Spleen controls upbearing and Stomach controls downbearing. Both Spleen and Stomach are the origin of food digestion and transport, and they enable the transformation of the fine essences and the engendering and transformation of qi and Blood (in this manner it is called the postnatal root). The meridians of Small Intestine and Large Intestine are entangled with Heart and Lung. The function of the separation of clear and turbid substances of Small Intestine and the function of carrying and transforming the food waste of Large Intestine are each a part of digestive power and they have a strong connection with the function of both Spleen and Stomach respectively.

Disorders of Spleen include Spleen qi deficiency, Spleen yang deficiency*1, centre qi deficiency*2, blood management failure*3, Stomach yang deficiency, Stomach yin deficiency*4, the counter-flow ascent of Stomach qi, persistent diarrhoea, and incontinence and constipation. Clinically, we recognize these as abnormal functions of digestion, absorption, and the carrying and distribution of essence and excretion.[Ref 10, Ref 11]

(Symptoms of *1 and *2 include white complexion and spiritual fatigue; of *1, abdominal pain relieved by warmth and pressure; of *3, bleeding such as hemafecia and metrorrhagia; and of *4, dry mouth, mirror tongue and constipation).

Lung is situated in the chest, connected with the throat, and opens at the nose. As it is the highest location among the viscera, it is called the canopy. The channel of the Lung connects to that of Large intestine; the former is interior and the latter is exterior. Its main function is to dominate the qi and control respiration. Lung qi faces the hundred blood vessels and channels, regulates the water passage, disperses essence externally to the skin and downy hair, and controls the surface defence qi of the whole body. In other words, Lung works as a respiratory system, but it also controls fluid regulation, the movement of qi and blood, and the defence system of whole body.

Abnormalities of Lung include the non-diffusion of Lung qi, impaired depurative downbearing of Lung qi, Lung qi vacuity, and Lung yin vacuity*1. Clinically, they appear mostly as dysfunction of the respiratory system, a part of the pathology of fluid metabolism and blood circulation (edema, urination abnormality), external contraction with superficial pathogens and some skin diseases like atopic dermatitis. They are treated based on the lung pathology. [Ref 12, Ref 13]

(*1 shows a dry cough with little phlegm)

The Kidney is located in the lower back on either side of the spinal column and opens into the ear and the two yins (the perineal ante-tract and post-tract). Its condition is reflected in the hair of the head. The meridian of Kidney (interior organ) connects to Bladder (exterior organ). The main function of Kidney is to store essential qi which is the basis of growth, development, reproduction and the maintenance of the physiological activity of all the viscera.

The function of Kidney of controlling the water and bone through the production of marrow is based on both Kidney essence and qi. Kidney yin and yang give yin and yang to all the viscera, which is called innate qi.[Ref 14] As the vacuity of the yin and yang of the other viscera influences Kidney, long-term disease is said to influence Kidney.

Kidney yang has a strong correlation with Spleen yang, as implied by the occurrence of Spleen–Kidney yang deficiency; similarly, Kidney yin has a strong correlation with Liver yin, as implied by the occurrence of "Liver–Kidney yin deficiency." It has been said that Kidney and Liver have the same source. Accordingly, when we coordinate Kidney yin and Kidney yang, we must take care to pay attention to the fact that Kidney yin and yang closely cooperate. The physiological function of Kidney includes the urogenital system, the reproductive system, internal secretion and partial cerebral function. Although the function of Bladder is to store and excrete urine properly, urinary retention, incontinence and enuresis are considered to be diseases of Kidney because of the strong correlation of Kidney yang and qi transformation.

Dysfunctions of Kidney include Kidney yin deficiency[*1], Liver–Kidney yin deficiency[*2], Heart–Kidney yin deficiency[*3], Lung–Kidney yin deficiency[*4], Kidney yang deficiency[*5], Spleen–Kidney yang deficiency[*6], the failure of Kidney to receive qi[*7], Heart–Kidney yang deficiency[*8], yang deficiency with water flood[*9], insufficiency of Kidney essence[*10] and insecurity of Kidney qi[*11]. We must treat these diseases based on their pathology.[Ref 15, Ref 16]

(Symptoms of *1,*2,*3 and *4 include feverishness, dizziness, tinnitus, dry pharynx and/or mouth, and lumbago; those of *3 are palpitation, insomnia, and excessive dreaming; of *4, dry cough and night sweats; of *5, *6, *8 and *9, dizziness, tinnitus, sensitivity to the cold, cold limbs and pale complexion with weak knees and lumbar region; of *10,deficient reproductive function, hair and tooth loss; of *11, enursis, polyurea and low back pain)

7. Transmutation among the five phases and viscera

The mutual influences among diseases of the viscera are called transmutation. This is based on the engendering relation, the "mother and child relation," and restraint-based overwhelm and rebellion[Ref 2].

7.1 Transmutation based on engendering

One case is where the mother's disease is transmitted to the child. Another case is where the child's disease is transmitted to the mother.

The former case is shown through the symptoms of lumbar vertebrae pain or languishing, tinnitus and nocturnal emission in Kidney yin deficiency. It starts to be accompanied by forgetfulness, insomnia, irritation and being easily angered in Liver yin deficiency or ascendant hyperactivity of the Liver yang.

But as nurture exists in the first case, the situation easily improves.

An example of the latter case (child to mother) is shown through Heart–Liver Fire effulgence. That is, Fire symptoms of Liver such as being easily angered, irritation, dizziness and headache, and following Heart fire symptoms such as insomnia, palpitation and inflammation of the mouth and tongue. The mother qi is stronger than that of the child, and so the mother's disease is apt to become aggravated.

7.2 Transmutation based on overwhelm and rebellion

Liver qi depression, with symptoms such as fidgetiness, being easily angered, and pain of the lateral costal region, begins to invade the stomach with symptoms of nausea, vomiting and abdominal fullness. In this case Wood overwhelms Earth. Before long, cough or hemoptysis appears, or Wood invades Metal, whilst in the viscera, Liver rebellions against Lung. As Liver should be restrained by Lung, symptoms are mild. If the viscera are weak, transmutation easily occurs; if not, it rarely occurs. However, in the case of acute disease this mechanism doesn't work.

8. Regulation of win qi and revenge qi among the five phases

In Su-wen, zhi-zhen-yao-da-lun-pian when one phase causes overwhelm to the corresponding phase, it is said to have "win qi". Once this happens, revenge energy to restrain it appears, (which is called revenge qi/Win Revenge). The more win qi there is, the more revenge qi there will be, and vice versa. After all, in the regulation process of win revenge qi, there exists the law of action and reaction, which means the volume of win qi equals that of the revenge qi. This is described in the Fig. 1[Ref 2].

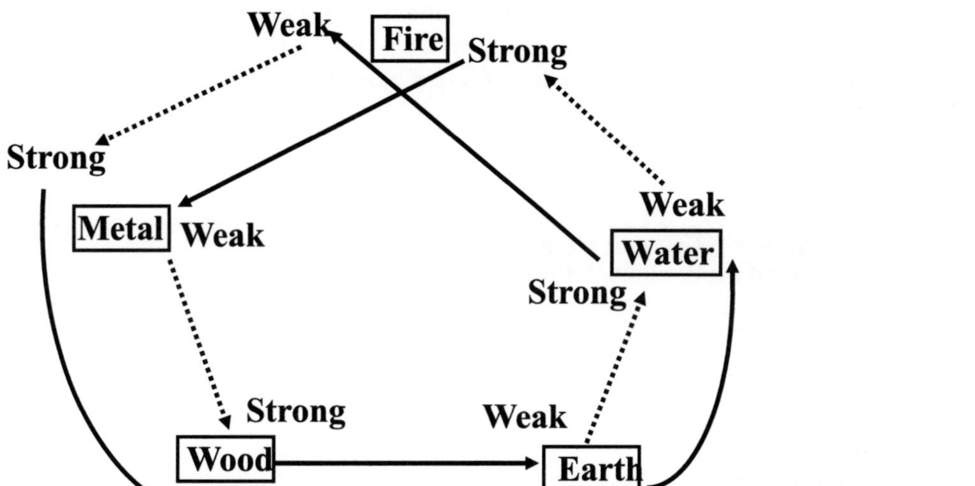

Fig. 1. Win qi and Revenge qi

Explained in terms of Fire in Fig.1, too much Fire qi overwhelms Metal qi → too much decline of Metal qi → Metal qi cannot regulate Wood qi → Wood qi gets excessive win qi → excessive decline of Earth qi → Water qi gets excessive win qi, which restrains Fire → the first excessive Fire qi is normalised. In case of a shortage of Fire qi → Metal gets excessive win qi → Wood qi declines → Earth qi gets excessive win qi → Water qi declines → Fire qi recovers to be normalised. It may be said this mechanism has a kind of feedback system.

When one phase (A) gets excessive qi and the phase which should restrain phase (A) cannot restrain it, the cooperation between these two phases is destroyed and the excessive qi of the phase (A) accumulates more qi while the declined phase is restrained by phase (A) and so declines further. This situation produces an abnormal condition of disorder.
Following Su-wen, in Liu-wei-da-lun-pian: "Once a harmful situation is produced, engendering transformation becomes terribly out of order. In Si-sheng-xin-yuan (wu-xing-sheng-ke-pian), engendering and restraining develop through qi transformation. The quality has no relation with these."

9. Treatments of diseases based on five-phase theory[Ref 2]

9.1 Restrain the transmission of pathological changes of viscera

Diseases develop through dysfunction of viscera, yin-yang and qi-blood.
Dysfunctions of the viscera produce abnormalities of engendering and restraining.
When we treat patients, we must pay attention not only to diseases themselves, but also to the transmission of pathological changes of viscera. We must regulate qi excesses and shortages of viscera based on the law of engendering, restraining, overwhelm and rebellion, by controlling the transmission of pathological changes of viscera and thereby maintaining normal function. For example, when Liver has a disease we must strengthen the function of Spleen and Stomach to protect them from transmission from Liver. Since, by the strengthening of the function of Spleen and Stomach, it is harder for the transmission of pathological change from Liver to Spleen to occur, the disease will be easier to cure.
In Nan-jing.qi-shi-qin-an, it is advanced that once Liver gets a disease, it will transmit it to Spleen. Accordingly, we must give qi to Spleen. The possibility of the transmission of pathological change depends upon the function of viscera. If the viscera qi is in vacuity, the transmission of pathological change will occur; if the viscera qi is in sufficiency, no transmission will occur.

9.2 Treatment rules and treatment methods

9.2.1 Treatment based on the law of engendering

This includes two cases. First there is that of the disease of the mother invading the child. Second, there is that of the disease of the child invading the mother. In Nan-jing (liu-shi-liu nan), it is written that if the child qi is in vacuity, the mother qi must be supplemented (mother qi supplementation), and if the mother qi is sufficient, the child qi must be reduced (child qi reduction).
Mother qi supplementation: In cases where the child qi is insufficient, the mother qi must be supplemented. A dysfunction between mother and child comes from deficiency.
Example
① A shortage of Kidney yin cannot enrich Liver/Wood followed by Liver yin shortage; the ascendant hyperactivity of Liver yang and the so-called Liver qi ascending counterflow will result.
Methods to enrich Water to moisten Wood: this is a therapeutic method to treat Liver yin deficiency by nourishing Kidney yin.
② Methods of engendering Metal-Kidney (enrich Lung and Kidney)

i. Lung deficiency causes circulation-dysfunction of fluids and humours such that Kidney is not enriched.

ii. Owing to the shortage of Kidney yin, Kidney essence qi can't rise, and this is followed by a failure of purification and the downsending of lung. This situation is characterized, for example, by dry cough, qi counterflow, hemoptysis, bone-steaming tidal fever, night sweat, and nocturnal emission etc.

③ Tonify Spleen to engender Lung qi

Tonify Spleen qi to tonify Lung qi. Usually, a continuing cough with plenty of clears puta, a small quantity of viscous sputa, appetite loss, pale tongue and weak pulse will appear.

Purge Child qi: When mother qi is in excess, the child qi should be purged. The dysfunction between mother and child comes from the existence of excess qi. In the case of a disease of Liver derived from excess qi, such as Liver fire or Liver fire flaming upward, Liver/Wood is the mother and Heart/Fire is the child. The treatment is to purge the Heart Fire and it helps to purge the Liver Fire. When a child's disease is caused by a deficiency, we must not only tonify child qi but also tonify mother qi so as to get engenderment from the mother.

9.2.2 Treatment based on the law of restraining

This refers to the treatment by which the weak phase is recovered either by restraining the strong side or else supporting the weak side. In other words, before the strong side can cause overwhelm, treatment to strengthen the energy of the weak side is started.

I Restraining the strong side is mainly applied to the morbidity in overwhelm and rebellion

A. When Liver overwhelms Spleen, treatment to pacify Liver is applied. In this case, Liver easily causes rebellion to Lung, which means that at one phase, such as overwhelm by Liver, rebellion to Lung easily happens at the same time. When we treat Liver, it means that Spleen and Lung are treated as well. In this case Yi-gan-san-jia-chen-pi-ban-xia (in Japanese :Yokukansankachinpihange) is often applied.

B. Depressed Spleen and Stomach qi → Rebellion from Spleen to Liver occur → Liver cannot do free-coursing and ordered reach, for which treatment to move Spleen-Stomach qi is applied.

II Supporting the weak side because of the shortage of restraining energy

① Method to soothe Liver and fortify Spleen

In Liver deficiency, when Spleen-Stomach transmission and transformation doesn't work, Liver is supplemented and pacified and the Spleen is fortified.

In Liver depression and Spleen deficiency, this method is used. Symptoms include an oppressive feeling in the chest, hypochondria and a distended feeling including pain, appetite loss, abdominal distension, loose passage, belching and gas. (Depressed Liver qi can't give proper restraining to Spleen).

② Method to cultivate Earth and suppress Water

In Spleen, with an abnormal function like weak restraining to Kidney, warming Spleen yang moves the qi and fortifies it to improve the controlling water of Kidney (Spleen restrains for Kidney so as not to get water flood; in other words, fortify Spleen yang in order to warm Kidney). Clinically, this is applied to Spleen deficiency, Spleen-Kidney yang deficiency and water flooding the body tissues with edema, distension and fullness. To this symptom Ren-shen-tan (in Japanese: ninjinto) and fu-zi (in Japanese: bushi) are applied.

③ Method to support Metal to restrain Wood (weak restrain to Liver by Lung). In other words, a method to purge Liver and clear Lung, or else regulate Lung to purify. and downsending to restrain Liver. Hypochondriac pain, a bitter taste in the mouth, nervousness, agony and a string-like, rapid pulse and a cough with hemoptysis are often observed.

④ Method to purge Fire and fortify Water

This means purging Heart Fire and fortifying Kidney water; in other words, to purge south and fortify north, or to nourish yin to move Fire down. With the combination of a shortage of Kidney yin and hyperactive Heart yang, so-called non-interaction between the Heart and Kidney occurs. Lumbago, nervousness, insomnia, nocturnal emission, palpitation, exhausting fever and night sweats are often observed. We must note the fact that Kidney belongs to Water and Fire (Kidney controls yin and belongs to Water, and the life gate that belongs to Kidney controls yang and belongs to Fire).

Kidney yin deficiency causes hyperactive fire, blind movement and functional acceleration, such as nocturnal emission, tinnitus, throat pain and dryness. These phenomena are the result of Kidney yin deficiency or yang hyperactivity of Kidney itself, but they have no relation to the fact that Water cannot restrain Fire.

However, when Kidney is weak to restrain Heart, tonify Kidney with yin and purge heart Fire which will support Kidney to restrain Heart.

We can use the law of the relations of engendering and restraining among viscera as a mental therapy. Sorrow is the emotion of Lung and belongs to Metal. Anger is the emotion of Liver and belongs to Wood. As Metal conquers Wood, sorrow conquers anger. Fright is the emotion of Kidney and belongs to Water. Joy is the emotion of Fire. As Water conquers Fire, fright conquers joy. Anger is the emotion of Liver and belongs to Wood. Thought is the emotion of Spleen and belongs to Earth. As Earth can conquer Water, thought defeats fright.

The modern cognition about the study with five-phase theory

In TCM theory, the core of health exists in the dynamic balance between the body and its circumstances; the destruction of this balance is the real cause of disease.

Accordingly, the main theme of the research and study of TCM is the pursuit of methods and remedies to restore degraded physical conditions to a balanced state.

The basic rule of treatment within TCM lies in the regulating of yin and yang, the reforming of tendencies and defects and the recovery of general physical balances.

In recent years, many monographs in cybernetics theory have been published which elucidate TCM theory. For instance, inhibition and the generation of the law of engendering and restraining within the five-phase theory reflect the self-control principle in the human body. With this law, the concept of feedback is included. The five-phase theory, which reflects the transformation law in the cause-and-effect rule, contains the programmatic control concept from cybernetics theory. Further, the method of classification in five-phase theory through the comparison of shapes is similar to the same class-system concept in cybernetics theory.

The five systems in five-phase theory have many routes and form a closed system, with feedback regulations at numerous levels, and thereby maintains the stability of a self-controlled system.

Further, the regulation of inhibition and the generation and regulation of win qi and revenge qi in five-phase theory exemplify the function of the five-phase system in performing automatic regulations.

Applying the five-phase theory to disease in modern medicines

① Examples of mother-child transmission in five-phase theory

- Between Kidney and Liver
- Prolonged dysfunction of Liver is often followed by Kidney dysfunction (Liver Kidney depletion)

- Several monographs have reported that human bone marrow cells, which belong to Kidney, are related to the improvement or progress of liver cell fibrosis. This pattern has been recognised in mice as well.[Ref 17, Ref 18]
- Between Kidney and Lung
  Goodpasture syndrome shows hemoptysis followed by acute glomerulonephritis, which means that the mother's disease (Lung) is transmitted to the child (Kidney) based on mother-child transmission.
- Between Liver and Heart
  In cardiac liver cirrhosis, liver cirrhosis is often derived from right heart failure. This is another case of transmission from the child to the mother.

② Examples of overwhelm and rebellion

- Between Liver and Spleen
  Nervous gastritis and functional gastrointestinal disorder are caused by stress (Liver qi abnormalities).
- Between Kidney and Heart
  In chronic heart disease, an important deteriorating cause is complication arising from Kidney disease; most likely, this will be accumulated Kidney evil resulting from Kidney disease, which will overwhelm Heart. In chronic Kidney disease, an important cause of death is the complication of Heart disease. This may be said to be a kind of rebellion from Heart to Kidney.
- Between Liver and Lung
  Hepatopulmonary syndrome: in chronic liver disease, like liver cirrhosis, telangiectasis or telangiectasia is often observed in the lung, followed by dyspnea. This may be rebellion from Liver to Lung.

Finally, various modern diseases, including incurable disease, have been recognised by five-phase theory and they have sometimes been successfully treated. Therefore, if five-phase theory is properly applied, chronic intractable diseases are sometimes successfully treated.

In particular, in routine life, we have many stresses that we can't avoid and which inflict pain on us. When we consider that those stresses make liver qi abnormalities, we can obtain clues to their improvement, as shown below.

In this chapter, I have applied the lecture Lu-Gan-Fu gave to his son Lu-xi*a, namely that "The evil qi accumulation in one viscus can overwhelm to the restraining viscus. If yang deficiency aggravated in a viscus, the evil qi equals cold pathogen, if heat accumulated enormously, the evil qi equals heat pathogen.

(*a:13th and 14th generation of Lu family noted for wen-bin in China. Their work appeared in the title "Traditional Chinese Medicines Improve the Course of Refractory Leukemic Lymphoblastic Lymphoma and Acute Lymphocytic Leukaemia."*Am.J.Chin.Med*, Vol XXIII, No. 2,pp195-211. 1995)

On applying five-phase theory to treatment, the most important point is to identify the viscera causing the various symptoms. Next is the decision of the order of appearance of the symptoms. Usually by this means we can speculate upon which viscus is at the root of the patient's disease. Next by comparing the various symptoms, we can speculate upon the existence of engendering, restraining, overwhelming, and rebellion among the viscera.[Ref 19] The "Organ pattern identification Table" is very useful and convenient[Ref 16] in this regard.

Below, eleven cases are discussed in detail and in terms of the correlations of medical diagnoses with TCM theory using five-phase theory. The formulas prescribed are shown in

"Chinese Herbal Medicine. FORMULAS & STRATAGIES (Bensky Balolet: published by East Land 1990)." Herbs are shown in *CHINESE HERBAL MEDICINE Materia Medica* 3rd Ed.: published by East Land 2004. To save space, their identification in TCM is described after the symptoms in parenthesis. Numerals in circles refer to the numerals in the respective figures. With Liver, ①, Heart,②, Spleen,③, Lung, ④ and Kidney,⑤are used. Peculiar Japanese prescriptions are explained in this text.

Susceptibility to common cold caused by Kidney deficiency

Case 1 A 60-year-old Japanese female
Chief complaint: Recent susceptibility to catching common colds
Present illness: She found herself prone to catching colds. She had been sensitive to the cold and suffers from frequent urination (Kidney yang deficiency). She has had a weak constitution (Spleen qi deficiency) since childhood. Two years ago, a feeling of throat stuffiness continued. A close examination revealed as the cause a benign thyroid tumour, which was left untreated. Upon her visit to my clinic, she reported that every time she felt tired, she caught a cold (Lung qi deficiency), which was unusual for her. Intake of ge-gen-tang (in Japanese Kakkonto) released the exterior muscle layer and exorcised the common cold within a few days, but she soon caught a cold again. She had looked after her mother at her home and paid much attention to both her husband and mother, which induced a great deal of stress (Liver qi depression) until two years ago when her mother died. In spite of the fact that she was freed from her mother's care, since that time she has become even more susceptible to colds and so visited my clinic.
Past history: She has suffered from dysmenorrhoea, for which total extirpation of the uterus was carried out (Liver qi depression with blood stasis). As she does not have enough stamina, she couldn't work hard (qi deficiency) and has been sensitive to the cold.
Present status: Height, 158cm; weight: 48kg; pulse, 74/min, fine, slippery, string-like, tongue body, pale with reddish limbic, tongue fur, whitish with thin centre (yin deficiency); sublingual vessel enlarged (blood stasis)
Identification: Kidney Yang deficiency, Lung qi deficiency
Treatment: Ba-wei-di-huang-wan (tonifies the yang and yin of Kidney, nourishes the blood)
Clinical course: With no change to her lifestyle and working conditions, she did not catch a cold for the 5 months or more since she started taking 30 pills of Ba-wei- di-huang-wan (common dosage: 60 pills/day).
Discussion: Susceptibility to colds indicates qi deficiency of Lung. The fact, especially, that her colds appeared when she had some trouble which caused her stress implies a rebellion of Liver against the Lung. But she felt her stress decreased after her mother's death two years ago. Accordingly, stress does not influence her frequent catching of colds, but the fact that intake of ba-wei-di-huang-wan decreased her frequency of catching colds implies that the qi deficiency of Lung was reversed by giving yang to Kidney, which was transmitted through their engendering relation.

Ulcerative colitis case

Case 2 A 29-year-old Japanese female who works for civil aviation.
Chief complaint: Diarrhoea, abdominal pain, bloody stool, lumbago, stress-induced insomnia
History of present illness: Her bloody stool had continued in spite of the administration of routine remedies including sufficient rest since 24th of Jan, X year. By continuing an

adrenocortical hormone for one month, the bloody stool stopped. She visited my clinic in June, X year as she hoped to stop the recurrence of her bloody stools. Nine years earlier, she had been diagnosed with ulcerative colitis, which was brought on by a lot of stress. Since then she had been taking 5-amino salicylate. At the beginning she suffered from only bloody stools, but more recently she has suffered from lumbago as well. From seven years earlier to the present, the ulcerative colitis had recurred about once a year. This recurrence was usually evoked by stress or working all night (Wood overwhelms Earth). Overwork often led to abdominal pain followed by bloody stools. She reported that she was routinely feeling abdominal fullness and gassy stomach. Overeating or coldness caused diarrhoea (Spleen yang deficiency ③, ③-②). She dislikes meats. Her digestive system easily gets cold (Spleen yang Deficiency. ③-②) when stressful things happen and Spleen qi deficiency occurred with the failure of controlling Blood (Liver overwhelms Spleen ①-②).

During childhood, she suffered from chilblains, disliked the air conditioner during the summer, wore too many clothes in the winter, and had cold limbs (Kidney yang deficiency ⑤). More recently, she became fatigued easily and perspired greatly during the summer (qi defficiency). She has an irregular period (Blood deficiency of Liver and Liver qi stagnation ①-①, ①-③) and menstrual pain (Liver qi stagnation and blood stasis ①-①).

Past history: She suffered from alopecia areata several times between the ages of ten and twenty-five years old

Present state: Height, 160cm; weight, 55kg; Pulse, 56/min, fine, sunken, slippery; teeth-marked tongue (retention of water.③-②) with a thin white fur; Blood Pressure (BP), 98/62 (mmHg).

Identification: Spleen failing to control the blood. Spleen and Kidney Yang deficiency with water flood. Bowels with damp and heat.

Treatment: Tonify Spleen qi to control the blood, spread Liver qi and relieve constraint. When stressors lead to insomnia, nourish the blood and yin and warm the Kidney to promote urination and stop diarrhoea.[Ref 16]

Prescriptions: ①Jia-wei-gui-pi-tang (in Japanese: Kamikihito) benefits the Spleen qi to control the blood. This equals gui-pi-tang supplemented with chai-fu (Bupleuri Radix) which spreads Liver qi to relieve constraint and clear heat; and zhi-zi (Gardeniae Fructus) which drains heat and eliminates irritability, clears heat, and eliminates dampness (decoction).[Ref 14] ② Zhen-wu- tang warms Kidney to promote urination and stop diarrhoea.

This prescription was made by TSUMURA & CO (http://www.tsumura.co.jp /english/index.htm) (Tokyo Japan).[Ref 20]

Clinical course: After starting herbal therapy, little by little her diarrhoea improved. Her bloody stools decreased in number as well. When she visited my clinic in May, two months after her first visit, she informed me that she had no diarrhoea and no bloody stool, but she would like to continue 5-mino salicylate to make sure. She continued one month's medicine and then stopped. One year and three months later, she visited my clinic to obtain the same herbal remedies for prevention. She told me she had had no symptoms, including diarrhoea and bloody stools, so far (Fig. 2).

Discussion: As the first bloody stool appeared following a stressful episode, the stressful event induced Liver qi depression which in turn overwhelmed Spleen leading to a failure to control Blood. In Jia-wei- gui-pi-tan, ren-shen, bai-chu, zhi-gan-zao, huan-qi worked to tonify the Spleen qi, to stop diarrhoea and bloody stool. Fu-ling, long-yan-rou and suan-zao-ren tonified and nourished Heart blood so as to tranquilise. The chai-fu worked to disperse stagnated Liver qi so that Liver would not overwhelm Spleen. The recent complication of lumbago may be a result of overwhelm from Spleen with excess coldness pathogen to Kidney. As mentioned already, a method to cultivate Earth and suppress Water, like Zhen-wu-tang, was prescribed. The zhi-zi (Gardeniae Fructus) likely supported the subsidence of the colitis. Zhen-wu-tang warmed the yang of Kidney and Spleen, thereby tonifying Spleen and Kidney, which stopped the progression of her lumbago and bloody stools.

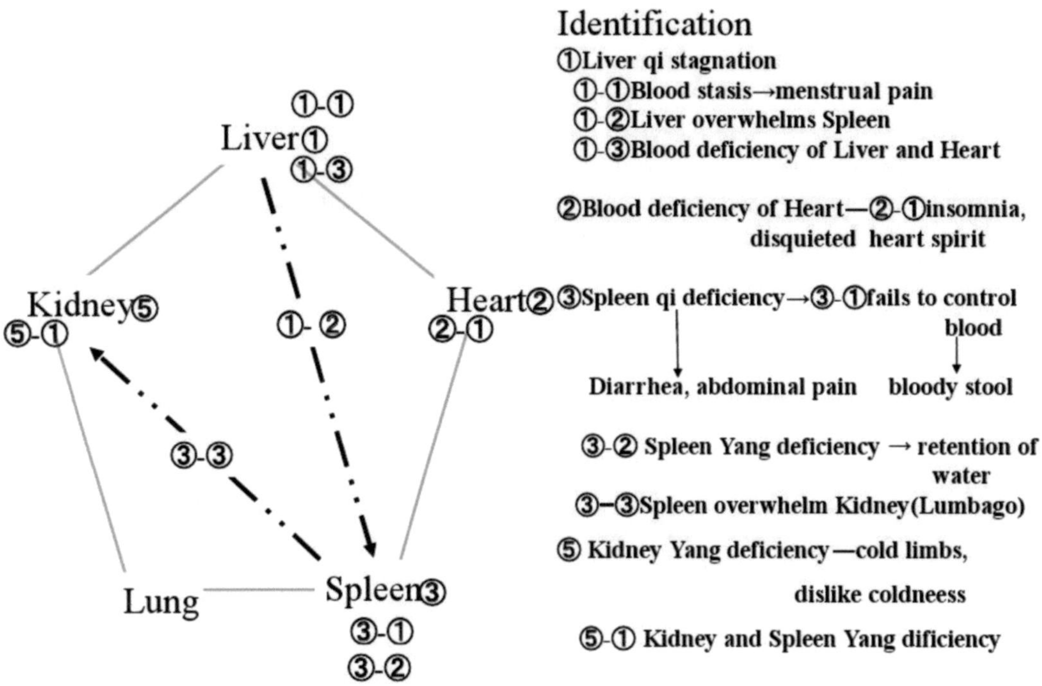

Fig. 2. Relations among viscra with five phase theory of Case 2

Great improvement after insertion of intra-cardiac pacemaker

Case 3 A 73-year-old Japanese housewife

Chief complaint (First visit): Dull feeling in Stomach, frequent cystitis, Kidney ptosis with vesical inertia, oversensitivity to the cold

History of present illness: She often had a dull feeling in her stomach. She could not take meats or fatty food. Coldness easily evoked abdominal pain or diarrhoea, and she felt that she easily got colds (Spleen Yang deficiency ③,③ Lung qi deficiency ④-①). She often saw purple spots without any reason. She has serious kidney ptosis and vesical inertia (sunken middle qi ③-①), frequent suffering from cystitis (Kidney yang deficiency ⑤-①), and continuing throat discomfort throughout winter (Lung qi deficiency④-①). She visited my clinic in February of X year to decrease the frequency of cystitis.

Present status: Height 140cm, Weight 41kg, Blood pressure 126/72mmHg, pulse, 70/min, weak

Past history: She reported to have had a weak constitution since childhood and often felt lassitude (qi deficiency). She had been oversensitive to the cold and has suffered from cystitis. Her digestive system was weak. Her throat discomfort had continued throughout the winter and she felt as if she had been catching a cold all winter. Her menopausal symptoms continued for more than ten years with lassitude and perspiration, for which she had to take a tranquiliser.

Identification before insertion of intra-cardiac pacemaker: Spleen and Kidney Yang deficiency, Heart qi deficiency, Lung yang and qi deficiency. Liver overwhelms Spleen

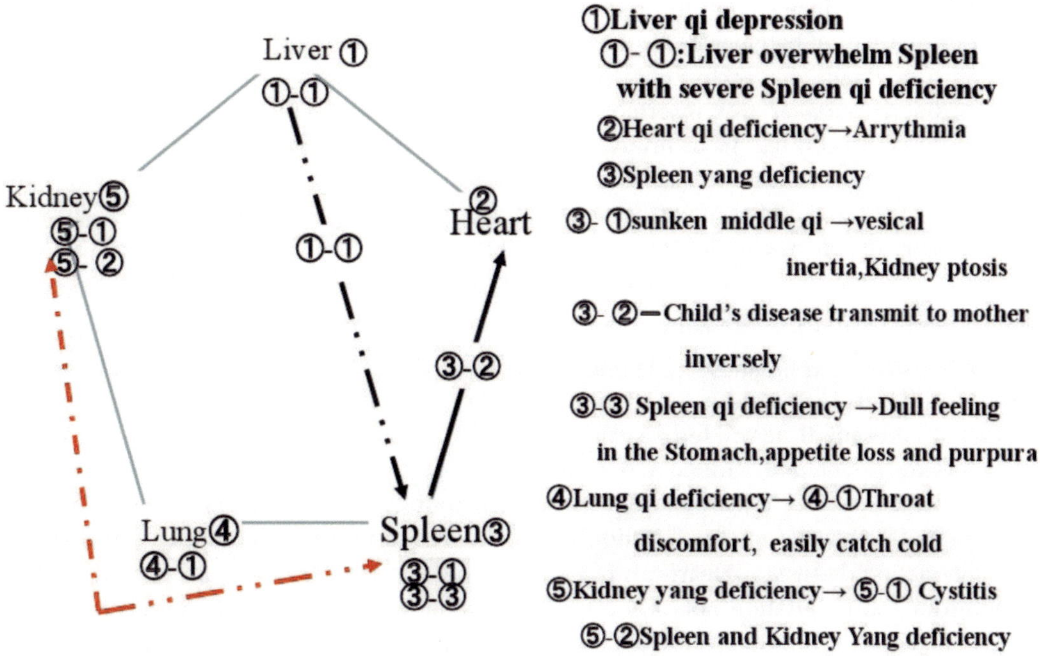

Fig. 3. Relations among viscera with five phase theory of case 3 (Just before insertion of intra-cardiac pacemaker)

Treatments: Warm the Kidney and Spleen yang, tonify Spleen, clear heat and moistness of bladder

Prescriptions:①bu-zhong-yi-qi-tang (in Japanese: Hochuekito) tonifies the qi of the middle burner and raises sunken yang, with fu-zi (Aconiti Radix) reviving and assisting the yang, warming the fire and dispersing cold, ba-wei-di-huang-wan (in Japanese: Hachimijiogan) warms and revives the yang and enriches the yin of Kidney. ③WTTCGE (*Wisteria floribunda* 2g, *Trapa natans* 2g, *Terminalia chebulae* 2g, *Coix lachryma-jobi* 4g, *Ganoderma lucidum* 4g, *Elfuinga applanata* 2g in dry weight/day: effective for herpes genitalis, labialis and chronic herpes viruses infectious diseases to increase the NK cell activity and prevent inflammation). [Ref21, Ref22]

Clinical Course: I prescribed bu-zhong-yi-qi-tang supplemented with fu-zi for yang deficiency of Kidney, ba-wei-di-huang-wan and hot water extracts of WTTCGE for continuing throat discomfort through the winter. The latter was combined with modified zhu-ling-tang (in Japanese: Chyoreito) in order to promote urination, clear heat, and nourish the yin for frequent cystitis. The cystitis improved but not perfectly. Her digestive system symptoms and purpura remained. Twelve years after her first visit, arrhythmia started -

sometimes 30~40/min - and caused instantaneous unconsciousness. Fourteen years after first visit, the insertion of an intra-cardiac pacemaker was carried out without changing the intake of herbal therapies. After this, her appetite loss and other associated symptoms of digestive system - including purpura - disappeared almost completely and the disease rate of cystitis dramatically decreased and has remained decreased up until the present.

Discussion: On her first visit, she did not have arrhythmia while her yang deficiency of Kidney and Spleen were long-term conditions. Twelve years later she had arrhythmia. This may mean that during the long duration of Spleen yang deficiency, based on the engendering relation between Heart and Spleen, the Spleen may have stolen her Heart qi in the long run. Finally, her arrhythmia continued. Fourteen years later after her first visit, an intra-cardiac pacemaker was inserted and the Heart qi was tonified and followed by the enrichment of Spleen qi. Accordingly, her purpura and digestive symptoms disappeared and her appetite was restored. As Kidney and Heart belong to the same lesser yin, with increasing Heart qi, Kidney qi was increased and Kidney yang was also increased allowing for Bladder to be warmed and being followed by the disappearance of Bladder inflammation. Her nervousness decreased, probably as a result of tonifying Heart.

Male climate period (Severe Autonomic nerve dysfunction syndrome)

Case 4. A 46-year-old Japanese male medicine wholesaler

Chief complaint: Tachycardia, palpitation, hypertension, a hot face and staggering

History of present illness: He began to suffer from a hot face, staggering, insomnia and hypertension (Liver and Kidney yin deficiency ①-①, ②, ⑤-⑤) in April. He had been doing aerobic exercise for a long time without any trouble. However, on September 25 of the same year, tachycardia and palpitation continued for more than one hour after aerobics (non-interaction between Heart and Kidney ((②-①). Furthermore, he suffered from tachycardia and palpitation not only after aerobics but also while resting, which led to his giving up aerobics. As he would sit, he felt palpitation and had a pale face and, upon standing up, he felt as though he was losing consciousness.

An intake of psychotropic medications for one week had no beneficial effect. His blood pressure had been high and unstable. On straining during working, his face would get hot and the temples would throb uncomfortably (Ascendant hyperactivity of Liver yang ①-①-①). His stiffness of shoulder, neck and back (Liver qi depression and blood stasis, interruption of meridian and collaterals ①-③) and heaviness of the occipital region (retention of dampness ⑤-②) continued. At his first visit on October 12, he felt something was heaving up from the epigastrium and his BP was 170/100mmHg (Kidney yin deficiency followed by ascendant hyperactivity of deficient fire:⑤-③).

On that day he started taking chai-hu-jia-long-gu-mu-li-tang (in Japanese: Saikokaryukotsuboreito - this unblocks the three yang stages, and sedates and calms the spirit: TSUMURA & CO)[Ref20] which aggravated his hotness of face and palpitations and so was stopped. Generally, his general fatigue was severe, his urination volume was large, and he experienced discomfort on rainy days (retention of dampness:⑤-②). He often had muddy stools (Spleen qi deficiency:③-①) and was irritated, got angry easily, experienced hotness of the face and had night sweats ascendant hyperactivity of Liver yang (①-①-①). When he was tired, his soles were hot with sweat (Kidney yin deficiency ⑤-③). He felt asthenopia, dim eyesight and dry eye (Liver blood deficiency ①-④). (Fig 4).

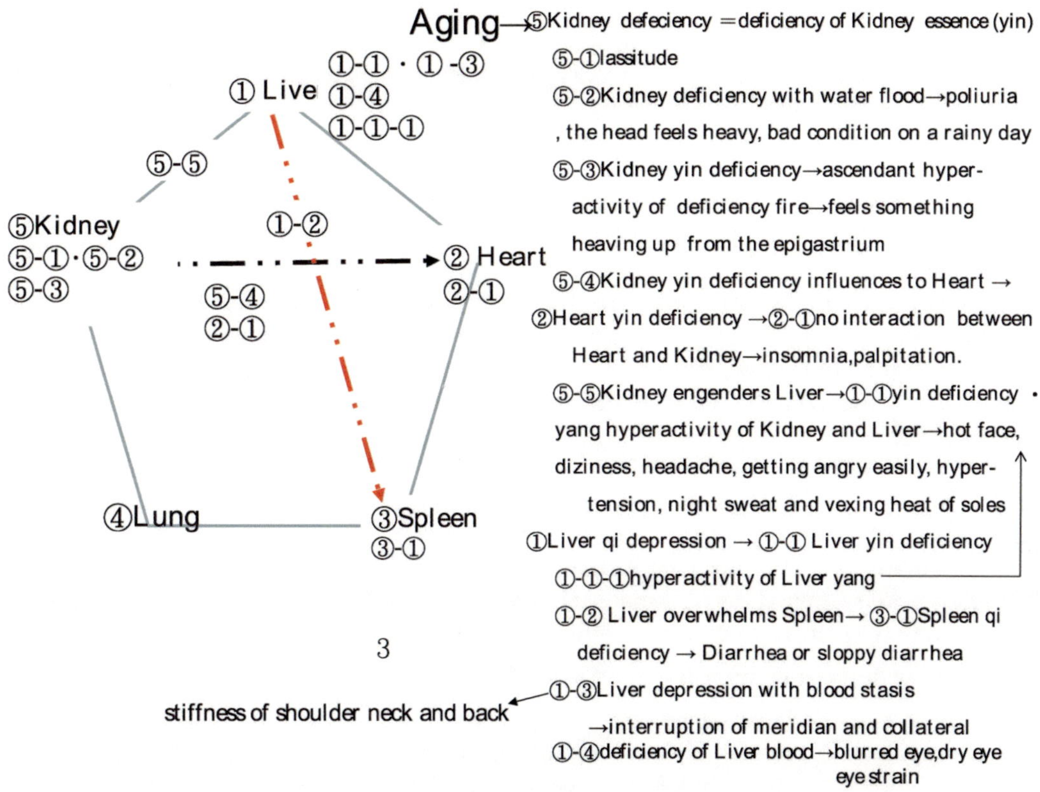

Fig. 4. Relations among viscera with five phase theory of case 4 (before treatment)

On October 25, he began an intake of gui-zhi-fu-ling-wan (in Japanese: Keishibukuryogan - this invigorates the blood and transforms blood stasis: TSUMURA & CO)[Ref 20] but only about 20% of his symptoms decreased. He visited a Kampo clinic and was administered zi-yin-jiang-huo-tang (in Japanese: Jiinkokato[Ref 20, Ref 24] - this tonifies yin:zhi-gan-zao, dang-gu, shao-yao, sheng-di-huang, tian-men-dong, mai-men-dong, bai-shu, chen-pi, huang-bo, zhi-mu, sheng-jiang, da-zao).[Ref.22]

On November 17, tachycardia, palpitation and discomfort started to decrease and his irritation and instances of getting angry decreased by around 50%. No further improvement occurred. On November 24, he visited my clinic and diagnosed as follows.

Identification: Liver qi depression with blood stasis, ascendant hyperactivity of Liver yang (①-①-①), Kidney and Liver yin deficiency(⑤-③,①-①), Kidney deficiency with water flood(⑤-②).

Treatments: Tonify Kidney yin and essence and Liver yin

Prescription: Turtle powder (whole body was treated with heat and dried: 2g/day) was added.

Clinical Course: One week later he had recovered completely. By mid-January of the following year, he could perform aerobics without any trouble, and the intake of all remedies except for turtle powder was stopped. He has been taking turtle powder since then, for several years, because if he stops he starts to feel strange and uncomfortable.

Discussion

During the male climacteric period, the male hormone decreases which means Kidney essence and yin decreases in TCM theory. It is reasonable that the prescription of zi-yin-jiang-huo-tang[Ref 23] caused symptoms to improve by 50%. The reason chai-hu-jia-long-gu-mu-li-tang worsened the situation is because his symptoms originated from the deficiency of Kidney essence and yin rather than by the inhibited three yang stages. This remedy tended to consume yin, which aggravated this situation. Shortage of Kidney yin caused Heart Fire effulgence (⑤-④. ②. ②-①), which means non-interaction between the Heart and Kidney.

My TCM teacher, Lu Xi told me that his father, Lu Gan-fu, taught him that overwhelmingness occurs from viscus with excess evil qi to the corresponding viscus. If this theory is applied to Kidney, it may be said that hyperactive Kidney yang based on Kidney yin deficiency overwhelms Heart. Accordingly, hyperactive Kidney yang and Heart fire can exist together.

Liver yin deficiency by engendering from Kidney (①-①), and ascendant hyperactivity of Liver yang (①-①-①) followed by overwhelm from Liver to Spleen (①-②.③-①), which were almost all resolved by prescribing the turtle powder.

There are many herbs for tonifying Kidney yin or essence, but when they are not effective; it is necessary to try animal-derived material in order to enrich Kidney yin or essence. Animal-derived materials are sometimes very effective for these cases.

Aged female depression after husband's death

Case 5: A 76-year-old Japanese female

Chief complaint: Depression with severe self-reproach, no vitality.

History of present illness: Since two years ago, when her husband died, she had been suffering from impatience, depression with a guilty conscience (Liver qi depression), and insomnia. She could not get to sleep easily and she routinely took tranquilizers. Upon awakening, she felt heavy depression. As her false teeth did not fit, she ate by grinding her food. She had cold forefeet and had difficulty in hearing. Though table tennis had been her hobby, she had stopped due to lack of vitality. Up until her husband's death, she had climbed one mountain (600m height) once a week.

Past history: She had been hospitalized after the great Hanshin earthquake. Menopause occurred at fifty-two years

Family history: Her brothers all died from TB.

Present status: Height, 156cm; weight, 48kg; BP, 138/78mmHg; pulse, 66/min. fine, slippery, sunken, with a weak chi/cubit pulse; tongue body, red; tongue fur, thin (Liver qi depression, Spleen qi deficiency (①, ①-②)

Identification: Qi deficiency, Liver qi depression, Deficiency of Kidney yin and yang

Treatment: Soothe Liver to release depression, tonify Spleen and Kidney

Prescription: ① bu-zhong-yi-qi-tang and ② soft-shelled turtle (tonifies yin and Kidney). Beginning on day thirty-eight nu-shen-san[Ref 24] (in Japanese: Nyoshinsan - dan-gui, chuan-xiong, gui-zhi, bai-chu, mu-xiang, huang-qin, huang-lian, ren-shen, gan-cao, xiang-fu-zi, da-huang, zong-lu-zi, ding-xiang soothes and tonifies Liver, clears heat, and warms the lower body)[*1. Ref 25] was added to her previous prescriptions.

Clinical course: Ten days after starting Kampo medicine (bu-zhong-yi-qi-tang, soft-shelled turtle) her mental irritation - including her depression with guilty conscience - decreased.

However, she still suffered occasionally from extreme depression. She continued with the same medicines. On day thirty-eight, a new prescription, nu-shen-san, was added. Three days after the addition of nu-shen-san, her feelings became more pleasant and her depression improved remarkably. She could go to the theatre and go shopping with a neighbouring housewife. She could not believe how depressed she had been. She continued for another thirty days with the same medicines and quit them all seventy-six days after starting Kampo medicine. She reported that she had completely recovered from her depression and could lead a satisfactory and normal life. Her insomnia disappeared as well.

Discussion: This patient's Kidney yang and yin were rather deficient because her forefoot was cold even in the summer; she felt hot in sole and she had difficulty in hearing. She liked drinking cold cow's milk and had a dry mouth. The body of her tongue was red and her tongue fur was thin (Kidney yin deficiency⑤-③). The soft-shelled-turtle tonifies yin and Kidney. By taking this, Kidney would be enriched. The enriched Kidney may have engendered the Liver, which likely played a role in improving the depression to some extent. Bu-zhong-yi-qi-tang - which tonifies Spleen qi and supports the upbearing of qi - also contributed to improving the depression. It is certain that these two medicines were partly effective in decreasing her depression, but her depression did not disappear completely and the addition of nu-shen-san improved the feeling of loss dramatically. Nu-shen-san soothed Liver and tonified it with other prescriptions, which engendered Heart, and was followed by the improvement of her insomnia and disappearance of her depression.

(*1: This prescription was created by Sohaku Asada during the period between the Meiji and Edo eras, and has been used for any flush and dizziness surrounding childbirth as well as coldness of the lower parts of the body, by soothing Liver, discharging heat, tonifying Liver and warming the lower parts).

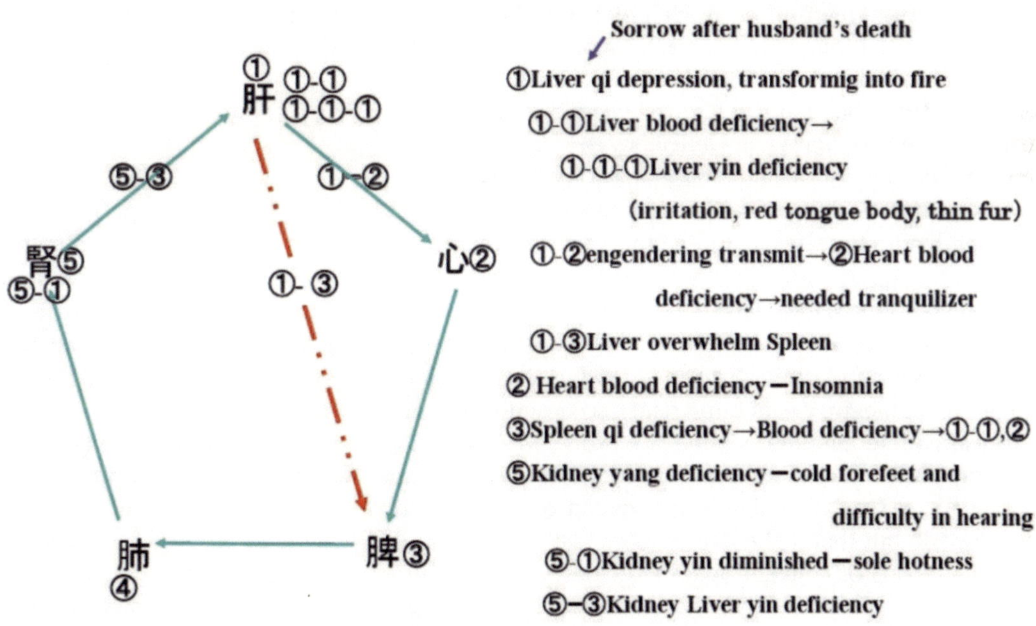

Fig. 5. Relations among viscera with five phase theory of case 5.

Interstitial Pneumonia

Case 6 : A 62-year-old Japanese female
Chief complaint: Cough, dyspnea and palpitation aggravated on motion, cold legs, frequent urination
History of present illness: Her dry cough continued until white sputa was discharged (Lung qi and yin deficiency ④) followed by palpitation. Her cough was aggravated on rainy days (Lung fails in purification and downbearing ④-①). Palpitation and dyspnea were severe (Lung influenced to Heart, Heart qi deficiency ②, ④-④). Recently, even in the summer, her ankles would get cold (the Mother's abnormality is transmitted to the child by way of engendering ④-③). The frequency of urination was more than ten times/day (Kidney yang deficiency: ⑤). In winter, her soles felt hot (yin deficiency ⑤-①). Recently, fatigue has increased (qi deficiency). Since menopause, she has experienced hot flashes and sensitivity to heat (yin deficiency with fire effulgence ①-①,⑤-①,⑤-②). She prefers a cold drink (⑤-②, ①-①). In spite of suffering from cataracts and glaucoma evoked by adrenal cortex hormones, she continues to take 4mg of adrenal cortex hormone (predonine). She had high intraocular pressure (Liver yin deficiency ①,①-①). She has a small gallstone (1 cm). (Liver qi stagnation ①).
Past history: When she was fifty-eight years old, she had such severe dyspnea and palpitation that she was hospitalised for two-and-a-half months. She was diagnosed with interstitial pneumonia and, for three years, adrenal cortex hormones were prescribed. Five years later, dyspnea and palpitation were aggravated again. She visited another doctor and re-started adrenal cortex hormones therapy, which proved ineffective. Various other kinds of treatments have not worked.
Family history: Her grandfather suffered from asthma
Present status: Height, 158cm, weight, 57kg. Pulse, sunken, fine, forceless, 60/min (Heart qi deficiency②); tongue body, pale dark, swollen sublingual collateral vessels (Liver qi stagnation→blood stasis①); BP, 120/78mmHg
Identification: Lung qi and yin deficiency, Heart qi deficiency, Phlegm obstructing the Lung, Kidney yin and yang Deficiency
Treatments: Tonify Lung qi and yin, Tonify Heart qi
Prescriptions: ① zhi-gan-cao-tang(in Japanese: Syakanzoto - this augments the qi, nourishes the blood, enriches the yin and restores the pulse) ② qin-fei-tang[Ref 25] (in Japanese: Seihaito - this clears lung inflammation in order to remove sputa and stop coughs; Wan-bin-gui-chun, written by Gong Ting xian)[*1Ref 24] supplemented with bai-he (Lilli Bulbus - this moistens Lung, clears heat to stop coughs, and enriches Lung yin), zhi-mu (Anemarrhenae Rhizoma - this clears heat and drains Fire and enriches the yin) and pi-pa-ye (Eriobotryae Folium - this transforms phlegm, clears Lung heat and downbears Lung qi).
Clinical course: She first visited my office on August 23, X year. Around seven days after starting herbal therapies, her conditions started to improve, and so she continued with taking them. On November 4 she visited our clinic and reported that she could do some housework, but that if she overworked, asthma occurred. As she felt a dry throat, owing to the side effects of conventional medicines, and I added zi-yin-jiang-huo-tang (in Japanese: Jiinkokato – this tonifies yin)[*2] and ma-xing-gan-shi-tang (in Japanese: Makyokansekito - this facilitates the flow of Lung qi and clears heat)[*3] for her asthma fits. Ma-xing-gan-shi-tang was quick to be effective. On her visit of November 30, she reported she could lead a normal life as a housewife and that her persistent cough and dry throat had disappeared.

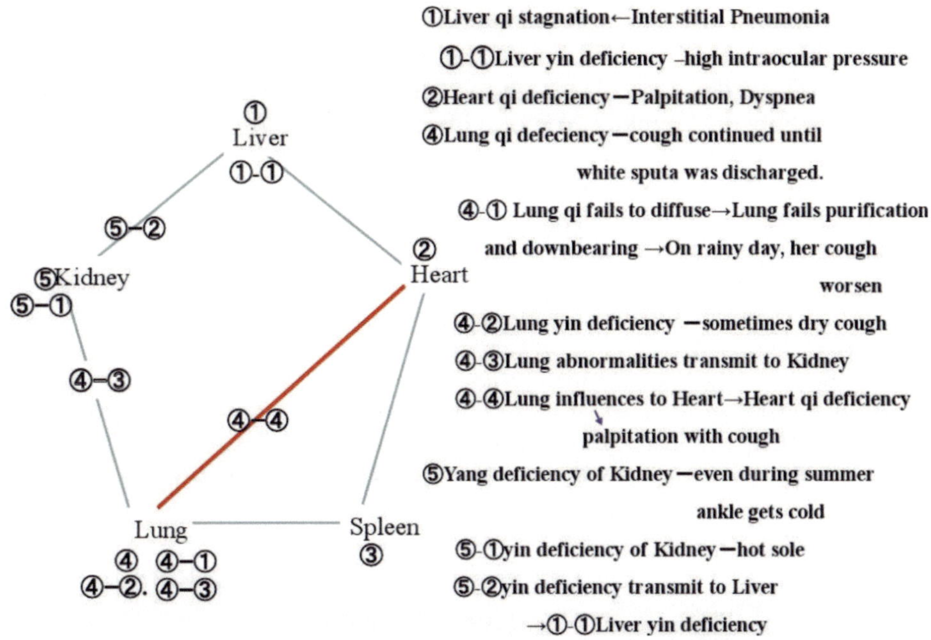

Fig. 6. Relations among viscera with five phase theory of case 6 (Interstitial Pneumonia before treatment)

Discussion: As the patient had not been so oversensitive to the cold in her previous healthy days, the existence of recent cold legs and frequent urination could be the result of the transmission of accumulated Lung abnormalities to Kidney, from Lung, through the engendering route. Her symptom's aggravation on rainy days implies that Lung yang (qi) deficiency leading to retention of moistness. However, Lung yin deficiency also existed, which was the cause of her severe dry cough. Qin-fei-tang and pi-pa-ye cleared the heat and phlegm of the Lung and tonified the yin of Lung along with bai-he and zhi-mu. Enriching the Lung yin strengthened the Lung qi. Zhi-gan-cao-tang tonified the Heart qi, together with Lung qi enrichment, and worked synergistically based upon the close relation between the two viscera. It was likely that this was the reason why she improved so quickly.

Her intraocular high blood pressure may have been due to the Liver yin deficiency transforming into Fire transmitted from the Kidney yin deficiency.

(*1 Qin-fei-tang: fu-lig, dang-gui, mai-men-dong, huang-qin, jie-geng, chen-pi, bei-mu, sang-bai-pi, zhi-zi, tian-men-dong, xing-ren, zhu-ru, da-zao. *1 *2,*3: these are all product of Tsumura Co.)

Pulmonary emphysema

Case 7 A 73-year-old Japanese male.

Chief complaint: Frequent cough with transparent sticky sputa, dyspnea on motion, difficulty in walking with powerless legs, and sensitivity to the cold.

History of present illness: He had serious dyspnea on motion (Lung qi deficiency ④). Taking just one step in walking made him feel like choking (Heart qi deficiency ②,②-①). He complained of powerless legs (Kidney qi deficiency ⑤). During the summer he didn't like air conditioning; instead, he dressed in heavy clothing and used a big futon ((⑤-①). He had feet that were cold to numbness (Kidney yang deficiency ⑤-①). He also had a groin

hernia. He had been light eater and sometimes he experiences stomach aches (Spleen qi deficiency ④-③,③).
The previous year, he had been diagnosed with serious pulmonary emphysema at a major hospital, but continued to smoke two pieces of cigarettes a day. He generally discharges a lot of transparent sticky sputa (phlegm obstructing the lung (④, ④-①).
Sometimes he discharges yellow sputa (localised inflammation in Lung). He told me that he usually discharges sputa around ten times/day (Lung qi deficiency ④, ④-①). As he easily catches colds during the winter, he rarely goes out.
Present Status: Height, 156 cm; weight, 41 kg; BP, 146/70mmHg, Pulse, 72/min, string-like, slippery, weak (Heart qi deficiency ②), purple-red tongue, white thick fur with spot defoliation (cold damp entering interior, stomach qi and deficiency③).
Past history: Between the ages of nineteen and twenty-four years, he was hospitalised with TB. About four years ago, a fever of more than 39°C continued for around fourteen days, causing him to be hospitalised. Since this time, he has noticed dypnea on motion. His frequent cough and oversensitivity to the cold have been a long-term problem.

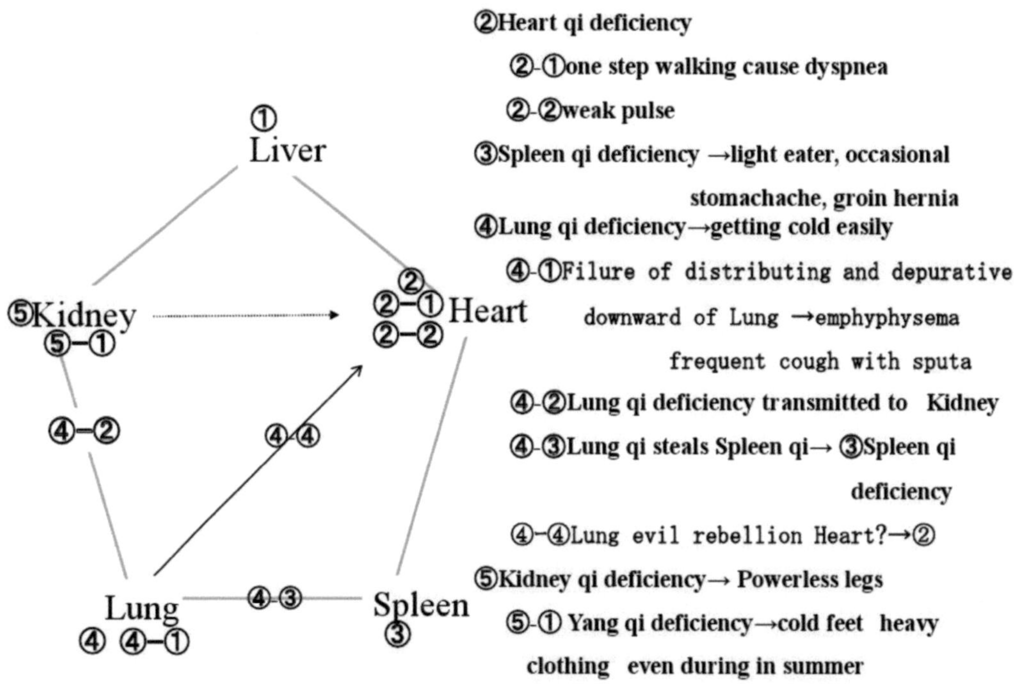

Fig. 7. Relations among viscera with five phase theory of case 7 (Pulmonary emphysema before treatment)

Identification: Qi deficiency of Lung and Heart, Failure of Lung in fluid distribution and depurative downbearing. Yang deficiency of Kidney.
Treatments: Tonify Lung and Heart qi.
Prescriptions: ① zhi-gan-cao-tang (TSUMURA & CO.: this augments the qi, nourishes the blood, enriches the yin and restores the pulse).*1 Ref 24 ② qin-fei-tang*2 with supplemental bai-he (Lilli Bulbus: this moistens Lung, clears heat to stop coughs and enriches Lung yin)
*1:Powder type - a product of Tsumura Co. *2:same as case 6)

Clinical course: When the patient visited my clinic on April 11 for the first time, he reported that he had taken preserved zhi-gan-cao-tang for three weeks but that his cough and sputum had not changed, even though he felt slightly better. I added the qin-fei-tang. On his second visit on April 30, he reported that he could walk and move without much trouble. On June 26, he reported that routine movement and walking were much improved, and that the volume of sputa had decreased. He continued taking the same remedies, and around one year later, he could lead a more relaxed life without much trouble. He continues to smoke two cigarettes a day and he plays "go" from time to time. His sensitivity to the cold has improved and he can walk without trouble. He has not caught a cold so far. He has taken only qin-fei-tang for one year, and has done fine on this reduced regimen.
Discussion: The patient suffered from TB during youth and he has continued smoking while playing "go" since then. That may be one of the reasons he suffered from pulmonary emphysema. The heavy abnormalities of Lung (Lung evil qi) were transmitted to Kidney, which depleted the qi further, leading to Kidney yang deficiency. Even in summer he was heavily clothed and used a thick coverlet. His Heart qi deficiency may have derived from Heart–Lung qi deficiency syndrome, or Lung qi abnormalities might have influenced the heart through the rebellion route. Spleen qi deficiency, such as being a light eater, experiencing occasional stomach aches or groin hernia, might have derived from the stealing of Spleen qi by the lung. Once Lung qi was restored, his coldness, stomach aches, groin hernia, and frequency of cough with sputa were remarkably decreased. It is clear that in his case Lung was the main organ that caused and aggravated his various symptoms.

Recurrence of metastatic kidney cancer in bladder

Case 8. A 52-year-old Japanese businessman
Chief complaint: Intractable metastatic kidney cancer, nose dryness
History of present illness: At age 51, the patient had noticed hematuria. Twelve months later, in April, X year, he was diagnosed with cancer of Kidney. A left nephroureterectomy was carried out in a national hospital in May. Partial cancer cell infiltration was recognised, which was resected without gross cancer tissues. Nose dryness has continued (yin deficiency of Lung ④-①).
Past history: He had been a heavy smoker. Since X-6 year, he suffered from hoarseness and pharyngitis (Lung yin deficiency④-①) and choking pressure in the chest (Heart blood obstruction with blood stasis ②-①). In X-4 year palpitations accompanied these symptoms (Heart qi deficiency ②) and his voice would become more hoarse, with a dry mouth and dry lips (Lung yin deficiency④-①). He usually took the drug for angina pectoris.
In spring of the X-3 year, when he looked backwards, dizziness occurred (obstruction with blood stasis, upper orifices interruption①, ②-①), which was much improved with exercise. In June, he again felt tightness of the chest and numbness from right shoulder to the arm (Heart blood stasis ②-①) and sometimes got edema of leg (Kidney qi deficiency, blood stasis ⑤). He occasionally suffered reflex vomiting from too much smoke.
In X-2 year, hematuria was detected. In February of X-1 year, a benign left tonsil tumour was extracted (Blood stasis of Lung meridian ④-②). He stopped smoking after the extraction of this tumour.
Family history: There have been no particular problems in his family regarding cancer or malignant tumours.
Present status: Height, 171cm; weight, 60kg; BP, 146/80mmHg. Right pulse, string-like and slippery; left pulse, string-like; the body colour of the tongue is pale and dark, tooth-

marked, and with a slimy yellowish fur (Dampness-heat of Spleen). There were no other particular problems.
Identification: Blood stasis in Kidney, Qi deficiency of Lung and Heart with fluid retention.
Treatments: Activate blood to remove stasis, clean heat, remove moistness and soothe liver, regulate qi.

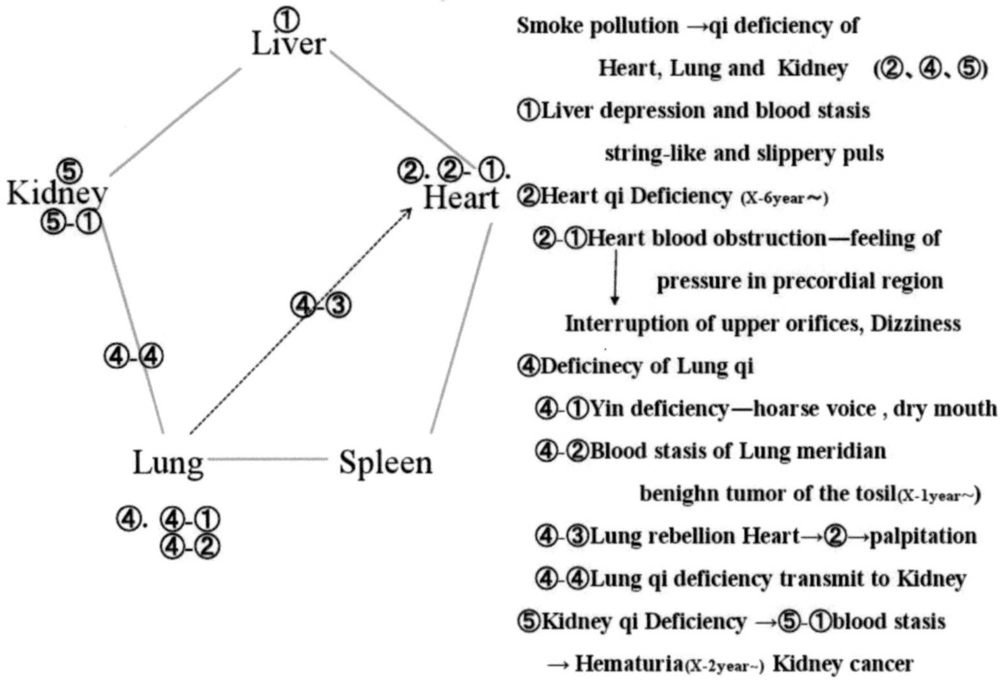

Fig. 8. Relations among viscera with five phase theory of case 8 (Reccurence of metastatic Kidney cancer in bladder)

Prescription: Prescription I composed of: ①Activate blood group: hong-hua (Carthami Flos 3), chuan-xion (Chuanxion Rhizoma 3), dan-shen (Salviae miltiorrhizae Radix 4), yu-jin (Curcumae Radix 3), san-qi (Notoginseng Radix 3, separately taken), she- chong (Eupolyphaga 3.5) and e-shu (Zedoariae Rhizoma 3); ①-②Activate the blood and clean the heat group: mu-tan-pi (Moutan Cortex 3); ② Clean heat and remove dampness group: huang-qin (Scutellariae Radix 3), Huan-bo (Phellodendri Cortex 1); ③ Tonify Spleen qi and drain dampness group: Fu-ling (Poria 5), Bai-shu (Atractylodis Rhizoma 4) and Zhu-ling (Polyporus 3); ④ Spread Liver qi and reduce fever group: chai-hu (Bupleuri Radix 1); ⑤ Tonify the qi, nourish the blood and calm the spirit, augment Heart qi group: ling-zhi (Ganoderma 2); ⑥ Warms and unblocks the channels and collaterals and assists the yang group: gui-zhi (Cinnamomi Ramulus 2) and ⑦ moderate, harmonise and tonify Spleen group: gan-cao (Glycyrrhizae Radix 1.5). The numeral at the end of parenthesis mean the daily used weight. All materials were decocted in hot water with the instrument on the market with the regular method.
Clinical course: From September 28, X year, the patient started the prescription mentioned above and stopped smoking after the operation. During a periodic follow-up at the end of

October, no tumour was detected._On November 25, three small tumours (diameter, 1 mm) and 1 larger tumour (diameter, 5 mm) were found. Until the middle of March of the next year, as intravesical instillation of an anticancer drug was carried out every two weeks(eight times in total) with prescription I . During the periodic follow-up of April 6,X+1 year, only the 5-mm tumor was discovered to have survived and this was excised.

To this situation, Prescription II was added to Prescription I. Prescription II was composed of bai-hua-she-she-cao (Hydyotis diffusae Herba which clears heat and resolves dampness and fire toxicity 4.5), wang-bu-liu-xing(Viccariae Semen which promotes the movement of blood 4.5) and shui-zhi(Hirudo which breaks up and drives out blood stasis and reduces fixed masses 4.5) and continued without any conventional therapies. As a recurrence was not recognised at the periodic check, the moiety of the decoction was halved from October X+1. In April X+2 year, he returned to work and continued to take the same volume of the decoction. From X+11 to X+13year, he reduced his dose at 1/6 of the initial volume, and since X+14 he stopped. Now, more than three years have passed since then and without any recurrence.

Discussion: A therapy of Prescription I with an anticancer infusion every two weeks for four months did not work to eradicate remaining one biggest cancer. Since then, Prescription I combined with Prescription II has been continued for fourteen years. After stopping this, more than three years has passed without a recurrence, so far, which will mean Prescription I and II worked to inhibit the recurrence. The fact that, by stopping smoking in X year before the first visit, the symptoms of Heart and Lung quickly disappeared would imply that these symptoms are all derived from smoking.

In X-6 year, Lung related symptoms (hoarseness and pharyngitis) appeared with Heart related symptoms (a feeling of tightness in chest) appearing in X-4 year; these symptoms have continued and aggravated with palpitations. In X-2 year, hematuria appeared for the first time during a yearly medical check. In X-1 year, benign tonsil tumour was resected. This could mean Lung abnormality rebels Heart when his palpitations started((④-③). Next abnormalities transmitted to Kidney through the engendering route from Lung to Kidney.

By stopping smoking before the first visit, the symptoms of the Heart and Lung had nearly all disappeared, but the abnormal situation of Kidney could not change.

Drugs for activating the blood and moving qi, cleaning the heat and removing dampness, and tonifying the qi, worked synergistically to restore satisfactory function of Kidney such that the cancers would not recur.

A case of depression

Case 9 A 38-year-old Japanese housewife and office worker (48 kg, 155cm)

First visit: On 16th of February in X year

Chief complaints: Depression, spiritlessness, a dull feeling in the stomach, menstrual pain

Clinical history: She began working at age twenty-one, and married at age twenty-five. At thirty-five years, she changed her job because it involved too much stress. She has been suffering from depression, spiritlessness (Liver qi depression and stagnation ①), stiffness of the shoulder and a blocked feeling of the blood vessels in the temple and at the base of the neck (Blood stasis ①-①). Stress creates a dull feeling in the stomach (Wood overwhelms Earth ①-④). Manual therapy improved her condition (freeing the collateral vessels), premenstrual nausea (③-③), and the blood-shot condition and mucus of her right eye

(Liver qi stagnation-transforming into heat ①-②). Other symptoms included a dry feeling of the skin and lip (①-②), coldness of the forefoot, constipation which improved by warming(Kidney yang deficiency ⑤-①). She suffered from profuse dreaming (disquieted heart mind ①-③), hot palms (yin deficiency - fever of three yin meridians of the hand), hay fever with rhinorrhea in fatigue (Spleen–Kidney yang deficiency → water dampness failing in transportation → cold fluid retention in Lung ⑤-②). She smokes ten cigarettes a day (arteriosclerotic progression, impaired viscera).

Past history: During primary school days, she often suffered from convulsions on falling asleep (her yin and yang couldn't copulate successfully). In the past, she has been pale, with a tooth-marked tongue (Spleen yang deficiency with dampness retention ③.③-②), and her sublingual collateral vessels showed blood stasis (Liver qi depression and blood stasis ①-①).

States Present: Height is 162cm; weight is 59kg; pulse is string like, slippery, fine, 72/min; tongue has a pale body and is teeth-marked (retention of water ③-①、③-②) with a thin white fur.

Sublingual blackish vessel is enlarged (blood stasis).

Identification: Liver qi depression and static blood, Liver overwhelms Spleen, Liver causes rebellion in Lung, Spleen–Kidney yang deficiency

Treatment: Soothe Liver. Harmonise Liver and spleen. Warm and free collateral vessels.

Prescriptions and herbs: Si-ni-san[Ref 26] (in Japanese: Shigyakusan*1 - soothes liver, regulates qi, harmonises liver and spleen) [Ref 26] together with xion-gui-tiao-xue-yin[Ref27] (in Japanese: Kyukichoketsuin*2 - this regulates qi, activates blood, tonifies blood/regulates menstruation; this originates from Wan- bin-gui-chun), ban-xia (Rhizoma Pinelliae Ternatae - this dries dampness and transforms phlegm), mahuang (Ephedrae Herba - this induces sweating and releases the exterior) and gui zhi (Cinammomi Ramulus - this releases the exterior and warms yang to unblock the meridian)

(*1: Si-ni-san: chai-fu, shao-yao, zhi-shi, gan-cao

*2: Xion gui tiao xue yin :dan-gui, chun-xiong, sheng-di-huang, bai-chu, fu-ling, chen-pi,

*3: wu-yao, xiang-fu-zi, mu-dan-pi, yi-mu-cao, da-zao, sheng-jiang, gan-cao)

Clinical course: A numerical Rating Scale (NRS) employing the patient's self-report of symptoms in numerals (with the worst condition experienced so far scored as 10 and with no symptoms scored as 0) was used to monitor the course (Fig 9), and the patient's disease situation was described with five-phase theory (Fig 10).

Discussion As shown in Figs. 9 and 10, herbal therapy decreased the NRS. Since I do not prescribe special medicines for Kidney, the improvement of foot coldness was not so successful.

However, other symptoms improved relatively well. Si-ni-san mainly worked to reduce Liver qi stagnation and, with xion-gui-tiao-xue-yin in collaboration, this removed the blood stasis and regulated qi. Furthermore, the rebellion in the lung from Liver must have decreased since, in spite of the absence of treatment for rhinorrhea in fatigue, it disappeared completely (data not shown). The dull feeling in the stomach evoked by stress decreased comparatively well, which means that overwhelm in the stomach disappeared. The simultaneous treatment of every imbalanced viscus often leads to quick recovery because every normalised viscus works simultaneously and synergistically..

The qi movement of each phase will be normalised by this treatment.

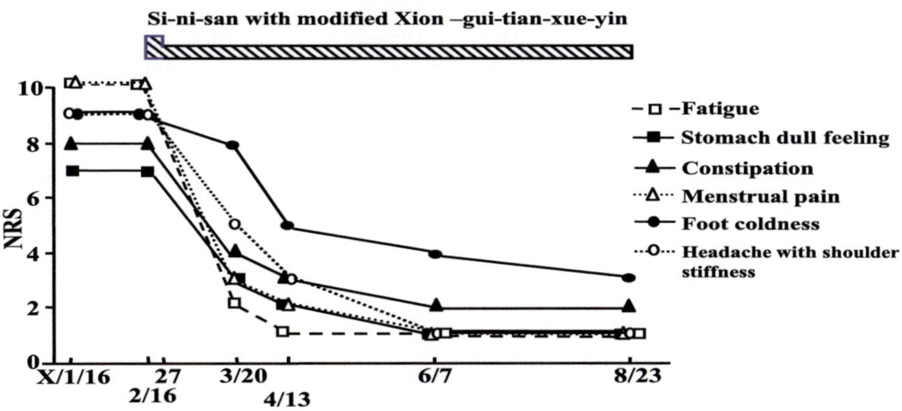

Fig 9 Clinical course of case 9 after taking Si-ni-san with Xion gui tian xue yin

Fig. 9. Clinical course of case 9 after taking Si-ni-san with Xion gui tian zue yin.

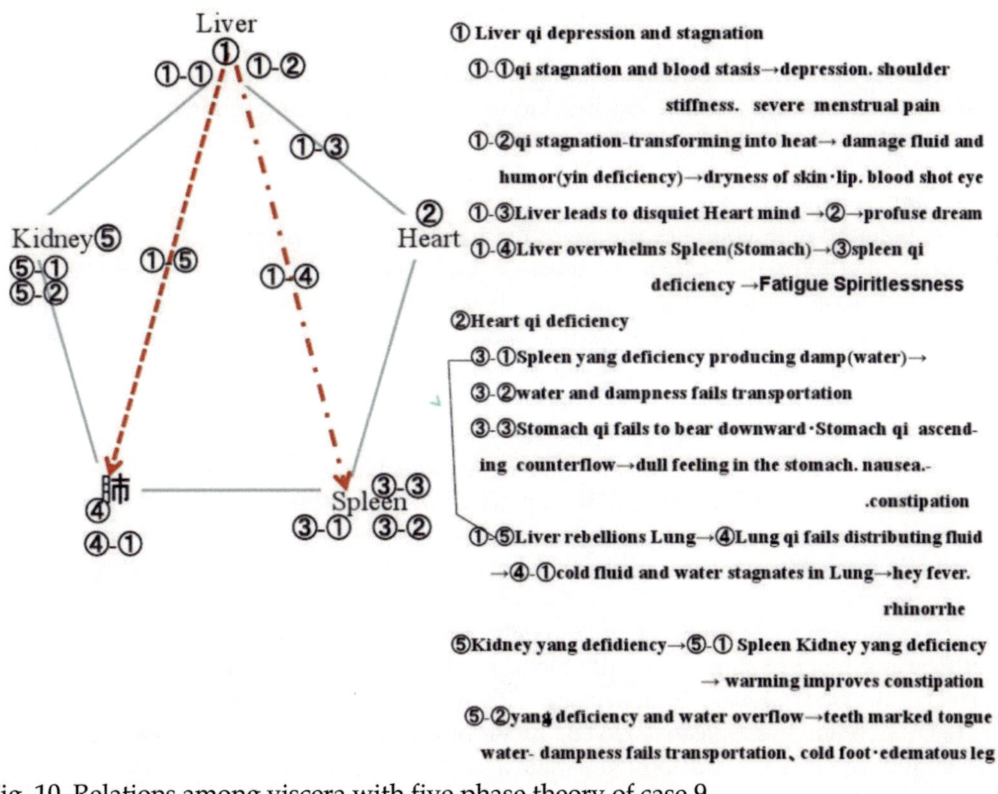

Fig. 10. Relations among viscera with five phase theory of case 9.

Asthma with dyspnea and general fatigue

Case 10 A 50-year-old Japanese female who works for a Japanese pub

Chief complaint: The patient finds it impossible to lie down, due to dyspnea and palpitation (Lung and Heart qi deficiency ②,④). She experiences suffocating dyspnea and general fatigue. Perfumes, cigars, cosmetics and other stimuli cause dyspnea. She has asthma and is sensitive to chemical substances (Lang qi deficiency ④).

History of present illness: For almost a year, beginning in the summer when her stress tremendously increased, she had been suffering from palpitation and suffocating dyspnea (Probably, Liver rebellions Lung, Heart and Lung qi deficiency ①-⑤.②,④), and she could not lie down or maintain a sitting posture with general fatigue (Lung qi deficiency ④). Furthermore, she had cold limbs, sensitivity to coldness, frequent urination during the night, and edema (Kidney Yang deficiency ⑤-①, ⑤-②) and condition worsens on rainy days. She doesn't want to drink water even though she feels thirsty (Kidney yang deficiency with water flood ⑤-①.⑤-②). She often had concentrated urine, her soles are hot during the night (Kidney yin deficiency ⑤-③). She experienced fullness in the abdomen after meals, has many stressors in her life, breast pain, and fullness of the chest around the time of menstruation (Liver depression and qi stagnation ①-①).

Additionally, she has had severe shoulder stiffness, enlargement of the sublingual vessel (blood stasis ①-①), asthenopia, dim eyesight, numbness of limbs (Blood deficiency of liver ①-②), headache, a short temper, facial hotness, and she prefers cold water (ascendant hyperactivity of liver yang ①-③). She cannot sleep easily, having insomnia, profuse dreaming, and a feeling of uneasiness (Heart blood and yin deficiency ②.②-①).

She is sensitive to various chemical substances, such as smoke, dust, insecticide, cosmetics, exhaust gas, and the smell of dishes (Lung qi deficiency ④). The adrenal cortex hormone that she takes causes eye pain, headache, skin irritation and choking (Lung qi deficiency ④).

At another clinic, yi-gan-san[Ref 28] (this pacifies liver to extinguish wind)[*1] added with banxia (Rhizoma Pinelliae Ternatae - this dries dampness, transforms phlegm), chen-pi (Citri reticulatae Pericarpium - this regulates qi, dries dampness, transforms phlegm), si ni san[Ref 26], qin-fei-tang[Ref 25] with xing-gan-shi-tang, chai-hu-gui-zhi-tang (in Japanese: Saikokeishito - this releases and harmonises lesser yang-stage disorders and releases the muscle layer and exterior), ban-xia-hou-po-tang (in Japanese: Hangekobokuto - this promotes qi movement, dissipates clumps, directs rebellious qi downward, and transforms phlegm) were prescribed with conventional drugs such as montelukast sodium, salmeterol xinafoate and procaterol, but these were not effective.

(*1 chai-fu, can-zao,dan-gui,bai-chu.fu-ling,diao-teng-gou)

Past history: She had suffered from alopecia areata, which is possibly stress-induced.

Present status: Height 162cm; weight 51.5kg; the tip of the tongue is red (Heart meridian has heat) and there is a fissure in the middle of the body of the tongue (Spleen yin deficiency); the tongue's fur is thin, pale and white; the sublingual vessel is blackish and enlarged (blood stasis).

Pulse: float and weak (Heart blood and yin deficiency)

Identification: Liver qi stagnation with blood stasis ((①-①), Blood deficiency of Liver and Heart ((①-②, ②-①), Liver yin deficiency with ascendant hyperactivity of Liver yang ((①-③). Liver overwhelms Spleen ((①-④), Liver rebellions Lung ((①-⑤). She had to use bronchodilators, such as salmeterol xinafoate and procaterol hydrochloride. She worked for long hours in the air conditioning and her limbs must have been cooled, causing the Kidney yang to decrease, which might be inversely transmitted to Lung and which may be one of the reasons for the aggravation of her asthma.

Treatments: Tonify Lung qi, soothe Liver, regulate qi, tonify Heart qi and blood,tonify qi, yin and yang of Kidney.

Prescriptions: ① zi-yin-zhi-bao-tang[Ref 29] (in Japanese: Jiinshihoto - this soothes Liver, regulates qi, tonifies Spleen and tonifies yin to clear Lung)[*a]; ② zhi-gan-cao-tang; ③ ba-wei-di-huang-wan (the same as in case 3)

([*a]:dang-gui, bai-shao, bai-chu, fu-ling, chen-pi, zhi-mu, bei-mu, xian-fu-zi, di-gu-pi, mai-men-dong bao-he, chai-fu, gan-cao.)

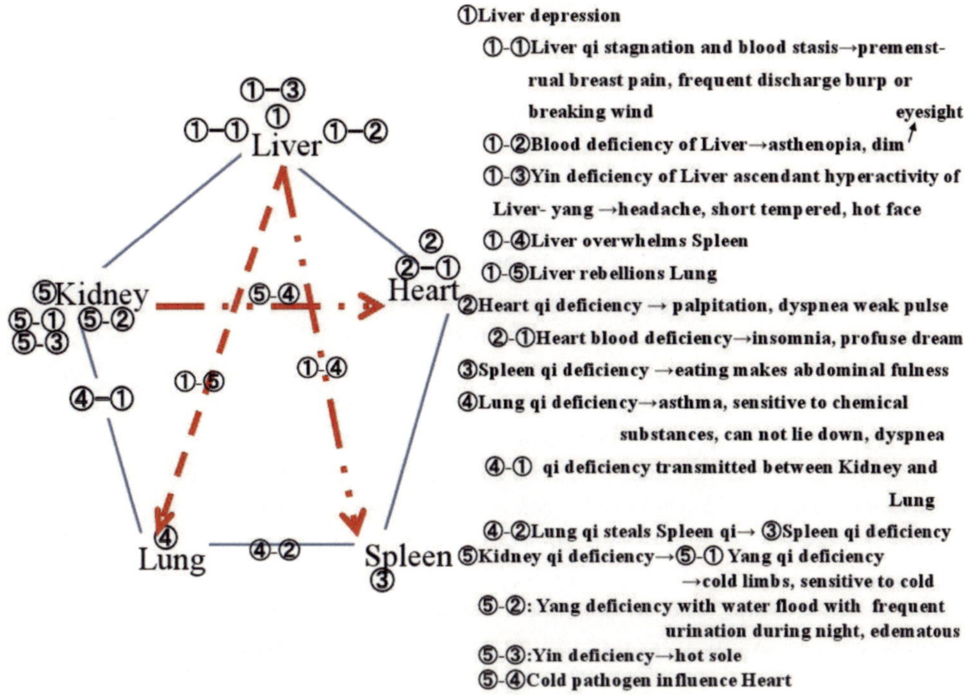

Fig. 11. Relations among viscera with five phase theory of case 10.

Clinical course Prescriptions were administered in late April. Ten days later, on May 11, she visited the clinic and reported that, although she was not completely cured, her condition was much improved and that she could resume working. The abnormal sensation of the Lung disappeared. Dyspnea during the day improved, but at night it was still not good. On May 31, she reported that daytime dyspnea had disappeared and that at night her asthma fits decreased and she did not need to use the bronchodilator. She could work without trouble. On June 17, she reported that she had stopped using two of her three bronchodilators and could pursue a routine life as in previous days when she was healthy. Only when she was tired would she use her bronchodilator in order to prevent fits.

Discussion: Her asthma fits began during the summer one year ago, before she visited my clinic. As she experienced much stress through her work, Liver qi stagnation may have played a role in this aggravation. However, many Liver-soothing formulas did not work. I supposed that her asthma was aggravated not only by rebellion from Liver but also from the

Lung qi deficiency brought about from Kidney yang deficiency that was transmitted inversely to Lung. This may be because, during the summer, she worked for long hours in the air conditioning and her limbs must have been cooled, causing Kidney yang to decrease, which was inversely transmitted to Lung. Moreover, she has been - by her nature - sensitive to coldness. Her deficiency of Heart qi may be a result of the mutual relation between the Lung and Heart. Some rebellion from the Kidney of yang deficiency may participate in the Heart qi deficiency. These included zi-yin-zhi-bao-tang for soothing the Liver and regulating qi, tonifying the Spleen and yin to clear the Lung[Ref 30], zhi-gan-cao-tang (Tsumura Co.) for augmenting the qi, nourishing blood, enriching the yin of Heart and restoring the pulse, and Ba-wei-di-huang-wan for warming and tonifying the yang of the Kidney. This means we treat all viscera at the same time. This is the reason she could recover so promptly from her disease and could work again. As a general rule, treating the dysfunction of all viscera to restore their qi at the same time will lead to a quick recovery, based on the smooth circulation of respective qi among viscera with synergy. If one of them were not to have been treated, the recovery would have been slower. (The treatment of this patient was carried out by Dr Shimizu Ishigaki, Director of Yasookodomo Clinic, Shizuoka Prefecture and the author).

Difficulty in walking with staggering for more than 1 year

Case 11: A 67-year-old Japanese housewife 160 cm, 68 kg

Chief complaint: Dizziness, staggering, difficulty in walking (Heart blood and qi deficiency,②-① → interruption of upper orifices), dyspnea, susceptibility to catching colds (Lung qi deficiency ④-①), edema of face and limb (retention of water produced by yang deficiency (③-①-①, ⑤-①), coldness from occipital region to the back (Coldness of Du Meridian: governor vessel), facial flush (stagnated Liver qi transforming into fire → Liver yin deficiency ①-②-①, ③-②), cold forefoot (Kidney yang deficiency ⑤), hand stiffness, numbness and pain on rising (Liver qi deficiency, blood stasis ①).

Clinical history: First visit: February 22 2006. Since more than two years ago, she has often pitched forward and has had a sensation of walking on air in spite of her paying close attention to her gait. Many thorough examinations by brain surgeons, and at several major hospitals, have produced no explanation for these symptoms. She had been suffering from insomnia, profuse dreams and amnesia (Liver, Heart blood deficiency. ①-③, ②-①), a feeling of stool stasis, abdominal fullness (Liver overwhelms Spleen, Spleen qi deficiency, gastric hyperacidity ①-④, ③), edema of face and limbs for several years (Spleen yang deficiency, retention of water and moisture ③-①-①), low blood pressure on rising, aggravated by warmth, shoulder stiffness (stagnated Liver qi and blood stasis ①,①-①), dry eyes, blood-shot eyes, heat in her palm (Liver depression transforming into fire → Liver yin deficiency ①-②-①), a heavy feeling in her legs (moisture retention by Kidney yang deficiency ⑤-⑤-①), back pain on catching a cold (Lung qi deficiency④, ④-①), and chronic pancreatitis based upon her being a kitchen drinker for the past seventeen years (Spleen dampness-heat ③). She had her menopause at age fifty-six.

Past history: She suffered from rotary dizziness with vomiting between the ages of around forty and fifty (③,③-①). She takes camost mesilate from time to time because of chronic pancreatitis.

Family history: Her older brother died from pancreatic cancer and her younger sister died from lung cancer. She has three children.

Present illness: 72/min, fine, slippery, sunken pulse (Heart qi deficiency ②); a pale red tongue with white fur; over-swelling of dark sublingual collateral vessels (blood stasis). Standing blood pressure 110/80, sitting pressure 140/80.
Identification: Liver depression with blood stasis, fluid retention with yang deficiency of Spleen and Kidney; Deficiency of Heart qi and blood; Interruption to upper orifices
Treatment: Soothe Liver and regulate qi, activate blood, free the collateral vessels, remove moisture and tonify Spleen.
Prescriptions: Bu-yang-huan-wu-tang (BYHWT: tonifies the qi, invigorates the blood, and unblocks the channels)[Ref 30 *a] combined with she-chong-yin (in Japanese: Sesyoin - this activates blood to solve stasis)[Ref 31 *b] included BYHWT, yan-hu-suo (this invigorates the blood and promotes the movement of qi), niu-xi (this invigorates the blood and dispel blood stasis), mu-tan-pi (this clears heat and invigorates and dispels the blood), gui-zhi (this releases the exterior, assists the yang, warms and unblocks the channels and collaterals). Further, gan-cao, wu-yao (this regulates qi, warms the Kidney) , xiang-fu-zi (this spreads and regulates Liver qi, regulates menstruation and alleviates pain), chai-fu(Bupleuri Radix which spreads Liver qi and reduce fever), jie-geng (Platycodi Radix - this opens up and disseminates the Lung qi, pushes out puss and opens up and raises Lung qi) and wu-ling-san (in Japanese: Goreisan - this promotes urination, drains dampness, warms the yang and resolves qi).were added.
([a:] bu-yang-huan-wu-tang:huang-qi, dang-gui, chuan-xion, chi-shao, tao-ren hong-hua and di-long.
[*b]: she-chong-yin: tao-ren, dan-gui, mu-tan-pi, chuan-xion, chi-shao, gui-zhi, yan-hu-suo, niu-xi,hong^hua.)
Clinical course: Her constipation disappeared after almost two-and-a-half months. Her dizziness, staggering, pain and the numbness of her hands also improved tremendously within around four months.

Discussion

This patient has had too much stress for a long time, as she became a kitchen drinker with pancreatitis seventeen years ago. Stress made Liver qi depression and blood stagnation - especially in upper orifice - will be the main reason for her dizziness, staggering, and difficulty in walking and probably for her low standing blood pressure (①-①). The excessive over-swelling of her sublingual vessel implies the occurrence of severe blood stagnation. As Liver overwhelmed Spleen, she displayed many symptoms through her digestive system relating to water retention, including pancreatitis. Furthermore, her stress was so enormous that she had dyspnoea, with coldness causing her back pain (Liver rebellions Lung). As she has Kidney yang deficiency, seen through cold feet with a stagger, as well as the retention of moisture (⑤, ⑤-①), this might be caused by overwhelm from Spleen cold evil to Kidney and aging. Enormous Liver abnormalities, transmitted to Heart to cause palpitation, arrhythmia, dizziness with a stagger and blood deficiency (②,②-①). Water or moisture retention may influence her dizziness and staggering to some extent.
I classified herb mixtures (BYHWT+she-chong-yin+others): Gr 1,to activate Blood in order to solve Blood stasis (chuan-xion,chi-shao, tao-ren, hong-hua yan-hu-suo, niu-xi, mu-tan-pi), Gr 2 so as to tonify Blood(dan-gui,chuan-xion); Gr 3 to tonify qi(huang-qi); Gr 4 to regulate Liver qi(chai-fu); Gr 5 to regulate qi(yan-fu-suo, xiang-fu-zi, wu-yao), and Gr 6 including others (gyu-zhi,gan-cao,jie-geng,di-long,wu-ling-san).
Gr-1, Gr-2, Gr-3 and Gr-4 will work to soothe Liver, regulate qi, activate stagnated blood and tonify blood of Liver and Heart. As a result, the transmission of abnormal qi to Heart

from Liver, rebellion to Lung from Liver and overwhelm to Spleen from Liver will all decrease. Gr 1, Gr 2, Gr 3, gui-zhi and gan-cao will also operate to tonify Kidney qi and for Spleen and Lung as well. Wu-ling-san would support disappearance of water retention.

As such, each of the five viscus qi is tonified which leads to smooth recovery of her symptoms. Notably, after around two years of taking herbs, she became symptomless and was able to stop two years later without recurrence more than three years.

I suppose main reason of her recovery will be the disappearance of stagnated blood in brain and other parts of the body.

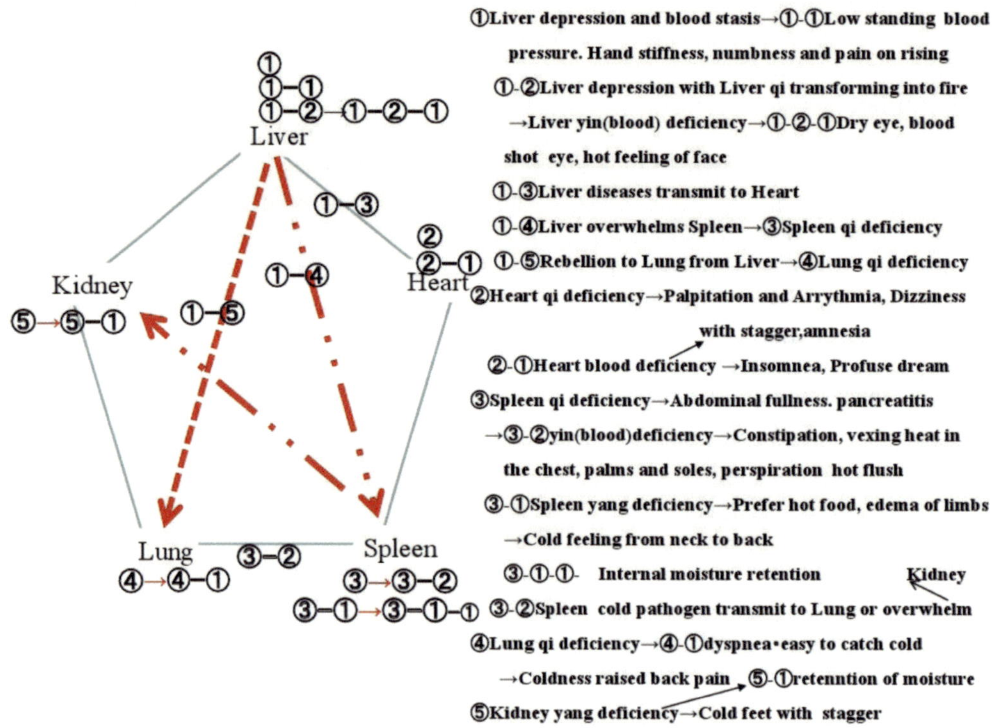

Fig. 12. Relations among viscera with five phase theory of case 11.

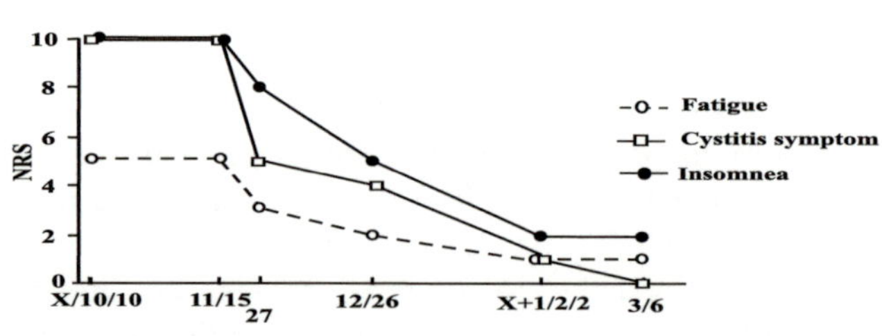

Fig14 Clinical course after taking herbal medecines of case 11

Fig. 13. Clinical course after taking herbal medecines of case 11.

10. Acknowledgement

Dr. Naoki Hirama MD.,Ph.D., director of Japanese Traditional Chinese Medicine and director of Hirama Clinic, for valuable suggestions and advices to this chapter.
Mr Hitoshi Matsunaga working for TSUMURA & CO. for valuable advices.
Xi Lu., lecturer of Traditional Chinese Medicine Foundation of Osaka. Member of Kobe Chuigaku Kenkyukai, for his instructive advices.
Yoko Takahashi, the visiting professor Shanghai University of Traditional Chinese Medicine for her instructive advices.
I am grateful to Dr. Dai Yong Sheng on literaturewhich I failed to include in the work because of failureto get them in time.

11. References

[1] *East Asian Medical Studies Society: Fundamentals Of Chinese Medicine.* Paradigm Publication:1985 p10-22
[2] (xiang-jie)zhong-yi-ji-chu-li-lun: Liu-yan-chi Gong-tian-bin-fu Zhang- rui-fu Jin-lian-rong. Toyogakujyutsusyuppan Kanagawaprefecture 1999 p36-58
[3] (xiang-jie) zhong-yi-ji-chu-li-lun: liu-yan-chi song-tian-bin-fu zhang- rui-fu jin-lian-rong. Toyogakujyutsusyuppan Kanagawaprefecture 1999. p48-50. This book was translated from [Liu-yan-chi"zhong-yi-ji-chu-li-lun-wen-da" Shang-hai-ke-ji-chu-ban-she] 1982.
[4] Song-lu-bing. pian, Chai-qi-ying-zi yi *Zhong-yi-bing-yin-bing-ji-xue* Toyogakujyutsu-syuppan Kanagawa prefecture 1998 p44-49
[5] *East Asian Medical Studies Society: Fundamentals of Chinese Medicine.* Paradigm Publication: 1985:79-84.
[6] *East Asian Medical Studies Society: Fundamentals of Chinese Medicine*. Paradigm Publication: 1985:p232-243.
[7] *East Asian Medical Studies Society: Fundamentals of Chinese Medicine.* Paradigm Publication: 1985: p233-242
[8] *East Asian Medical Studies Society: Fundamentals of Chinese Medicine.* Paradigm Publication: 1985:p67-72
[9] *East Asian Medical Studies Society: Fundamentals of Chinese Medicine.* Paradigm Publication: 1985:p204-211
[10] *East Asian Medical Studies Society: Fundamentals of Chinese Medicine.* Paradigm Publication: 1985:p74-78
[11] *East Asian Medical Studies Society: Fundamentals of Chinese Medicine.* Paradigm Publication: 1985:p218-232
[12] *East Asian Medical Studies Society: Fundamentals of Chinese Medicine.* Paradigm Publication: 1985:p70-73
[13] *East Asian Medical Studies Society: Fundamentals of Chinese Medicine.* Paradigm Publication: 1985:p211-218
[14] *East Asian Medical Studies Society: Fundamentals of Chinese Medicine.* Paradigm Publication: 1985:p184-187
[15] *East Asian Medical Studies Society: Fundamentals of Chinese Medicine.* Paradigm Publication: 1985:p243-249

[16] *East Asian Medical Studies Society: Fundamentals of Chinese Medicine.* Paradigm Publication: 1985:p250-263
[17] Nikeghbalian S, Pournasr B, Aghdami N et al., Autologous transplantation of bone marrow-derived mononuclear and CD133(+) cells in patients with decompensated cirrhosis. *Arch Iran Med.* 2011 Jan;14(1):p12-17
[18] Takami T, Terai S, Sakaida I, Novel findings for the development of drug therapy for various liver diseases: current state and future prospects for our liver regeneration therapy using autologous bone marrow cells for decompensated liver cirrhosis patients. *J.Pharmacol. Sci*. 2011;115(3):p274-278
[19] *East Asian Medical Studies Society: Fundamentals of Chinese Medicine.* Paradigm Publication: 1985:p203-249
[20] Yasui H, APPENDIX - Composition and Indications of 148 Prescriptions. T*he Journal of Kampo, Acupuncture and Integrative Medicine* (KAIM) Volume 1, Special Edition.November 2005 P14
[21] Hijikata Y, Tsukamoto Y, Effect of herbal therapy on herpes labialis and herpes genitalis. *Biotherapy*. 1998;11:p235-240.
[22] Yasuhara A, Yuka Y, Hijikata Y, Effect of herbal therapy on chronic herpes virus infections. *Alternative Therapies in Health and Medicine.* 9(5): 2003 p132-136
[23] Yasui H, APPENDIX-Composition and Indications of 148 Prescriptions. Zi-yin-jiang-huo-tang, *The Journal of Kampo, Acupuncture and Integrative Medicine* (KAIM) Volume 1, Special Edition. November 2005 p101.
[24] Yasui H, APPENDIX-Composition and Indications of 148 Prescriptions. Nu-shen san. *The Journal of Kampo, Acupuncture and Integrative Medicine* (KAIM) Volume 1, Special Edition.November 2005 p92
[25] Yasui H, APPENDIX-Composition and Indications of 148 Prescriptions. Qin-fei-tang. *The Journal of Kampo, Acupuncture and Integrative Medicine* (KAIM) Volume 1, Special Edition.November 2005 p87
[26] Yasui H, APPENDIX-Composition and Indications of 148 Prescriptions. Si-ni-san. *The Journal of Kampo, Acupuncture and Integrative Medicine* (KAIM) Volume 1, Special Edition.November 2005 p89
[27] Yasui H, APPENDIX-Composition and Indications of 148 Prescriptions. Xion gui tiao xue yin *The Journal of Kampo, Acupuncture and Integrative Medicine* (KAIM) Volume 1, Special Edition.November 2005 p99
[28] Yasui H, APPENDIX-Composition and Indications of 148 Prescriptions. Yi-gan-san. *The Journal of Kampo, Acupuncture and Integrative Medicine* (KAIM) Volume 1, Special Edition.November 2005 p93
[29] Yasui H, APPENDIX-Composition and Indications of 148 Prescriptions. Zi-yin-zhi-bao-tang. *The Journal of Kampo, Acupuncture and Integrative Medicine* (KAIM) Volume 1, Special Edition.November 2005 p101
[30] Bensky D, and Barolet R, *Formulas that Warm the Menses and Dispel Blood Statis. Chinese Herbal Medicine - Formulas & Strategies, Eastland Press*; 1990; p320-321
[31] Gagawa Genetsu, *Sanron* (describing the delivery of a baby) Saiseikan 1775

4

An Approach to the Nature of Qi in TCM–Qi and Bioenergy

Xing-Tai Li[1] and Jia Zhao[2]
[1]*College of Life Science, Dalian Nationalities University, Dalian*
[2]*Norman Bethune College of Medicine, Jilin University, Changchun*
China

1. Introduction

Traditional Chinese medicine (TCM), has been practiced for more than five thousand years, is a complete ancient medical system that takes a deep understanding of the laws and patterns of nature and applies them to the human body. TCM believes that the human body is a microcosm of the Universal macrocosm. Therefore, humans must follow the laws of the Universe to achieve harmony and total health. Even today TCM practitioners use these essential theories to understand, diagnose and treat health problems. In TCM, "harmony" is the ultimate goal. So, when nature's Qi undergoes change as it does seasonally, a person's internal Qi will respond automatically. If, for any reason, it can't make a smooth transition to the energy of the next season, TCM understands that illness will result. Often Western Complementary and Alternative Medicine (CAM) practitioners and their patients or clients derive their understanding of TCM from acupuncture. However, acupuncture is only one of the major treatment modalities of this comprehensive medical system based on the understanding of Qi or vital energy. These major treatment modalities are Qigong, herbal therapy, acupuncture, foods for healing and Chinese psychology.

Meridians, or channels, are invisible pathways through which Qi flows that form an energy network that connects all parts of the body, and the body to the universe. The ancient medical text 'The Yellow Emperor's Inner Canon (Nei Jing)' states: "The function of the channel (meridian) is to transport the Qi and blood, and circulate yin and yang to nourish the body". The energy practice of Qigong, with its postures and movements, also affects the flow of Qi. The energy pathways and the Organ Systems they link provide TCM with a framework for identifying the root cause of health problems and the diagnoses to heal them. Meridians work by regulating the energy functions of the body and keeping it in harmony. If Qi stagnates for too long in any meridian, it can become blocked and eventually turn into matter, setting the stage for conditions that can create a physical mass. TCM Meridian Theory states: "As long as Qi flows freely through the meridians and the Organs work in harmony, the body can avoid disease".

The study of Qi phenomena may help bridge some of the apparent difference between Western and Eastern culture. Several years ago, I was lucky to notice that some scientists contributed novel experimental works on Qi, and subsequently, the papers by Ohnishi *et al.*(2005) (Ohnishi first attended the school of Nishino Breathing Method in Tokyo over 10 years ago, and 3 years later, the collaboration with Mr Nishino started in order to find a scientific basis for Qi) stimulated the philosophical discussion by Flowers (2006). As Flowers beautifully described, in the Christian West, God was the center of everything as opposed to Qi being the center of everything in the East. Qi may be another name of 'life', Qi may represent the entity of life itself (Ohnishi *et al.*, 2007). Then, the understanding of Qi may shed light on other aspects of biological sciences. These articles prompted us to write this chapter covering the nature of Qi as well as its philosophical aspects and the significance in the modern civilization because the true foundation of TCM is Qi.

2. The history and concept of Qi

2.1 Qi in China

Qi (in Chinese, equivalent to Ki in Japanese) has been used as a healing technique in China for 4000 years. In Japan, Qi has been known to have a healing effect at least for 1500 years (Ohnishi *et al.*, 2007). The origin of the character of Qi was traced back to 3500 years ago. Confucius (who lived approximately 2500 years ago), taught moral and ethical behavior. In his Analects, the character of Qi appeared in four locations. It expressed the concept related to breathe, food and vitality. Taoism, which was founded by Lao-Tze (who was believed to have lived around the time of Confucius or 100 years later), have had more influence on Qi and Qigong. In the book 'Zhuangzi', which compiled the thoughts of Lao-Tze in the third century BC, the character of Qi appeared 39 times. What it explained was: 'Qi exists throughout the universe. When it assembles, it appears as a human life. When it disassembles, the human will dies. Therefore, do not worry about life and death. Live naturally and freely as you are'. The concepts of Qi, Yin/Yang and meridians formed the foundation of Chinese medicine.

A central medical classic, The Yellow Emperor's Inner Canon teaches us: 'It is from, calm, indifference, emptiness, and nondesiring that true Qi arises. If the spirit is harboured inside, whence can illness arise? When the will is at rest and wishes little, when the heart is at peace and fears nothing, when the body labours but does not tire, then Qi flows smoothly from these states, each part follows its desires, and the whole gets everything it seeks'. The Chinese philosopher, Mencius (372–289 BC) described Qi in terms of moral energy, related to human excellence. This reinforces the argument that Qi is contextual, fluid in nature and not a fixed entity.

Qi is pronounced "chee". You may see it spelled "Chi" or even "Ki" in Japanese, but they all carry the same meaning. What is meant by Qi? The concept of Qi is based on the ancient Chinese initial understanding of natural phenomena. That is, Qi is the most basic substance of which the world is comprised. Everything in the universe results from the movements and changes of Qi. Man depends on nature for his production and growth and must observe the common laws of the world. As everything in the world comes from the interaction of Heaven Qi and Earth Qi, man must breathe to absorb Heaven Qi and eat to absorb Earth Qi. Qi was originally a philosophic concept. The ancient Chinese philosophy holds that Qi is the most basic substance constituting the world. This concept was introduced into TCM and became one of its characteristics. Accordingly, TCM also believes that Qi is the most fundamental substance in the construction of the human body and in the maintenance of its life activities. After a comprehensive survey of the statements on Qi in TCM documents, we have come to the conclusion that the meaning of Qi in TCM has two aspects. One refers to the vital substances comprising the human body and maintaining its life activities. The other refers to the physiological functions of viscera and bowels, channels and collaterals. For example, clean Qi, turbid Qi, and the Qi of water and food (food essence) are substantial Qi, while the Qi of the heart, liver, spleen, kidney, stomach, and the Qi of the channels and collaterals are functional Qi. In TCM, Qi is considered to be the force that animates and informs all things. In the human body, Qi flows through meridians, or energy pathways. Qi is the most basic substances that constitute the human body and maintain its functional activities. Generally speaking, Qi is an essential substance that is full of vigor and flows fast. Qi is attributed to Yang, because it is mobile and functions to move and warm. In this sense, Qi is also named Yang Qi.

2.2 Qi in other countries

Qi, that which defies definition, is the key concept in Eastern medicine, Eastern philosophy, as well as in martial arts (Yuasa, 1993). It naturally follows that Qi is an important element in complementary and alternative medicine (CAM). Many authors have presented work on the effects and nature of Qi (Chang, 2003; Lee, 2003; Chen, 2004; Olalde, 2005; Hankey and McCrum, 2006; Shinnick, 2006; Weze *et al.*, 2007; Abbott *et al.*, 2007). For the pre-modern Chinese, Qi comprised both yin and yang, with duality and interdependence in operation. In this thinking, to narrowly define Qi is considered unnecessary. The workings of nature were explained as the workings of Qi. Qi was all encompassing. Humans were subject to the workings of Qi as well as being agents of Qi, every person being so in different ways and at different times. Still, we can not precisely describe Qi. We cannot objectively say 'Look! This is Qi'. When Western people talk about Qi in terms of the healing arts, Qi seems to be understood as 'vitality' or 'life-energy'. For those who are studying Chinese medicine, Qi is presented as being a substance flowing in our body along the 'meridians'. In the view of martial artists, Qi is a source of spiritual strength for winning. When an Eastern philosopher defines Qi, it is a function of life, which permeates through the life of an individual and the life of the universe. Physicists see it as a new kind of 'energy', and still, brain physiologists approach it as 'information' or 'entropy' (Ohnishi and Ohnishi, 2009a). Thermographical studies demonstrated that skin temperature was raised by 3–4°C when exposed to Qi emitted from Qigong healers (Machi, 1993). When Qi was received from Nishino, instructors of his school or from students who practice for many years, a warm sensation was felt. This again supports the idea that Qi has an infrared radiation component (Ohnishi *et al.*, 2007). Depending upon one's profession, discipline and necessity, Qi is understood differently, this looks like reports from many blind persons touching different parts of an elephant.

Qi has energy and entropy aspects. While it is often described in the West as energy, or vital energy, Qi is the energy of the body, of the meridians, of food, of the universe. The term Qi carries a deeper meaning. Qi has two aspects: one is energy, power, or force; the other is conscious intelligence or information. Many believe Qi is an 'energy'. However, it is interesting to note that there is a subtle difference in understanding between the Chinese and the Japanese. The former seems to believe that it is a 'substance' or 'matter' flowing in and through our bodies, and that it can be emitted from the body of a Qigong healer. In contrast, the Japanese considers that it is a form of energy. An interesting concept was published by Shinagawa's group that treats Qi as a form of 'information' (Shinagawa, 1990). Flowers considers Qi as being about 'relationships and patterning'. These concepts are another way of describing 'information'. The most interesting practice in Nishino Breathing Method (NBM) is called the Taiki-practice (a method developed by Kozo Nishino, the founder of the NBM, to develop the level of individual's Qi through the Qi communication between an instructor and a student). Through the study on the Taiki-practice, Ohnishi *et al.* (2006) raised the possibility that Qi-energy may carry information, and that the information is in a form of 'entropy'. If Qi consists of simple energy, then, Qi effects might be mimicked by an instrument. However, if Qi involves entropy, it may be difficult to artificially reproduce the entire Qi effect.

China has, in recent decades, spent an inordinate amount of resources on experiments to determine the existence and nature of Qi. China is easing up on this research for lack of concrete breakthroughs. But the quest to define Qi continues, with there being no breakthroughs that we know of. Whether someone in China or anywhere has the Holy Grail hidden from view I cannot say, but in the report by Ohnishi, it is claimed that the effects of Qi energy can be measured. The question is also posed of what Qi actually is. Qi acts as Subtle Energy? We have still not defined Qi.

3. The formation of Qi

Qi of the human body comes from the combination of three kinds of Qi, Primordial Qi inherited from parents, the fresh air inhaled by the Lung and the refined food Essence transformed by the Spleen. Primordial Qi is derived from the Congenital Essence of the parents and is the primary substance to produce an embryo. So it forms the basis of the human body and its life activities. Without Congenital Essence, there can be no human body. After birth, the congenital Essence is stored in the Kidney to promote development and to control the reproductive activity of the human body. The refined food Essence is generated by the food which is taken in after birth and is distributed all over the body to produce nutrients and Qi and Blood under the action of the Spleen and Stomach. Fresh air is inhaled by the Lung after birth and is the main source of Qi of the human body.

From the process of formation of Qi, we can see that Qi of the human body is closely related to the functional activities of the Kidney, the Spleen and Stomach, and the Lung, in addition to the congenital constitution, food and nutrients, and the environment. Only when these organs function properly can the Qi of the body flourish. Conversely, dysfunction of any of these organs will influence the formation of Qi and the physiological function of Qi. For example, dysfunction of the Lung will weaken respiration, leading to failure of fresh air to be inhaled and the turbid Qi of the body to be exhaled, with the resultant inadequate formation of Qi. The transformation and transportation of the Spleen and Stomach play a particular role in the formation of Qi, for man relies on the nutrients transformed and transported by the Spleen and Stomach for his life after birth. On one hand, the Spleen sends up nutrients to the Lung to be dispersed, on the other hand, it sends down nutrients to the Kidney to supplement Kidney Essence. So, hypofunctioning of the Spleen and Stomach influences all three elementary substances that produce Qi.

4. The functions of Qi

Generally speaking, different kinds of Qi have different functions. Qi of the human body serves several vital functions within the body. When imbalances arise, they are seen as disruptions in the functions of Qi. A prolapse, for example, is seen as a disruption in the ability of Qi to provide the raising and stabilizing function on a particular organ. The main functions of Qi within the body are listed below:

4.1 Promoting function

Qi is a sort of essence full of vitality. It can promote the growth and development of the human body, promote the physiological functions of each viscera, bowel, channel, collateral, tissue and organ and speed up the formation and circulation of blood and the metabolism of body fluid as well. For example, if the above functions are weakened as a result of the deficiency of Qi (vital energy), the following will occur: late and slow growth and development of the human body or senilism; weakened functions of viscera and bowels, channels and collaterals, tissues and other organs; insufficient blood formation or stagnation in blood vessels; and disturbance in the metabolism of body fluid. After birth, the Genuine Qi generated from Kidney Essence determines the growth and development of the human body. After middle age, Genuine Qi gradually declines, so a person grows old. If his Genuine Qi is deficient, a person's development will be poor.

The physiological functions of viscera and bowels and Channels and Collaterals of the human body all depend on the pushing of Qi as well as the nourishing of Blood. The vigor and the ascending, descending, exit and entry movements of Qi play a very important role in promoting the functional activities of viscera and bowels and Channels and Collaterals. Therefore, when Qi is deficient, hypofunctioning of viscera and bowels will ensue. For instance, deficient Lung Qi often leads to feeble breathing, a lower voice, lassitude, weak pulse, etc. Qi also promotes the generation, distribution and discharge of the Blood and Body Fluids. As Yin substances, Blood and Body Fluids depend on Qi's activities to be generated. In other words, generation of these substances relies on the activities of Qi of the Spleen and the Stomach, the Lung and the Kidney. Besides, Qi is a vigorous substance, so it can activate the flow of Blood and Body Fluids, as well as transform them into various secretions and excretions. For this reason, Qi Deficiency often leads to an impeded flow of Blood or stagnation of Blood, or retention of Body Fluids in the body, which, in turn, causes Phlegm or edema.

In TCM theory, blood and Qi are inseparable. Blood is the "mother" of Qi; it carries Qi and also provides nutrients for its movement. In turn, Qi is the "commander" of the blood. This means that Qi is the force that makes blood flow throughout the body. Losing too much blood causes an overall Qi deficiency. When there is a Qi deficiency, the body cannot function properly.

4.2 Warming function

Qi, as a Yang substance, is rich in heat, which can warm viscera and bowels, Channels, skin, and muscles and tendons, to maintain normal body temperature and the normal functional activities of these organs and tissues. Qi helps to control homeostasis and provides warmth for the body. Yellow Emperor's Inner Canon says: "Qi has a warming action". Qi is the main source of the heat needed by the human body. The body keeps its constant temperature mainly through the warming action of its Qi. Motion produces heat, so the heat carried by Qi is in fact, a result of the constant movement of Qi, and the body temperature is maintained by the constant movement of Qi. In addition, Qi's warming function contributes to the movement of Blood and Body Fluids. The warming effect of Qi is an imperative condition for the free flow of Blood and Body Fluids within the body.

Pathologically, disorders of Qi in its warming function are mainly manifested as two kinds: one is a cold manifestation due to Deficiency of Qi, which results mostly from the deficient

Qi failing to produce adequate Heat to warm the body, marked by aversion to cold and a desire for warmth, cold limbs, lower body temperature and sluggish flow of Blood and Body Fluids. A deficiency of Qi can cause lowered body temperature, intolerance to cold and cold limbs. The other is the manifestation of Heat due to stagnation of Qi, which is usually caused by sluggish flow of Qi in a local area.

4.3 Defending function

The defensive ability of the body results from the combined action of a number of physiological functions, of which the function of Qi plays a particularly important role. The defensive effect of Qi mainly indicates that Qi can defend the body from external pathogens. The defending action of Qi is shown in two aspects. One is to guard the surface of the skin against the exopathogen. The other is to combat the invading exopathogen so as to ward it off. Defensive Qi functions to protect the body surface, and control the opening and closing of the pores, so it can prevent the invasion of external pathogens. If the defensive function of Qi is deficient, the resistance of the body against the invasion of these factors will be weakened, and as a result, susceptibility to such diseases as the common cold is likely to occur. When the defending function of Qi is normal, the exopathogen has difficulty in invading the body. When the defending function of Qi becomes weaker, when the ability of the human body to fight the exopathogen is lowered, the body is easily invaded and diseases are caused. And what is more, these diseases are hard to cure.

4.4 Consolidating and governing function

By "consolidating and governing action", we mean that Qi holds organs in their place, keeps Blood in the vessels, governs the removal of fluids. Qi can keep blood flowing within the vessels; control and adjust the secretion and excretion of sweat, urine and saliva, and prevent the body fluid from escaping; consolidate and store sperm and prevent emission and premature ejaculation; hold the organs so as to prevent them from descending. A decrease in the above functions of Qi may cause various kinds of hemorrhage, spontaneous perspiration, polyuria, salivation, spermatorrhea, premature ejaculation, prolapse of the stomach, kidney and uterus. When Qi is deficient, Yin Fluids will be profusely lost. For example, failure of Qi to control Blood will cause various kinds of bleeding; inability of Qi to control Body Fluids will cause spontaneous sweating or profuse sweating, incontinence of urine or profuse urine; and failure of Qi to control emission will cause nocturnal emission, premature ejaculation, or seminal emission. The controlling effect of Qi and the pushing effect of Qi are opposite and supplement each other. On one hand, Qi promotes the distribution and discharge of Blood and Body Fluids; on the other hand, Qi controls the flow of these Yin substances to prevent their unnecessary loss. Only when these two opposite aspects are harmonized can the normal flow and discharge of the Yin substances and the metabolism of Blood and water be maintained.

4.5 Promoting metabolism and transformation

This refers to various conversions occurring along with the movement of Qi. It includes the changes of Qi during its movement and the generation and metabolism of Essence, Blood and Body Fluids and their transformation. "Qi hua" is a specific term in the science of TCM. It refers, in general, to various kinds of changes taking place in the body under the action of Qi. Specifically, it refers to the metabolism of fundamental substances, Qi, blood and body fluid, and the transformations which can occur between them. For example, Qi, blood and body fluid are formed in the following manner: ingested food is changed into food essence, and food essence is, in turn, transformed into Qi, blood or body fluid, and these can then be changed into any one of the others according to the physiological need of the body. All these are the specific manifestations of the action of the activity of Qi. The dysfunction of Qi in performing its action will affect the whole metabolism of the body. That is to say, it will affect the digestion, absorption, transformation and transportation of food: the formation, movement and transformation of Qi, blood and body fluid; and the excretion of feces, urine and sweat; thus causing various symptoms associated with abnormal metabolism. In short, the process in which Qi performs its functions is the process in which the substances in the body are metabolized, and in which the substances and energy are transformed. Qi assists in the formation and transformations within the body, for example the transformation of food into Qi and Blood. Qi is the foundation of all movement and growth in the body.

Although the above mentioned five functions of Qi differ from each other, they are all based on the basic property of Qi and enjoy close cooperation and mutual support.

5. The movement of Qi

As a whole, Qi in the cosmos takes two patterns of existence, diffused Qi and coagulated Qi. The former is more vigorous, cannot be detected directly and exists everywhere. The latter is manifested as various kinds of things that can be seen or that have certain shapes. In order to survive, coagulated Qi must communicate with diffused Qi and its generation as well as its ending results from movement of the diffused Qi. The movement of Qi is called Mechanism of Qi, which can be generalized as four aspects: ascending, descending, exiting and entering movements, which are based on directions. Ascending refers to the movement from below; descending, from above; exiting, from the interior; and entering from the exterior.

The various functions of Qi are all performed by its movement. The physiological function of viscera and bowels is often reflected on their Qi's ascent, descent, exit and entry movements. Qi flows throughout the whole body because of its strength and vigor. Although the activities of the human body are multiple, they can all be summarized as these four aspects. For example, the dispersing effect of the Lung is a manifestation of the exit and ascent of Qi, while its descending effect is a manifestation of the descending and entering movements of Qi. These movements of Qi are vital to life. Once they stop, life comes to an end. The four movements of Qi have to be kept in harmony. Only in this way can the physiological functions of the human body remain norma1 in TCM, the physiological state in which the four basic movements of Qi are coordinated and balanced is called "harmonious functional activities of Qi".

Qi has four main states of disharmonies: Qi deficiency, Qi stagnation, sinking Qi and rebellious Qi. These disharmonies may affect many parts of the body at once or within a particular meridian, organ or area. Deficiency of Qi, for example, may affect the Lungs with symptoms of shortness of breath, the Stomach/Spleen with symptoms such as poor appetite and the body in general with symptoms of fatigue and weakness. The ascent, descent, exit and entry movements of Qi are of prime importance in human life. The Kidney Essence, the food Essence transported and transformed by the Spleen and Stomach and the fresh air inhaled by the Lung, will not be distributed over the body to perform their physiological functions if they do not make ascent, descent, entry and exit movements.

6. The classification of Qi

As the most basic substance that constitutes the world, Qi can be used to name everything in the world, so it is hard to classify it. However, Qi mentioned here is something concrete. Qi of the human body also has two patterns of existence. The coagulated Qi is manifested as various visible or structural components of the body, such as viscera, body figure, sense organs, Blood, Body Fluids and Essence; the diffused Qi is manifested as the Qi that flows in the body, but takes no certain form, such as Primordial Qi, Pectoral Qi, Nutritive Qi and Defensive Qi that is classified according to its distribution, origin, and function.

6.1 Primordial Qi (yuan Qi)

Primordial Qi is also called "Inborn Qi", "Primary Qi" or "genuine Qi". It is the most important and fundamental of all, originates from the congenital essence (the innate essence stored in the kidney). But it also depends on the supplement and nourishment of the acquired essence developed in the spleen and stomach. It is received from heaven and combined with food essence to nourish the body. It commences from "the vital gate", the portion between the two kidneys, passes the triple warmer and circulates throughout the body. It goes inward to the five viscera and six bowels and outward to the superficial layer of the body. It goes everywhere and acts on all parts of the body. The primordial Qi has the functions of both activating growth and development and promoting the functional activities of all the viscera and bowels, channels and collaterals, tissues and other organs. Therefore, it is the motivating power of the vital activities of the human body. If Primordial Qi is deficient due to a congenital defect or improper feeding after birth, the functional activities of the whole body will become weakened.

6.2 Pectoral Qi (zong Qi)

Pectoral Qi is also termed Great Qi, it accumulates in the thorax where Qi of the whole body converges. So the thorax is also known as "the sea of Qi". Pectoral Qi is a combination of the fresh air inhaled by the lung and the food essence derived by the spleen and stomach from water and grain. It is stored in the chest and poured into the channels of the heart and lung just as Miraculous Pivot (Lingshu), says: "It goes out of the lung and circulates through the larynx and pharynx. This is the reason why it exits when being exhaled and enters when being inhaled." The book Classified Canon compiled by Zhang Jiebin in 1624 A.D. says: "It goes down to the elixir field to be stored, and fills the Point Qijie of the yangming Channel from which it continues to go downward to the feet." Pectoral Qi has two main functions. One is that it flows through the respiratory tract to promote the respiratory movement of the lung and is involved in the loudness or softness of voice and words. The other is that it fills the heart channel to promote and adjust its beat, and to promote and adjust the circulation of blood and Qi. It also exerts an influence on the warmth and activities of the limbs. In short, it has the function of nourishing the lung and the heart, thus promoting respiration and blood circulation.

Generally speaking, when Pectoral Qi is sufficient, the pulse will be moderate and forceful, and the Heart will beat rhythmically and evenly. If Pectoral Qi is deficient, the pulse will be swift, irregular, feeble or scattered. Pectoral Qi is usually considered a link connecting the functional activities of the Heart and those of the Lung. In the clinic, Deficiency of Pectoral

Qi in most cases indicates Deficiency of Lung Qi leading to Deficiency of Heart Qi and ensuing Blood Stasis. For example, when a patient suffering from chronic bronchitis develops pulmonary Heart disease, which is marked by shortness of breath, a low voice, palpitation, a purplish face, running or intermittent pulse, etc., he or she can be diagnosed as having deficient Pectoral Qi.

6.3 Nutritive Qi (ying Qi)

Nutritive Qi refers to the Qi circulating within the blood vessels and having a nourishing function. As it flows through the vessels with blood, it has such a close relationship with the latter that TCM often mentions them in a combined way "nourishing blood". In TCM, Blood consists mainly of two parts: Nutritive Qi and Body Fluids. Compared with defensive Qi, nourishing Qi belongs to yin, so it is also called "nourishing yin". Nutritive Qi comes mainly from the food essence transformed and transported by the spleen and stomach. After its formation, Nutritive Qi is sent to the Channels to flow in the order of the Twelve Regular Channels. This is why a chapter on Arthralgia-Syndrome of Plain Questions (Suwen) says: "What is nutritive Qi? It is actually the essence Qi transformed from food and water". Nutritive Qi originates from the middle warmer and enters the channels by way of the lung. It circulates throughout the body along one after another of the fourteen channels. The main functions of Nutritive Qi are to generate Blood and to nourish the whole body. That is, it flows into the channels through the lung and becomes a component of blood, and nourish the whole body for the physiological activities of all the viscera and bowels, channels and collaterals, tissues and other organs. Plain Questions says: "Nutritive Qi secretes its fluid, which enters the channels and turns into blood, thus nourishing the four extremities, the five viscera and the six bowe1s".

6.4 Defensive Qi (wei Qi)

Defensive Qi is the Qi moving outside the conduits and having protective functions. Compared with nourishing Qi, it belongs to yang, so it is also known as "defensive yang", it also comes from the food essence transformed and transported by the spleen and stomach. It is characterized by braveness in defence. That is why a chapter on Arthralgia-Syndrome of Plain Questions says: "Defensive Qi is a brave kind, which is produced by food and water." The distribution of Defensive Qi has two features: the flow following Nutritive Qi and free flow. The former indicates that Defensive Qi also goes along the Twelve Regular Channels, while the latter indicates that Qi is distributed all over the body. Defensive Qi circulates not within but outside the channels. Being vaporized to the diaphragm and scattered in the chest and abdomen, it travels between the skin and flesh. In spite of circulating outside the channels, it still leans against the channels when moving. Defensive Qi has three functions. The first is guarding the surface of the body against exopathogen. The second is keeping a relatively constant body temperature by controlling the opening and closing of the muscular striae and adjusting the excretion of sweat due to its permeation to the muscular striae. The third is nourishing the viscera, bowels, muscles, skin and hair. When defensive Qi is insufficient, the defending function of the human body is weakened, the exopathogen invades the body easily, and the disease is hard to cure. Abnormal circulation of defensive Qi may cause sleep disorders. When defensive Qi is deficient, spontaneous sweating will occur.

Nutritive Qi and defensive Qi have the same source. The former circulates within the channels, has the nourishing function and belongs to yin, whereas the latter circulates outside the channels, has the function of guarding the exterior of the body and belongs to yang. Only when they coordinate with each other can the opening and closing of the pores be kept normal, the body temperature constant, and the defending ability strong.

7. Modern investigations on Qi

In China, Qi has been known for 4000 years. In Japanese literature, the documentation of Qi goes back 1500 years. This is not limited to the East. In the West, Biblical literature suggests that curing sickness by extending a hand was practiced by a gifted individual. Since then, thousands of accounts have been published, and millions of people have talked about Qi-energy. Practical, clinical, philosophical and scientific studies on Qi have been actively reported in journals of complementary and alternative medicine (CAM). However, no reasonable mechanism, which can be examined or refuted from the scientific point of view, has been presented (Ohnishi and Ohnishi, 2009b).

Scientific investigations of Qi started about 30 years ago, but we still know very little and have so much to learn. Flowers (2006) mentioned that the speed of Qi investigation seems to have slowed down in recent years. Now the question comes as to what is the nature of Qi? As to the nature of Qi, Chinese and Japanese scientists have already reported that it involves infrared radiation. It was also reported that other forms of energy may be involved in Qi which include electromagnetic waves, electrostatic energy, magnetic energy, sound waves and so on (Kiang, 1978; Yuasa, 1993; Machi, 1993; Shinagawa, 1990). However, in the study of Qi, one difficult problem encountered. Namely, Qi can't be measured quantitatively with modern technology now (Ohnishi and Ohnishi, 2009a). We do not even know the qualitative nature of Qi yet, not to mention quantitative methods of measuring it. One of the pitfalls in the study on Qi is obviously that there seems to be no 'scientific' objective measure to evaluate its 'quantity'. Thus, the concept of Qi would be as important and effective, and also as difficult to quantify, as the concept of 'stress'.

7.1 The effects of Qi-therapy on health

External Qi-therapy (QT) is a process by which Qi is transmitted from a Qi master to another person for the purpose of preventing and curing disease, as well as protecting and improving health through regulation of mind and body. This may be a very useful intervention. Research studies have shown that QT is effective for relief of pain, relaxation of stress states and increasing immunity (Lee *et al.*, 2001a–c). Several studies attempted to reveal a specific effect of external Qi by modern biochemical and immunological methods (Chien *et al.*, 1991; Fukushima *et al.*, 2001; Lee *et al.*, 2001a and b; Shah *et al.*, 1999). Chien *et al.* (1991) reported that facilitating Qi from a Qigong masters increased the rate of cell growth and DNA synthesis. Lee *et al.* (2001a and b) reported psychoneuroimmunological effects of *in vivo* QT on humans and stimulatory effect on natural killer (NK) cell activity *in vitro* by emitted Qi. QT has an acute stimulatory effect on neutrophil superoxide generation (Lee, 2003). The studies show that Qi positively affect human innate immunity.

TCM considers chronic fatigue to reflect a disharmony and depletion in the supply of Qi, with blockage, stagnation, imbalance or change in the pattern or organization of Qi resulting in disease (Shin, 2002; Xing, 1987). Disruption to Qi manifests in symptoms such as pain, fatigue and mood disturbances. TCM practitioners consider that chronic fatigue reflects a disharmony and depletion in the supply of Qi in the body. Qigong is one of the traditional complementary interventions used to strengthen Qi through self-practice, and to manage the state of Qi to prevent and cure disease. Qigong seems to improve factors related to chronic fatigue such as sleep, pain, mental attitude and general mobility after 3 and 6 months. Qigong's positive effects indicate that it represents a potentially safe method of treatment for chronic fatigued patients (Mike Craske, 2009).

People attempt to find the mechanism behind the healing effects of Qi. Why do students of NBM continue to attend the class (many of them once a week, but some of them more often) for 10 or even 15 years? Because they feel healthier, or because they have a more youthful feeling than before. Through their study, students were shown to have higher immune activity and lower stress levels (Kimura *et al.*, 2005). Some students overcame cancer themselves by attending the class almost everyday to lift their Qi level. This experience may be related to *in vitro* results that Qi inhibited the growth of cancer cells (Ohnishi *et al.*, 2005). As to the anti-aging effect of NBM, Mr Nishino has long proposed that Qi may stimulate mitochondria to become more active, and thus, to provide more energy to the cells. Ohnishi *et al.* (2006) demonstrated that in isolated rat liver mitochondria, the respiratory control ratio was protected from deterioration by Qi, and lipid peroxidation was inhibited by Qi. These results suggest that Qi may inhibit apoptosis of the cells in our body, thereby inhibiting aging. Some students were shown to have higher bone density than their age- and gender-matched contemporaries who do not practice NBM (Nishino, 2006). Through *in vitro* tests, Ohnishi *et al.* found that Qi may be beneficial in preventing osteoporosis (Ohnishi *et al.*, 2007). They are accumulating data on health-related benefits of NBM, and also, trying to correlate this with the molecular and cellular mechanisms of Qi effects.

7.2 The effects of Bu-Zhong-Yi-Qi-Tang on health

TCM, with its long history of clinical practice, occupies an important place among the "alternative medicine" that has been gaining attention in recent years. Because of the general mildness in nature and the emphasis on relief, balance and harmonization rather than forceful suppression, a good many Chinese medicines are particularly suited for the frail, the elderly, the very young and those already weakened by diseases. Bu-Zhong-Yi-Qi-Tang, a basic prescription as an Qi tonic (Chinese medical concept: Bu-Qi) and a general health tonic, also one of the typical formulae in Japanese Kampo which is prescribed for people with the Qi deficient conditions in order to enhance their Qi (Terasawa, 2004; Li, 1992; Kawakita and Nomoto, 1998), composed of Astragali radix, Ginseng radix, Atractyloidis rhizoma, Glycyrrhizae radix, Angelicae sinensis, Aurantii pericarpium, Cimicifugae rhizoma and Bupleurum radix, has been prescribed for the alleviation of fatigue and depressed vitality as well as the improvement of gastroenteric circulation (Shih *et al.*, 2000). It has been reported to possess anti-tumor (Ito and Shimura, 1985), anti-bacterial (Li *et al.*, 1992), anti-nociceptive and anti-depressive activities (Koshikawa *et al.*, 1998), and to have some effects on impairment of hematopoietic organs (Ikeda *et al.*, 1990), stress incontinence (Murakami, 1988) and male infertility (Ishikawa *et al.*, 1992), to reduce the extent of radiation-induced apoptosis and protect the jejunal crypt (Chai *et al.*, 2009) and improve health status in general but slows down or partially reverses aging in particular (Shih *et al.*, 2000).

7.3 The effects of Qi on health

Qi is the concept of the state of the mind/body as a whole. It is thus not a 'subjective' state, which can only be known introspectively. From the clinical experience, the Qi deficiency state is diagnosed very 'objectively': those with 'Qi deficiency' are weak in voice, have no 'strength' in their eyes and their posture is poor. In this sense, Qi is a very objective entity. It is not an abstract and subjective entity like soul or spirit. Practitioners of TCM can judge a patient's Qi state by just glancing at their skin condition. Those people healthy in mind-body, or with good Qi, have bright and 'full' skin. Though difficult to quantify, these are 'objective'. Qi can be approached 'objectively'. There is thus a definite possibility that we can elaborate on the concept of Qi as an objective 'scientific' term. It is a basic East Asian 'philosophy' of health/disease that those with a good Qi state are highly immune to diseases (Kobayashi and Ishii, 2005). It is very nice to see that Western clinical researchers such as Irwin have undertaken the challenge to tackle this difficult problem of Qi or mind-body unity. Now is an exciting era, when for the first time it has became possible for a western psychiatrist and an Eastern dermatologist to work together towards reconciling this fundamental difference between the medicines of the East and the West.

In Asia, the use of Qi in enhancing one's vitality and improving health is employed even today. For example, Qigong therapies are popular in China as Qi-therapies are in Japan. More recently, similar healing techniques were known in Europe as the working of mesmerism or hypnosis. Unfortunately, these techniques are not well accepted as a branch of today's main-stream sciences, especially in the Western hemisphere. Many people consider them as folk medicine. Some people believe that they are 'supernatural' and 'para-psychological' phenomena. In fact, Qi is neither a paranormal nor para-psychological phenomenon but is a normal phenomenon. Since it is a normal phenomenon, Qi can be studied by modern scientific methodology. Only a limited number of investigators have been studying them as the object of scientific, medical investigation for the past 30 years.

In the past 30 years, many Chinese scientists regarded 'Qi' as a real substance flowing in our body, which can be represented by mass. On the contrary, most Japanese scientists treated 'Qi' as energy, except for Shinagawa who considered it to be information. Although neither Qi itself nor the mechanism of its effects is understandable or explicable within any paradigm of modern medical science, its effects on the human body are apparent and some studies have been tried to find the underlying mechanism with laboratory experiments (Ohnishi, 2007).

Ohnishi *et al.* are demonstrating that so-called 'Qi-energy' is a natural phenomenon, and therefore, it can be analyzed by rigorous scientific and objective investigations. A 'breathing method' was developed by a Japanese leading Qi-expert, Kozo Nishino, Since 'breathing' is directly related to oxygen respiration, he has long proposed that mitochondria may play a key role in maintaining vitality and health (Nishino, 1997;2004). This led them to undertake the project to explore a possible relationship between Qi-energy and mitochondrial function (Ohnishi *et al.*, 2006). Kozo Nishino has hypothesized for many years that the breathing method would increase oxygen delivery in the body, activate cell metabolism including mitochondrial function, thereby bringing us tangible health benefits (Kimura *et al.*, 2005; Ohnishi *et al.*, 2005). Recently, Ohnishi *et al.* found that his Qi protected isolated rat liver mitochondria from heat-induced deterioration, possibly by reducing the production of reactive oxygen species (ROS). The protection of mitochondria and the reduction of ROS generation would produce more energy from the nutrients and would result in healthier cells and organs. The protection of mitochondria from adverse effects of ROS would reduce the likelihood of premature apoptosis, and therefore would contribute to the longevity of the practitioners. His prediction that mitochondria would play key roles in maintaining health and longevity seems to be supported by these experiments (Ohnishi *et al.*, 2006).

Isolated rat liver mitochondria are a well-established model for studying biophysical and biochemical aspects of energy metabolism. The simplest marker for the integrity and intactness of mitochondria is a respiratory control ratio (RCR, which is the ratio between State-3 and State-4 respiration) (Chance and Williams, 1955). Ohnishi *et al.* measured the RCR and analyzed the degree of lipid peroxidation in the mitochondria by measuring the amount of TBARS (thiobarbituric acid reactive substances). Using this model, they found that a heat treatment (incubation at 39°C for 10 min) decreased the RCR by about 60%. While the Qi-energy emitted from the fingers of Nishino could inhibit the decrease. They also attempted to find the mechanism for the Qi-effect. After the early work by Boveris and Cadenas (1975), ROS has been recognized as an important factor to damage mitochondrial functions. In order to test whether Qi-energy could reduce the ROS production, they measured the amount of mitochondrial lipid peroxidation after the heat treatment using a well-known assay technique for TBARS. Lipid peroxidation was increased during the heat deterioration, suggesting that mitochondria were exposed to oxidative stress. Lipid peroxidation is known to damage the mitochondrial membrane. However, lipid peroxidation was inhibited by Qi-energy, and the mitochondrial integrity was preserved.

From the standpoint of health and longevity, their results may have the following significance: (i) Qi-energy may protect mitochondria from oxidative injury. If the same reaction takes place in the practitioners' body, then mitochondria may produce more energy, and therefore, it has beneficial effects on cellular metabolism. (ii) Mitochondria are known to play key roles in apoptosis of many cell types. If cytochrome c and other apoptosis-inducing factors (AIF) are released from mitochondria, they activate a series of cascade reactions to cause apoptotic cell death (Green and Reed, 1998; Narita *et al.*,1998; Susin *et al.*, 1999; Lorenzo *et al.*, 1999; Shimizu *et al.*, 1999). Although apoptosis is a fundamental feature of almost all animal cells and it is indispensable for the normal development of tissues, organs and immune systems (Jacobson *et al.*, 1997), excessive apoptosis could cause diseases (Thompson, 1995). Therefore, protecting mitochondrial integrity would help prevent cytochrome c release, thereby inhibiting inappropriate apoptosis from taking place. In conclusion, Qi-energy maintains mitochondrial membrane integrity during the heat deterioration process. Mitochondria are constantly exposed to the danger of ROS-induced oxidative injury. The effect of Qi seems to be related to the inhibition of oxidative injury on mitochondrial membranes caused by ROS. Therefore, Qi would have a beneficial effect on protecting mitochondria; thus, it would maintain efficient cellular metabolism and decrease the chance of unnecessary apoptosis.

'Qi-energy', which can be enhanced through the practice of Nishino Breathing Method (NBM), was reported to have beneficial health effects. It has been known for 20 years that the practitioners of Qi experienced beneficial health effects (Yumi, 2005). It was shown that the practice increased immune activity and decreased the stress level of the practitioners (Kimura *et al.*, 2005). From the collaboration with Master Nishino, Ohnishi *et al.* showed that 'Qi' is not a paranormal or parapsychological phenomenon, but a natural phenomenon. An interesting observation from the standpoint of CAM was that the Qi-energy, which inhibits

cell division of cultured cancer cells (Ohnishi *et al.*, 2005) or protects isolated mitochondria from oxidative injury, was the same as that which could move other individuals in the Taiki-practice (Ohnishi and Ohnishi, 2006). This suggests that the training gained from the Taiki-practice may produce beneficial health effects. This is the reason why they are studying the mechanism behind the Taiki-practice.
Ohnishi *et al.* explain the philosophical and psychological background of Qi, emphasize that the unique aspects of Eastern philosophy are 'non-linearity' and 'holistic' approach and then present physics aspect of Qi. Their experiments demonstrated that a 'Qi-beam' carries 'entropy' (or information), which is different from 'energy' (Ohnishi and Ohnishi, 2009a). We believe that the human will uncover the secret of Qi in the near future with the rapid development of modern life science.

8. The significance of studying Qi

The difference between the cultures in the West and the East may be described by the difference between 'linear philosophy' and 'nonlinear philosophy'. Since Qi phenomena are essentially nonlinear, a straightforward application of linear philosophy may not be effective in its study. We hope that the study of Qi phenomena may help bridge some of the apparent difference between Western and Eastern culture. As Flowers mentioned, in the Christian West, God was the center of everything as opposed to Qi being the center of everything in the East. Qi may be another name of 'life'. As Flowers beautifully described, Qi may represent the entity of life itself (Flowers, 2006). Then, the understanding of Qi may shed light on other aspects of biological sciences. We hope that the study of Qi might help to unite more aspects of Eastern and Western philosophy.
Understanding of Qi will help bridge Western and Eastern viewpoints, According to Eastern thought, the universe has 'life' and the function of 'life' is represented by Qi. Qi flows and circulates throughout the universe and through each human being. Qi is a non-linear phenomenon, and therefore, it can function as an essential element of life and the universe (both of which are non-linear). If Western people could understand Qi more, they would incorporate holistic Eastern philosophy into their own philosophical system. Then, mind and body, as well as life and its environment, will be viewed as a unified entity, and the world would finally become a better place to live.
The concept of Qi would be of great value towards this direction, as it is understood as a kind of 'energy' of mind/body as a whole. If, therefore, there was some concrete method to enhance (strengthen) Qi, it would become one of the cornerstones of holistic medicine of the future. Thus, from the medical point of view, Qi can be seen as the totality of the body's healing systems or defense mechanisms which include the immune system as their essential part. Qi has both energy and entropy (information) aspects. The practice of breathing to enhance the Qi level may in-essence help to restore the original ability of human beings. Therefore, it may contribute to improve our health, wellness and life itself.
Qi phenomenon seems to be characteristic to the nonlinear nature of life. If so, the study of Qi may help deepen our understanding on our life and the universe itself. Since Qi is related to our life activity, the understanding of Qi would contribute to the elucidation of the beautiful nature of life itself. Further development and understanding of Qi may help round out our belief in technology-oriented modern science which lacks humanistic aspects. This may help to transform the 'Century of Death' to the 'Century of Life'. The 19th century was the age of the 'industrial revolution' which was symbolized by an invention of a steam

engine. The 20th century is the age of 'nuclear energy'. Then, what would make the 21st century more humanistic so that history might regard it as a century of life? The pursuit of studies on Qi might be a positive step. In conclusion, Qi phenomenon is not paranormal. It is a normal and real phenomenon and can be the object of rigorous scientific study. If the question is posed, 'Why do you study Qi?' We will answer, as a famous mountain climber once said, 'Because it is there!' We believe that further analysis of Qi may open up a new horizon in life science.

9. The comparisons between Qi and bioenergy

Qi, an important category in the ancient Chinese philosophy, is a simple understanding of natural phenomena. According to ancient Chinese philosopher, Qi is the most basic material that constitute the world, the everything in the universe were produced by the motion of Qi, and it is roughly similar to the concept material of Western philosophy. The theory of Qi in ancient philosophy was introduced into the medical field, the basic theory of Qi in traditional Chinese medicine (TCM) was formed, i.e., the concept of Qi in TCM was established during the mutual penetration between the materialist philosophy and medicine in ancient China, it is a concept of material. In TCM, Qi is constantly in motion, is the subtle substance with a strong vitality which constitute the human body and maintain the activities of human life, is one of the most basic material, it is also known as the "essence Qi". When the concept Qi in TCM was used to discuss the human body, it often has the meaning of both life material and physiological functions. Therefore, Qi in TCM is one of the most important basic concepts. Bioenergetics research in life sciences have played an important role, Mitchell's chemiosmotic theory earned the 1978 Nobel Prize in Chemistry, as the coupling between electron transport in the respiratory chain and adenosine diphosphate (ADP) phosphorylation which is caused by electrochemical gradient of protons between internal and external mitochondrial membrane was expounded; Nobel Prize in Chemistry in 1997 was awarded academician PD Boyer in the U.S. Academy of Sciences for elucidating generation mechanism of adenosine triphosphate (ATP)—the most important energy molecules. The work was closely related to the energy production and consumption which is required for life activities, and the binding-changes and rotation-catalytic mechanism of ATP synthase was proposed. ATP synthase is the smallest molecular motor in the world. In this paper, the relationship between Qi and bioenergy was approached to.

9.1 The generation of Qi and ATP

9.1.1 The generation of Qi

Qi in TCM, constitute the body and maintain life activities, has the following three sources and is a combination of them. (i). Congenital essence: This essence, which is born before the body, is the basic material of life, is intrinsic from the parents. (ii). Acquired essence: is acquired from the diet to obtain nutrients from the transportation and transformation through the spleen and stomach, that is, the essence of water and food. (iii). The clear air in the nature: the fresh air inhaled through the breathing exercise of lungs.

From the generation process of Qi, Qi depends on the normal function of the organs and tissues of the body, but the physiological functions of the viscera kidney, spleen and stomach, lungs are closely related to it. The lung, being the dominator of Qi, operates the Qi of the whole body; spleen and stomach, being the acquired foundation, their function of

transformation and transport is particularly important in the Qi generation process; kidney, being the source of Qi generation and the congenital foundation, store the essence of life which includes congenital and acquired essence. For example, Qi, blood and body fluid are formed in the following manner: ingested food is changed into food essence, and food essence is, in turn, transformed into Qi, blood or body fluid, and these can then be changed into any one of the others according to the physiological need of the body. The waste from the eaten food and the products produced in the course of metabolism are changed, separately, into feces, urine and sweat which are ready to be removed from the body.
The Qi in the human body is different in classification and formation. But, generally speaking, it has no more than two sources. One is the innate vital substance one inherits from one's parents before birth. The other is the food essence and fresh air one receives from air, water and food in the natural world. The materials obtained in the two ways above have to be processed and transformed by the viscera and bowels before becoming the Qi of the human body. The process for Qi to be formed is as follows: The innate vital substance acted on by the kidney comes out of the gate of life (the portion between the two kidneys) and goes up to the middle warmer. There it combines with the food essence coming from the spleen and continues upwards until it combines with the fresh air inhaled by the lung. The food essence transformed and transported by the Spleen must be sent up to the Lung to combine with fresh air to produce the nutrients necessary for man's life activities. Finally it turns into Qi. It is easy to see from the above that the Qi of the human body is formed through the joint work of the kidney, the spleen, the stomach and the lung in combining the innate vital substance taken from one's parents, the food essence received from water and food, and the fresh air obtained from nature.

9.1.2 The generation of ATP

The major function of mitochondria is the generation of ATP, the energy currency of the cell, by oxidative phosphorylation. Essential mechanisms of energy production, signaling, biosynthesis and apoptosis are contained within mitochondria, and their orchestration plays a determinant role in cell physiology (Benard *et al.*, 2006; Bailey *et al.*, 2005). Since mitochondria generate between 80% and 90% of all ATP produced in the cell, the rest of the energy was provided from anaerobic glycolysis and the conversion of creatine phosphate (PCr) by creatine kinase (CK) (Papa, 1996; Radda *et al.*, 1995), it is understandable that in tissues like the cardiac muscle and liver (each hepatocyte contains 1000–2000 mitochondria) these organelles occupy 20–30% of the cell volume, having mitochondrial function, or dysfunction, a critical role in the performance of these tissues (Smith *et al.*, 2008; Yang *et al.*, 2010). An adult needs about 3000 kcal, or 400 mol ATP (about 200 kg) every day. Mitochondrial oxidative phosphorylation (OXPHOS) enzymes including 5 oligomeric protein complex, i.e. complex I (NADH dehydrogenase), complex II (succinate ubiquinone reductase), complex III (cytochrome c reductase), complex IV(cytochrome c oxidase, COX) and complex V(H^+-ATP synthase). Complex I and II capture electrons from the reduced coenzyme I (NADH) and succinate respectively, and transfer them to coenzyme Q (CoQ), CoQ is oxidized by complex III and IV. These complexes (except complex II) are coupled electron flow to proton pump and to ensure that the generated proton driving force was used by complex V to form ATP from ADP and phosphate (Pi) coupling reaction, each complex is composed by different subunits, and complex I, II, III and IV contain several redox active prosthetic groups (Papa, 1996).

Bio-energy materials - ATP generation process in modern medicine is as follows: ATP, the "Universal Currency" of bioenergy in the cell, is a direct provider of energy required for the body, provide efficient energy for any endergonic reactions. Therefore, life is basically dependent on the activities of ADP -ATP cycle. There are two types of ATP-generating mechanisms: substrate level phosphorylation in the original fermentation pathway and photophosphorylation and OXPHOS that use electron transport system in the evolutionary pathways. The efficiency for generating ATP of the latter is about 20 times compare to the former, the key reasons for high efficiency in photophosphorylation and OXPHOS system depend on the proton pumps and ATP synthase in biomembrane, for example, ATP synthase catalyze endergonic reaction by binding the protons that accumulated in one side of the membrane: ADP + Pi (phosphate) → ATP. Then, proton pump coupled with the electron transport system to generate energy.

Now, let's look at the overview of the mitochondrial ATP production. Mitochondria are intracellular organelles mainly devoted to energy production. From the point of the main generation process of bio-energy substance-ATP, at first, the three major nutrients carbohydrates, lipids and proteins are decomposed into the simple sugars, fatty acids and amino acids respectively by different enzymes in the body. Then pyruvate was generated from glucose by glycolysis, acetyl coenzyme A (CoA) was then formed from pyruvate through the pyruvate dehydrogenase complex, acetyl-CoA, can also be generated in mitochondria from fatty acids by β-oxidation, then enter the Krebs cycle, and the 20 kinds of standard amino acids that make up proteins can be decomposed in the body to generate acetyl-CoA, oxaloacetate, fumarate, succinyl-CoA and α-ketoglutaric acid and other substances to enter the citric acid cycle. The hydrogens stripped off in the Krebs cycle were accepted by nicotinamide adenine dinucleotide (NAD^+) or flavin adenine dinucleotide (FAD) to enter in the respiratory chain of inner mitochondrial membrane through a series of electron carriers (low potential to high potential), the electrons were finally transported to oxygen accompanied by the phosphorylation of ADP to generate ATP.

The following describes the basic processes occurring in a typical normal cell, using glucose as a major source of energy. The breakdown of glucose into water and CO_2 includes two steps, namely, glycolysis (the anaerobic phase) taking place in the cytoplasm, and OXPHOS (the aerobic phase) occurring in the mitochondria. Of the total yield of 38 ATP per mole of glucose, two are produced in the glycolysis process and 36 during the OXPHOS. It is important to note that oxygen availability in the mitochondrion is a critical factor for the normal ATP production in the cell. Glycolysis depends on the entrance of glucose from the capillary into the cell via the glucose transporter. The end product of glycolysis, pyruvate, is transported into the mitochondria by a specific carrier protein. The pyruvate is transformed, in the matrix of the mitochondria, into acetyl coenzyme A that activates the tricarboxylic acid (TCA) cycle. In the mitochondria, the TCA cycle generates NADH which enters the electron transport chain (ETC) leading to the OXPHOS that generates ATP (Mayevsky, 2009).

The mitochondrial respiratory chain consists of four enzyme complexes (complexes I–IV), and two mobile carriers (coenzyme Q and cytochrome c) along which the electrons liberated by the oxidation of NADH and $FADH_2$ are passed, and ultimately transferred to molecular oxygen. This respiratory process generates the electrochemical gradient of protons used by the F_1F_o ATP synthase (i.e., complex V) to phosphorylate ADP and produce ATP. Briefly, nutrients such as glucose, amino acids and fatty acids are transformed by intermediary metabolism into their reduced equivalents (NADH, H^+ or $FADH_2$), which are further oxidized by the mitochondrion to generate ATP. Mitochondria of normal tissues typically oxidize combinations of these energy substrates (fatty acids, the glycolysis end product pyruvate and amino acids) to establish the electrochemical gradient of protons ($\Delta\mu H^+$) used by the F_1F_o-ATP synthase to produce ATP (Benard *et al.*, 2010). In this regard, mitochondria play a pivotal role by producing almost all the cellular energy (Freyre-Fonsecaa *et al.*, 2011). It is quite evident that the generation of ATP requires both acquired essence —the essence of water and food (which can be regarded as decomposition products of the three major nutrients—monosaccharides, fatty acids and amino acids) and the clear Qi in the nature - the fresh air (mainly oxygen, around 90% oxygen inhaled by the body was consumed by the process of ATP production through mitochondrial electron transport), mitochondria are also needed. But modern biochemical research show that human mitochondria are maternally inherited, that is, mitochondria of everyone are from the mother genetically, and this can be called the congenital essence. Therefore, the Qi and ATP have common sources.

9.2 The functions of Qi and bioenergy

Generally speaking, Qi of the human body has five functions: promoting, warming, defending, consolidating and governing, promoting metabolism and transformation, these functions of Qi are consistent with those of energy metabolism. All cells in the body depend on a continuous supply of ATP in order to perform their different physiological and biochemical activities (Mayevsky, 2009). In modern medicine, all the physiological activities of the body are dependent on bio-energy source (ATP) generated by substance metabolism (including oxygen metabolism), various forms of physiological functions can be played by ATP through different effectors to maintain all life activities. Large amounts of ATP are used in muscle contraction, nerve impulse conduction, compound biosynthesis or other biological processes (Benard *et al.*, 2010).

Qi is a vigorous substance that flows fast in the human body. So it promotes the growth and development of the body, the movement, distribution and discharge of Blood and Body Fluids, and the physiological functional activities of viscera and bowels, channel, collateral, tissue and organ. Qi, as a Yang substance, heat source of the body, is rich in heat, which can warm viscera and bowels, channels, skin, and muscles and tendons, to maintain normal body temperature and the normal functional activities of these organs and tissues. This Qi function is of important to physiological significance of the human body. "Qi hua" is a specific term in the science of TCM. It refers, in general, to various kinds of changes taking place in the body under the action of Qi. Specifically, it refers to the metabolism of fundamental substances, Qi, blood and body fluid, and the transformations which can occur between them, it is actually material conversion and energy conversion process. Although the above mentioned five functions of Qi differ from each other, they enjoy close cooperation and mutual support. Qi is the foundation of all movement and growth in the body.

According to TCM, "if Qi gets together, it will result to the birth; if Qi is harmonious, then the human body is healthy; if Qi is disordered, the human will be sick; if Qi is depleted, the human will die." According to the modern life science, energy metabolism is the center for life activity, if the energy metabolism is normal, the body can carry out normal vital activities, If no bio-energy is supplied for the body, the life activities cease immediately. Therefore, Qi and bioenergy have identical functions.

10. The effects of QIHM and QRHM on energy metabolism—An experimental perspective

ABSTRACT Aims: TCM practitioners usually compose prescriptions made up of Qi-invigorating herbal medicines (QIHM) or Qi-flow regulating herbal medicines (QRHM) for Qi system diseases, and have accumulated abundant clinical experience for a long time. To approach to the nature of Qi in TCM from bioenergetics, the effects of QIHM (ginseng, astragalus root, pilose asiabell root, white atractylodes rhizome) and QRHM (immature bitter orange, magnolia bark, green tangerine and lindera root) on oxidative phosphorylation (OXPHOS), bioenergy level and creatine kinase activities were investigated.

Methods: QIHM and QRHM were administered by oral gavage daily for 10 days. Mice liver mitochondria were isolated by differential centrifugation. The effects of QIHM and QRHM on energy metabolism were studied from the production, regulation, and storage of bioenergy. Mitochondrial OXPHOS curve was determined by Clark oxygen electrode method. The levels of adenosine triphosphate (ATP), adenosine diphosphate (ADP) and adenosine monophosphate (AMP) in liver cells were determined by reversed-phase high performance liquid chromatography (RP-HPLC), adenylate energy charge (AEC), total adenylate pool (TAP) were calculated. The creatine kinase (CK) activities in mice skeletal muscle were determined by a commercial monitoring kit. The regularity of action of QIHM and QRHM were analyzed and concluded.

Results: Ginseng and astragalus root can decrease oxygen consuming rate and respiratory control ratio (RCR) of liver mitochondria obviously, we consider this is appearance of lowering standard metabolic rate and is a kind of protective adaptation. QRHM can increase P/O ratio and RCR. Both QIHM and QRHM can stimulate activity of CK significantly in the storage of energy, and QRHM is stronger than QIHM. But it is worth notice that all the four QIHM can increase levels of ATP, AEC and TAP; on the contrary, all the four QRHM can decrease levels of ATP, AEC and TAP in liver cells. In a word, QIHM and QRHM increase and decrease bioenergy level of liver cells respectively *in vivo*. Therefore, Qi is closely related to bioenergy.

Conclusion: Qi and bioenergy have common sources and identical functions. QIHM and QRHM are able to improve and decrease the energy state of the body respectively. Qi and bioenergy have general characteristics in many aspects. The experiments provide scientific evidence for Qi in TCM is bioenergy.

Key words: Qi; bioenergy; Adenosine triphosphate; qi-invigorating herbal medicine; qi-regulating herbal medicine.

According to TCM theory, Qi (vital energy) refers to a kind of refined nutritive substance within the body. Qi is one of the most basic, the most important, and the most complicated concept in TCM. We propose a hypothesis that Qi is closely related to bioenergy according to the ancient concept of Qi and modern bioenergetics. TCM practitioners usually compose prescriptions made up of Qi-invigorating herbal medicines (QIHM) or Qi-flow regulating herbal medicines (QRHM) for Qi system diseases, and have accumulated abundant clinical experience for a long time. QIHM is a kind of herbal medicines which can invigorate Qi and treat syndromes of Qi deficiency, they have the effects of invigorating Qi, promoting the production of body fluid and tonifying the spleen and lung etc. QRHM is a kind of herbal medicines which can induce the flow of Qi, regulate the Qi system diseases and treat the syndromes of stagnation of Qi or rebellious Qi etc. They can activate Qi to reduce pain, depress upward-reverse flow of Qi, break the stagnant Qi to remove masses etc. QIHM and QRHM have similar nature and atributive channels, but their flavours are different significantly. QIHM taste sweet while QRHM taste acrid-bitter, and their compositions are also different. Although Qi of TCM is similar to the concept of modern medical bioenergy in some aspects, the energy nature of Qi still lacks convincing evidence. Therefore, we take it as our basic point to approach the characteristics of QIHM and QRHM on energy metabolism. We have approached the rules of QIHM and QRHM from the production (oxidative phosphorylation), storage (creatine kinase activity) and regulation (adenylate energy charge) of bioenergy (ATP). Since there is no direct detection method on Qi, the widely used QIHM (ginseng, astragalus root, pilose asiabell root, white atractylodes rhizome) and QRHM (immature bitter orange, magnolia bark, green tangerine and lindera root) were selected to study the effect on energy metabolism to approach to the nature of Qi in TCM.

Sasang constitutional medicine (SCM) is a unique traditional Korean therapeutic alternative form of medicine. In both SCM and TCM theories, Qi is the most essential element, the 'driving force' that constitutes the body and maintains the activities of life, visceral functions and metabolism. In a generalized scope, the essence of Qi in SCM can be compared with that of energy in modern physiology. The metabolic process in physiology provides energy, kinetic and potential energies, whereas metabolism in SCM produces and regulates Qi. Since catabolism breaks own complex molecules into simple ones and releases kinetic energy, this pathway can be compared with the process of consuming Qi in SCM. Similarly, anabolism, which links together simple molecules to form more complex molecules and stores potential energy, is comparable with the process of producing and storing Qi in SCM. In terms of interior–exterior exchange, the process of taking up raw materials from the external environment to produce Qi in SCM (function of the spleen) corresponds to the process of digestion and absorption of food and water and inhaling air in physiology (Kim and Pham, 2009). To approach to the nature of Qi in TCM from bioenergetics, the effects of QIHM and QRHM on oxidative phosphorylation (OXPHOS), bioenergy level and creatine kinase (CK) activities were investigated.

Materials and methods

Animals and materials

Male Kunming mice (Grade II, Certificate No 2002-5), weighing 22±2.0 g each, were purchased from Experimental Animal Center, Dalian University. All mice were cared for according to the Guiding Principles in the Care and Use of Animals. The experiment was approved by Medical College Council on Animal Care Committee of Dalian University (China) in accordance with NIH guidelines (NIH, 2002). Rodent laboratory chow and tap water were available *ad libitum* during the period. Spherisorb C_{18} reversed-phase chromatographic column (4.6 mm×250 mm, 5 μm particle size) was produced by Dalian Institute of Chemistry and Physics, Chinese Academy of Sciences. Adenosine triphosphate (ATP), adenosine diphosphate (ADP), adenosine monophosphate (AMP), 2-Thiobarbituric acid (TBA), and 1,1,3,3-tetraethoxypropane (TEP) were from Sigma Chemical (St Louis, MO, USA). N-2-Hydroxyethylpiperazine-N'-2-ethane sulfonic acid (HEPES) was from Merck (Darmstadt, Germany). Coomassie Brilliant Blue G-250 (CBBG-250) was purchased from Fluka (Bushs SG, Switzerland). Bovine serum albumin (BSA) was from Boehringer Mannheim Corp. (Indianapolis, IN, USA). Tris(hydroxymethyl)aminomethane (Tris) was from Gibco BRL

(Grand Island, NY, USA). A commercial creatine kinase monitoring kit [N-acetyl-L-cysteine(NAC)-activated] was from Beijing Zhongsheng High-Tech Bioengineering Company (Beijing, China). All other chemicals and solvents used in the study were of analytical grade made in China. Ginseng, astragalus root, pilose asiabell root, white atractylodes rhizome, immature bitter orange, magnolia bark, green tangerine and lindera root, are *Panax ginseng* C.A. Mey (Tongrentang red ginseng), *Astragalus membranaceus* (Fisch.) Bge.var. mongholicus (Bge.) Hsiao, *Codonopsis pilosula* (Franch.) Nannf, *Atractylodes macrocephala* Koidz, *Citrus aurantium* L, *Magnolia officinalis* Rehd et Wils, *Citrus reticulate* Blanco and *Lindera aggregate* (Sims) Kosterm respectively, were purchased from Beijing Tongrentang Drugstore, and identified by professor Li Jiashi at Beijing University of Traditional Chinese Medicine.

Preparation of the aqueous extracts of QIHM and QRHM

Powdered dry ginseng, astragalus root, pilose asiabell root, white atractylodes rhizome, immature bitter orange, magnolia bark, green tangerine and lindera root were immersed in distilled water (the ratio of the drug and distilled water was 1:10) for 0.5 hour and extracted thrice with distilled water for 0.5 hour each in a boiling water bath. The filtrate was collected after filtration with gauze, mixed and condensed to 0.2 g crude drug/ml.

Animal groups

Mice in each QIHM and QRHM group (n=10) were administered respective aqueous extracts (4 g crude drug/kg/day) by oral gavage and mice in the control group received an equivalent volume of normal saline for 10 days, there are nine groups all together. All the mice were maintained with free access to food and drinking water.

Isolation of liver mitochondria

Mitochondria were isolated by differential centrifugation using a modified version of the protocol of Michele *et al.* (1992). Mice were dislocated and their livers were removed immediately and placed in an ice-cold isolation medium (containing 0.25 M sucrose, 0.5 mM EDTA and 3 mM HEPES, pH 7.4). Livers were homogenized with a motor-driven Teflon pestle in wet ice at 0°C. Following homogenization, samples were centrifuged at 1,000 g for 10 min. This, and all other centrifugation steps, used a Beckman JA-25.50 rotor and Beckman J_2-MC centrifuge at 4°C. Supernatants were removed and centrifuge at 12,000 g for 10 min. The pellets were washed twice in the isolation medium, and respun at 12,000 g. Following the final wash, mitochondria were resuspended in the same medium. Protein determinations were carried out using Bradford (1976) method.

Measurement of oxidative phosphorylation curve of liver mitochondria

Respiratory control ratio (RCR) of liver mitochondria was measured using the method described by Estabrook (1967). Oxygen consumption was measured at 30°C in a closed, stirred, and thermostatted glass vessel equipped with a Clark-type oxygen electrode in 2.0 ml respiration buffer. The respiration buffer (pH 7.4) consisted of sucrose 225 mM, EDTA 1 mM, $MgCl_2$ 5 mM, KCl 15 mM, KH_2PO_4 15 mM, Tris 50 mM, L-glutamic acid 5 mM, DL-malate 10 mM, and mitochondrial protein 5 g/L. Respiratory state 3 (S_3) was the oxygen (O_2) consumption by mitochondria in the presence of substrate after the addition of 0.25 mM adenosine diphosphate (ADP, ADP is a potent stimulator of mitochondrial respiration). Respiratory state 4 (S_4) was the oxygen consumption when all the ADP has been phosphorylated. S_3 and S_4 can be calculated according to the oxidative phosphorylation

(OXPHOS) curve. Respiration rates were expressed in nanomoles atom O per minute per milligram of protein. RCR was the ratio of S_3 to S_4 respiration. P/O ratio is the number of ADP molecules phosphorylated per oxygen atom reduced.

Determination of creatine kinase activity

Mice were killed via dislocation, and skeletal muscle from the hind leg was rapidly removed, weighed and made into 1% homogenates with normal saline at 0°C. 2.0 ml homogenate was centrifuged at 2,000 g for 5 min, 100 µl supernatant was added to 900 µl normal saline and mixed, 10 µl of which was used for determination of creatine kinase (CK) activity. CK activity was measured by using a commercial CK monitoring kit [N-acetyl-L-cysteine(NAC)-activated], following the manufacturer's protocol.

Measurement of ATP, ADP, and AMP in liver cells by HPLC

Mice were killed via dislocation, and livers were rapidly removed, weighed and made into 10% homogenates with normal saline at 0°C, 1 ml of ice-cold 0.3 M perchloric acid was added to 1 ml of 10% liver homogenates that were kept on ice for an additional 5 min. Harvested materials were centrifuged at 15,000 g at 4°C for 10 min. The supernatant was neutralized with 80 µl of 3 M KOH, and tubes were kept on ice for an additional 30 min. The resulting precipitate was removed by centrifugation, and the supernatant was stored at -80°C until it was analyzed. 10 µl of neutralized cell extract was used for determination of ATP, ADP, and AMP in liver cells, which was carried out by gradient RP-HPLC (reversed-phase high performance liquid chromatography) with ultraviolet detector at room temperature and with mobile phase at a rate of 0.8 ml/min. Mobile phases used for the gradient system were buffer A (0.05 M KH_2PO_4-K_2HPO_4, pH 6.0) and buffer B, consisting of buffer A plus 10% methanol (*v/v*). All buffers and solutions used for HPLC analysis were filtered and degassed through a 0.45 µm filter. Gradient elution procedure: buffer A was used as mobile phase between 0 and 3 min, buffer A was changed from 100% to 0% and buffer B from 0% to 100% between 3 and 6 min, buffer B was mobile phase between 6 and 9 min, buffer A was the mobile phase after 9 min, all the running time was 12 min, the detection wavelength was set at 254 nm. ATP, ADP and AMP quantitation in liver cells was calculated by computing the peak area of them, identification and quantitative measurements of nucleotides were carried out by the injection of standard solutions of nucleotides with known concentrations. Standard curves were plotted for individual compounds and were used to determine the contents of ATP, ADP, and AMP in each sample. Total adenylate pool (TAP) and adenylate energy charge (AEC) were calculated by the following formulas respectively: TAP = [ATP] + [ADP] + [AMP], AEC = ([ATP] + 0.5[ADP])/TAP. AEC represents a linear measure of the metabolic energy stored in the adenine nucleotide system.

Statistical analysis

Data were expressed as means±SD and statistical differences between groups were analyzed by Student's *t* test which was performed using SPSS 16.0 statistical software (SPSS Inc., Chicago, Illinois, USA). The probability (*P*) values <0.05 were considered to be statistically significant.

Results

The effects of QIHM and QRHM on OXPHOS of liver mitochondria

The liver is known to be the hub of the metabolism; it plays a major role in controlling glucose storage and flux. It is also known that, during heat stress, both lipids and carbohydrate stores can be mobilized for energy generation to attenuate the stress response (Manoli *et al.*, 2007). In addition, many biochemical studies have been performed using mitochondria from liver cells. The rate of ATP synthesis and oxygen consumption (respiratory state 3) driven by complex I substrates, the respiratory control ratio (RCR) and P/O ratio were reduced in liver mitochondria by ginseng and astragalus root, but there were no significant effect on state 4 ($P > 0.05$) (Table 1). It showed that the efficiency of ATP production via ADP phosphorylation was decreased. In perfectly coupled mitochondria, there would be no proton leak across the inner mitochondrial membrane, and the entire gradient generated by the respiratory chain would be used to generate ATP (Boudina and Dale Abel, 2006). Control of oxidative phosphorylation (OXPHOS) allows a cell to produce only the precise amount of ATP required to sustain its activities. Recall that under normal circumstances, electron transport and ATP synthesis are tightly coupled. The value of P/O ratio (the number of molecules of Pi consumed for each oxygen atom reduced to H_2O) reflects the degree of coupling observed between electron transport and ATP synthesis (Mckee and Mckee, 1999). Oxygen consumption increase dramatically when ADP is supplied. The control of aerobic respiration by ADP is referred to as respiratory control. Substrate oxidation accelerates only when an increase in the concentration of ADP signals that the ATP pool needs to be replenished. This regulation matches the rates of phosphorylation of ADP and of cellular oxidations via glycolysis, the citric acid cycle, and the electron-transport chain to the requirement for ATP (Horton, *et al.*, 2002).

Ginseng and astragalus root can decrease oxygen consuming rate and RCR of liver mitochondria obviously, I consider this is appearance of lowering standard metabolic rate and is a kind of protective adaptation. Qi deficiency patients need nutritional supplements, adequate rest, and should reduce energy consumption, ginseng and astragalus root can just achieve this goal, while the effect of other QIHM is not obvious. All the four QRHM can increase RCR and P/O ratio (Table 1).

The effects of QIHM and QRHM on creatine kinase activities

Although ATP is the instantaneous donor of bio-energy in the body, it can not be stored, but phosphocreatine (PCr) can. Among the energy metabolism enzymes in the muscle cells, creatine kinase (CK, EC 2.7.3.2) plays a significant role in energy homeostasis. CK is distributed in skeletal muscle, heart, brain and other tissues and catalyzes the reversible conversion from ATP and creatine (Cr) to ADP and phosphocreatine (PCr, high energy phosphate able to supply ATP on demand) (Zhao *et al.*, 2007; Brancaccio *et al.*, 2007). CK performs a pivotal physiological role in high energy consuming tissues, by acting as an energy buffering and transport system between the sites of ATP production and consumption by ATPases (Bessman and Geiger, 1981). Creatine kinase rapidly provides ATP to highly energy-demanding processes, the rate of transfer of the phosphoryl group from PCr to ADP by CK is greater than the maximum rate of ATP generation by OXPHOS, and this ensures rapid resynthesis of ATP (Wallimann *et al.*, 1998). High tissue CK activity, whether constitutive, induced, or both, may rather directly enhance contractile responses by enhancing cellular energy and contractile reserve (Brewster *et al.*, 2007). Greater CK activity could bind more ADP and increase the rate of the conversion of ADP to ATP, which could reduce the relative levels of local ADP at the contractile proteins (Clark, 1994). CK enhances ATP buffer capacity. We believe that high CK activity may be quite beneficial for rapid and dynamic energy demand. Thus, increased CK activity in muscle tissue might lead to hyperdynamic activity. Both QIHM and QRHM can stimulate activity of CK significantly in the storage of energy, and QRHM is stronger than QIHM (Table 1).

Group	State 3 (nmol /min/mg)[d]	State 4 (nmol /min/mg)[d]	RCR	P/O	CK (U/μg)[e]
Control	83±11	19.4±2.6	4.2±0.6	2.61±0.28	2.25±0.28
Panax ginseng	66±11[b]	18.3±1.9	3.6±0.4[a]	2.21±0.30[b]	2.58±0.26[a]
Astragalus membranaceus	68±13[a]	18.0±2.5	3.7±0.4[a]	2.32±0.24[a]	2.60±0.29[a]
Codonopsis pilosula	80±15	18.3±2.2	4.3±0.6	2.66±0.26	2.59±0.29[a]
Atractylodes macrocephala	81±14	19.1±1.8	4.2±0.7	2.60±0.28	2.63±0.32[a]
Citrus aurantium	91±10	18.5±2.9	4.9±0.4[b]	2.89±0.27[a]	3.32±0.27[b]
Magnolia officinalis	99±13[b]	19.0±2.1	5.1±0.5[b]	2.92±0.34[a]	3.20±0.44[b]
Citrus reticulate	96±12[a]	19.3±2.2	4.9±0.6[a]	2.88±0.22[a]	3.09±0.49[b]
Lindera aggregate	86±16	16.6±2.3[a]	5.2±0.7[b]	2.93±0.31[a]	3.23±0.35[b]

[d] nanomole O_2 per minute per milligram protein (nmol O_2 min^{-1} mg $protein^{-1}$). [e] Unit of CK activity per microgram protein (U μg $protein^{-1}$). [a] $P<0.05$ *vs* Control. [b] $P<0.01$ *vs* Control.

Table 1. Effects of QIHM and QRHM on respiratory function of liver mitochondria and CK activities *in vivo* (n=10, mean ± standard deviation).

The effects of QIHM and QRHM on energy state of mice hepatocyte in vivo

Adenylate energy charge (AEC) is a sign parameter of cellular energy state (the higher [ATP], the larger the AEC, the higher [AMP], the smaller the AEC), when the tissue's ATP level increased, the pathway for generating ATP would be inhibited; When ATP levels drop due to over consumption of energy by the body, the pathway for generating ATP would be stimulated. AEC represents a linear measure of the metabolic energy stored in the adenine nucleotide system. AEC remained at a fairly narrow range of changes, just like pH value in the cells, energy charge also has a buffering effect, AEC of the most cells fluctuate in the 0.8-0.95 range. Ginseng is commonly known as a high-level herb for tonifying Qi, according to our former study, *Panax ginseng* polysaccharide could increase levels of ATP, TAP and AEC in liver cells under chronic hypoxia condition, therefore, improving energy status, protect mitochondria by inhibiting mitochondrial swelling (Li *et al.*, 2009). It is worth notice that all the four QIHM can increase levels of ATP, AEC and TAP, the effect of ginseng is the most potent; on the contrary, all the four QRHM can decrease levels of ATP, AEC and TAP in liver cells. All the four QIHM can't affect the levels of ADP and AMP; while all the four QRHM can decrease levels of ADP, and increase levels of AMP in liver cells. In a word, QIHM and QRHM increase and decrease bioenergy level of liver cells respectively *in vivo*. Therefore, Qi is closely related to bioenergy. This result shows that the decreased energy state of the body can be improved by taking QIHM and the effect of QRHM is contrary to that of QIHM. Therefore, the effects on energy regulation of two types of Qi system drugs are different (Table 2).

The similarities and differences in natures, tastes, channel tropism and compositions

Qi is an important concept in physiology and pathology of TCM, directed towards the two main therapeutic principles of Qi—qi-invigoration and qi-flow regulation are self-evidently extreme important. The two therapeutic principles are closely related, complementary and two-way adjustable, and difficult to substitute by others. If they are used properly, they will play an important clinical role in overcoming various difficult diseases. Since there is no direct detection method on Qi, the widely used QIHM (ginseng, astragalus root, pilose asiabell root, white atractylodes rhizome) and QRHM (immature bitter orange, magnolia bark, green tangerine and lindera root) were selected to study the effect on energy metabolism to approach to the nature of Qi in TCM, Comparison of the regulatory role of QIHM and QRHM are summarized as follows.

Group	ATP/ (mmol·L^{-1})	ADP/ (mmol·L^{-1})	AMP/ (mmol·L^{-1})	TAP/ (mmol·L^{-1})	AEC
Control	1.02±0.28	0.78±0.20	0.09±0.07	1.89±0.33	0.745±0.021
Panax ginseng	1.41±0.36^{a}	0.86±0.24	0.07±0.05	2.34±0.46^{a}	0.786±0.031^{b}
Astragalus membranaceus	1.36±0.31^{a}	0.84±0.23	0.11±0.05	2.31±0.38^{a}	0.770±0.026^{a}
Codonopsis pilosula	1.33±0.22^{a}	0.85±0.25	0.12±0.08	2.30±0.32^{a}	0.763±0.015^{a}
Atractylodes macrocephala	1.25±0.19^{a}	0.81±0.26	0.10±0.06	2.16±0.28	0.764±0.016^{a}
Citrus aurantium	0.70±0.26^{a}	0.53±0.14^{b}	0.25±0.12^{b}	1.48±0.27^{b}	0.651±0.024^{b}
Magnolia officinalis	0.71±0.23^{a}	0.61±0.13^{a}	0.19±0.09^{a}	1.51±0.23^{b}	0.673±0.033^{b}
Citrus reticulate	0.75±0.25^{a}	0.49±0.14^{b}	0.27±0.12^{b}	1.51±0.26^{a}	0.660±0.028^{b}
Lindera aggregate	0.61±0.22^{b}	0.47±0.16^{b}	0.29±0.13^{b}	1.37±0.21^{b}	0.618±0.027^{b}

All values are mean±SD (n=10). $^{a}P<0.05$, $^{b}P<0.01$ versus Control group. Each value expressed in mmol·L^{-1} (ATP, ADP, AMP, TAP) or as a ratio (AEC). ATP: adenosine triphosphate; ADP: adenosine diphosphate; AMP: adenosine monophosphate; TAP: total adenylate pool; AEC: adenylate energy charge

Table 2. The effects of QIHM and QRHM on energy status of mice hepatocytes *in vivo* (n=10, mean ± standard deviation).

The channel tropism of QIHM and QRHM are all the spleen, lung and stomach channel, this shows that they have common target sites in the body. The natures of QIHM are mild or warm, and QRHM are warm, the properties of the two kinds of medicines are similar. QIHM are sweet taste, medicines with sweet taste have the effects of invigoration, normalizing the function of the stomach and spleen, and buffering emergency, etc. they are usually used for tonifying deficiency, easing the pain, and harmonizing the property of different drugs, they are mostly moist and good at nourishing and moistening dryness evil. QRHM are bitter and/or hot tastes, medicines with bitter taste have the effects of purgation and drying the wetness evil etc. medicines with hot taste have the effects of dispersing, promoting the circulation of qi and blood. Therefore, QIHM and QRHM have obviously different effects due to the different tastes. All the QIHM contain more water-soluble carbohydrate due to the sweet taste, and almost all QRHM don't contain or contain less water-soluble carbohydrate composition, most of them contain volatile components (Zheng *et al.*, 1998). Therefore, QIHM and QRHM have obviously different components due to the different tastes (Table 3).

Effects	Items	QIHM	QRHM
Same or similarities	1. channel tropism	spleen, lung and stomach	spleen, lung and stomach
	2. natures	mild or warm	warm
	3.CK activity	increase	increase
Cross effects	1. RCR	decrease or no effect	no effect or increase
	2. oxygen consumption rate	decrease or no effect	no effect or increase
Differences	1. tastes	sweet	bitter and/or hot
	2. compositions	more carbohydrate	volatile components
	3. bioenergy level	increase	decrease

Table 3. Comparisons of the regularity between QIHM and QRHM

11. Conclusion

Qi, is the most basic, the most important and the most nebulous concept, and can be called the biggest enigma in TCM. Research on the nature of Qi in TCM has important theoretical and clinical significance. By analyzing and concluding generation process and function of Qi and bio-energy (ATP), and the effects of Qi-invigorating herbal medicines (QIHM) and Qi-regulating herbal medicines (QRHM) on energy metabolism, the following conclusions can be drawn: Qi and bioenergy have common source and identical functions. Regulation on energy metabolism by QIHM and QRHM showed significant differences due to the different chemical compositions and flavors, QIHM and QRHM are able to improve and decrease the energy state of the body respectively. QIHM invigorate "Qi" through increased intracellular ATP level; and QRHM regulate "Qi" by reducing intracellular ATP levels. Thus, there are many common natures between Qi and bio-energy. Studies on the nature of Qi in TCM should be carried out in other areas of life science due to the wide implications for Qi. With the rapid development of modern life science, we believe that mankind will reveal the truth of the enigma in the near future, it would be better for clinical services.

Without having a scientific model, we cannot advance the research. A future step in Qi research would be to set up effective model to assess Qi effect and identify the effect of Qi on energy metabolism which plays the central role in life activities. If such a model is found, then, the next task might be to find the mechanism of how Qi act. We have a long way to go, but at least, we now have a model which is based upon biochemical pharmacology. With this, we can advance our search to understand the mechanisms of Qi-related phenomena and Qi-healing processes, which have been known for 4000 years.

12. References

Abbott RB, Hui K-K, Hays RD, Li M-D, Pan T. A randomized controlled trial of tai chi for tension headaches. Evid Based Complement Alternat Med 2007; 4: 107 - 113.

Bailey SM, Landar A, Darley-Usmar V. Mitochondrial proteomics in free radical research. Free Radic Biol Med 2005; 38: 175–188.

Benard G, Bellance N, Jose C, Melser S, Nouette-Gaulain K, Rossignol R. Multi-site control and regulation of mitochondrial energy production. Biochim Biophys Acta 2010; 1797: 698–709.

Benard G, Faustin B, Passerieux E, Galinier A, Rocher C, Bellance N *et al.* Physiological diversity of mitochondrial oxidative phosphorylation, Am J Physiol Cell Physiol 2006; 291: C1172–C1182.

Bessman SP, Geiger PJ. Transport of energy in muscle: the phosphorylcreatine shuttle. Science 1981; 211: 448–452.

Boudina S, Dale Abel E. Mitochondrial uncoupling: A key contributor to reduced cardiac efficiency in diabetes. Physiology 2006; 21:250-258.

Boveris A, Cadenas E. Mitochondrial production of superoxide anions and its relationship to the antimycin-insensitive respiration. FEBS Lett 1975; 54:311–314.

Bradford MM. A rapid and sensitive method for the quantation of microgram quantities of protein utilizing the principle of protein-dye binding. Anal Biochem 1976; 72:248–254.

Brancaccio P, Maffulli N, Limongelli FM. Creatine kinase monitoring in sport medicine. Br Med Bull 2007; 81-82: 209–230.

Brewster LM, Clark JF, van Montfrans GA. Is greater tissue activity of creatine kinase the genetic factor increasing hypertension risk in black people of sub-Saharan African descent? J Hypertens 2007; 18: 1537–1544.

Chai C, Kou J, Zhu D, Yan Y, Yu B. Mice exposed to chronic intermittent hypoxia simulate clinical features of deficiency of both Qi and Yin syndrome in traditional Chinese medicine. Evid Based Complement Alternat Med 2009; doi:10.1093/ecam/nep226

Chance B, Williams GR. Respiratory enzymes in oxidative phosphorylation. I. Kinetics of oxygen utilization. J Biol Chem 1955; 217:383–393.

Chang SO. The nature of touch therapy related to Ki: practitioners' perspective. Nurs Health Sci 2003; 5: 103 - 114.

Chen K. An analytic review of studies on measuring effects of external QI in China. Altern Ther Health Med 2004;10:38 - 50.

Chien CH, Tsuei JJ, Lee SC, Huang YC , Wei YH. Effect of emitted bioenergy on biochemical functions of cells. Am J Chin Med 1991; 19: 285–292.

Clark JF. The creatine kinase system in smooth muscle. Mol Cell Biochem 1994; 133–134:221–232.

Estabrook RW. Mitochondrial respiratory control and the polarographic measurement of ADP:O ratios. Methods Enzymol 1967; 10: 41-47.

Flowers J. What is Qi? Evid-based Complement Altern Med 2006; 3:551–552.

Freyre-Fonsecaa V, Delgado-Buenrostroa NL, Gutiérrez-Cirlosb EB, Calderón-Torresa CM, Cabellos-Avelarb T, Sánchez-Pérezc Y *et al.* Titanium dioxide nanoparticles impair lung mitochondrial function. Toxicology Letters 2011; 202: 111–119.

Fukushima M, Kataoka T, Hamada C, Matsumoto M. Evidence of Qigong energy and its biological effect on the enhancement of the phagocytic activity of human polymorphonuclear leukocytes. Am J Chin Med 2001; 29: 1–16.

Green DR, Reed JC. Mitochondria and apoptosis. Science 1998; 281: 1309–1312.

Hankey A, McCrum S. Qigong: life energy and a new science of life. J Altern Complement Med 2006; 12:841 - 842.

Horton HR, Moran LA, Ochs RS, Rawn JD, Scrimgeour KG. Principles of Biochemistry (third edition), New Jersey: Science Press and Pearson Education North Asia Limited, 2002.

Ikeda S, Kaneko M, Kumazawa Y, Nishimura C. Protective activities of a Chinese medicine, Hochu-ekki-to, to impairment of hematopoietic organs and to microbial infection. Yakugaku Zasshi 1990; 110: 682–687.

Ishikawa H, Manabe F, Zhongtao H, Yoshii S, Koiso K. The hormonal response to HCG stimulation on patients with male infertility before and after treatment with hochuekkito. Am J Chin Med 1992; 20: 157–165.
Ito H, Shimura K. Studies on the antitumor activity of traditional Chinese medicine. Gan-To-Kagaku-Ryoho 1985; 12: 2145–2148.
Jacobson MD, Weil M, Raff MC. Programmed cell death in animal development. Cell 1997; 88: 347–354.
Kawakita T, Nomoto K. Immunopharmacological effects of Hochu-ekkito and its clinical application. Prog Med 1998; 18: 801–807.
Kiang T. Chinese 'Nature Magazine': Chinese style. Nature 1978; 275: 697.
Kim JY, Pham DD. Sasang constitutional medicine as a holistic tailored medicine. Evid-based Complement Altern Med 2009; 6(S1):11–19.
Kimura H, Nagao F, Tanaka Y, Sakai S, Ohnishi ST, Okumura K. Beneficial effects of the Nishino Breathing Method on the immune activity and stress level. J Altern Complement Med 2005;11:285 - 291.
Kobayashi H, Ishii M. Mind–body, Ki (Qi) and the skin: Commentary on Irwin's 'Shingles immunity and health functioning in the elderly: Tai Chi Chih as a behavioral treatment'. Evid-based Complement Altern Med 2005; 2(1):113–116.
Koshikawa N, Imai T, Takahashi I, Yamauchi M, Sawada S, Kansaku A. Effect of Hochuekki-to, Yoku-kan-san and Saiko-ka-ryukotsu-borei-to on behavioral despair and acetic acid-induced writhing in mice. Meth Findings Exp Clin Pharmacol 1998; 20: 47–51.
Lee M. Effects on *in vitro* and *in vivo* qi-therapy on neutrophil superoxide generation in healthy male subjects. Am J Chin Med 2003; 31:623 - 628.
Lee MS, Huh HJ, Jang HS, Jeong SM, Ryu H, Chung HT. Effects of Qi-therapy on *in vitro* natural killer cell cytotoxic activity. Am J Chin Med 2001a; 29: 17–22.
Lee MS, Huh HJ, Jang HS, Ryu H, Chung HT. Psychoneuroimmunological effects of Qi-therapy: preliminary study on the level of anxiety, mood, cortisol and melatonin, and cellular function of neutrophil and natural killer cell. Stress and Health 2001b; 17: 17–24.
Lee MS, Yang KH, Huh HJ, Kim HW, Ryu H, Lee HS *et al.* Qi-therapy as an intervention to reduce chronic pain and to enhance mood in elderly subjects: a pilot study. Am J Chin Med 2001c; 29: 237–245.
Li XT, Chen R, Jin LM, Chen HY. Regulation on energy metabolism and protection on mitochondria of Panax ginseng polysaccharide. Am J Chin Med 2009; 37(6): 1139-1152.
Li XY, Takimoto H, Miura S,Yoshikai Y, Matsuzaki G, Nomoto K. Effect of a traditional Chinese medicine, Bu-zhong-yi-qi-tang (Japanese name: Hochu-ekki-to) on the protection against Listeria monocytogenes infection in mice. Immunopharmacol Immunotoxicol 1992; 14: 383–402.
Lorenzo HK, Susin SA, Penninger J, Kroemer G. Apoptosis inducing factor (AIF): a phylogenetically old, caspase-independent effector of cell death. Cell Death Differ 1999; 6:516–524.
Machi Y. The Science of Ki. Tokyo: Tokyo Denki University Press, 1993 (in Japanese).
Manoli I, Alesci S, Blackman MR, Su YA, Rennert OM, Chrousos GP. Mitochondria as key components of the stress response. Trends Endocrinol Metabol 2007; 18: 190–198.
Mayevsky A. Mitochondrial function and energy metabolism in cancer cells: Past overview and future perspectives. Mitochondrion 2009; 9: 165–179.

Mckee T, Mckee JR. Biochemistry: An Introduction (second edition). New York: McGraw-Hill Companies, Inc. 1999.

Michele AS, Jhon Z, Alain YF, Lee CP. Ischemic injury to rat forebrain mitochondria and cellular calcium homeostasis. Biochim Biophys Acta 1992; 1134:223–232.

Mike Craske NJ, Turner W, Zammit-Maempe J, Lee MS. Qigong ameliorates symptoms of chronic fatigue: A pilot uncontrolled study. Evid-based Complement Altern Med 2009; 6: 265 - 270.

Murakami, Y. Clinical effect of hotyuekkito (bu-zhong-yi-qi-tang) on symptoms due to renal ptosis and stress incontinence. Hinyokika Kiyo 1988; 34: 1841–1843.

Narita M, Shimizu S, Ito T, Chittenden T, Lutz RJ, Matsuda H *et al.* Bax interacts with the permeability transition pore to induce permeability transition and cytochrome c release in isolated mitochondria. Proc Natl Acad Sci USA 1998; 95:14681–14686.

Nishino K. The Breath of Life: Using the Power of Ki for Maximum Vitality. Tokyo, New York, London: Kodansha International, 1997.

Nishino K. Nishino Breathing Method: Activation of Life Energy. Tokyo: Kodansha, 2004 (in Japanese).

Nishino K. The Nishino Breathing Method (in Japanese). In: Arita H, (ed). The Dictionary of Respiration. Tokyo: Asakura Book Publishing Co., 2006; 678 - 697.

Ohnishi ST. Ki: A key to transform the century of death to the century of life. Evid-based Complement Altern Med 2007; 4: 287–292.

Ohnishi ST, Nishino K, Uchiyama K, Ohnishi T, Yamaguchi M. Ki-energy (life-energy) stimulates osteoblastic cells and inhibits the formation of osteoclast-like cells in bone cell cultured models. Evid-based Complement Altern Med 2007; 4: 225–232.

Ohnishi ST, Ohnishi T. The Nishino breathing method and Ki-energy (Life-energy): A challenge to traditional scientific thinking. Evid-based Complement Altern Med 2006; 3: 191–200.

Ohnishi ST, Ohnishi T. Philosophy, psychology, physics and practice of Ki. Evid-based Complement Altern Med 2009a; 6(2): 175–183.

Ohnishi ST, Ohnishi T. How far can Ki-energy reach?—A hypothetical mechanism for the generation and transmission of Ki-energy. Evid-based Complement Altern Med 2009b; 6(3): 379–391.

Ohnishi ST, Ohnishi T, Nishino K. Ki- Energy (Life-Energy) protects isolated mitochondria from oxidative injury. Evid-based Complement Altern Med 2006; 3: 475–482.

Ohnishi ST, Ohnishi T, Nishino K, Tsurusaki Y, Yamaguchi M. Growth inhibition of cultured human carcinoma cells by Ki-energy (Life Energy): Scientific study of Ki-effect on cancer cells. Evid-based Complement Altern Med 2005; 2: 387–393.

Olalde JA. The systemic theory of living systems and relevance to CAM. Part I: The theory. Evid Based Complement Alternat Med 2005; 2: 13 - 18.

Papa S. Mitochondrial oxidative phosphorylation changes in the life span. Molecular aspects and physiopathological implications. Biochim Biophys Acta 1996; 1276:87-105.

Radda GK, Odoom J, Kemp G, Taylor DJ, Thompson C, Styles P. Assessment of mitochondrial function and control in normal and diseased states. Biochim Biophys Acta 1995; 1271:15-19.

Shah S, Ogden AT, Pettker CM, Raffo A, Itescu S, Oz MC. A study of the effect of energy healing on *in vitro* tumor cell proliferation. J Altern Complement Med 1999; 5: 359–365.

Shih HC, Chang KH, Chen FL, Chen CM, Chen SC, Lin YT *et al.* Anti-aging effects of the traditional Chinese medicine Bu-Zhong-Yi-Qi-Tang in mice. Am J Chin Med 2000; 28: 77-86.

Shimizu S, Narita M, Tsujimoto Y. Bcl-2 family proteins regulate the release of apoptogenic cytochrome c by the mitochondrial channel VDAC. Nature 1999; 399: 483–487.

Shin MS. Brief view of chi and alternative therapy. Orient Pharm Exp Med 2002; 2: 1 - 16.

Shinagawa Y. The Science of Qigong (in Japanese). Tokyo: Kobunsha, 1990.

Shinnick P. Qigong: where did it come from? Where does it fit in science? What are the advances? J Altern Complement Med 2006; 12: 351 - 353.

Smith JR, Matus IR, Beard DA, Greene AS. Differential expression of cardiac mitochondrial proteins. Proteomics 2008; 8: 446–462.

Susin SA, Lorenzo HK, Zamzami N, Marzo I, Brothers G, Snow B *et al.* Molecular characterization of mitochondrial apoptosis-inducing factor. Nature 1999; 397: 441–446.

Terasawa K. Evidence-based reconstruction of Kampo medicine: part II—the concept of Sho. Evid Based Complement Alternat Med 2004; 1: 119–123.

Thompson CB. Apoptosis in the pathogenesis and treatment of disease. Science 1995; 167: 1456–1462.

Wallimann T, Dolder M, Schlattner U, Eder M, Hornemann T, O'Gorman E *et al.* Some new aspects of creatine kinase (CK): compartmentation, structure, function and regulation for cellular and mitochondrial bioenergetics and physiology. Biofactors 1998; 8 :229–234.

Weze C, Leathard HL, Grange J, Tiplady P, Stevens G. Healing by gentle touch ameliorates stress and other symptoms in people suffering with mental health disorders or psychological stress. Evid Based Complement Alternat Med 2007; 4: 115 - 123.

Xing C. Chinese Acupuncture and Moxibustion. Beijing, China: Foreign Languages Press, 1987.

Yang L, Tan GY, Fu YQ, Feng JH, Zhang MH. Effects of acute heat stress and subsequent stress removal on function of hepatic mitochondrial respiration, ROS production and lipid peroxidation in broiler çhickens. Comparative Biochemistry and Physiology, Part C, 2010; 151: 204–208

Yuasa Y. The Body, Self-Cultivation and Ki-energy (translated by S. Nagatomo and M.S. Hull). Albany, NY: State University of New York Press, 1993.

Yumi K. The Ultimate Example of Nishino Breating. In: Nishino K. (ed). Method: Everyday of Yumi Kaoru with Slim and Bouncing Body. Tokyo: TAKE Shobo Pub. Co., 2005 (in Japanese).

Zhao TJ, Yan YB, Liu Y, Zhou HM. The generation of the oxidized form of creatine kinase is a negative regulation on muscle creatine kinase. J Biol Chem 2007; 282: 12022–12029.

Zheng HZ, Dong ZH, Yu J. Modern Studies and Application of Tradional Chinese Herbal Medicine. Beijing: Xueyuan Press, 1998 (in Chinese).

Part 2

Clinical Practice

5

Hyperspectral Imaging Technology Used in Tongue Diagnosis

Qingli Li
Key Laboratory of Polor Materials and Devices, East China Normal University
China

1. Introduction

Traditional Chinese Medicine (TCM) is a range of medical practices used in China for more than four millenniums, a treasure of Chinese people (Lukman, He, & Hui, 2007). The important role of TCM and its profound influence on the health care system in China is well recognized. The West also has drawn the attention towards various aspects of TCM in the past few years (Chan, 1995). TCM consists of a systematized methodology of medical treatment and diagnosis (Watsuji, Arita, Shinohara, & Kitade, 1999). According to the basic concept of TCM, the different body-parts, zang-viscera and fu-viscera, the meridians of the body are linked as an inseparable whole. The inner abnormality can present on outer parts, while the outer disease can turn into the inner parts (Bakshi & Pal, 2010). Therefore, some diseases can be diagnosed from the appearance of the outer body. As the significant component part of TCM theory, TCM diagnostics includes two parts: TCM Sizhen (the four diagnosis methods) and differentiation of syndromes. The TCM physician experience the gravity of health condition of a sick person by means of the four diagnosis methods depending on the doctor's body "sensors" such as fingers, eyes, noses etc. Generally, TCM Sizhen consists of the following four diagnostic processes: inspection, auscultation and olfaction, inquiry, and pulse feeling and palpation (Nenggan & Zhaohui, 2004).

In the inspection diagnostic process, TCM practitioners observe abnormal changes in the patient's vitality, colour, appearance, secretions and excretions. The vital signs encompass eyes, tongue, facial expressions, general and body surface appearance. The inter-relationship between the external part of the body such as face and tongue and the internal organ(s) is used to assist TCM doctors to predict the pathological changes of internal organs. In the auscultation and olfaction process, the doctor listen the patient's voice, breathing, and coughing used to judge the pathological changes in the interior of the patient's body. Inquiry diagnosis method is refer to query patient's family history, feelings in various aspects, such as chills and fever, perspiration, appetite and thirst, as well as pain in terms of its nature and locality. Palpation approach involves pulse diagnosis (Siu Cheung, Yulan, & Doan Thi Cam, 2007). The palpation diagnosis has been accepted as one of the most powerful method to give information for making diagnosis from ancient time till now. The pulse waves are measured at six points near the wrists of both hands. The waves are different each other and give us information about different organs (Hsing-Lin, Suzuki, Adachi, & Umeno, 1993). Tongue diagnosis is another inspection diagnostic method which observes the abnormal changes in the tongue proper and the tongue coating to diagnose diseases. This method offers many advantages, such as non-invasive, simple and inexpensive. Tongue diagnosis is one of the most precious and widely used diagnostic methods in TCM, as well as it is great valuable in both clinic applications and self-diagnosis (Bo Pang, Wang, Zhang, & Zhang, 2002). Human tongue is one of the important organs of the body, which carries abound of information of the health status. The information often include tongue colour, tongue fissures or cracks, sublingual veins, tongue coating, etc. There are close relations between these information and our health conditions (Siu Cheung et al., 2007). Whenever there is a complex disorder full of contradictions, examination of the tongue can often quickly clarify the main pathological processes. The tongue's appearance is also a useful gauge for monitoring the improvement or deterioration of a patient's condition (B Pang, Zhang, & Wang, 2005). Therefore, tongue diagnosis is one of the few diagnostic techniques that accord with the most promising direction in the 21st century: no pain and no injury (B. Pang, Zhang, & Li, 2004).

As a convenient and non-invasive method, there are some significances of tongue diagnosis such as judge the exuberance or decline of the genuine Qi, distinguish the nature of disease, detect the location of disease, and infer the tendency of disease (Bakshi & Pal, 2010). However, traditional tongue diagnosis method has inevitable limitations that impede its medical applications. First, the clinical competence of tongue diagnosis is determined by the experience and knowledge of the TCM doctors which has the problem of objectification and standardization. Second, tongue diagnosis is usually based on the detailed visual discrimination, which depends on the subjective analysis of the examiners, makes the diagnostic results unreliable and inconsistent. Thirdly, traditional tongue diagnosis is intimately related to the identification of syndromes, and it is not very well understood in Western medicine and modern biomedicine (B. Pang et al., 2004). Finally, the change of the inspection circumstance like a light source affects the diagnosis result a lot (Kim, Do, Ryu, & Kim, 2008). Therefore, it is necessary to develop some quantitative and objective diagnostic standard for tongue diagnosis.

Nowadays, the rapid progress of information science and technology promotes the automatization of tongue diagnosis based on modern image processing and pattern recognition approaches (B. Pang, David, & Wang, 2005). There has been some work on computerized tongue diagnosis, and many issues of standardization and quantification have been resolved. In recent years, some computer-aided tongue diagnosis systems based on the texture, colour and other proper of tongue image have been developed (Wenshu, Shenning, Shuai, & Su, 2009). These systems include the Computerized Tongue Diagnosis System in TCM (Jiang, Chen, & Zhang, 2000), Automatic Recognition System of TCM Tongue Diagnosis, TID-2000 TCM Tongue Diagnosis Expert System (X. Yu et al., 1994), Tongue Imaging Analysis Instrument (Shen et al., 2003), Automatic Tongue Diagnosis System (Lun-chien, Hou, Ying-ling, Chiang, & Cheng-chun, 2009), computer aided tongue diagnosis system (CATDS) (Zhang, Wang, Zhang, Pang, & Huang, 2005), a prototype of tongue diagnosis support system (Ikeda, Fujiwara, & Yoshida, 2006), and Imaging System for Tongue Inspection (Yang, 2002), etc. In addition, Hong Kong Institute of Technology and Harbin Institute of Technology had made progresses in TCM automatic analysis of tongue image and had built a database with more than 5000 instances of tongue images (X. Yu et al., 1994). Some image processing and pattern recognition algorithms based on these tongue images have also been presented. On automated tongue body segmentation, Li, et al. proposed an improved snake algorithm (W. Li, Zhou, & Zhang, 2004). David Zhang, et al.

have presented a series of tongue body segmentation algorithms such as the Bi-elliptical deformable contour (REDC) algorithm (Bo Pang et al., 2002; B Pang et al., 2005), the combination of polar edge detection and active contour model (Zuo, Wang, Zhang, & Zhang, 2004), etc. Yang, et al. presented the colour active contour models to segment the tongue body (S. Yu, Yang, Wang, & Zhang, 2007). Some other algorithms also have been presented to analyze the tongue color (C. H. Li & Yuen, 2002; Y. G. Wang, Yang, & Zhou, 2007; Zhang, Wang, & Jin, 2005), tongue shape (Z. Liu, Jing-Qi, Tao, & Qun-Lin, 2006; Xu, Tu, Ren, & Zhang, 2008), sublingual veins (Chiu, Lan, & Chang, 2002; Yan, Wang, & Li, 2009; Yan, Yu, Wang, & Li, 2008), tongue fissures and cracks (L. L. Liu & Zhang, 2007; L. L. Liu, Zhang, Kumar, & Wu, 2008; Yue Zhou, Li Shen, & Jie Yang, 2002), tongue coating (Kim et al., 2008; Wu, Zhang, Li, Wang, & Yang, 2008), etc. These studies prove that the accurate segmentation of tongue body and extraction of tongue features is important for computerized tongue diagnosis. Although many issues of standardization and quantification problems have been resolved by these methods, there are still some difficulties because of the limitations of images captured by traditional CCD cameras. For example, the principal difficulties are that when these images are used it is difficult to distinguish in RGB colour space between the tongue and neighbouring tissues that have a similar colour. It is difficult to distinguish between tongue coating and tongue substance and to discrimination the colour automatically and quantificationally. The thickness and transparence of the sublingual mucosa covering the sublingual veins may change due to the different degrees of varicosity. For these reasons, current methods of tongue feature extraction or diagnosis perform well only on tongue images acquired under some special conditions and often fail when the quality of image is less than ideal. Therefore, automatic tongue diagnosis becomes difficult due to the limited information of common digital images, the variation of the illumination, etc. This will undoubtedly limit the applications of these approaches in clinical medicine.

Hyperspectral imaging technology, which comes from the remote sensing field (Chiou, 1984; Harsanyi & Chang, 1994), may offer a solution for these constraints. Hyperspectral remote sensing exploits the fact that all materials reflect, absorb, and emit electromagnetic energy, at specific wavelengths, in distinctive patterns related to their molecular composition (Manolakis & Shaw, 2002). If we introduce this technology to the biomedical diagnosis field, some pathological changes of organism or tissues can be detected and quantificationally analysed in a new way. Actually, hyperspectral imaging of human tissue have been used for many years for characterization and monitoring of applications in biomedicine (Chaudhari et al., 2005; Demos & Ramsamooj, 2003; Timlin J A, 2004). In our previous work, we have developed a microscopic pushbroom hyperspectral imaging system (MPHI) and apply it to analyse the rat retinal sections (Qingli Li, Wang, Zhang, Xu, & Xue, 2010; Qing Li Li, Xue, Xiao, & Zhang, 2007), human blood cells(Qingli Li, Dai, Liu, & Liu, 2009), etc. All these studies show that the hyperspectral imaging technology has significantly advanced in the area of biomedical imaging and early diagnosis. According to the electromagnetic theory, pathological changes of the object surface have a close relationship with its spectrum (Irigoyen & Herraez, 2003; Somosy, Bognar, Thuroczy, & Koteles, 2002). If hyperspectral imaging technology is introduced to computerized tongue diagnosis, both spatial and spectral data, which contain the pathological information of the tongue surface, can be obtained. Therefore, new algorithms should be developed to take advantage of the rich hyperspectral data not found in traditional CCD-based images. In this chapter, an acousto-optic tunable filter (AOTF) based hyperspectral tongue imaging system as well as its applications in computerized tongue diagnosis are presented. The remainder of the chapter is organized as follows. In Section 2 we describe the setup of the hyperspectral tongue imaging system (HTIS). Section 3 proposes the hyperspectral tongue images and the data preprocessing method. Section 4 briefly introduces the tongue body segmentation method based on hyperspectral tongue images. In Section 5, we describe the tongue colour analysis algorithm based on HTIS. In Section 6, tongue cracks extraction algorithm is presented. In Section 7, sublingual veins extraction algorithm based on the new system is proposed. Our conclusions are presented in Section 8.

2. Hyperspectral tongue imaging system

Most contemporary research on computerized tongue analysis focuses on operations in the gray-scale or colour [red-green-blue (RGB)] images (K. Q. Wang, Zhang, & Li, 2001). These images are captured by traditional charge coupled device (CCD) cameras which can only provide the spatial and colour information of tongue surface. The information contained in the CCD based images may not sufficient for computerized tongue diagnosis. Different from the traditional CCD cameras, hyperspectral imaging sensors in the reflective region of the spectrum (sometimes referred to as imaging spectrometers) can acquire digital images in many contiguous and very narrow spectral bands that typically span the visible, near-infrared, and even mid-infrared portions of the spectrum. This enables the construction of an essentially continuous radiance spectrum for every pixel in the scene. Thus, hyperspectral data exploitation makes possible the automatization and quantification of tongue diagnosis based on their spatial and spectral signatures.

In the past few years, we have developed the pushbroom hyperspectral tongue imaging (PHTI) system and found some useful applications in tongue diagnosis (Qingli Li, Liu, Xiao, & Xue, 2008; Q L Li, Xue, & Liu, 2008; Q. L. Li, Xue, Wang, & Yue, 2006). This PHTI system can capture tongue images from 400 nm to 800 nm with spectral resolution at 5 nm. The number of the efficient pixel is 652*620 for each single band image. However, this system needs pushbroom in one of the spatial dimensions to get the hyperspectral image of the whole scene, which makes the process time-consuming. To overcome this problem, we developed an acousto-optic tunable filter (AOTF) based hyperspectral tongue imaging system recently. AOTF is a rapid wavelength-scanning solid-state device that operates as a tunable optical band pass filter. The acoustic wave is generated by radio-frequency signals, which are applied to the crystal via an attached piezoelectric transducer (Inoue & Penuelas, 2001). When such a filter is placed in the optical train of a camera, different wavelengths can pass through it as a function of time. Unlike in a grating based instrument, no motion of the imager or object is required to obtain a complete image cube (Gupta, 2003). This new system offers the advantage of having no moving parts, having simple and compact structure, and can be scanned at very high rate which is more suitable for tongue imaging than the pushbroom one.

The instrument hardware of the AOTF based HTIS is shown in figure 1. The system consists of a camera lens (Nikon AF-S DX 18-200 mm VR II lens), an AOTF (Brimrose, CVA-200), an AOTF controller (radio-frequency drive unit), a CCD camera (Beijing JionHope Technology Ltd., AM1530), a data collection board, and a computer. From the figure we can see that the instrument has similar configuration compared with the standard CCD cameras commonly used by most contemporary research except that an AOTF adapter was coupled between camera lens and CCD in the new system. The dimension of the AOTF based HTIS is 408 mm

(L) × 77 mm (H) × 77 mm (W) as the size of Nikon AF-S DX 18-200 mm VR II lens is 96 mm (L) × 77 mm (Φ), AOTF adapter is 254 mm (L) × 60 mm (H) × 67 mm (W), and CCD is 58 mm (L) × 58 mm (H) × 58 mm (W). The AOTF adapter with Brimrose synthesizer electronics can provide narrow bandwidth, rapid wavelength selection, and intensity control. The high spatial resolution of the AOTF camera is ≥ 100 line pair/mm @ 532 nm. The designed wavelength ranges is 400 - 1000 nm and the spectral resolution is 2 - 6 nm (2 nm @ 543 nm; 5 nm @ 792 nm). The minimum wavelength selection sweep interval of the AOTF is 20 ns, which can meet the imaging speed demand of tongue. The block diagram of the computer controlled experimental setup for the AOTF-based HTIS is shown in figure 2. The tongue surface is illuminated by the light sources under the control of computer. The reflected light by tongue surface are firstly collected via the camera lens, then diffracted by the AOTF adapter, and imaged on the CCD detector at last. The new system can capture image scenes in contiguous but narrow spectral bands under the control of the AOTF controller. The hyperspectral tongue images provided by the instrument can be visualized as a 3D cube (Figure 3) because of its intrinsic structure, where the cube face is a function of the spatial coordinates and the depth is a function of wavelength. In this case, each spatial point on the face is characterized by its own spectrum (often called spectral signature). This spectrum is directly corresponds to the amount of energy that the tongue represented, as hyperspectral sensors commonly utilize the simple fact that a tongue can emits light in certain frequency bands. Consequently, the hyperspectral tongue image data provides a wealth of information about an image scene which is potentially very helpful to tongue diagnosis.

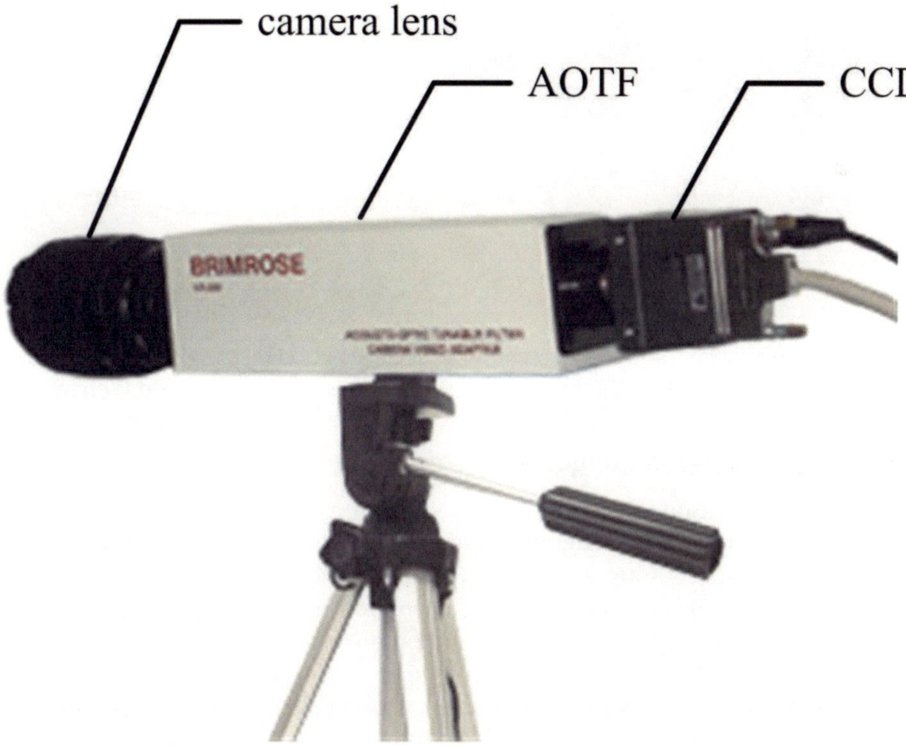

Fig. 1. Actual picture of HTIS

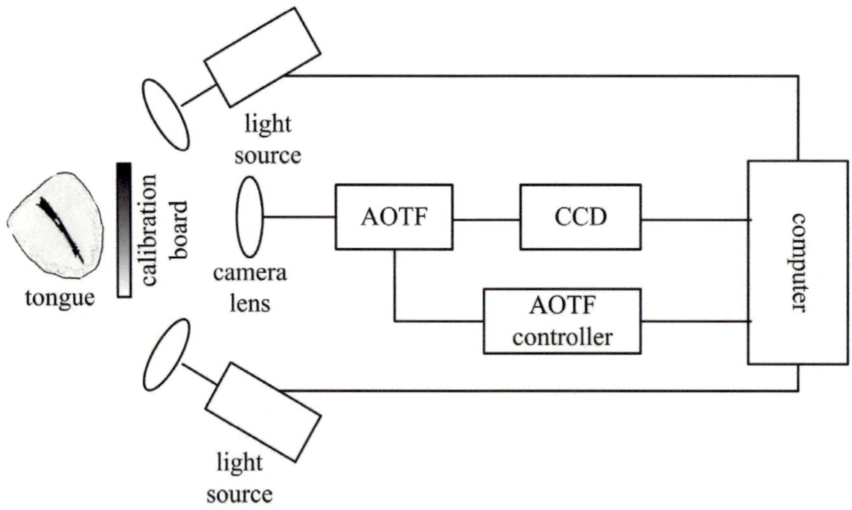

Fig. 2. Diagram of AOTF-based hyperspectral tongue imaging system

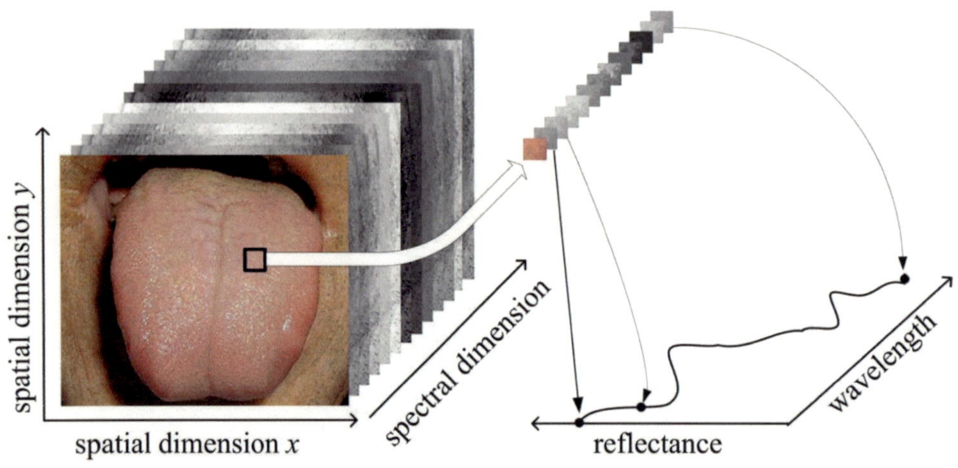

Fig. 3. The hyperspectral tongue imagery data cube (the cube face is a false colour image with the 758 nm, 634 nm, and 430 nm single-band images as the R, G, and B channels)

3. Hyperspectral tongue images and pre-processing

3.1 Hyperspectral tongue images

As one of the most important diagnostic methods in traditional Chinese medicine (TCM), tongue diagnosis inspects tongue to examine the physiological function and pathological changes of human body (Yan et al., 2009). Therefore, it is very important to capture the whole information of tongue surface for computerized tongue diagnosis. Most existing computerized tongue diagnosis methods are using tongue images captured by traditional CCD cameras (colour-based imaging methods). These colour-based images are commonly captured and displayed as a set of three black and white images collected with red (R), green (G), and blue (B) light, i.e., at wavelengths of approximately 630 nm, 545 nm, and 435 nm, respectively (Ballard & Brown, 1982). These wavelengths are chosen to match the spectral response of the human eye (Irigoyen & Herraez, 2003; Ornberg, Woerner, & Edwards, 1999). The relationship between the hyperspectral tongue images and the colour-based RGB images can be presented by figure 4. From the figure it can be seen that the hyperspectral tongue images not only contain the whole information that RGB images contained, but also can provide some information that the RGB images not contained. Although the colour-based tongue image processing is not a very difficult task, it may be neglect some details that dose not exist in the original RGB image in some cases. When the hyperspectral tongue images are used in tongue diagnosis, all bands which cover the wavelength range from 400 nm to 1000 nm will participate in the process. So the hyperspectral-based method can get more information than the colour-based imaging methods. In addition, this is not the only reason that we introduce hyperspectral imaging technology to computerized tongue diagnosis. The technology may also have some other good applications in this field, such as tongue body segmentation, tongue colour discrimination, tongue coating analysis, tongue sublingual veins recognition, etc. Therefore, hyperspectral imaging technology is more useful than traditional CCD cameras in modernization of TCM. Figure 5 illustrate a representative subtotal of hyperspectral images captured at various wavelengths of tongue surface and sublingual veins using the AOTF-based HTIS, respectively. From the figures it can be seen that there are different tongue features in different single band images.

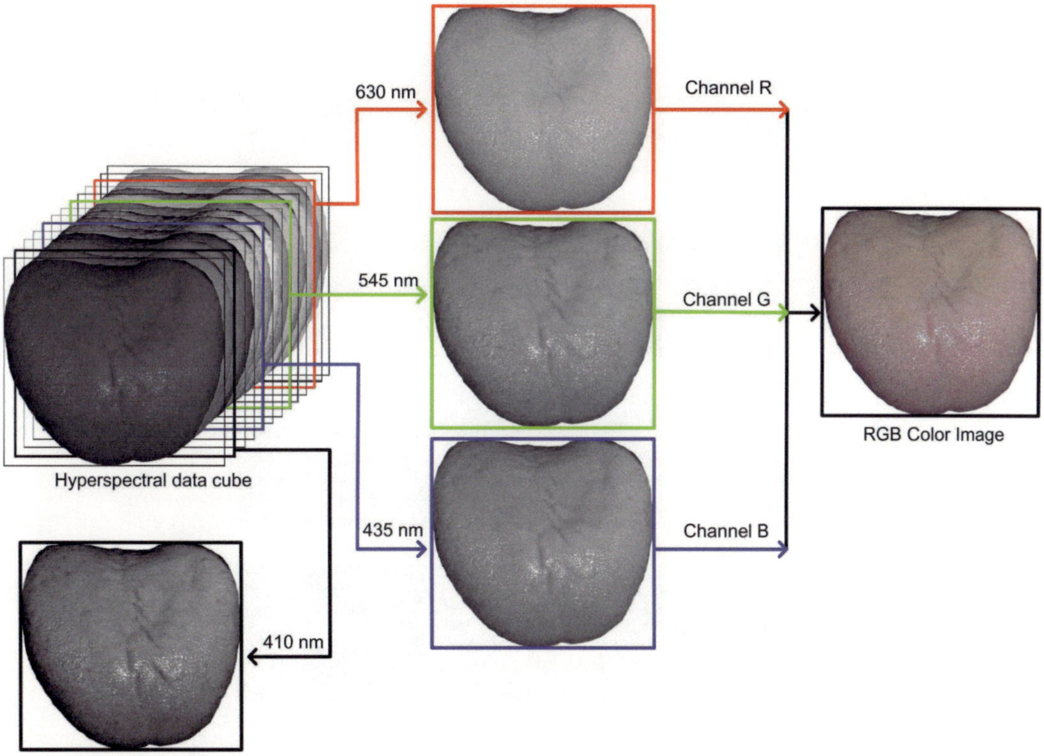

Fig. 4. Relationship between hyperspectral images and colour-based RGB images

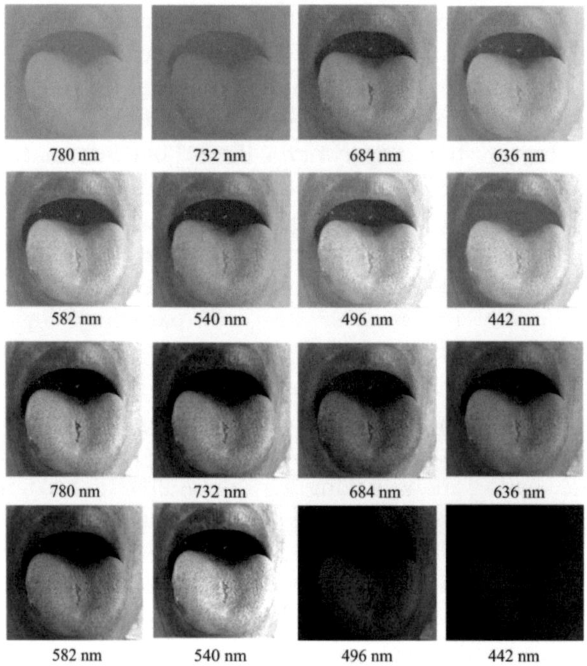

(a)

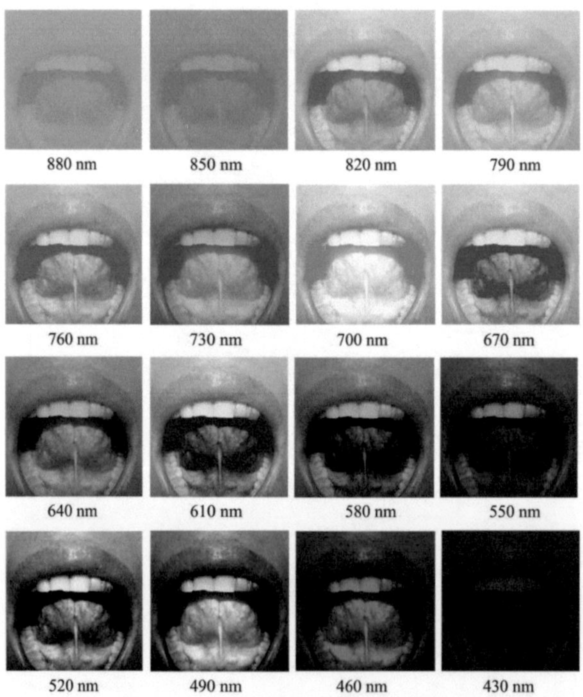

(b)

Fig. 5. Single band images of (a) tongue surface and (b) sublingual veins

3.2 Spectral response calibration

One of the big advantages of the HTIS over conventional imaging techniques is the fact that it is capable of acquiring both spatial and spectral information of tongue surface. The spectral response range of the hyperspectral tongue images covering the whole visible wavelength, it can provide more information than the RGB images captured by the traditional CCD. Therefore, it is possible to identify tongue features automatically based on spectral signatures extracted from the hyperspectral tongue images. As the spectral response of the HTIS is inhomogeneous, some data pre-processing procedure should be performed before the spectra extraction. To calibrate the spectral response of the HTIS, a white plane made of Teflon is selected to be the reference plane. Before tongue image collection, a scene of hyperspectral images of the reference plane is captured. Figure 6 shows a typical intensity curve of a pixel extracted from the hyperspectral data of the reference white plane. This curve can be used to represent the spectral response of the HTIS to some extent according to its optical model and sensor model. We define the gray correction coefficient to calibrate the spectral response of the system. The gray correction coefficient $k\ (i, j; \lambda)$ of each pixel can be calculated by the following formula:

$$k(i,j;\lambda) = \frac{DN(i,j)}{DN(i,j;\lambda)} \tag{1}$$

where $k\ (i, j; \lambda)$ is the gray correction coefficient of pixel (i, j) in band λ; $DN(i, j; \lambda)$ is the gray value of pixel (i, j) in band λ of the reference hyperspectral data; $DN(i, j)$ is the average gray value of pixel (i, j) in all bands, it can be calculated according to the following formula:

$$DN(i,j) = \left(\sum_{\lambda=1}^{N} DN(i,j;\lambda)\right) / N \tag{2}$$

where N is the total band number of the hyperspectral data. Then, the hyperspectral data of tongue can be calibrated with the gray correction coefficient and the true intensity curve can be extracted. The calibration formula is as follows:

$$DN'(i,j;\lambda) = DN(i,j;\lambda) \cdot k(i,j;\lambda) \tag{3}$$

where $DN'\ (i, j; \lambda)$ is the gray value of pixel (i, j) at wavelength λ after calibration. In order to assess the efficiency of the calibration method, another white plane is selected as the sample and the hyperspectral data is collected under the same working conditions with the reference plane. Figure 7 shows an intensity curve of the same pixel extracted from the hyperspectral data of the sample white plane before and after calibration respectively. From the figure it can be seen that the intensity curve of the sample white plane is close to the theoretical value after calibration. Then we can get the real tongue intensity curve from the hyperspectral tongue images with the spectral response calibration method.

4. Tongue body segmentation

Currently there are two main issues in computerized tongue analysis. One is the objective representation of tongue's colour, texture and coating with the help of image analysis technology (Zheng, Yang, Zhou, & Wang, 2006). The other is automatic tongue body segmentation. Tongue body segmentation is the primitive work of tongue image analysis. Recently, the main segmentation algorithms are threshold segmentation algorithm, region grow method, watershed algorithm, BEDC algorithm (B Pang et al., 2005), active contour model (for example the snake method (W. Li et al., 2004)), etc. However, these methods can not give satisfied results in the tongue segmentation application. The reason is that the automatic segmentation of anatomical structures in traditional monochromatic images is often performed using model-based nonrigid registration methods. That is to say, an automatic segmentation of a certain structure can be obtained by registering a labelled model, typically generated in a manual segmentation process, to another data set containing the structure of interest. This registration is difficult and laborious (Crum, Hartkens, & Hill, 2004). This is a problem that might be solved if the variability in the spectra of different tissue types could be used to distinguish between the human tongue and the nontongue biological substances in hyperspectral image space (Z. Liu, Yan, Zhang, & Li, 2007).

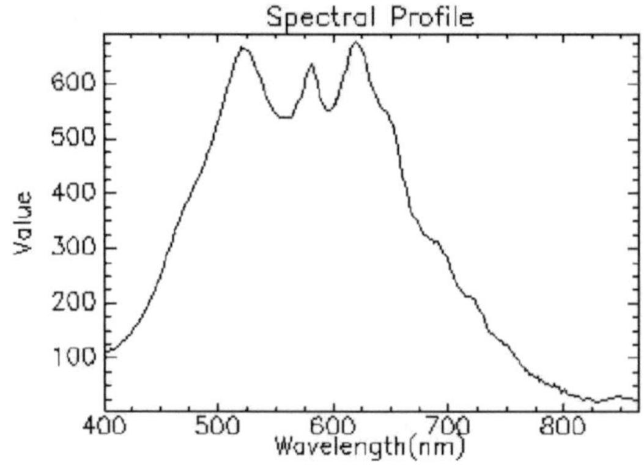

Fig. 6. An intensity curve extracted from the hyperspectral data of the white plane.

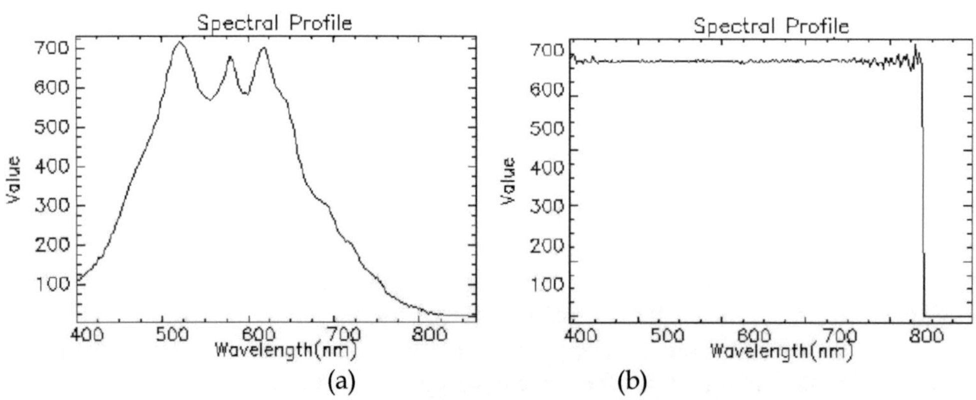

Fig. 7. Spectral response calibration result (a) before calibration and (b) after calibration.

After capture the hyperspectral tongue images, an algorithm which can simultaneously utilizes both the spatial and spectral information of the hyperspectral tongue imagery data can be used to segment the tongue body. To evaluate the effectiveness of the hyperspectral based method, we use a spectral angle mapper (SAM) based automatic tongue segmentation algorithm to segment tongue body. The SAM is an automated method for directly comparing image spectra to known spectra (usually determined in a lab with a spectrometer) (Kruse, Lefkoff, & Boardman, 1992). This method treats both spectra (the questioned and known) as vectors and calculates the spectral angle between them. This method is insensitive to illumination since the SAM algorithm uses only the vector direction and not the vector length. Figure 8 show the core of the SAM based automatic tongue segmentation algorithm. First, a transformed image cube (the SAM cube) is constructed by applying the SAM algorithm with each pixel in the original *N*N* cube with each and every other pixel in the original hyperspectral tongue imagery data cube. In other words, band 1 of the transformed SAM cube contains the spectral angle of the spectrum in pixel location (sample 1, line 1) with every other spectrum in the cube. Band 2 of the SAM cube contains the spectral angle of the spectrum in pixel location (1, 2) with every other spectrum in the original cube, etc. Thus, a 'spectrum' from the SAM cube contains information about tongue edge. The spectra of the SAM cube are then analyzed, each in turn, for edge detection. In other words, a one-dimensional edge detection technique is applied to the one-dimensional data of each SAM cube spectrum. The SAM cube spectrum band number corresponds to pixel address in the original hyperspectral tongue imagery data cube. Thus, when an edge is detected in the analysis of an SAM cube spectrum, the 'band number' of the edge is converted to the (sample, line) address of the original hypspectral tongue imagery data cube and a point is plotted on a separate output plane indicating the presence of the edge (Resmini, 2004). So the SAM based automatic tongue segmentation algorithm converts a two-dimensional kernel-based edge detection problem into a series of one-dimensional edge detection problems.

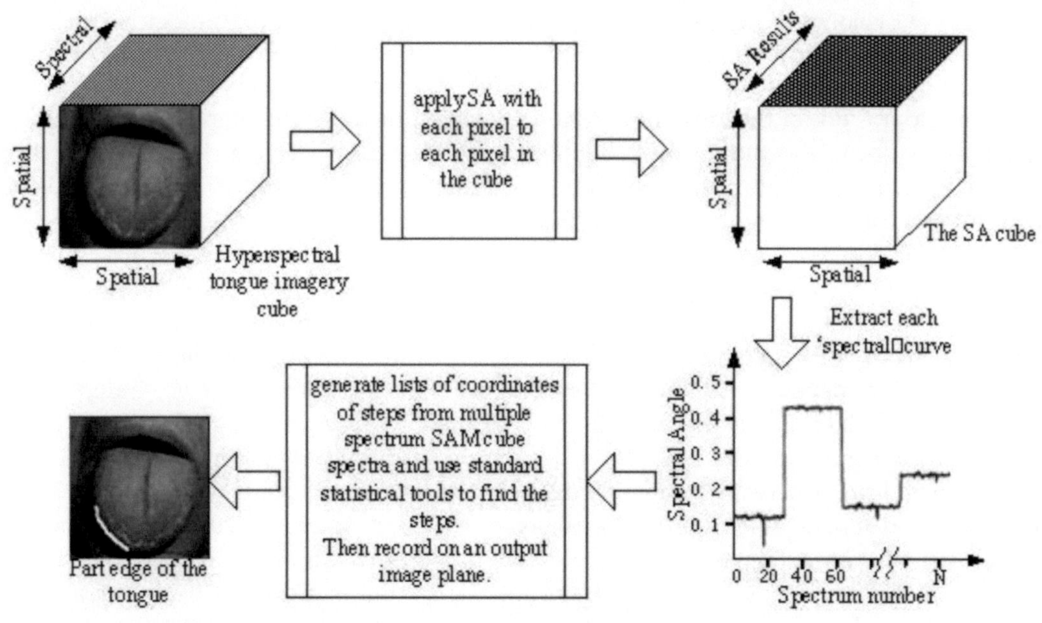

Fig. 8. The core of the SAM based automatic tongue segmentation algorithm

To evaluate the new automatic tongue body segmentation method, several hyperspectral tongue images were captured by the AOTF based system. After the pre-processing and calibration of the hyperspectral data, we can extract the transmittance spectra of each pixel in the whole scene. Then the SAM based automatic tongue segmentation algorithm was used to segment tongue body from the hyperspectral images. Figure 9 shows the segment results by the new algorithm. The results demonstrate the efficiency of this approach.

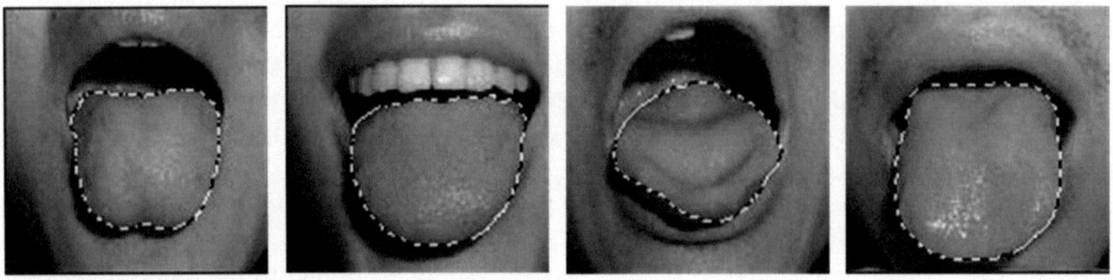

Fig. 9. Tongue body segmentation results

5. Tongue colour analysis and discrimination

In the area of computer-assisted medical diagnosis, colour image analysis can be a useful aid in standardization and automation. Colour image analysis has been applied to assess the power of new drugs on the spreading of skin erythema (Nischik & Forster, 1997), to the identification of skin tumour border (Hance, Umbaugh, & Moss, 1996), assessment and tracking of wound severity (Hansen, Sparrow, & Kokate, 1997), and matching tongue colour images for tongue diseases diagnosis (C. H. Li & Yuen, 2002), etc. These researches show that different colours of organism have some relationship with its physiological functions and changes. So the colour retrieval from images automatically and quantitatively is very important for the purpose of disease diagnosis and prognosis assessment.

Tongue colour is one of the most important pathological features for computer aided tongue diagnosis system. By the use of digital imaging and processing technology, some physiological information of human body condition can be retrieved by analyzing colour features and colour differences extracted from tongue images (X. Wang & Zhang, 2010). For the CCD based RGB colour tongue images, colour image matching can be performed using colour coordinates or based on colour histograms of images in different colour spaces. Therefore, in order to get consistent and standard colour perception of tongue images for tongue analysis, further colour correction to determine the mapping algorithm between its unknown device-dependent RGB colour spaces and a particular known device-independent colour space is necessarily needed. In the past few years, some algorithms in colour correction of tongue images have been developed, such as polynomial-regression-based algorithm and support-vector regression (SVR)-based algorithm (Zhang, Wang, & Jin, 2005), the optimized tongue colour correction scheme (X. Wang & Zhang, 2010), etc. Although these methods can extract some tongue colour features, there are still some difficulties because of the limitations of RGB images captured by the traditional CCD cameras. The principal difficulties are first that when these images are used it is difficult to distinguish in RGB colour space between the tongue and neighbouring tissues that have a similar colour, second it is difficult to distinguish between tongue coating and tongue substance, and third it is also difficult to discrimination the colour automatically and quantificationally. Finally, colour distortion of tongue image, which is often caused by the inconstancy of lighting conditions, can seriously affect the validity of diagnosis results and furthermore, impair the interchange ability among tongue images captured by different devices. For these reasons, current methods of tongue colour calibration or recognition perform well only on tongue images acquired under some special conditions and often fail when the quality of image is less than ideal (Y. G. Wang et al., 2007). So tongue colour analysis becomes difficult due to the limited information of common digital images, the variation of the illumination, etc.

According to the principle of physics, colours of an object surface have close relationship with its spectrum (Irigoyen & Herraez, 2003). As spectra of an organism in the range of wavelengths of the visible light (among 400 nm–750 nm approximately) completely includes the RGB colour space, spectra can be used to retrieve tongue colours more accurately. When the HTIS is used in tongue diagnosis, new automatic tongue colour calibration and discrimination method based on hyperspectral images can be used to recognize and classify tongue colours according to the spectral signatures rather than the colour values in RGB colour space. As different tongue colours have different reflectance spectral signatures, we use the SAM algorithm to classify tongue colours. This method is insensitive to illumination since the SAM algorithm uses only the vector direction and not the vector length. The result of the SAM tongue colour classification is an image showing the best match at each pixel. Then different tongue colours can be classified accurately by the SAM algorithm.

In the experiment, 230 scenes hyperspectral tongue images are selected for colour recognition test. The colours of tongue substances are quantized into six classes: light white, pale red, red, maroon, purple and reddish purple, while the colours of tongue coatings include four categories: white, light yellow, yellow and gloom. To evaluate the performance of the tongue colour classification method, four experienced doctors have been asked to label the reference samples, classify all of the 230 tongues using naked eyes, and evaluate the experimental results. Due to the discrepancy between inspection results of different doctors, we treated the consensus as the ground truth. The numbers of tongues corresponding to each category of substances and coatings were given in Tables 1

	color	light white	pale red	red	maroon	purple	reddish purple	Overall
recognize results	light white	25	1				1	
	pale red	2	53	3	1			
	red	1	4	30	3	1	1	
	maroon		2	1	45	1		
	purple		1	1	2	23	2	
	reddish purple		1			3	22	
	Number of tongues	28	62	35	51	28	26	230
	Rate of correctness (%)	89	85	86	88	82	85	86

Table 1. Colour recognition results and rates of correctness for different categories of substances

and Tables 2. The rate of correctness for each category of substances or coatings was defined as the percentage of the number of tongues classified correctly by the proposed method to the number of tongues in this category (Qingli Li & Liu, 2009). From Tables 1 and Tables 2 it can be seen that the proposed method has good performance in terms of the rates of correctness for colour recognition of coatings and substances. Therefore, hyperspectral tongue images can be used to tongue colour analysis and discrimination. This method is effective to reduce the colour difference between images captured using different cameras or under different lighting conditions, as the method recognize and classify tongue colours using their spectral signatures rather than their colour values in RGB colour space.

	color	white	light yellow	yellow	gloom	Overall
recognize results	white	35	3			
	light yellow	3	108	3		
	yellow	2	9	45	2	
	gloom		2	2	16	
Number of tongues		40	122	50	18	230
Rate of correctness (%)		88	89	90	89	89

Table 2. Color recognition results and rates of correctness for different categories of coatings

6. Tongue cracks extraction and classification

According to the TCM theory, human tongue carries abundant information about the health status of a person. Among the information that collected from tongue surface, the appearance of cracks has been known to have the greatest clinical importance. A crack tongue, also known as a scrotal tongue, is a benign condition characterized by deep grooves (fissures) in the dorsum of the tongue. Tongue cracks refer to the surface of the tongue covered with all kinds of cracks or lines in deep or shallow shape, which are induced by the fusion or separation of the ligular papillae. Normally, the tongue surface should be smooth and soft and show no cracks. When obvious cracks appear on the tongue surface, it suggests the deficiency of *Qi*-blood and the consumption of *Yin* by excessive heat and, sometimes, the blood stasis. For instance, a deep crack in the center reaching to the tip reflects hyperactivity of Heart fire (L. L. Liu & Zhang, 2007). In the past few years, many studies have been conducted on tongue cracks extraction and classification methods based on gray or colour images. Pham and Cai (Pham & Cai, 2004) constructed an algorithms to calculate six features on a tongue in order to analyze different types of tongue disease. These features include roughness, amount of fissures, a* and b* (chromatic dimensions of L* a* b* colour space), energy, and entropy functions computed from the gray level cooccurrence matrix. Liu and Zhang et al. (L. L. Liu & Zhang, 2007; L. L. Liu et al., 2008) presented a tongue crack detection scheme based on the wide line detector (WLD) algorithm. There are also other tongue cracks extraction algorithms, such as the multiscale edge detection algorithm (Shen et al., 2003), the 2D Gabor wavelet transform coefficient energy (GWTE) algorithm (Y Zhou, L Shen, & J Yang, 2002), and the tongue texture analysis method based on the gray covariance matrix model (B. Pang et al., 2004). Although these methods can extract tongue texture or cracks correctly from tongue images, some difficulties still exist in analyzing these features in detail because of the limitations of images captured by traditional CCD cameras.

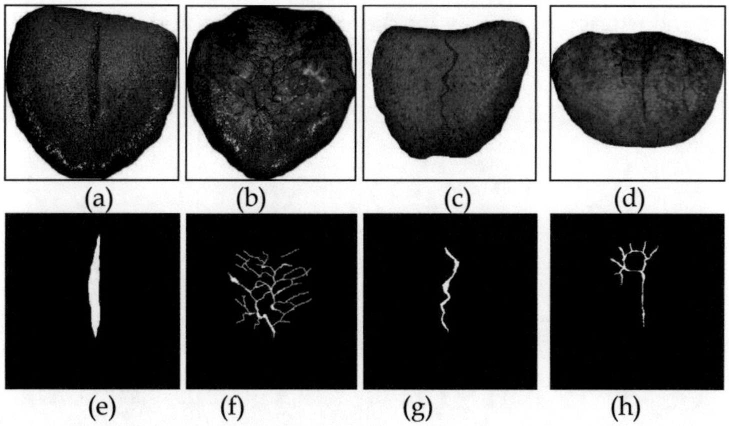

Fig. 10. Tongue cracks extraction results: (a)-(d) single band images, (e)-(h) extraction results by the hyperspectral-based method

In TCM, the appearance of obvious cracks on the tongue surface suggests the development of some pathological changes. According to electromagnetic theory, pathological changes of the object surface have a close relationship with its spectrum (Somosy et al., 2002). If hyperspectral imaging technology is introduced to computerized tongue diagnosis, both spatial and spectral data, which contain the pathological information of the tongue surface, can be obtained. Therefore, tongue cracks can be extracted by some new algorithms which can take advantage of the rich hyperspectral data not found in traditional CCD images (Q. L. Li, Wang, Liu, Sun, & Liu, 2010). Generally, there are three steps in a typical tongue cracks extraction procedure, which is finding, tracking, and linking (L. L. Liu & Zhang, 2007). For hyperspectral tongue images, the spectral signatures should be added to the three stages to improve the extraction accurate. In the cracks finding stage, a target-constrained interference-minimized filter (Ren & Chang, 2000) is used to perform the extraction. The filter casts the detection of a foreground signature mixed with background signatures, as a linearly constrained adaptive beam-forming problem. This technique can be used to determine a vector operator that suppresses the undesired background signatures while enhancing that of the known target signature. After perform the cracks finding procedure, we can get a gradient image with tongue cracks seed images and some noisy pixels. Although the gradient image displays most connected cracks, some isolated spots and misidentified areas still exist in the image. So the tracking and linking process is performed to track the cracks candidates obtained in the first step. As tongue cracks commonly refer to the surface of the tongue covered with all kinds of connected cracks or lines in deep or shallow shape, a roving window of the Hueckel's operator (Ballard & Brown, 1982) is used to prolong or link the bright pixels on the histogram-sliced image. Then postprocessing is performed to reduce the misclassified pixels. Two morphological characteristics of tongue cracks are selected in this algorithm: length and area. The threshold values of them are set to 10 pixels and 100 pixels according to the evaluation standard commonly used by TCM doctors. Then the extracted cracks will be discarded if its length is very short or its area is too small. The final result shows a binary image to represent the extracted tongue cracks which can be classified easily. In the tongue cracks extraction experiment, four scenes of hyperspectral tongue images with different kind of cracks were selected and processed.

Figure 10 shows the extraction results by the proposed method. From the figure it can be seen that the hyperspectral-based tongue cracks extraction method is effective.

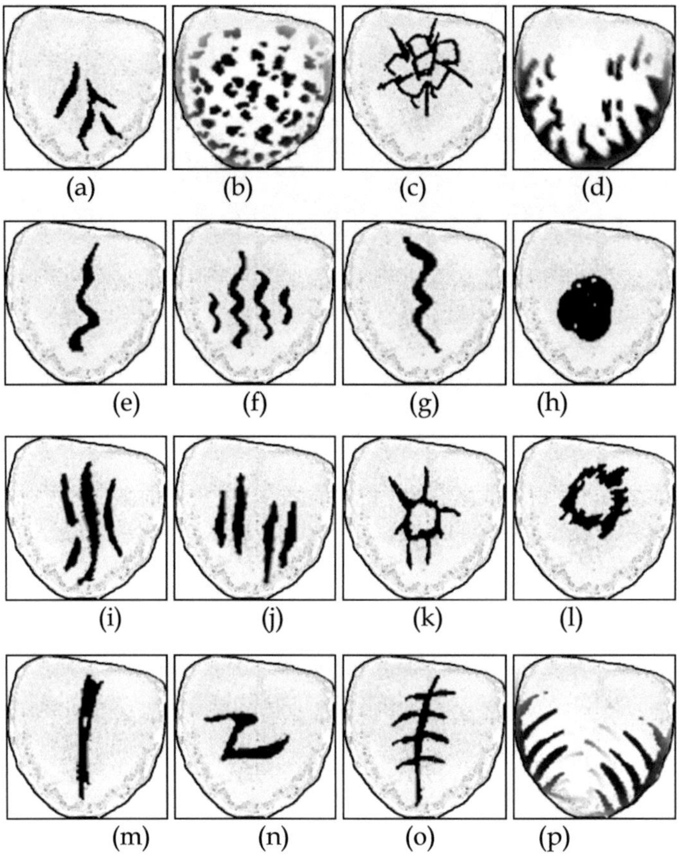

Fig. 11. Typical tongue crack categories

After tongue cracks extraction, they should be classified into several categories to help doctors to diagnose disease. According to the TCM theory, there are 16 kinds of typical tongue cracks as shown in figure 11 (named as Ba zi, Duo dian, Gui, Ju chi, Lai she, Qu chong, Qu she, Shi xin, Shui zi, Si zhi, Tai Yang, Xuan zhen, Yi zi, Yu gu, and Zuoyou pie cracks, respectively). These typical tongue cracks can be regarded as objects with different shapes which commonly observed in the clinical tongue diagnosis in TCM. We can classify these cracks by a shape classifier which comprises a feature extraction stage and a shape matching stage. Shape classification is a basic problem in computer vision. Its application has been found in various areas such as industrial part identification, target identification, character recognition, and medical diagnosis (He & Kundu, 1991). Shape can be represented either by its contour or by its region. Contour-based descriptors such as curvature, chain codes, Fourier descriptors, etc. have been widely used as they can preserve the local information that is important in classification of complex shapes (Thakoor, Gao, & Jung, 2007). Tongue cracks can be assumed to be formed by various segments, each of which has a constant curvature. Therefore, curvature can be chosen as the feature of contour-based shape descriptors and the hidden Markov model (HMM) (Thakoor et al., 2007) can be used as the framework of tongue cracks modelling and classification. Then the generalized probabilistic descent (GPD) method (Katagiri, Juang, & Lee, 1998) was used as a training algorithm for the tongue cracks classifier. At last, tongue cracks can be classified into different typical categories. To evaluate the hyperspectral based tongue cracks classify method, 480 scenes of hyperspectral tongue images were captured by the HTIS from in-patients in hospital. These tongue cracks can be divided into 16 typical classes named Class 1 ~ Class 16 which corresponding to figure 1 (a) ~ (p), respectively. The 16 typical tongue cracks are chosen according to the diagnostic criteria commonly used by TCM doctors (S. Wang, Wang, & Wang, 2001). The numbers of tongue cracks corresponding to each category classified by the proposed algorithm was given in Table 3 (the confusion matrix of classification). The rate of correctness for each category of cracks is defined as the percentage of the number of tongues classified correctly by the proposed method to the number of tongues in this category. From the table it can be seen that the proposed method has good performance in terms of the rates of correctness for tongue cracks classification. As a preliminary research, we just use the most simple classify method here. To classify tongue cracks more accurately, some other

Cracks type	C 1	C 2	C 3	C 4	C 5	C 6	C 7	C 8	C 9	C 10	C 11	C 12	C 13	C 14	C 15	C 16	Overall
Classification results																	
C 1	23				1												
C 2		12					2									1	
C 3	1		22						1				1				
C 4				50			1					2				1	
C 5				1	30									1			
C 6						38				2	1				1		
C 7							33							1			
C 8			1					25	4				4				
C 9		1			2			3	43			1				1	
C 10						2				17	1				1		
C 11	1		1								13						
C 12				1				1				29				2	
C 13			1									1	27				
C 14						3	1				1			16	1		
C 15		1				1			1						12		
C 16				2												32	
Number of tongues	25	14	25	54	33	44	37	29	49	19	16	33	32	18	15	37	480
Rate of correctness (%)	92	86	88	93	91	86	89	86	88	89	81	88	84	89	80	86	88

Table 3. Tongue cracks classification results and rate of correctness for each category

classification method such as support vector machines (SVM) should be used in the future as SVM is a more accurate classifier than the maximum likelihood method and can efficiently analyze hyperspectral data directly in the hyperdimensional feature space without the need for any feature-reduction procedure (Melgani & Bruzzone, 2002).

7. Sublingual veins analysis

According to TCM diagnostics theory, sublingual veins collateral stem from the base of tongue and connect directly with visceras, especially the heart, spleen, liver and kidney. Under normal conditions, they are bluish purple in colour and moist. These veins travel naturally without meandering, distending or exhibiting any varicosity. The sublingual veins are sensitive indicators of the blood stasis and show the activity of the blood circulation (Chiu et al., 2002). Inspection of sublingual veins can provide valuable insights into the healthy status of human body (Yan et al., 2009). However, the subjective characteristics of the traditional method impede this objective because sublingual vein diagnoses are usually based on detailed visual discrimination, which mainly depends on the subjective analysis of the examiners. Therefore, a quantitative analysis should produce the possibility of evaluating and classifying the severity of blood stasis in a less subjective way and deriving an automatic diagnostic procedure.

In recent years, some studies have shown that the accurate extraction of tongue features is important for computerized tongue diagnosis (Bakshi & Pal, 2010; Qingli Li & Liu, 2009; B. Pang et al., 2005; B. Pang et al., 2004). The automatic extraction of sublingual veins from complex scenes should also be foremost solved due to the qualities of segmentation directly influencing the subsequent feature extraction and recognition. Some experiments have been conducted on sublingual images acquired by an ordinary camera under a visible light source or an infrared light source for the extraction of sublingual veins. Takeichi and Sato (Takeichi & Sato, 1997) performed computer-assisted image analyses on the colour of the tongues of 95 medical students to enhance the accuracy and objectivity of sublingual veins inspections for determining blood stasis. This is a prior research on colour of sublingual veins. Then, Chiu et al. (Chiu et al., 2002) developed a computerized inspection system and presented a method to extract the chromatic and geometrical properties of sublingual veins quantitatively. Their system is also a colour based method that can extract the length, width, area, and colour information from the sublingual veins. Afterwards, Yan et al. (Yan et al., 2008) used monochrome industrial CCD with enhanced near infrared sensitivity to capture sublingual vein images. More recent studies by them (Yan et al., 2009) have focused on the pixel-based sublingual vein segmentation algorithm and adaptive sublingual vein segmentation algorithm for colour sublingual images with visible and low contrasts. Although many issues on the standardization and quantification of sublingual veins have been resolved, there are still some difficulties because of the limitations of these kinds of images (Q. Li, Wang, Liu, Guan, & Xu, 2011). For example, the thickness and transparence of the sublingual mucosa covering the sublingual veins may change due to the different degrees of varicosity. This change may lead to the sublingual veins being clear in some sublingual images but blurry in others, the contours of the sublingual veins are difficult to extract.

If the HTIS were used to capture the sublingual vein images, it can provide both the spectral and spatial information of the sublingual veins. The spectra extracted from the hyperspectral sublingual images can be represented as a non-stationary sequence of feature vectors, and the spectral correlation and band-to-band variability can be characterized using some models. For example, the SAM or the hidden Markov model (HMM) can be used to extract the sublingual veins from hyperspectral images. Unlike existing approaches, the new method can recognize sublingual veins using their spectral signatures rather than their gray values. To evaluate the effectiveness of the HTIS on sublingual veins analysis, some scenes of hyperspectral sublingual images were captured. Figure 5 (b) shows some single band images of sublingual veins. Here we use the improved spectral angle mapper algorithm to segment the sublingual veins. Spectral angle mapper (SAM) algorithm is a tool that permits rapid mapping of spectral similarity of one image spectrum to another spectrum (Kruse et al., 1992; Park, Windhama, Lawrencea, & Smitha, 2007). The algorithm determines the spectral similarity between two spectra by calculating the 'angle' between them. The angle between the endmember spectra vector and each pixel vector in N-dimensional space is compared. Smaller angles represent closer matches to the reference spectra. This algorithm can extract the target from hyperspectral images effectively by mapping the spectral similarity. However, the wavelengths often shift several bands with the influence of noise in the real HTIS which lead to some extraction errors. To overcome this disadvantage, an improved spectral angle mapper (ISAM) algorithm is used to extract the sublingual veins. The ISAM algorithm calculate the spectral angle (SA) not only between the reference spectral vector and the testing spectral vector, but also between the reference spectral vector and the testing spectral vector with shift 2 bands both forward and backward, respectively. Then the maximum was selected as the real SA value between the two vectors as the following formula

$$SA = Max\left(\alpha\left(\vec{T}_j, \vec{R}\right)\right) = Max\left(\cos\left(\sum_{i=1}^{N} t_{i+j} r_i \Big/ \sqrt{\sum_{i=1}^{N} t_{i+j}^2 \sum_{i=1}^{N} r_i^2}\right)\right) \quad (4)$$

where j = -2, -1, 0, 1, 2.

This method is insensitive to illumination since the ISAM algorithm uses only the vector direction and not the vector length. It also can reduce the wavelengths shift errors effectively. Figure 12 shows the extraction results by the ISAM algorithm with SA = 0.1. From the figure it can be seen that the ISAM algorithm can segment the sublingual veins accurately. As sublingual veins may be correlated with certain diseases (Pham & Cai, 2004), defining several quantitative features for classification in a computer-aided tongue disease diagnosis is necessary. According to the diagnostic standards of experienced doctors, two quantitative features can be selected after sublingual vein extraction, that is, the breadth feature and the chromatic feature. The breadth feature denotes the breadth measurement of the segmented sublingual veins, the value of which is the indicator of a special disease (Yan et al., 2009). The chromatic feature is another important pathological feature of sublingual veins. The colours used as diagnostic measurements in sublingual vein disease diagnoses are usually compounds of several colours due to the complex disorder caused by some pathological processes. The existing colour analysis mainly utilizes the RGB triple values or hue values of single pixels or the mean of the tongue texture block (C. H. Li & Yuen, 2002; B. Pang et al., 2004), which is difficult due to the limited information of these kinds of images. As presented in the previous section, we can use spectra to retrieve organism colours, as the wavelength range of the hyperspectral tongue imaging system covering the whole visible light includes the RGB colour spaces. Therefore, different colours of sublingual veins can be represented by the corresponding reflectance spectral curves. With these quantitative sublingual vein features, some classifiers, such as Bayesian networks, neural networks, and support vector machines, can be used to model the relationship between these quantitative features and diseases.

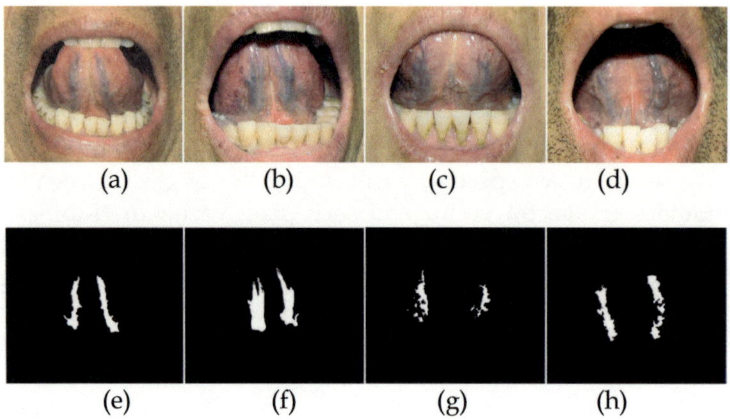

Fig. 12. Sublingual veins extraction results. (a)~(d) false colour images composed by single band images at 630 nm, 540 nm, and 430 nm as R, G, and B channels. (e)~(h) the extraction results by the ISAM algorithm.

8. Conclusion

Among the four diagnostic processes of TCM: inspection, auscultation and olfaction, inquiry, and pulse feeling and palpation, the examination of tongue is one of the most important approaches for getting significant evidences in diagnosing the patient's health conditions. However, owing to its drawbacks in quantification and standardization, the development of tongue diagnosis is stagnated (Zhang, Wang, Zhang et al., 2005). Computerized methods for TCM allow researchers to identify required information more efficiently, discover new relationships which are obscured by merely focusing on Western medicine, and bridge the gaps between Western Medicine and TCM (Lukman et al., 2007). Therefore, getting the overall information about tongue surface is very important for computerized tongue diagnosis system. In this chapter, an AOTF based HTIS which can capture hyperspectral images of human tongue at a series of wavelengths is developed and used in tongue diagnosis. The basic principles and instrumental systems of the new system, the data pre-processing method as well as some applications are presented. Compared with the pushbroom hyperspectral tongue imager used in our previous works (Q. Li et al., 2008; Q. L. Li et al., 2006), this new type of hyperspectral tongue imaging system has the advantage of having no moving parts and can be scanned at very high rates. As the hyperspectral tongue images can provide more information than the CCD based images, we can find some successful applications in computerized tongue diagnosis such as tongue body segmentation, tongue colour analysis and discrimination, tongue cracks extraction and classification, sublingual veins analysis, etc. Preliminary experiments show that the AOTF-based hyperspectral tongue imaging system is superior to the traditional CCD based methods because the hyperspectral images can provide more information about the tongue surface. In future studies, we will extract the quantitative features of the tongue surface and find some methods to model the relationship between these features and certain diseases.

9. Acknowledgment

This work is supported in part by the National Natural Science Foundation of China (NSFC) (grants 61177011, 60807035, 60976004)), the Specialized Research Fund for the Doctoral Program of Higher Education of China (grant 200802691006), the project supported by the Shanghai Commission of Science and Technology (SCST) China (grant 09JC1405300), the Fundamental Research Funds for the Central Universities, and the Project supported by the State Key Development Program for Basic Research of China(Grant No. 2011CB932903). We are grateful for the assistance and support provided by Mrs Ivona Lovric and the Editorial Board of this book.

10. References

Bakshi, D., & Pal, S. (2010, 16-18 Dec. 2010). *Introduction about traditional Tongue Diagnosis with scientific value addition.* Paper presented at the Systems in Medicine and Biology (ICSMB), 2010 International Conference on.

Ballard, D. H., & Brown, C. M. (1982). *Computer Vision*: Prentice Hall.

Chan, K. (1995). Progress in traditional Chinese medicine. *Trends in Pharmacological Sciences, 16*(6), 182-187.

Chaudhari, A. J., Darvas, F., Bading, J. R., Moats, R. A., Conti, P. S., Smith, D. J., et al. (2005). Hyperspectral and multispectral bioluminescence optical tomography for small animal imaging. *Physics in Medicine and Biology, 50*(23), 5421-5441.

Chiou, W. C. (1984). Dynamic descriptors for contextual classification of remotely sensed hyperspectral image data-analysis. *Applied Optics, 23*(21), 3889-3892.

Chiu, C.-C., Lan, C.-Y., & Chang, Y.-H. (2002). Objective assessment of blood stasis using computerized inspection of sublingual veins. *Computer Methods and Programs in Biomedicine, 69*(1), 1-12.

Crum, W. R., Hartkens, T., & Hill, D. L. G. (2004). Non-rigid image registration: theory and practice. *British Journal of Radiology, 77*, S140-S153.

Demos, S. G., & Ramsamooj, R. (2003). Hyperspectral imaging of cells: toward real-time pathological assessment. In K. M. Iftekharuddin & A. A. S. Awwal (Eds.), *Photonic Devices and Algorithms for Computing V, Proceedings of the SPIE* (Vol. 5021, pp. 133-137). San Diego, CA, USA.

Gupta, N. (2003). A no-moving-parts UV/visible hyperspectral imager. *Chemical and Biological Standoff Detection, 5268*, 89-95.

Hance, G. A., Umbaugh, S. E., & Moss, R. H. (1996). Unsupervised color image segmentation: with application to skin tumor borders. *IEEE Eng. Med. Biol. Mag., 15*(1), 104-111.

Hansen, G. L., Sparrow, E. M., & Kokate, J. Y. (1997). Wound status using color image processing. *IEEE Trans. Med. Imaging, 16*(1), 78-86.

Harsanyi, J. C., & Chang, C. I. (1994). Hyperspectral image classification and dimensionality reduction-an orthogonal subspace projection approach. *IEEE Transactions on Geoscience and Remote Sensing, 32*(4), 779-785.

He, Y., & Kundu, A. (1991). 2-D shape classification using hidden markov model. *IEEE Transactions on Pattern Analysis and Machine Intelligence, 13*(11), 1172-1184.

Hsing-Lin, L., Suzuki, S., Adachi, Y., & Umeno, M. (1993, 25-29 Oct. 1993). *Fuzzy theory in traditional Chinese pulse diagnosis.* Paper presented at the Neural Networks, 1993. IJCNN '93-Nagoya. Proceedings of 1993 International Joint Conference on.

Ikeda, N., Fujiwara, Y., & Yoshida, H. (2006, 18-21 Oct. 2006). *Tongue diagnosis support system.* Paper presented at the SICE-ICASE, 2006. International Joint Conference.

Inoue, Y., & Penuelas, J. (2001). An AOTF-based hyperspectral imaging system for field use in ecophysiological and agricultural applications. *International Journal of Remote Sensing, 22*(18), 3883-3888.

Irigoyen, J., & Herraez, J. (2003). *Electromagnetic spectrum and color vision.* Paper presented at the Proceedings of the 3rd International Symposium on Image and Signal Processing and Analysis, ISPA 2003.

Jiang, Y., Chen, J., & Zhang, H. (2000). Computerized system of diagnosis of tongue in Traditional Chinese Medicine. *Chinese Journal of Integrated Traditional and Western Medicine, 20*(2), 145-147.

Katagiri, S., Juang, B.-H., & Lee, C.-H. (1998). Pattern recognition using a family of design algorithms based upon the generalized probabilistic descent method. *Proceedings of the IEEE, 86*(11), 2345 - 2373.

Kim, K. H., Do, J. H., Ryu, H., & Kim, J. Y. (2008, 23-26 Nov. 2008). *Tongue diagnosis method for extraction of effective region and classification of tongue coating.* Paper presented at the Image Processing Theory, Tools and Applications, 2008. IPTA 2008. First Workshops on.

Kruse, F. A., Lefkoff, A. B., & Boardman, J. W. (1992). *The spectral image processing system (SIPS)-software for integrated analysis of AVIRIS data.* Paper presented at the Summaries of the 4th Annual JPL Airborne Geoscience Workshop, Pasadena.

Li, C. H., & Yuen, P. C. (2002). Tongue image matching using color content. *Pattern Recognition, 35*(2), 407-419.

Li, Q., Dai, C., Liu, H., & Liu, J. (2009). *Leukemic cells segmentation algorithm based on molecular spectral imaging technology* Paper presented at the International Symposium on Photoelectronic Detection and Imaging 2009: Advances in Infrared Imaging and Applications, Beijing, China.

Li, Q., Liu, J., Xiao, G., & Xue, Y. (2008). Hyperspectral tongue imaging system used in tongue diagnosis, *The 2nd International Conference on Bioinformatics and Biomedical Engineering, 2008. ICBBE 2008.* (pp. 2579-2581). Shanghai.

Li, Q., & Liu, Z. (2009). Tongue color analysis and discrimination based on hyperspectral images. *Computerized Medical Imaging and Graphics, 33*(3), 217-221.

Li, Q., Wang, Y., Zhang, J., Xu, G., & Xue, Y. (2010). Quantitative analysis of protective effect of Erythropoietin on diabetic retinal cells using molecular hyperspectral imaging technology. *IEEE Transactions on Biomedical Engineering, 57*(7), 1699-1706.

Li, Q., Wang, Y. T., Liu, H. Y., Guan, Y. N., & Xu, L. A. (2011). Sublingual vein extraction algorithm based on hyperspectral tongue imaging technology. *Computerized Medical Imaging and Graphics, 35*(3), 179-185.

Li, Q. L., Wang, Y. T., Liu, H. Y., Sun, Z., & Liu, Z. (2010). Tongue fissure extraction and classification using hyperspectral imaging technology. *Applied Optics, 49*(11), 2006-2013.

Li, Q. L., Xue, Y. Q., & Liu, Z. (2008). A novel system for tongue inspection based on hyperspectral imaging system. *Journal of Biomedical Engineering, 25*(2), 368-371.

Li, Q. L., Xue, Y. Q., Wang, J. Y., & Yue, X. Q. (2006). Application of hyperspectral imaging system in tongue analysis of traditional Chinese medicine. *Journal of Infrared and Millimeter Waves, 25*(6), 465-468.

Li, Q. L., Xue, Y. Q., Xiao, G. H., & Zhang, J. F. (2007). New microscopic pushbroom hyperspectral imaging system for application in diabetic retinopathy research. *Journal of Biomedical Optics, 12*(6), 1-4.

Li, W., Zhou, C., & Zhang, Z. (2004, June 15-19). *The segmentation of the body of tongue based on the improved snake algorithm in traditional chinese medicine.* Paper presented at the Proceedings of the 5th World Congress on Intelligent Control and Automation, Hangzhou.

Liu, L. L., & Zhang, D. (2007). Extracting tongue cracks using the wide line detector. In *Medical Biometrics* (Vol. 4901, pp. 49-56): Springer Berlin / Heidelberg.

Liu, L. L., Zhang, D., Kumar, A., & Wu, X. (2008). *Tongue line extraction.* Paper presented at the Pattern Recognition, 2008. ICPR 2008. 19th International Conference on, Tampa, FL.

Liu, Z., Jing-Qi, Y., Tao, Z., & Qun-Lin, T. (2006, 13-16 Aug. 2006). *Tongue Shape Detection Based on B-Spline.* Paper presented at the Machine Learning and Cybernetics, 2006 International Conference on.

Liu, Z., Yan, J. Q., Zhang, D., & Li, Q. L. (2007). Automated tongue segmentation in hyperspectral images for medicine. *Applied Optics, 46*(34), 1-7.

Lukman, S., He, Y. L., & Hui, S. C. (2007). Computational methods for Traditional Chinese Medicine: A survey. *Computer Methods and Programs in Biomedicine, 88*(3), 283-294.

Lun-chien, L., Hou, M. C. c., Ying-ling, C., Chiang, J. Y., & Cheng-chun, H. (2009, 17-19 Oct. 2009). *Automatic Tongue Diagnosis System.* Paper presented at the Biomedical Engineering and Informatics, 2009. BMEI '09. 2nd International Conference on.

Manolakis, D., & Shaw, G. (2002). Detection algorithms for hyperspectral Imaging applications. *Ieee Signal Processing Magazine, 19*(1), 29-43.

Melgani, F., & Bruzzone, L. (2002). Support vector machines for classification of hyperspectral remote-sensing images, *Geoscience and Remote Sensing Symposium, 2002. IGARSS '02. 2002 IEEE International* (Vol. 1, pp. 24-28).

Nenggan, Z., & Zhaohui, W. (2004, 10-13 Oct. 2004). *TCM-SIRD: an integrated aided system for traditional Chinese medicine Sizheng.* Paper presented at the Systems, Man and Cybernetics, 2004 IEEE International Conference on.

Nischik, M., & Forster, C. (1997). Analysis of skin erythema using true color images. *IEEE Trans. Med. Imaging, 16*(6), 711-716.

Ornberg, R. L., Woerner, B. M., & Edwards, D. A. (1999). Analysis of stained objects in histological sections by spectral imaging and differential absorption. *The Journal of Histochemistry & Cytochemistry, 47*(10), 1307-1331.

Pang, B., David, Z., & Wang, K. Q. (2005). Tongue image analysis for appendicitis diagnosis. *Inf. Sci., 175*(3), 160-176.

Pang, B., Wang, K., Zhang, D., & Zhang, F. (2002, 2002). *On automated tongue image segmentation in Chinese medicine.* Paper presented at the Pattern Recognition, 2002. Proceedings. 16th International Conference on.

Pang, B., Zhang, D., & Li, N. M. (2004). Computerized tongue diagnosis based on bayesian networks. *IEEE Trans. On Biomedical Eng., 51*(10), 1803-1810.

Pang, B., Zhang, D., & Wang, K. Q. (2005). The bi-elliptical deformable contour and its application to automated tongue segmentation in chinese medicine. *IEEE Transactions on Medical Imaging, 24*(8), 946-956.

Park, B., Windhama, W. R., Lawrencea, K. C., & Smitha, D. P. (2007). Contaminant Classification of Poultry Hyperspectral Imagery using a Spectral Angle Mapper Algorithm. *Biosystems Engineering, 96*(3), 323-333.

Pham, B. L., & Cai, Y. (2004). *Visualization techniques for tongue analysis in traditional Chinese medicine.* Paper presented at the roceedings of the SPIE.

Ren, H., & Chang, C. (2000). Target-constrained interference-minimized approach to subpixel target detection for hyperspectral images. *Optical Engineering, 39*(12), 3138-3145.

Resmini, R. G. (2004). Hyperspectral/spatial detection of edges (HySPADE): An algorithm for spatial and spectral analysis of hyperspectral information. *Algorithms and Technologies for Multispectral, Hyperspectral, and Ultraspectral Imagery X, 5425*, 433-442.

Shen, L., Wei, B., Cai, Y., Zhang, X., Wang, Y., Chen, J., et al. (2003). Image analysis for tongue characterization. *Chinese Journal of Electronics, 12*(3), 317-323.

Siu Cheung, H., Yulan, H., & Doan Thi Cam, T. (2007, 10-13 Dec. 2007). *Machine learning for tongue diagnosis.* Paper presented at the Information, Communications & Signal Processing, 2007 6th International Conference on.

Somosy, Z., Bognar, G., Thuroczy, G., & Koteles, G. J. (2002). Biological responses of tight junction to ionizing radiation and electromagnetic field exposition. *Cellular and Molecular Biology, 48*(5), 571-575.

Takeichi, M., & Sato, T. (1997). Computerized color analysis of "xue yu" (blood stasis) in the sublingual vein using a new technology. *Am J Chin Med, 25*(2), 213-219.

Thakoor, N., Gao, J., & Jung, S. (2007). Hidden markov model-Based weighted likelihood discriminant for 2-D shape classification. *IEEE Transactions on Image Peocessing, 16*(11), 2707-2719.

Timlin J A, S. M. B., Haaland D M, et al. (2004). Hyperspectral imaging of biological targets: the difference a high resolution spectral dimension and multivariate analysis can make. *IEEE International Symposium on Biomedical Imaging: Macro to Nano, 2*, 1529-1532.

Wang, K. Q., Zhang, D., & Li, N. M. (2001). *Tongue diagnosis based on biometric pattern recognition technology*. Singapore: The World Scientific Publishers.

Wang, S., Wang, P., & Wang, h. (2001). Tongue texture and hepatocirrhosis. *J. Gansu College of TCM, 18*(4), 36-38.

Wang, X., & Zhang, D. (2010). An Optimized Tongue Image Color Correction Scheme. *IEEE Transactions on Information Technology in Biomedicine*, 1355-1364.

Wang, Y. G., Yang, J., & Zhou, Y. (2007). Region partition and feature matching based color recognition of tongue image. *Pattern Recognition Letters, 28*(1), 11-19.

Watsuji, T., Arita, S., Shinohara, S., & Kitade, T. (1999, 1999). *Medical application of fuzzy theory to the diagnostic system of tongue inspection in traditional Chinese medicine.* Paper presented at the Fuzzy Systems Conference Proceedings, 1999. FUZZ-IEEE '99. 1999 IEEE International.

Wenshu, L., Shenning, H., Shuai, W., & Su, X. (2009, 3-5 Nov. 2009). *Towards the objectification of tongue diagnosis: Automatic segmentation of tongue image.* Paper presented at the Industrial Electronics, 2009. IECON '09. 35th Annual Conference of IEEE.

Wu, Z.-z., Zhang, X.-l., Li, Y.-h., Wang, J.-g., & Yang, M. (2008, 12-14 Dec. 2008). *Exploration of tongue coating protein based on proteomics assessment and bioinformatics analysis.* Paper presented at the IT in Medicine and Education, 2008. ITME 2008. IEEE International Symposium on.

Xu, J., Tu, L., Ren, H., & Zhang, Z. (2008, 16-18 May 2008). *A Diagnostic Method Based on Tongue Imaging Morphology.* Paper presented at the Bioinformatics and Biomedical Engineering, 2008. ICBBE 2008. The 2nd International Conference on.

Yan, Z., Wang, K., & Li, N. (2009). Computerized feature quantification of sublingual veins from color sublingual images. *computer methods and programs in biomedicine, 93*(2), 192-205.

Yan, Z., Yu, M., Wang, K., & Li, N. (2008). Sublingual vein segmentation from near infrared sublingual images. *Journal of Computer Aided Design & Computer Graphics 20*(12), 1569-1574.

Yang, C. (2002, 2002). *A novel imaging system for tongue inspection.* Paper presented at the Instrumentation and Measurement Technology Conference, 2002. IMTC/2002. Proceedings of the 19th IEEE.

Yu, S., Yang, J., Wang, Y., & Zhang, Y. (2007, 6-8 July 2007). *Color Active Contour Models Based Tongue Segmentation in Traditional Chinese Medicine.* Paper presented at the Bioinformatics and Biomedical Engineering, 2007. ICBBE 2007. The 1st International Conference on.

Yu, X., Tan, Y., Zhu, Z., Suo, Z., Jin, G., Weng, W., et al. (1994). Study on method of automatic diagnosis of tongue feature in Traditional Chinese Medicine. *Chinese Journal of Biomedical Engineering, 13*(4), 336-344.

Zhang, H. Z., Wang, K. Q., & Jin, X. S. (2005). *SVR based color calibration for tongue image.* Paper presented at the Proceedings of 2005 International Conference on Machine Learning and Cybernetics.

Zhang, H. Z., Wang, K. Q., Zhang, D., Pang, B., & Huang, B. (2005, 2005). *Computer Aided Tongue Diagnosis System.* Paper presented at the Engineering in Medicine and Biology Society, 2005. IEEE-EMBS 2005. 27th Annual International Conference of the.

Zheng, Y. J., Yang, J., Zhou, Y., & Wang, Y. Z. (2006). Color-texture based unsupervised segmentation using JSEG with fuzzy connectedness. *Journal of Systems Engineering and Electronics, 17*(1), 213-219.

Zhou, Y., Shen, L., & Yang, J. (2002). Feature analysis method of tongue image by Chinese medical diagnosis based on image processing. *Infrared and Laser Engineering, 31*(6), 490-494.

Zhou, Y., Shen, L., & Yang, J. (2002). Feature analysis method of tongue image for Chinese medical diagnosis based on image processing. *Infrared Laser Engineering, 31*(6), 490-494.

Zuo, W., Wang, K., Zhang, D., & Zhang, H. (2004, 18-20 Dec. 2004). *Combination of polar edge detection and active contour model for automated tongue segmentation.* Paper presented at the Image and Graphics, 2004. Proceedings. Third International Conference on.

6

Advances in Chinese Medicine Diagnosis: From Traditional Methods to Computational Models

Arthur de Sá Ferreira
Centro Universitário Augusto Motta,
Brazil

1. Introduction

Ancient Chinese medicine practitioners deduced about 5,000 years ago that the exterior appearance of the body was closely related to the functions of the internal organs and viscera. They sought for explanations for this interior-exterior connection by establishing relationships between human beings and Nature. Other natural philosophers also applied such reasoning, *e.g.* Aristotle [384-322 BC], Leonardo Da Vinci [1452-1519], and René Descartes [1596-1650]. Although it is not possible to say that Chinese medicine practitioners were unique in this task, they organized those relationships in a pioneer manner long before their Western counterparts. Chinese and Western physicians were not distinct in their conceptual framework, but their respective medical practices evolved on different cultures and historical contexts. Therefore, it is expected that the advances on medical knowledge represent this cultural divergence.

Many efforts have been made to integrate the ancient, traditional knowledge of Chinese medicine into contemporary, Eastern medical practice. Diagnosis is a key element in this integration of medical systems since it links the patient's needs to the available therapeutic resources. The art of Chinese medicine diagnosis was enriched throughout history but it main traditional aspect remains unchanged: the exclusive use of information available to the naked senses. Clinical information provided by vision, hearing, smelling, and touching is interpreted in a framework of Chinese medicine theories of physiology. No equipment or instrument was developed with specific diagnostic purposes or based on Chinese medicine theories. However, advances in computation and biomedical instruments allowed more powerful analysis of clinical data and quantification of parameters otherwise assessed only in a qualitative fashion. As a consequence, computer models for diagnosis in Chinese medicine were developed and tested in the last few decades and are promising tools in the clinical environment.

This chapter introduces the traditional methods of diagnosis in Chinese medicine and introduces their evolution into computational models. Current methods for validation of computational model by the assessment of their diagnostic accuracy and possible sources of errors are also presented. Finally, perspectives on the issue of computational diagnosis are discussed.

2. Science and art in Chinese medicine diagnosis

Science may be understood as the common sense refinement through a prospective effort to transform sensorial impressions into sequential, logic facts with intra- and inter-experimental relationships subjected to verification and reproducibility at a certain level of confidence. Such relationships should minimize the quantity of basic principles while maximize the explained medical events. Such an organized knowledge has been guiding clinical practice in China since early times and may have interacted with other cultures on a reciprocal manner, either by knowledge transmission or acquisition. Ancient textbooks present extensive details regarding the empirical search for a cause-effect relationship, as well as the necessary training to become a physician. As a matter of fact, Chinese medicine practitioners held distinct positions in old China (Tao, 1953b). Systematization of Chinese medical knowledge allowed the accumulation of "positive" trial-and-error results, the discussion of "negative" results for therapy improvement, and the transmission of medical knowledge. Accordingly, new methods for diagnosis and intervention were developed in consonance with this systematization. In this sense, Chinese medicine is thus composed of scientific knowledge since its wide theoretical framework differentiates it from the popular knowledge.

Such scientific approach of medical theories is also reflected in the diagnostic field. From the historical point-of-view, diagnostic methods probably started with the simple need to answer dichotomous questions, such as "Is the subject dead or alive?". From this starting point, diagnostic methods evolved into more complex methods capable of identification of several constitutional aspects, different aetiologies and their relationships, as well as the differentiation of multiple morbid or comorbid states. Descriptions of prognosis based on the patient's examination reflect this high evolution of diagnostic methods since accurate prognosis depends on accurate diagnosis and extensive theory-based practice.

The main approach to scientific research on Chinese medicine has been to explain the observed phenomena by means of its experimental verification. By doing this, the validity of the Chinese medical knowledge is indirectly assessed by observing physiologic or therapeutic responses to acupuncture or herbs prescriptions. An interesting, alternative approach is to seek for the scientific evidence that corroborate or not data reported by Chinese medicine practitioners - ancient and contemporary ones included. Such an integrative approach is a very attractive strategy for development of robust methods in the diagnostic field.

3. Recognition of morbid states and the concept of pattern

Apparently, the first group of morbid conditions to be recognized were infections. As early as the Chin [221-207 BC] and Han [206 BC-219 AD] dynasties, outbreaks of epidemics led to the differentiation of infections and classification of their symptoms. In sequence, disorders of the digestive system were recognized and also named according to key-symptoms. Neurologic, metabolic, cardiovascular, and ophthalmic disorders are among the other early-recognized conditions (Tao, 1953a). Progressively, other morbid conditions were identified in the field of nutrition, paediatry, otorhinolaryngology, stomatology, dermatology, urologic obstetrics and gynaecology (Tao, 1958a; Tao, 1958b). The recognition of new diseases, as well as the improvement of information regarding manifestations, diagnosis and prognosis were continuous developed until nowadays.

The definition of morbid conditions in Chinese medicine differs from its counterpart in Western medicine. A pattern (or syndrome, *zheng*) is the morbid entity of Chinese medicine and can be derived from any physiologic theory: *Ba-gan, Zang-fu, Liu-jing, Wei-qi Ying-xue, San-jiao, Bing-yin, Qi-xue, Jin-ye, Wu-xing, Jing-luo* (Zaslawki, 2003). A pattern is a set of manifestations that are absent or present depending on individual, social and environmental conditions. This set of manifestations is similar to a "cluster of symptoms" in Western medicine (Dodd et al., 2001). Each pattern presents a wide description of manifestations including its onset, duration, location, progression and severity, collectively known as pattern dynamism (Zaslawki, 2003). Manifestations are not limited to signs and symptoms, but also body characteristics and shape, psychological statuses, personality, emotional conditions, interaction with environmental climate, and behaviours. The term "manifestation profile" describes a subset of all possible manifestations related to the pattern presented by a patient. Hence, different patients may present different manifestation profiles and yet get the same pattern as a diagnosis. As a corollary, the same manifestation profile exhibited by different patients may be related to different patterns.

Several types of patterns are distinguished, namely single, complex and multiple patterns. Single patterns are those related to a unique affected internal system (*zangfu*) or channel (*jingmai*). For instance, *Shen-yin* deficiency and *Gan-xue* deficiency are both single patterns. Complex patterns consist of two or more affected internal systems or channels and often share aetiologies or risk factors, being an example the *Gan-Dan* damp-heat. Multi-patterns are those in which several single patterns are observed due to either to pattern transmission or exposure to multiple aetiologies. For an example of multi-patterns, consider the following transmission, *Shen-yin* deficiency leading to *Gan-yang* rising.

Notice that the concept of pattern is not strictly related to diseases or syndromes in the Western medicine (Lu & Chen, 2009). In contemporary Chinese medicine literature, diseases were assigned to patterns based on matched 'signs and symptoms' to integrate both medical practices (O'Connor & Bensky, 1987; Auteroche & Navailh, 1992; Maciocia, 1996; Ross, 2003). Indeed, the scientific approach has been to assess the pair disease/pattern model. In this context, the same disease may be related to several patterns as well as the same pattern may be observed in several diseases. It is very important to observe this disease/pattern interaction because of the implications to statistical analysis and consequently data interpretation. Very often, a study sample is firstly selected from individuals with disease already diagnosed and secondly is subjected to the traditional Chinese medicine diagnostic procedure. Hence, statistical inference and data interpretation cannot be extrapolated to the overall population - implying limited external validity - but is limited to the disease under investigation.

4. Diagnosis as a pattern differentiation process

Ancient Chinese medicine literature does not to explicitly discuss diagnostic reasoning (Yang & Li, 1993; Luo, 1995; Yang, 2003; Flaws, 2004; Yang & Chase, 2004). Contemporary literature reports that Chinese medicine practitioners apply only the differentiation reasoning for decision-making (Maciocia, 1996; Zaslawki, 2003). The diagnosis in Chinese medicine is obtained through a process named "pattern differentiation" or "syndrome differentiation" (*bian zheng*). In such a process, the practitioner examines the patient to seek for meaningful manifestations that indicate a single, a complex or an even a multi-pattern condition. Recently, Chinese medicine diagnosis started to incorporate other strategies from Western medicine (Zhou & Zhang, 2006; Zhu et al., 2006; N.L. Zhang et al., 2008), such as the deductive-inductive reasoning, tests that confirm a target hypothesis, eliminate an alternative hypothesis, or discriminate among competing ones (McSherry, 1999).

Pattern differentiation is performed in a three-stage process, namely: information gathering, data interpretation, and decision-making:

- Information gathering: refers to the assessment of manifestations present or absent in patients using traditional examination, possibly in coadjutant with contemporary methods. It is highly dependent on the physician's ability to recognize manifestations and to consider those reported by the patient.
- Data interpretation: involves the understanding of the acquired clinical information and its consideration. Also, it encompasses the selection of the best physiologic theory to explain the patient's manifestation profile. If a particular theory does not explain the interaction among manifestations (and possibly patterns), another theory - more general or specific - can be selected in the next stage.
- Decision-making: is the process of identification of a pattern among other possible ones. If it was possible, practitioners should rely on pathognomonic manifestations to perform pattern differentiation. However, not all patterns exhibit such a feature, and many patterns share common manifestations. Moreover, patterns have several manifestations that can be present or not depending on individual constitution and environmental factors.

It is worth notice that pattern differentiation is "always possible" due to the wide concept of manifestation and the diversity of physiologic theories to better differentiate the true pattern (or patterns) from possible ones.

5. Traditional examination methods in Chinese medicine

In the medical diagnostic context, "traditional" refers to methods, knowledge, skills, and beliefs indigenous to different cultures applied to health obtainment, maintenance and restoration. Often, when adopted by different cultures it is termed "alternative" or "complimentary" medicine (WHO, 2008). For information gathering, the traditional methods are still applied nowadays and are essentially similar to those practiced by Western physicians (Peterson et al., 1992).

The traditional Chinese ontology of examination is named "Four Examinations" (*sizhen*). It consists of the sequential application of inspection (*wang*), auscultation and olfaction (*wen*), inquiry (*wen*), and palpation (*qie*) (Tao, 1958a). Several classic authors discussed detailed information regarding this sequence of examination and its impact on diagnostic errors and potential cure rates. For instance, a "superior" Chinese medicine practitioners collect data from patients according to the Four Examinations and interpret those manifestations using medical theories, obtaining a cure rate of 90%; "mediocre" and "inferior" doctors have cure rates of 70-80% and 60% patients, respectively (Yang & Li, 1993; Luo, 1995; Yang, 2003; Flaws, 2004; Yang & Chase, 2004). Recently, it was shown that individual examination methods provide diagnostic accuracies compatible with "inferior doctors" (Ferreira, 2008) and are significantly improved after cumulative application of all Four Examinations (Ferreira, 2009).

According to such ontology, the naked senses are considered sufficient to the trained, skilled practitioner to recognize and label patterns. While elaborated instrumentation was invented and developed for acupuncture and moxibustion treatment - including different types and shapes of needles, moxa presentations - not an instrument was developed for diagnostic purposes. This subjective, personal practice inputs an extremely high dependency in the examiner's knowledge and the applied procedures.

Several contemporary textbooks are devoted to the patient's examination following that ontology and will not be explored here. Some categories worth mention regarding each examination method (Zhou et al., 2004; Ferreira, 2008). Inspection is performed to collect information regarding the patient's: general aspect; face aspect; tongue body, fur, and movement; body constitution; gait; urine and stools aspect. Children under 2-3 years old must have their throat, orifices, finger veins, and *luo* channels inspected (S.C. Wang et al., 2002). Auscultation and olfaction are executed to collect information on the patient's: breath; speech; cough; secretion; and excretions. Inquiry is conducted to observe the patient's preferences; cold and fever; transpiration; head and body; chest and abdomen; pain; excretions; diet and appetite; sense organs; sleep; medical history; habits; and quality of life ("present dignity, past obscurity"). Palpation is performed to identify: painful areas; skin temperature; points; cubital skin; and pulse images.

Some criticism may arise from the sequence of the traditional ontology for examination. As a corollary of the holistic approach of Chinese medicine, the order in which Examination methods are applied does not change the pattern differentiation outcome. Assuming that practitioners always use the Four Examinations and are successful in this task, they conclude their screening procedure with the same manifestation profile no matter the applied order. This must not be confused with the timeline of onset of manifestations because when at screening, the patient presents simultaneously all manifestations. Although each Examination contributes differently for reducing pattern differentiation errors, it seems that the order in which the Four Examinations are used is just a matter of keeping a rigid routine to ensure that every aspect of screening was performed (Ferreira, 2011).

6. Introduction to computational models for pattern differentiation

With the advance in computing techniques and equipment, the pattern differentiation process is properly evolving into a computer-based procedure. The rapid evolution of mathematical methods based on computational algorithms allowed the implementation of diagnostic techniques derived from simple to complex routines. Additionally, study designs, statistical methods for data analysis, and guideline reports are also available for assessment of diagnostic accuracy and epidemiologic performance of automated methods. However, the computerization of Chinese medicine cannot overlook its theoretical foundation since it provides the basis for intervention.

6.1 Attributes of computational models for pattern differentiation

It is not difficult to build computational models for diagnostic purposes - the difficulty lies in making them good and reliable. An idealized pattern differentiation model should perform as a "superior" practitioner or even better. Thus, a computational model of pattern differentiation must present the following attributes:

- Respectful concerning the theoretical framework of Chinese medicine;
- Robust performance across a variety of suitable physiologic theories with minimal computational cost;
- Ability to perform despite having different amounts of manifestations in the manifestation profile;
- Ability to identify exams composed of single, complex and multi-patterns;
- Ability to merge manifestations that correspond to the same pattern;
- Ability to split manifestations that correspond to more than one pattern;
- Ability to decompose multiple patterns despite "noisy" manifestations and biological variability;

- Minimal use of arbitrary thresholds and minimal sensitivity to any required thresholds;
- Multi-pass algorithm to allow classification context to grow iteratively;
- Valid stopping criteria for iterative process;
- Ability to decouple low-assignment rate versus low-error rate trade-off as much as possible;
- Accuracy and completeness of pattern differentiation;
- Ability to supply some measurement of confidence regarding the pattern differentiation results.

6.2 Dataset of computational models for pattern differentiation

Despite the use of different approaches to perform pattern differentiation, some elements are common to those methods, such as the usage of knowledge datasets, training and testing databases, and questionnaires. As far as the manual insertion is the most frequent method applied, some discussion is needed on this topic.

Although many efforts have been made to standardize medical terms, currently there is no standard dataset for patterns and manifestations. In general, datasets have been generated by manual insertion of terms collected from literature (Ferreira, 2008; Ferreira, 2009, Ferreira, 2011) or by data mining algorithms (refer to Lukman et al., 2007 for a revision on mining methods applied to Chinese medicine; Zhou et al., 2010). Patterns on database must be mutually exclusive and collectively exhaustive (Harding, 1996), *i.e.*, for each manifestation there is at least one possible pattern, and there is no pattern without manifestations. Manual insertion leads datasets subjected to common errors of:

- Typography: typos, case-sensitive letters, and medical synonymous;
- Manifestation redundancy: for the same pattern, typing a manifestation twice or more in the same examination method or among different methods regarding the same pattern;
- Pattern label redundancy: typing the same pattern's label twice in the dataset, making such label not unique and possibly with different descriptions;
- Pattern description redundancy: typing the same pattern's description twice in the dataset yet with distinct labels, making their content not mutually exclusive (in this case, both patterns are indeed the same pattern).

The errors described above can be minimized or even eliminated with the use of simple routines for intra-pattern and inter-pattern exploratory analyses using common string search algorithms. It is strongly recommended running such routines for quality control of manually inserted datasets before model validation, especially when dealing with large datasets or even multiple datasets simultaneously. For instance, intra-pattern consistency can be obtained by excluding any repetitions of manifestations in the same examination method, as well as among the Four Examinations describing the respective pattern (Ferreira, 2008). Inter-pattern consistency can be obtained by ensuring that two patterns were not described with the same complete manifestation profile (Ferreira, 2008; Ferreira, 2009). Analysis of dual pattern similarity by means of the Jaccard coefficient (Jaccard, 1901) and associated confidence interval (Real, 1999) is an alternative to check for pattern redundancy (Ferreira, 2011). The use of a controlled vocabulary from dataset avoids the typos, eliminates language ambiguity and ensures that every one is using the same terms to mean the same attribute which limits the use of synonymous.

7. Computational models for pattern differentiation

The application of objective rules for pattern differentiation may help diminish diagnosis variability (G.G. Zhang et al., 2005; G.G. Zhang et al., 2008) dependent on the practitioner's expertise. A large amount of computational methods have been published, too many to list them all. Some of them were developed and tested against simulated and real cases, in different disease models, and are discussed here. In chronological sequence, this work includes the Traditional Chinese Medicine *Sizheng* Integrated Recorder and Aided Syndrome Differentiator (TCM-SIRD), modified Greedy Bayesian Pattern Search algorithm (GBPS*), Information Management System of Traditional Chinese Medicine Syndrome Project based on Prior Knowledge Support Vector Machine (P-SVM), Chinese Medical Diagnostic System (CMDS), Pattern Differentiation Algorithm (PDA), and Multi-Label k-Nearest Neighbour (ML-kNN).

7.1 Traditional Chinese Medicine *Sizheng* Integrated Recorder and Aided Syndrome Differentiator (TCM-SIRD)

Zheng and Wu (2004) developed the Traditional Chinese Medicine *Sizheng* Integrated Recorder and Aided Syndrome Differentiator (TCM-SIRD). This system performs information gathering based on sensors (image, pulse and odor signal acquisition) and text information. A computational routine, namely "Integrated *Sizheng* Information Application", merges the data transferred from sensors and provides assistant diagnosis service by means of data interpretation. The provided output (such as type of tongue coating, face image, and pulse) is used to form a primary differentiation of syndromes by the "*Sizheng* Expert Decision", the decision-making modulus based on rules extracted from Chinese medicine experts' experience. The objective rules extracted from expert practitioners were not described, neither their computational implementation.
The authors described methods to be implemented for an objective assessment of diagnostic with description of a single test case. Although the model for pattern differentiation was not detailed described, the authors advocated the use of the Four Examinations. No description was given on how the information was processed for diagnosis. No result regarding its diagnostic accuracy was reported.

7.2 Modified Greedy Bayesian Pattern Search algorithm (GBPS*)

X. Wang et al. (2004) designed a self-learning expert system with a novel hybrid learning algorithm based on Bayesian networks, called the modified greedy Bayesian pattern search algorithm (GBPS*). The proposed pattern differentiation model was based on the GBPS algorithm (Spirtes & Meek, 1995) with a modified version in the search procedure algorithm. The maximum accuracy of 88% obtained for pattern differentiation was estimated by pseudo-random generation of a sample. The authors discussed the high dimensionality of patient instances represented by multiple manifestations and diagnostic hypotheses. Their results suggested the use of most frequent attributes to reduce such dimensionality and consequently increase diagnostic accuracy.
The authors developed based on the "united system of syndrome differentiation" characterized by two characteristics. The first characteristic, the "key elements for syndrome differentiation", was abstracted from keywords in medical theories and grouped in two categories (the place where diseases occur; and the pathological state of the body or possible causes that make disease break out). As each key element usually exhibits a variable

strength of association to manifestations, the pattern identification could be performed according to whether the key element is present or not. The second characteristic, the "standard syndrome-name database," was used to solve the problem that a pattern could be assigned with different labels by different practitioners. In the database, a standard pattern label includes at least one of the key elements described above. A dataset of 800 cases from real patients was used to train the Bayesian classifier.

The complete system for pattern differentiation is designed in modulus and its architecture consists of three parts: (1) input of the system, thereof one is sample database with attributes of symptoms and key elements, the other two are key-elements database and database of clinical observations to be diagnosed; (2) Analysis and diagnosis part, that is, the kernel part of the system, including: module for variable selection, module for discovering dependency relationship, module for learning classifiers, module for syndrome differentiation, module for mining frequent sets among key elements, and module for modification by experts; and (3) user interface, through which users and the system can interact with each other.

The computational model for pattern differentiation proceeds in two phases and its pseudo-code was provided (X. Wang et al., 2004). During the first phase, the key elements present by a patient are identified. The second phase searches the standard syndrome-name database, inquiring whether the corresponding patterns consist of these identified key elements. The algorithm considers all the attributes (including manifestations, key elements and patterns) as Boolean variables that take only two values: absent and present. The module for syndrome differentiation used the learned classifier to compute the posterior probability of every key element with Bayes theorem, and output those elements whose probability exceeds the threshold set by experts. Then the module queries and outputs the names of those patterns containing these key elements from standard pattern-name database. Furthermore, the module computes occurrence probability of each pattern by multiplying the probabilities of its corresponding key elements, under the assumption that these key elements are independent. Finally, the module selects the patterns with the probability excess diagnosis threshold.

7.3 Information Management System of Traditional Chinese Medicine Syndrome Project based on Prior Knowledge Support Vector Machine (P-SVM)

Yang et al. (2005) developed the Information Management System of Traditional Chinese Medicine Syndrome Project based on Prior Knowledge Support Vector Machine (P-SVM). SVM aims to process training and generalization with limited information provided by the sample data set without consideration of knowledge from application background. In the framework of limited sample data set learning, SVM makes maximum use of the information provided by sample data set theoretically regardless the application related knowledge. The authors reported an accuracy rate of 95% with the trained P-SVM to classify a sample set of 2,000 simulated records.

The general principle of the method is described here, and its pseudo-code was provided (Yang et al., 2005). A pattern dataset is used to train and test the P-SVM model. The test procedure consists of: a) generation of an expert knowledge dataset; b) description of the expert knowledge as rules to train the dataset to create the scale of confidence values; c) input data with confidence values to the Platt's Sequential Minimal Optimization (P-SMO) algorithm; d) comparison of the accuracy rates under different amount of training samples. The pattern dataset included the literature from 1978 to 2004 with approximately 400,000 entries and its ontology was organized with the entries: author, origin, title, subject heading, subheading, key word, and abstract. In the classification system of SVM with prior knowledge, the classifier will learn the traits of the certain thematic information from the corresponding prior knowledge. Therefore, based on the prior knowledge, the classifier is able to find out the appropriate literary information from the massive data.

No description of how the cases were simulated is available; thus, it is not possible to repeat the simulation procedure and to compare accuracy results. Moreover, the P-SVM theory was not discussed in light of the mode-of-thinking of Chinese medicine experts.

7.4 Chinese Medical Diagnostic System (CMDS)

Huang and Chen (2007) developed the Chinese Medical Diagnostic System (CMDS) for pattern differentiation of diseases related to the digestive system. It uses a Web interface and expert system technology in diagnosing 50 types of digestive system diseases. The authors compared the diagnosis of 20 simulated cases made by CMDS and diagnosticians and found the results satisfactory; however, they did not report either simulation procedures or statistical validity. The authors also stated that the Four Examinations were necessary for achieving a correct diagnosis. The authors reported 'high reliable and accurate diagnostic capabilities' in 95% of 50 simulated cases without any description of either how cases were simulated or possible sources and types of error.

The CMDs departed from an ontology-based model, in which the proposed ontology was derived from the traditional one but focused on digestive diseases and patterns. The whole system is composed by three main components: a) Java Expert System Shell (JESS); b) Database set; and c) knowledge extractor. The routine for pattern differentiation in depicted in the inference engine modulus of the JESS and automatically matches facts (user's entries) against patterns and concludes which rules are fired in CMDS. Two databases (general and knowledge databases) are used to store all information and rules necessary for pattern differentiation, respectively.

7.5 Pattern Differentiation Algorithm (PDA)

Ferreira (2008) proposed the pattern differentiation algorithm (PDA) based on an objective criterion developed to account for pattern holism (Guang, 2001). A second criterion was proposed and provided a significant increase in diagnostic accuracy of the model, being up to 94.7%(sensitivity = 89.8%; specificity = 99.5%) with the Four Examinations for *Zangfu* patterns (Ferreira, 2009). This method allowed testing the impact of different combinations of the Four Examinations and the amount of available information presented by patients on PDA's statistical performance. Also, it's associated method of model validation uncovered types of diagnostic errors otherwise not assessed by other computational models (Ferreira, 2011). Clinically, PDA was applied to patients with arterial hypertension and help understand that *Zangfu* patterns associated to this disease are indeed evidence of the progression of target-organ damage (Luiz et al., 2011).

PDA works in a three-stage schema and its pseudo-code was provided elsewhere (Ferreira, 2009). The first stage - data collection and dataset search - uses the data entry from patient's exam to search for free terms and quoted phrases, *e.g.*, *headache* and *"headache"*. The former term recalls patterns with *headache* within its manifestations profile (*ocular headache, occipital headache,* etc.); the latter term recalls patterns with the exact term. Combinatorial procedure (Zuzek et al., 2000) was used after data collection because the diagnosis does not depend on the sequence of the results obtained during the exam (Wolff, 2006). Manifestations were described as specifically as possible including onset ("palpitation in the morning", "palpitation in the evening"), duration ("acute headache", "chronic headache"), location ("occipital headache", "ocular headache") and severity ("dry tongue", "slight moist tongue", "moist tongue"), as well as any other characteristic that may be necessary to allow the pattern differentiation. Manifestations that co-occur in two or more patterns were assigned with the same term to increase the accuracy of string search algorithm.

At the second stage - selection of candidate patterns - a pattern is considered as a 'candidate' if it presents at least one manifestation collected at the exam. Patterns with no manifestations recognized were not used for further analysis. The "strength" of such indication of the candidate pattern is calculated as an objective criterion $F_{\%,K}$. This is an important stage since it recalls any possibility ($F_{\%,K}>0$) within the dataset and increases the sensitivity of the algorithm. Since patterns maybe described by different quantities of manifestations, the available information must be normalized to allow comparison among them and hence was used as a second objective criterion, $N_{\%,K}$,. It is expected that the occurrence of a successful pattern differentiation increases with decreasing $F_{\%,K}$. It is also expected that the occurrence of a successful pattern differentiation increases with increasing $N_{\%,K}$. However, as the accuracy of a diagnostic test is expected to decrease with either lower or higher cutoff values, it is appropriate to subtract a cutoff values from $N_{\%,K}$ to dislocate the accuracy curve to its optimum operating point. As such, the maximum accuracy is associated with the minimum $N_{\%\text{-}cutoff,K}$. Hence, the candidate patterns simultaneously ranked in descending order of $F_{\%,K}$ and ascending order of $N_{\%\text{-}cutoff,K}$ represent a list of diagnostic hypotheses.

The last stage - pattern differentiation - identifies the diagnosis. The diagnostic algorithm receives the manifestation profile and outputs for each tested profile: a) the identified diagnosis; b) the list of diagnostic hypotheses. Pattern differentiation is considered successful in either of two situations: 1) if PDA founds a unique diagnostic hypothesis that explains simultaneously all collected manifestations, *i.e.* $F_{\%,K}$=100%; or 2) if there is one pattern among all diagnostic hypotheses with a highest, unique $F_{\%,K}$ value and lowest, unique $N_{\%\text{-}cutoff,K}$ value. Otherwise, if multiple diagnostic hypothesis were found with equal values of $F_{\%,K}$ and not unique values of $N_{\%,K}$ the procedure is considered unsuccessful since differentiation among competing patterns was not possible. In this case, physicians have access to the diagnostic hypotheses list and may want to revise the collected manifestations, continue examination of the patient to search for other manifestations, replace the collected symptoms/signs with more specific ones, or even subjectively chose a pattern.

PDA's average time for pattern differentiation of each case with the Four Examinations is estimated in less than 0.1s, which is suitable for clinical applications. There is no need to train PDA, which is a mathematical process already subject to bias. PDA's method is simple, and both criteria can be calculated even manually by a Chinese medicine practitioner (for a low number of candidate patterns). It's reasoning is entirely based on the actual process executed by Chinese medicine experts and thus reduces the error in data collection and analysis. PDA is more stable than other learning algorithms because the final diagnosis does not depend on the initial guess or sequence of manifestations used during the learning phase (Ferreira, 2009).

However, PDA is dependent on the pattern dataset. PDA's dataset was built in a form of open base, in which new information can be added (or modified) to the knowledge database

to increase statistical performance of the criterion. As a corollary, the proposed methodology relies on human experts, not only to select the knowledge, but also to provide the database organization. To reduce the implications of the manual insertion of information, computational routines for inter-pattern and intra-pattern consistency were implemented.
The major limitation of PDA is that it was tested only for *Zangfu* single patterns (Ferreira, 2008; Ferreira, 2009; Ferreira, 2011). Such case is the simplest one found in clinical practice for *Zangfu* patterns since the pathological process just begun to promote changes in homeostasis. The same subject may present several patterns simultaneously that are not mutually exclusive. Additionally, common etiologies and pattern transmissions among *Zangfu* are contributing factors to limit the model's performance. Finally, other theories are often used to perform diagnosis and were not yet evaluated (Maciocia, 1996).

7.6 Multi-Label k-Nearest Neighbour (ML-kNN)

Liu et al. (2010) obtained up to 78% accuracy using only the Inquiry method (n=185 manifestations) for identification of multi-patterns (based on 6 ZFSPs) related to coronary heart disease obtained from real cases. The pseudo-code of the ML-kNN was provided by the authors.
The kNN is an algorithm that searches for the nearest point in a training data set. This theory regards an instance as a point in synthesis space; thus, the label of a test instance is probably similar to those of several nearest points. The data set for pattern differentiation of coronary heart disease belongs to multi-label; whereas kNN only processes single label data sets, so the collected data set should be split into many groups of single label to be calculated. In the multi-label data, there is much relationship among each label, so simple splitting inevitably result in data loss. For this reason, multi-label learning algorithms are developed so as to better reveal the correlation of the labels, of which multi-label kNN (ML-kNN) is a popular technique. ML-kNN is a lazy multi-label learning algorithm developed on the basis of kNN. Based on the theory of kNN, ML-kNN aims to find k nearest instances for each test instance. In ML- kNN, the labels of test instances are judged directly by nearest instances, which is different from kNN.

8. Validation of computational models for diagnosis in Chinese medicine

For the model to be useful, expert practitioners must have confidence in the results and predictions that are inferred from it. Verifying or validating the model can provide such confidence. In principle, model validation is done by comparing the model's behaviour with the patient's and evaluating the difference. In the diagnostic field, the computational model is compared to either a gold-standard or a reference-standard method.

8.1 Model validation with "gold-standard" and "reference-standard"

The main issue related to diagnostic accuracy tests it he need for a "gold-standard" method or at least a "reference-standard" method to compare the results obtained with the model being tested. The gold-standard method for diagnosis is the one that provides the *true* health status of a person while the reference-standard method for diagnosis is the one that provide the health status *closest to the true one*. Obviously, gold-standard methods are preferred for model validation and assessment of a model's diagnostic accuracy. However, it is almost impossible to test clinical diagnostic models with gold-standard methods since the true health status is unknown a priori. In this case, a diagnostic model with known statistical properties is applied to obtain a result that is used as the reference-standard.

Patterns identified by a panel of expert Chinese medicine practitioners has been used as the standard for diagnostic accuracy tests of computational models using data from population samples (Zhou & Zhang, 2006; Zhu et al., 2006; N.L. Zhang et al., 2008). This method presents a major drawback since the real diagnosis is not known and samples may be biased (hospital patients, community subjects, etc.). Moreover, the agreement in diagnosis among practitioners may be low (31.7%; 27.5–35%) (G.G. Zhang et al., 2005), despite some improvement after training (73%; 64.3–85.7%) (G.G. Zhang et al., 2008). The Standards for Reporting Interventions in Controlled Trials of Acupuncture (STRICTA) (MacPherson et al., 2010) recommend that the experience of Chinese medicine practitioners should be reported in clinical studies because such experience may influence diagnosis. As such, new diagnostic tests should not be compared to diagnoses made by Chinese medicine practitioners but with methods that guarantee correct diagnosis.

For the determination of the accuracy of Chinese medicine diagnostic tests, a large number of patients with possible combinations of the manifestations for each pattern must be generated. Thus, it is virtually impossible to estimate the diagnostic accuracy without computer methods. Stochastic simulation models have been used for research in health sciences. A well-known simulation method is the Monte Carlo (Metropolis & Ulam, 1949), in which the basic idea is to stochastically generate examples of a numerical variable and then evaluate the outcome of the model under evaluation. With stochastic methods, simulated patients can have their health status characterized by a computational model. The simulation of cases fixes both issues by randomly selecting manifestations only from the selected single pattern (Ferreira, 2009). Stochastic method allows a focus on the properties of manifestation profiles instead of individual manifestations. This procedure generates a large number of examples of any given pattern (stochastic process) and then examines the relative proportion of successes of the diagnostic test (deterministic process). Some modifications of the original Monte Carlo method are needed to enable stochastic methods to process nominal variables. Because cases are simulated from all possible manifestations of each pattern in the dataset, the output of the computational model can be compared to the actual name of the simulated pattern in the dataset. Thus, simulation of cases can be considered as a gold-standard method. Moreover, patient simulation models can be composed of independent algorithmic codes (i.e., there is no code sharing), so the results of the identification are blinded to the simulation parameters.

Currently, the computational model for simulating patients and testing diagnostic accuracy is the Manifestation Profile Simulation Algorithm (MPSA) (Ferreira, 2008; Ferreira, 2009, Ferreira, 2011). MPSA generates the study population according to different strategies to create case (true positive) and control (true negative) groups, as well as a proposal for identifying and handling missing cases. The inclusion criterion is the simulation of cases representing a single pattern in the knowledge dataset. For simulation purposes, MPSA assumes that the probability of each manifestation in the general population is given from previous studies or, if unknown, it is suggested to follow a uniform distribution (Ferreira, 2009). The comparison between the simulated pattern and the identified diagnosis yields the binary classification of the proposed method for pattern differentiation.

In MPSA, true positive (TP) cases of a pattern K are simulated by selecting from the dataset a random quantity of manifestations $N_{R,K}$. Each sorted manifestation is excluded from the set of possible manifestations to prevent multiple occurrences of the same manifestation at the respective simulated case. This iterative process continued until the $N_{R,K}$ manifestations were sorted to generate the manifestation profile. To obtain a true negative (TN) control for the same pattern *K*, two alternatives were proposed. In the first alternative, this respective pattern *K* is removed from the dataset and the same quantity $N_{R,K}$ is selected from the entire dataset and respective examination methods (Ferreira, 2008; Ferreira, 2009). The second alternative is to sort $N_{R,K}$ manifestations from another pattern pseudo-randomly chosen in the dataset after exclusion of pattern *K* (Ferreira, 2011). In both alternatives, the procedure allows a quantitative pair-wise comparison between TP and TN profiles with respect to the available information for pattern K, $N_{\%,K}$. Although the TP pattern was removed from the dataset, its manifestations that co-occur in other patterns are still present and could be selected to compose a TN manifestation profile. Since patterns may not present manifestations for some of the examination methods, empty manifestation profiles related to these examination methods represent missing cases and were excluded from analysis.

Despite the main advantage of knowing a priori the true pattern and methodological blinding, some limitations need to be mentioned. Manifestations may be sampled multiple times within the same run, resulting in less variation of manifestations profile than it would be expected to see in real patients. Also, manifestations may not be chosen at all, resulting in not tested data. However, large simulated samples from the dataset diminished these limitations (Ferreira, 2008). To assess the quality of the simulated cases and controls, a routine can be implemented to check if all manifestations were used for simulation of manifestations profiles. The algorithm performs a 'reverse engineering' by recreating the dataset from all simulated true positive cases. The algorithm searched among all manifestation profiles simulated for each pattern and grouped the manifestations present at least once among the simulated cases into a temporary dataset. After comparison with the original dataset, the algorithm reports whether the patterns that were completely simulated (*i.e.* all manifestations were used for analysis), partially simulated and not used for simulation (Ferreira, 2011).

8.2 Detection and classification problems

In general, the diagnostic process is designed to detect if the subject is healthy or ill. In this case, two groups of subjects with known true conditions are used: a group of individuals in which the condition to be tested is truly present; and a group o individuals in which the condition to be tested is truly absent. Adapted to Chinese medicine framework, a "healthy pattern" diagnosis must be described in the same manner as the "ill" patterns. For instance, the "liver-blood deficiency" pattern should have the mutually exclusive counterpart "liver-blood healthy" pattern. The description of such health-related patterns is possible because pattern differentiation process is not limited to assessing presence/absence of manifestations (e.g. asymptomatic individuals may be also have their patterns identified). A completely healthy person will present all healthy patterns simultaneously. However, in clinical practice it is difficult to find a patient that is completely healthy and thus the pattern differentiation process must be applied to patients. In this case, the diagnostic model must recognize the underlying pattern (or patterns) and not the healthy or ill statuses.

8.3 Sample sizes, participant recruitment and sampling

A important issue in diagnostic accuracy studies is the sample sizes determination, which can be estimated based on equations derived for detecting differences in accuracy tests using receiver operating characteristic (ROC) curves (Hanley & McNeil, 1982). For calculations, it is necessary the expected difference in accuracy between the reference and the index test, the level of significance (usually α=5%, $Z\alpha$=1.645, one-sided), and the power of the test (usually β=90%, $Z\beta$=1.28). The equation designed to real cases can be used in simulated ones provided that the absolute consistency between original and recreated datasets is proved as described before. This is an important issue related to the quality control in this study and should not be omitted in other simulations studies were pattern differentiation outcomes are assessed (Ferreira, 2011).

8.4 Estimating the diagnostic accuracy of a diagnostic model

Diagnostic models present domains of validity, *i.e.* they should not be used outside the validation scope since there is no estimation concerning its performance. The implications range from underestimation to overestimation of the model's diagnostic accuracy. The Standards for Reporting of Diagnostic Accuracy (STARD) (Bossuyt et al., 2003) summarized the necessary steps for conducting scientific works to determine diagnostic accuracy of models. Although not specified in the STARD, such methodology can be also be adopted by studies in which computational models perform diagnosis, even in case of simulated patients. The validity of a new diagnostic model is obtained by comparison of the new model's results with the actual result. However, very often the actual value is not known most commonly due to absence of gold-standard diagnostic methods.
Accuracy, sensitivity, specificity, positive and negative predictive values are the most common measures of a model's performance. Accuracy is defined as the proportion of true results in the population. Sensitivity is the probability that the test is positive given that the patient is sick (Altman & Bland, 1994a), while specificity is the probability that the test is negative given that the patient is not sick (Altman & Bland, 1994a). Positive and negative predictive values are proportions of true positives and true negatives out of all positive results, respectively (Altman & Bland, 1994b). All those estimators are obtained from 2×2 confusion matrices (Table 1) made from classification of simulated and identified diagnosis (Jekel, 1999; Altman & Bland, 1994a; Altman & Blend, 1994b). Departing from Table 1 and adapting the epidemiological concepts to Chinese medicine framework, computational models can be evaluated with estimations of:

		Gold-standard test result	
		Simulated pattern (Case)	Other pattern (Control)
New test result	Identified pattern	True positive (TP)	False positive (FP)
	Other pattern	False negative (FN)	True negative (TN)

Table 1. Confusion 2×2 matrix for assessment of diagnostic accuracy between the reference test and pattern differentiation algorithm.

a. Accuracy: proportion of successful pattern differentiation (true results) in the population (equation 1). Diagnostic accuracy indicates the total sum of corrected assigned cases.

$$Accuracy = \frac{TP+TN}{TP+FN+TN+FP} \times 100\%; \qquad (1)$$

b. Sensitivity: proportion of successful pattern differentiations correctly predicted by PDA in cases (equation 2).

$$Sensitivity = \frac{TP}{TP + FN} \times 100\%; \qquad (2)$$

c. Specificity: proportion of successful pattern differentiations correctly predicted by PDA in controls (equation 3);

$$Specificity = \frac{TN}{TN + FP} \times 100\%; \qquad (3)$$

d. Negative predictive values: proportion of unsuccessful pattern differentiation correctly predicted by PDA (equation 4).

$$Negative \quad predictive \quad value = \frac{TN}{TN + FN} \times 100\%; \qquad (4)$$

e. Positive predictive values: proportion of successful pattern differentiation correctly predicted by PDA (equation 5).

$$Positive \quad predictive \quad value = \frac{TP}{TP + FP} \times 100\%. \qquad (5)$$

ROC plots are used to visualize and estimate accuracy of the model's classification. Those estimators are readily available from 2x2 crosstabs obtained from simultaneous classification of the results regarding the "gold-standard" and the new model under evaluation. In ROC plots, the smallest cutoff value is the minimum observed test value minus 1, and the largest cutoff value is the maximum observed test value plus 1. All the other tested cutoff values were the averages of two consecutive ordered observed test values (Hanley & McNeil, 1982; Hanley & McNeil, 1983; Altman & Bland, 1994c).

8.5 Comparing diagnostic accuracy of two computational models

Consider now the situation where two computational models can be used. It is of interest to select the best model in terms of diagnostic accuracy. Such a comparison can be performed based on a pair of 2×2 confusion matrices (Table 2) made from classification of simulated and identified diagnosis simultaneously by the two computational models.

	True negative				True positive		
	Model 1	-	+		Model 1	+	-
Model 2	-	A	B	Model 2	+	a	b
	+	C	D		-	c	d

Table 2. Confusion 2×2 matrices for comparison of binomial proportions between the two diagnostic tests. (+) and (-) indicate positive and negative test results respectively. B is the number of TN cases classified correctly by test 2 and falsely by test 1 and conversely for C cases and analogously for the TP group.

The 95% confidence interval (95%CI) for the binomial proportions p (accuracy, sensitivity, specificity, negative predictive value, positive predictive value; equations 1-5) can be calculated with Wilson's method (Agresti & Coull, 1998). If both models are to be evaluated on the same samples of TP and TN cases, an adaptation of McNemar's test for correlated proportions is applied (Linnet & Brandt, 1986). The TP and the TN profiles are divided into four parts according to their test responses (Table 2). Estimations related to ROC curves (AUC and respective 95%CI) can be obtained with the nonparametric Wilcoxon statistic (Hanley & McNeil, 1982; Hanley & McNeil, 1983).

Since the Four Examinations provide the basic ontology for pattern differentiation, it is of interest to study the partial contribution of each Examination as well as their cumulative, sequential application. Hence, the diagnostic accuracy may be studied in terms of the following sets of the Four Examinations:

1. Inspection;
2. Auscultation & Olfaction;
3. Inquiry;
4. Palpation;
5. Inspection, Auscultation & Olfaction;
6. Inspection, Auscultation & Olfaction, Inquiry;
7. Inspection, Auscultation & Olfaction, Inquiry, Palpation.

Indeed, as manifestations are closely related to the interdependent internal organs, combined Examination methods are preferable since they cover several forms of presentation of the same pattern.

8.6 Recognition of diagnostic errors in pattern differentiation

All models have a certain domain of validity. This may determine how exactly they are able to describe the system's behavior. It is hazardous to use a model outside the area it has been validated for. Reports of errors for Chinese medicine practitioners are available from ancient literature (Yang & Li, 1993; Luo, 1995; Yang, 2003; Flaws, 2004; Yang & Chase, 2004) including non-skilled practice, misdiagnosis and mistreatment; however, little contemporary literature is available on this subject. Evidence shows that subjectivity of manifestations or limited detection of clinical features is the major causes of unreliable pattern differentiation made by Chinese medicine practitioners (Kim et al., 2008; O'Brien et al., 2009). While diagnostic errors can never be eliminated, they can be minimised through understanding factors related to the pattern differentiation process.

Recognition of factors related to the performance of diagnostic methods is relevant to the development of reliable methods that can be implemented for clinical and research purposes. The first limitation to pattern differentiation algorithms is that the user must possess a certain level of knowledge to discriminate or interpret the patient's complains (Harding, 1996). Therefore, an implicit assumption to all current computational models is that the patients are capable of reporting their symptoms and that the Chinese medicine practitioners are able to correctly identify manifestations.

Pattern similarity is intrinsic to Chinese medical knowledge. Pattern similarity introduces errors in the pattern differentiation process, as the patient's true pattern may not be properly assigned. Dual pattern similarity has moderate, statistically significant effect on pattern differentiation outcome but cumulative application of the Four Examinations progressively reduces the strength of significant association between pattern similarity and diagnostic errors (Ferreira, 2011).

Currently three pattern differentiation outcomes can be distinguished, namely (a) identification of the true pattern (correct diagnosis), (b) identification of a pattern that is not the true pattern (misdiagnosis) and (c) no identification of pattern at all (undiagnosis). For discrimination of those types of diagnostic errors, 2x3 crosstabs (Table 3) are used to differentiate among correct diagnosis, misdiagnosis and undiagnosis.

		Gold-standard test result	
		Simulated pattern (Case)	Other pattern (Control)
New test result	Identified pattern	Correct (TP)	Erroneous (FP)
	Other pattern	Erroneous (FN)	Correct (TN)
	No pattern identified	Absent	Absent

Table 3. Crosstabs (2x3) for investigation of diagnostic errors of computational models.

The distinction of error types in this study is possible if the manifestation profiles of true negative controls are any other true pattern that was not its true positive counterpart, and not just random manifestations from all patterns in dataset as in other studies. This modification expands the interpretation of false negative cases from one wide option ('it can be any other pattern, no pattern at all, or it was not possible to uniquely identify any pattern K') into two separate options ('it is pattern *K'* or 'it was not possible to uniquely identify any pattern in dataset'). With this true condition made known a priori it is possible to distinguish misidentification from no identification among unsuccessful outcomes (Ferreira, 2011).

9. Future directions

Although validated diagnostic models are available, several issues limit their application in patient care. For instance, almost all computational models deal with single patterns - a condition rarely seen in clinical practice - or a single disease. Complex and multiple patterns present additional difficulties in the diagnostic task since there are several combinations of two or more patterns that could result in the same diagnosis. Multiple patterns decomposition is then an open field of research with direct clinical applications and should be investigated.

Standardization of treatment prescription is possible since well-defined, consistent diagnosis can be achieved with computational models. Current trends focus in computer-aid to perform diagnosis and treatment. It is believed that the combination of traditional methods and modern resources may improve the efficacy of Chinese medicine intervention.

Suggested topics for future research on computational models for pattern differentiation:

- Construction of an internationally available Chinese medicine ontology and web-based knowledge dataset with patterns and manifestations.
- Use of qualitative, "fuzzy-like" scales developed in Eastern medicine. Ex.: tongue fur.
- Discovery of which subsets of manifestations lead to a more accurate diagnosis Determination of the distribution of manifestations in each pattern (and patterns in the dataset) to improve the simulation of manifestation profiles.
- Incorporation of common etiologies and pattern transmissions into computational models to extend its application in general clinical practice.

10. References

Agresti, A.; & Coull, B.A. Approximate is better than "exact" for interval estimation of binomial proportions. *The American Statistician*, Vol. 52, No. 2, (May 1998), (119-126), ISSN 0003-1305.

Altman, D.G.; & Bland, J.M. Diagnostic tests 1: Sensitivity and Specificity. *British Medical Journal*, Vol. 308, (June 1994a), (1552), ISSN 0959-535X.

Altman, D.G.; & Bland, J.M. Diagnostic tests 2: predictive values. *British Medical Journal*, Vol. 309 (July 1994b), (102), ISSN 0959-535X.

Altman, D.G.; & Bland, J.M. Diagnostic tests 3: receiver operating characteristic plots. *British Medical Journal*, Vol. 309 (July 1994c), (188), ISSN 0959-535X.

Auteroche, B.; Navailh, P. (1992). *O Diagnóstico na Medicina Chinesa*. Andrei, ISBN 978-85-747-6070-6, São Paulo, Brazil.

Bossuyt, P.M.; Reitsma. J.B.; Bruns, D.E.; Gatsonis, C.A.; Glasziou, P.P.; Irwig, L.M.; Moher, D.; Rennie, D.; de Vet, H.C.W.; & Lijmer, J.G. The STARD statement for reporting studies of diagnostic accuracy: explanation and elaboration. *Annals of Internal Medicine*, Vol. 138, No 1, (January 2003), (W1-W12), ISSN 0003-4819.

Dodd, M.; Janson, S.; Facione, N.; Faucett, J.; Froelicher, E.S.; Humphreys, J.; Lee, K.; Miaskowski, C.; Puntillo, K.; Rankin, S.; & Taylor, D. Advancing the science of symptom management. *Journal of Advanced Nursing*, Vol. 33, No. 5, (March 2001), (668-676), ISSN 0309-2402.

Ferreira, Ade. S. Statistical validation of strategies for Zang-Fu single pattern differentiation. *Zhong Xi Yi Jie He Xue Bao*, Vol. 6, No. 11, (November 2008), (1109-1116), ISSN 1672-1977.

Ferreira, A.S. Diagnostic accuracy of pattern differentiation algorithm based on traditional Chinese medicine theory: a stochastic simulation study. *Chinese Medicine*, Vol. 4, (December 2009), (24), ISSN 1749-8546.

Ferreira, A.S. Misdiagnosis and undiagnosis due to pattern similarity in Chinese medicine: a stochastic simulation study using pattern differentiation algorithm. *Chinese Medicine*, Vol. 6, (January 2011), (1), ISSN 1749-8546.

Flaws, B. (translator). (2004) *Nán Jīng (The Classic of Difficulties)*. Blue Poppy Press, ISBN 1-891845-07-1, Denver, United States of America.

Guang, J.Y. The mode of thinking in Chinese clinical medicine: characteristics, steps and forms. *Clinical Acupuncture and Oriental Medicine*, Vol. 2, No. 1, (March 2001), (23-28), ISSN 1461-1449.

Hanley, J.A.; & McNeil, B.J. The meaning and use of the area under a receiver operating characteristic (ROC) curve. *Radiology*, Vol. 143, (April 1982), (29-36), ISSN 0033-8419.

Hanley, J.A.; & McNeil, B.J. A method of comparing the areas under receiver operating characteristic curves derived from the same cases. *Radiology*, Vol. 148, (September 1983), (839-843), ISSN 0033-8419.

Harding, W.T. Compilers and Knowledge Dictionaries for Expert Systems: Inference Engines of the Future. *Expert Systems with Applications*, Vol. 10, No. 1, (1996), (91-98), ISSN 0957-4174.

Huang, M.J.; & Chen, M.Y. Integrated design of the intelligent web-based Chinese Medical Diagnostic System (CMDS): systematic development for digestive health. *Expert Systems with Application*, Vol. 32, No. 2, (February 2007), (658-673), ISSN 0957-4174.

Jaccard, P. Étude comparative de la distribution florale dans une portion des Alpes et des Jura. *Bulletin del la Société Vaudoise des Sciences Naturelles*, Vol. 37, (1901), (547-579).

Jekel, J.F.; Elmore, J.G.; & Katz, D.L. (1999). *Epidemiologia, Bioestatística e Medicina Preventiva*, Artmed, ISBN 8536302968, Porto Alegre, Brazil.

Kim, M.; Cobbin, D.; & Zaslawski, C. Traditional Chinese medicine tongue inspection: an examination of the inter- and intrapractitioner reliability for specific tongue characteristics. *The Journal of Alternative and Complementary Medicine*, Vol. 14, No. 5, (June 2008), (527-536), ISSN 1075-5535.

Linnet, K., & Brandt, E. Assessing diagnostic tests once an optimal cutoff point has been selected. *Clinical Chemistry*, Vol. 32, (July 1986), (1341-1346), ISSN 0009-9147.

Liu, G.P.; Li, G.Z.; Wang, Y.L.; & Wang, Y.Q. Modelling of inquiry diagnosis for coronary heart disease in traditional Chinese medicine by using multi-label learning. *BMC Complementary Alternative Medicine*, Vol. 10, (2010), (37), ISSN 1472-6882.

Lu, A.P.; & Chen, K.J. Integrative Medicine in Clinical Practice: From Pattern Differentiation in Traditional Chinese Medicine to Disease Treatment. *Chinese Journal of Integrative Medicine*, Vol. 15, No. 2, (April 2009), (152), ISSN 1993-0402.

Luiz, A.B.; Cordovil, L.; Barbosa Filho, J.; & Ferreira, A.S. Zangfu zheng (patterns) are associated with clinical manifestations of zang shang (target-organ damage) in arterial hypertension. *Chinese Medicine*, Vol. 6 (June 2011), (23), ISSN 1749-8546.

Lukman, S.; He, Y., & Hui, S.C. Computational methods for Traditional Chinese Medicine: A survey. *Computer Methods and Programs in Biomedicine*, Vol. 88, No. 3, (December 2007), (283-294), ISSN 0169-2607.

Maciocia, G. (1996). *Fundamentos da Medicina Tradicional Chinesa: Um texto abrangente para acupunturistas e fitoterapeutas*. Roca, ISBN 85-7241-150-X, Rio de Janeiro, Brazil.

MacPherson, H.; Altman, D.G.; Hammerschlag, R.; Youping, L.; Taixiang, W.; White, A.; Moher D; & STRICTA Revision Group. Revised STandards for Reporting Interventions in Clinical Trials of Acupuncture (STRICTA): extending the CONSORT statement. *PLoS Medicine*, Vol 7, No. 6, (June 2010), (e1000261), ISSN 1549-1277.

McSherry, D. Strategic induction of decision trees. *Knowledge-Based Systems*, Vol. 12, No. 5, (October 1999), (269-275), ISSN 0950-7051.

Metropolis, N.; & Ulam, S. The Monte Carlo method. *Journal of the American Statistical Association*, Vol 44, No. 247, (September 1949), (335-341), ISSN 0162-1459.

O'Brien, K.A.; Abbas, E.; Zhang, J.; Guo, Z.X.; Luo, R.; Bensoussan, A.; & Komesaroff, P.A. Understanding the reliability of diagnostic variables in a Chinese medicine examination. *The Journal of Alternative and Complementary Medicine*, Vol. 15, No. 7, (July 2009), (727-734), ISSN 1075-5535.

O'Connor, J. & Bensky, D. (1987). *Acupuncture a Comprehensive Text.* Eastland Press, ISBN 0-939616-00-9, Seattle, United States of America.

Peterson, M.C.; Holbrook, J.H.; Von Hales, D.; Smith, N.L.; & Staker, L.V. Contributions of the history, physical examination, and laboratory investigation in making medical diagnoses. *Western Journal of Medicine*, Vol. 156, No. 2, (February 1992), (163-165), ISSN 1476-2978.

Real, R. Tables of significant values of Jaccard's index of similarity. *Miscellània Zoològica*, Vol. 22, No. 1, (June 1999), (29-40), ISSN 0211-6529.

Ross, J. (2003). *Combinação Dos Pontos de Acupuntura: a Chave para o Êxito Clínico*, Roca, ISBN 85-7241-417-7, São Paulo, Brazil.

Spirtes, P., & Meek, C. (1995). Learning Bayesian networks with discrete variables from data. *Proceedings of the First International Conference on Knowledge Discovery and Data Mining*, pp. 294–299, ISBN 978-0-929280-82-0, Menlo Park, California, USA, August 20-21, 1995.

Tao, L. Achievements of Chinese medicine in the Chin (221-207 BC) and Han (206 BC-219 AD) dynasties. *Chinese Medical Journal*, Vol. 71, No. 5, (September-October 1953a), (380-386), ISSN 0366-6999.

Tao, L. Achievements of Chinese medicine in the Sui (598-617 A.D.) and Tang (618-907 A.D.) dynasties. *Chinese Medical Journal*, Vol. 71, No., (July-August 1953b), (801-820), ISSN 0366-6999.

Tao, L. Achievements of Chinese medicine during the Ming (1368-1644 A.D.) dynasty. *Chinese Medical Journal*, Vol. 76, No. 2, (February 1958a), (178-198), ISSN 0366-6999.

Tao, L. Chinese medicine during the Ming dynasty. *Chinese Medical Journal*, Vol. 76, No. 3, (March 1958b), (285-301), ISSN 0366-6999.

Wang, S.C., Li, Y.G., & Guo, X.M. (2002). *Pediatrics of Traditional Chinese Medicine - A Newly Compiled Practical English-Chinese Library of Traditional Chinese Medicine*, Shanghai University of Traditional Chinese Medicine, ISBN 7-81010-653-8, Shanghai, China.

Wang, X.; Qu, H.; Liu, P.; & Cheng, Y. A self-learning expert system for diagnosis in traditional Chinese medicine. *Expert Systems with Applications*, Vol. 26, No. 4, (May 2004), (557-566), ISSN 0957-4174.

Wolff, J.G. Medical diagnosis as pattern recognition in a framework of information compression by multiple alignment, unification and search. *Decision Support Systems*, Vol. 42, No. 2, (November 2006), (608-625), ISSN 0167-9236.

World Health Organization. Traditional medicine. Fact sheet nº 134. Revised November 2008. Available from http: //www.who.int/mediacentre/factsheets/fs134/en/

Luo, X.W. (translator). (1995) *Jīnkuì Yāoluè (Synopsis of Prescriptions of the Golden Chamber with 300 Cases)*. New World Press, ISBN 7-80005-291-5, Beijing, China.

Yang, S.Z.; & Li, J.Y. (translators). (1993). *Pí Wèi Lún (Treatise on the Spleen & Stomach)*, Blue Poppy, ISBN 0-936185-41-4, Denver, United States of America.

Yang S.Z. (translator). (2003). *Zhōng Zàng Jīng (Master Hua's Classic of the Central Viscera),* Blue Poppy, ISBN 0-936185-43-0, Denver, United States of America.

Yang, S.Z.; & Chace, C. (translators). (2004). *Zhēn Jiǔ Jiǎ Yǐ Jīng (The Systematic Classic of Acupuncture & Moxibustion),* Blue Poppy, ISBN 0-936185-29-5, Denver, United States of America.

Yang, X.B.; Liang, Z.H.; Zhang, G.; Luo, Y.J.; & Yin, J. (2005). A classification algorithm for TCM syndromes based on P-SVM. *Proceedings of 2005 International Conference on Machine Learning and Cybernetics*, pp. 3692-3697, ISBN 0-7803-9091-1, Piscataway, New Jersey, USA, August 18-21, 2005.

Zaslawki C. Clinical reasoning in traditional Chinese medicine: implications for clinical research. *Clinical Acupuncture and Oriental Medicine,* Vol. 4, No. 2-3, (2003), (94-101), ISSN 1461-1449.

Zhang, G.G.; Lee, W.; Bausell, B.; Lao, L.; Handwerger, B.; & Berman, B. Variability in the Traditional Chinese Medicine (TCM) Diagnoses and Herbal Prescriptions Provided by Three TCM Practitioners for 40 Patients with Rheumatoid Arthritis. *The Journal of Alternative and Complementary Medicine,* Vol. 11, No. 3, (July 2005), (415-421), ISSN 1075-5535.

Zhang, G.G.; Singh, B.; Lee, W.; Handwerger, B.; Lao, L.; & Berman, B. Improvement of Agreement in TCM Diagnosis Among TCM Practitioners for Persons with the Conventional Diagnosis of Rheumatoid Arthritis: Effect of Training. *The Journal of Alternative and Complementary Medicine,* Vol. 14, No. 4, (May 2008), (381-386), ISSN 1075-5535.

Zhang, N.L.; Yuan, S.; Chen, T.; & Wang, Y. Statistical Validation of Traditional Chinese Medicine Theories. *The Journal of Alternative and Complementary Medicine,* Vol. 14, No. 5, (June 2008), (583-587), ISSN 1075-5535.

Zheng, N.; & Wu, Z. (2004). TCM-SIRD: an integrated aided system for traditional Chinese medicine Sizheng. *Proceedings of 2004 IEEE International Conference on Systems, Man and Cybernetics,* pp. 3864-3868, ISBN 0-7803-8566-7, The Hague, The Netherlands, October 10-13, 2004.

Zhou, C.L; & Zhang, Z.F. Progress and prospects of research on information processing techniques for intelligent diagnosis of traditional Chinese medicine. *Zhong Xi Yi Jie He Xue Bao,* Vol. 4, No. 6, (November 2006), (560-566), ISSN 1672-1977.

Zhou, X.; Chen, S.; Liu, B.; Zhang, R.; Wang, Y.; Li, P.; Guo, Y.; Zhang, H.; Gao, Z.; & Yan, X. Development of traditional Chinese medicine clinical data warehouse for medical knowledge discovery and decision support. *Artificial Intelligence in Medicine,* Vol. 48, No. 2-3, (February-March 2010), (139-152), ISSN 0933-3657.

Zhou, X.Z.; Wu, Z.H.; Yin, A.N.; Wu, L.C.; & Fan, W.Y.; Zhang, R. Ontology development for unified traditional Chinese medical language system. *Artificial Intelligence in Medicine,* Vol. 32, No. 1, (September 2004), (15-27), ISSN 0933-3657.

Zhu, W.F.; Yan, J.F.; & Huang, B.Q. Application of Bayesian network in syndrome differentiation system of traditional Chinese medicine. *Zhong Xi Yi Jie He Xue Bao,* Vol. 4, No. 6, (November 2006), (567-571), ISSN 1672-1977.

Zuzek, A.; Biasizzo, A.; Novak, F. Sequential diagnosis tool. *Microprocessors and Microsystems*, Vol. 24, (2000), (191-197), ISSN 0141-9331.

7

Application and Effect of Acupuncture and Moxibustion for Analgesia in Perioperative Period of Total Knee Arthroplasty

Bang Jian He and Peijian Tong
Zhejiang Traditional Chinese Medicine University, China

1. Introduction

As patients going to take total knee arthroplasty(TKA) lying in bed for a long time, eating less, bowel movements Slowing down, then influencing defecation.And they will come up with tension and fearness.At the same time, their lifestyle is changing. Epidemiological survey of constipation displaying: tension, anxiety and depression are the dangerous factors of constipation. Eating less, Diet low in fiber content are easily leading to constipation. In addition, lots of patients aren't used to defecate in bed for a long time, which will also making the defecation difficult. While constipation may cause whole body and partial illness, we should pay more attention to it.

Total knee replacement surgery has become the ultimate effective treatment for the disease. However, this surgical method is associated with severe postoperative pain, including severe pain 60%, 30% moderate pain, not only to patients with pain, but also to varying degrees, affect the circulatory, respiratory, digestive, endocrine, immune and other function of each system that may lead to various postoperative complications, serious impact on early postoperative functional rehabilitation and treatment. Postoperative pain not due to early exercise, active physical therapy, so prone to deep vein thrombosis, pulmonary embolism, infection and other complications. Patients within the environment can also lead to disorder, anxiety is not conducive to sleep and rest, short-term deterioration in the quality of life of patients. Severe pain due to joint dysfunction caused by anxiety, depression, most patients need a year of health care in order to get the final improveing. Almost all patients are expected to be their smallest incision, postoperative pain and satisfaction with the lightest of functional recovery. Therefore, adequate postoperative analgesia, especially for sports is not just pain relief, but also to help patients get out of bed early, active physical therapy, as much as possible to restore knee activity and the prevention of deep vein thrombosis formation and other complications. In addition, effective postoperative analgesia reduces stress response, so that patients in a stable environment, and reduce patient anxiety, sleep and rest help to improve the quality of life in patients with short-term..

Early postoperative pain caused by stress response, significantly increased the secretion of stress-quality alcohol, so that myocardial contractility, heart rate, cardiac output increased, liver and kidney blood vessels and gastrointestinal vasoconstriction, myocardial oxygen consumption significantly increase induced myocardial oxygen supply/oxygen ratio disorders, but also make the body insulin sensitivity, glucose uptake and utilization of energy for the oxidation of reduced capacity. These will affect the perioperative and postoperative quality of life of patients recovered as soon as possible. Therefore, postoperative pain and reduce the body's stress response, the promotion of early postoperative recovery has a positive effect.

2. Mechanism of acupuncture analgesia in the perioperative period of total knee arthroplasty

The current total knee arthroplasty analgesia strategies, mainly compound of preemptive analgesia and multimodal analgesia. Postoperative analgesia with epidural administration, intravenous, intra-articular administration, local continuous joint cryotherapy, oral drug therapy. Today, we discuss mainly the total knee replacement surgery perioperative analgesic mechanism of acupuncture, as follows:

2.1 Nerve

2.1.1 Central mechanism

Signal is acupuncture acupuncture analgesia and pain signals in the central nervous system interactions, processing and integration of the results. Studies have shown that the central nervous system from spinal cord to the cerebral cortex at all levels are involved in this interaction. Acupuncture analgesia is a multi-channel, multi-level synthesis process. Spinal cord of the central segment of the downstream modulation and high modulation is the main mechanism of acupuncture analgesia.

2.1.1.1 Spinal cord injury is acupuncture signal and primary signal integration hub. Acupuncture both hyperalgesia induced by dorsal horn neurons produce inhibitory postsynaptic potentials (IPSP), but also caused depolarization of the spinal cord and peripheral transmission occurs presynaptic inhibition. Therefore, the level of acupuncture in the spinal cord can produce analgesia, the mechanism involves both presynaptic inhibition, postsynaptic inhibition is also involved.

2.1.1.2 The structure of the spinal cord above the mechanism of acupuncture analgesia in the spinal cord above the central thalamic structures including nuclear-forebrain loop-the loop parafascicular nucleus, the brain-the edge of pain loop, descending inhibitory system under the central nucleus and thalamus-ventrolateral orbital cortex-in the periaqueductal gray pathway. ① central thalamus in the nucleus-forebrain loop-the loop parafascicular nucleus: acupuncture causes the central nuclear signals resulting from the impulse may be excited by forebrain circuits (caudate nucleus, pillow core, cortex and thalamic reticular nucleus) to reach the parafascicular nucleus, activity of pain-sensitive neurons produce inhibitory modulation.② in the brain-the edge of pain loop: the limbic system in the midbrain periaqueductal gray (PAG), nucleus accumbens, amygdala and habenula, these neural pathways between nuclei with each other to form a circular path. The loop to 5-HT and enkephalin as neurotransmitters. Acupuncture to the releasing of brain 5-HT and enkephalin, promote analgesic effects loop rotation. ③ descending inhibitory system: Acupuncture information can be passed from brain PAG nucleus raphe magnus (NRM) to reach the spinal cord or trigeminal plexus, the information produced inhibition of pain modulation. (Liu Xiang, 1996) The following line suppression system, the main initiation site, the medullary NRM neurons, and one of the seam - spinal neurons as an indicator of unit discharge was observed acupoint electric stimulation PAG, nucleus accumbens and caudate nucleus can activate NRM neurons inhibition of spontaneous discharge and damage response; and electrolysis damage to these brain areas are able to block the analgesic effect of EA. Prompt the activation of descending inhibitory systems in play a major role in acupuncture analgesia. ④under the central thalamic nucleus - ventral lateral orbital cortex - in the periaqueductal gray matter: Teachers (Tang, Jing-shi &Yuanbing, 2002) research group studies have shown that the hypothalamus under the central nucleus (Sm)-ventrolateral orbital cortex (VLO)-PAG is not only a central feeling pain, but also constitute an important in pain modulation negative feedback loop, through the activation of the brainstem descending inhibitory system, the level of modulation in the spinal cord and trigeminal nociceptive transmission. The fine fiber loop in the excitement generated by acupuncture analgesia play an important role. Sm neurons they observed the response to acupuncture, as well as damage to Sm or VLO, or Sm injection of local anesthetic effect of acupuncture. The results show that acupuncture can activate neurons in rat Sm activity, these neurons respond to noxious mechanical stimulation was not found on non-noxious stimulation of neurons. Further studies have shown, bilateral electrolytic damage can be significantly reduced Sm or VLO strong electro-acupuncture (5.0 mA) on rat tail flick reflex inhibition, while the weak-pin (0.5mA) of the inhibitory effect no significant effect. Tip strong electro-acupuncture analgesia produced fine fibers excited by activation of Sm-VLO-PAG pathway. Sm microinjection in the local anesthetic lidocaine can significantly weaken the strong EA (5-6 mA) of the rat spinal dorsal horn nociceptive neurons in response to the inhibitory effect, while the weak-pin (1mA) had no effect on the effects of. The results for the Sm-VLO-PAG pathway involved in the fine fibers provides further proof of the analgesic.

2.1.2 Peripheral mechanisms

Peripheral nerve needle nerve signal transmission, the types of acupuncture by or to the types of fiber conduction problems, had long been in dispute. After a large number of experiments, now that: electric acupuncture(EA) of varying intensity, a different transmission fibers can be excited. Low-intensity electro-acupuncture (2 V) major excitatory I, II class and some III (Aδ) class crude fiber transmission through the integration of the role of pain in spinal cord segments to achieve analgesia, but also on the mechanism involved in the spinal cord, the analgesic effect showed limited of the specificity; and high-intensity electric acupuncture(EA) 18 V (over C fiber threshold, equivalent to noxious stimulation) is mainly excited III (Aδ), especially IV (C) class small transmission fibers, the spinal cord through the activation of negative feedback on the NRM pain adjustment mechanism to play a wide range of effects long after the analgesic effect of this analgesic effect without showing broad specificity. These facts prove that acupuncture is a noxious stimulus, transmission of C fibers in acupuncture analgesia play an important role. Capsaicin (Cap) effective selective damage to a descendant of C fibers, in recent years to use it in a sense of electric acupuncture(EA)-human transmission have done a lot of research. (Fangzong Ren, et al 1992 & Liu Xiang, et al, 1997) observed that after peripheral nerve with capsaicin treatment, significantly reduced the analgesic effect of EA, clear that the peripheral nerve C fibers are the main ingredients involved in acupuncture analgesia.(Xu Rong et al, 1993) will be a direct effect of capsaicin in the rat sciatic nerve, its pain threshold was significantly higher; electric acupuncture(EA) capsaicin treatment side of the "ring dance" of the analgesic effect, significantly lower than prior to treatment and control side effects Tip a capsaicin-sensitive C fiber transmission of information not only involved in pain transmission, but also involved in acupuncture analgesia an essential component of information transmission.

2.1.3 Neurotransmitters

Acupuncture analgesia by the brain to complete a number of neurotransmitters in the joint, and neurotransmitters in acupuncture analgesia mechanisms of acupuncture analgesia is the most extensive and deep areas.

2.1.3.1 Endogenous opioid peptides (EOP) acupuncture is mainly dominated by activating the endogenous opioid peptides in pain modulation system and analgesic effects, so the EOP is an important material basis for acupuncture analgesia.

(Wang Hongbei et al, 1998) at different frequencies of electroacupuncture on acute adjuvant arthritis (AA) in rats with pain and tissue reaction of β-endorphin (β-EP) Content of the study, observed two 5 Hz and 100 Hz frequencies for the AA rats were significantly power analgesic effect, but also significantly increased the hypothalamic content of β-EP, the two frequency electroacupuncture analgesia are related to hypothalamic β-EP levels were significantly elevated positive correlation, but both the frequency and electro-acupuncture analgesia between elevated β-EP levels in the hypothalamus no significant difference in the role. (Chen et al, 2004) further found that acupuncture can promote β-EP precursor POMC original (POMC) mRNA expression increased to further enhance the β-EP levels to analgesic effect. This not only immediate effect of acupuncture analgesia, there are more significant after-effects,. (Wang Sheng Xu et al, 1999) studies have shown that acupuncture can Jiaji AA levels in rat spinal cord dorsal horn of the original before dynorphin (PPD) mRNA expression was significantly increased, suggesting that EA may activate the dynorphin system resistant to injury, the level of inflammation in the spinal cord and hyperalgesia is modulated. (Huang Yong, 2004)A method of acupuncture in the study satisfied leucine enkephalin on the AA effects in rabbits, and found that satisfied a method and routine acupuncture can significantly improve the AA rabbit serum in the hypothalamus and brain leucine enkephalin (LEK) level of analgesic effect. LEK for the regulation of serum, Na A is better than routine acupuncture

Acupuncture can not only promote the release of central E0P can also make local E0P inflammation increases the synthesis and release, to achieve peripheral analgesia. (Zhao chang huan &Zhou jun, 2002)positions AA rats in the study of electricity for local opioid peptide gene expression observed when the EA in the AA rats increased the pain threshold, but also promote inflammation in local immune cells POMC and preproenkephalin (PENK) mRNA expression increased, to achieve peripheral pain modulation. Inflammation in AA rats while local injection of β-EP and LEK antisera may antagonize the analgesic effect of electro-acupuncture, in which β-EP antiserum stronger effect, suggesting that β-EP and LEK are involved in EA's peripheral towns pain in the process (Yangjie Bin et al, 1999), different acupuncture on peripheral analgesic mechanism of AA rats in the study, using electro-acupuncture, moxibustion, Bloodletting and four methods of acupoint-injection can increase the pain threshold of AA rats to electro-acupuncture, point injection is excellent, its peripheral analgesic mechanism may promote inflammation in local analgesic substances by β-EP and LEK increased, causing physical pain prostaglandin E2 (PGE2), histamine, 5 - hydroxytryptamine (5-HT), norepinephrine (NE) reduction achieved.

2.1.3.2 Monoamine neurotransmitter monoamine neurotransmitters are important bioactive substances in vivo, the relationship with acupuncture analgesia, the study is more 5-HT, NE and dopamine (DA). (Wang Sheng Xu et al, 1999) were observed in the EA Jiaji of AA in peripheral blood and the spinal cord content of monoamine neurotransmitters, studies show that: EA AA rats after the platelet 5-HT, and plasma 5-- HIAA (5-HIAA, 5-HT, the end product of catabolism) were significantly increased, indicating that acupuncture in the promotion of platelet 5-HT increased absorption, but also the blood of free accelerated catabolism of 5-HT involved in analgesia, electro-acupuncture to peripheral NE and DA were significantly decreased, which may be respectively enhanced sympathetic activity and inhibition of autonomic nervous activity. In the spinal cord, EA Jiaji AA rats significantly increased spinal 5-HT and 5-HIAA levels, while 5-HIAA increased significantly more than the 5-HT, indicating that electro-acupuncture analgesia Jiaji mechanism downstream activation of 5-HT, 5-HT on pain control system synthesis, release and use also increased, but synthesis faster than the speed of the release and use, so 5-HT content increased, indicating that 5-HT, is involved in spinal pain modulation important neurotransmitter; EA Jiaji spinal cord NE and DA content were significantly decreased, indicating that the NA and DA are involved in the mechanism of electroacupuncture analgesia in the spinal cord. These results suggest that peripheral and spinal cord monoamine neurotransmitters are involved in inflammatory pain modulation in rats during electroacupuncture analgesia. (Liang fan long et al 2001)prosperity AA rats in the study of electricity for local inflammation in 5-HT, NE, DA content in, they get the same results, and show some of the after-effects.

2.1.3.3 Substance P(SP), (Wang Sheng Xu et al, 2000), electro-acupuncture in the study of AA Jiaji effect of substance P in rat spinal cord found that EA can make the AA rat spinal cord lumbar enlargement of SP-positive cells in the immune response to a further increase in Tip EA Jiaji inhibit adjuvant-induced spinal cord dorsal horn release of SP, the SP storage increases, the mechanism through the spinal cord and spinal analgesic effect.

2.1.3.4 Nitrogen monoxidum(NO) is a neurotransmitter of new neurons found at different levels play an important role in pain modulation. (Tian Jin Hua et al, 1996) confirmed that NO can not only promote the formation of the spinal cord level and development of hyperalgesia, and pain in the brain caused by the role. （Pan Huijuan et al, 2002） also experiment found that acupuncture can significantly increase the pain threshold of AA rats, and has obvious after-effects; AA rats while significantly reducing the NO content in brain tissue, resulting in analgesia.

2.2 Psychology

2.2.1 Release of endorphins within the brown skin is a neuromodulator class of chemicals that can alter or adjust the postsynaptic neuron function, sexual and emotional pain control has an important role. Because of its role in pleasure and pain regulation and control, known as the "key to enter heaven." Researchers have checked out the course of acupuncture in reducing pain, endorphins at least part of the role (Fields & Levine, 1984; Murray, 1995; Watkins & Mayer, 1982), which is similar to opium and coffee, with the same receptors in the brain

2.2.2 Distracting mental process of the importance of the pain experience can be used to illustrate two extreme examples: First, do not feel physical pain stimulus, and second, when stimulated by a strong pain did not feel pain. Feelings of pain that occur will be pain response scenarios and habits of the impact of acquisition, so by distracting, resulting in appropriate information to enhance the contrast stimuli ability to overcome pain. Mel Zach (Ronald Melzack, 1973, 1980) proposed gated background theory that describes the psychological impact of pain perception, the theory that the cells in the spinal cord, as cut off as the door and prevent some of the pain signals into the brain, while allowing other signals into the brain and spinal cord to receptors in the skin send information to open or closed, the information provided from the brain of pain experienced by the background scene. Acupuncture treatment by applying an external stimulus, distracted the attention of patients, pain in the affected area so that it no longer focus on the scene. Psychology from the Chinese point of view, this should be easy to therapy empathy through the spirit of the transfer, change the patient's point of Love within the guilty to distraction emotions, changes in aspirations, in order to treat pain caused by emotional factors.

2.2.3 Since the perceived control of pain experience and decided on the physiological and psychological factors, to successfully deal with the pain factor is the establishment of another major source of stress, perceived control, that can change the event or experience for the process or result of faith. If you believe you can influence some of the symptoms of discomfort or pain of the daily process, you may better adapt to the symptoms of these disorders. Good results of acupuncture analgesia trust the doctor before administering treatment to give patients confidence so that patients have to reduce or cure the pain beliefs, and thus affect the perceived control of pain through the process. Therefore, the confidence of patients and doctors who stress indoctrination is extremely important. Chinese psychology to love wins love with this therapy or a fit of the Department.

2.2.4 Social and environmental support to provide social support is a resource for others to tell someone he is loved, cared for and respected, he lives in contact with each other and help each other a social network (Cohen & Syme, 1985). Acupuncture analgesia in the treatment of this social support mainly from doctors and family members, doctors information support, such as on the cause of the disease, information, recommendations on the effects of uncertainty, as well as doctors and their families emotional support, etc. Many researchers have pointed out that social support's role in mitigating damage when given to patients can rely on a sense, they are better able to cope with stress, pain and suffering, it can promote the individual has been diagnosed with the disease from rehabilitation. For pain patients, acupuncturists and differentiation before administering treatment information and emotional support in the treatment of the point of the eye. At the same time when the clinic environment, differentiation, treatment of mental quiet position also helps patients self-control and regulation. Enlighten the language of psychology, medicine therapies, including delight joyful way, way clear up doubts, and doubts therapy is also suggested that social support. But rather God Seishi therapy is a supportive environment, through meditation or repose, to achieve "without thinking of the suffering inside and outside workers are not shaped at all" to a read on behalf of the Wan study results.

2.2.5 Catharsis chronic pain damage to human health, its immune function, neurotransmitter, autonomic nervous system, mental and psychological adverse effects will be, it allows patients with physical pain, mental distress, reduce outdoor activities and social interaction, and gradually form a "sleep a fatigue, insomnia and a pain in a troubled one, "the vicious circle of pain in patients with enlarged and somatization. Therefore, so that patients get the emotional drain should have a good health benefits. Doctor to listen to on the one hand, and the course of treatment by acupuncture to relieve tension and calm the mind the body can have a relaxation response, which is an effective response to combat stress, muscle tension, cortical excitability, heart rate and blood pressure have decreased, the pain eased. This was reflected in the Chinese psychology along the intelligence from For therapy, the patient's compliance ideas, emotions, mind and body to meet the needs of patients, but the patient's psychological interpretation of the cause

In summary, the psychological mechanism of acupuncture analgesia can not be questioned. And the role of acupuncture analgesia in acupuncture, in place of a body from the outside and thoughtful hub at all levels, involving the nervous, endocrine and immune interactions of multiple factors, including anti-pain and pain caused by two aspects of the unity of opposites complex dynamic integration process. In this process, the nervous system and neurotransmitters as well as between various neurotransmitters, nerve, endocrine and immune systems are not isolated individual, but rather complement each other, interact, participate in the modulation of acupuncture on pain role. Although the mechanism of acupuncture analgesia in recent years made great progress in the study, but the mechanism of acupuncture analgesia has still not clear, need from multi-disciplinary, multi-level, multi-angle in-depth study in order to promote the town of acupuncture mechanism of pain and to promote the wider use of acupuncture in clinical.

3. Preoperative eletroacupuncture for postoperative pain

The clinical practice of acupuncture is growing in popularity world-wide. In parallel, interest in the scientific basis of acupuncture has been increasing, as reflected by a dramatic rise in the number of scientific publicationson acupuncture and related techniques (ART) in the recent decade. After 40 years of extensive studies, compelling evidence has been obtained to support acupuncture as a useful tool for treating a spectrum of diseases.In fact, more than 40 disorders have been endorsed by the World Health Organization (WHO) as conditions that can benefit from acupuncture treatment. Pain is particularly sensitive to acupuncture. Postoperative pain management remains a significant challenge for healthcare providers. Many patients experience pain after surgery, with about 86% reporting moderate, severe, or extreme pain. Opioids remain the mainstay for postoperative pain control. However, opioid analgesics are associated with undesirable side-effects, including nausea, vomiting, pruritus, sedation, dizziness, and decreased gut motility which can lead to delayed post-operative recovery. The use of adjunct analgesics that provide opioid-sparing effects and decrease the incidence of opioid-related side-effects is therefore useful. Acupuncture, a component of traditional Chinese medicine, is a well-known and widely used treatment for pain and other conditions that has been employed in China for more than 3000 yr. There have been increasing numbers of clinical trials evaluating the efficacy of acupuncture and related techniques as an adjuvant method for postoperative analgesia. Paul F, et al. designed a randomized, double-blind, sham-controlled study, which was used to compare three prophylactic acustimulation treatment schedules: preoperative—an active device was applied for 30 min before and a sham device for 72h after surgery;postoperative—a sham device was applied for 30 min before and an active device for 72h after surgery;and peri-operative—an active device was applied for 30 min before and 72 h after surgery (n 35 per group). All patients received a standardized general anesthetic, and on dansetron 4mg IV was administered at the end of surgery.The incidence of vomiting/retching and the need for rescue antiemetics were determined at specific time in tervals for up to 72 h after surgery. Nausea scores were recorded with an 11-point verbalrating scale.Other out come vari-ablesassessed included discharge times(for outpatients), resumption of nor malactivities of daily living, complete antiemetic response rate, and patient satisfaction with

Antiemetic therapy and quality of recovery.Perioperative use of the Relief Band significantly increased complete responses(68%)compared with use of the device before surgery only(43%).Median postoperative nausea scores were significantly reduced in the peri- and post-operative (versus preoperative) treatment groups.Finally, patient satisfaction with the quality of recovery (83± 16 and 85± 13 vs 72± 18) and antiemetic management (96± 9 and 94± 10 vs 86±13) on an arbitrary scale from 0 worst to 100 best was significantly higher in the groups receiving peri- or postoperative (versus preoperative) acustimulation therapy. For patients discharged on the day of surgery, the time to home readiness was significantly reduced (114± 41 min versus 164±50 min; P< 0.05) when acustimulation was administered perioperatively (versus preoperatively). In conclusion, acustimulation with the Relief Band was most effective in reducing postoperative nausea and vomiting and improving patients'satisfaction with their antiemetic therapy when it was administered after surgery. Sun er al.conducted a systematic review to quantitatively evaluate the efficacy of acupuncture and related techniques as adjunct analgesics for acute postoperative pain management. The authors concluded that perioperative acupuncture might be a useful adjunct for acute postoperative pain management.there are few Literatures about preoperative eletroacupuncture for postoperative pain after total knee arthroplasty, in our hospital, patients who takes the operation of total knee arthroplasty will be received preoperative eletroacupuncture at bilateral points (LI4–LI11, LR3–ST36, PC6–TE5) for 30 min with alternating frequencies of 3 and 15 Hz., postoperative range of motion(ROM)Of knee joint and Hospital for Special Surgery(HSS)score were recorded. two weeks after operation the initiative ROM and the HSS score were improved, so Applying preoperative eletroacupuncture in perioperative period Of knee joint replacement is favorable for alleviating postoperative pain, decreasing narcotic consumption, and promoting early rehabilitation.

Many studies have supported the effectiveness of acupuncture for postoperative pain relief However, the mechanism of acupuncture analgesia remains unclear. Acupuncture theory is based on two conditions:"yin", which is considered feminine, passive, dark, and cold, and "yang", which is masculine, aggressive, bright, and hot, as well as "qi, " which is considered thevitalenergy that flows and cycles throughout the body.The acupuncture theory is to harmonize any imbalance in yin-yang and qi in a human body to restore the body to a healthy condition.Acupuncture is thought to unblock any obstruction to the flow of qi and, thereby, relieves pain.The acupuncture technique that has been most often studied scientifically involves penetrating the skin with thin, solid, metallic needles that are manipulated by the hands or electrical stimulation. Although in the past scepticism has been voiced over the effects claimed for acupuncture, in recent years the effect of acupuncture on different conditions (pain and diseases) has been studied from a Western scientifc perspective, and the results have demonstrated that acupuncture has both physiological and psychological impacts. Needle insertion into the skin and deeper tissues, in addition to subsequent stimulation of the needles, results in aparticular pattern of afferent activity in peripheral nerves, mainly the A-delta and possibly also the C fibres. Acupuncture stimulation has been demonstrated to activate inhibitory systems in the spinal cord, which results in segmental inhibition of the sympathetic outfow and pain pathways, as predicted by the gate control theory. EA releases endogenous opioids and oxytocin, which seem to be essential in the induction of functional changes in different organ systems In this respect, particular interest has been dedicated to β-endorphin-an endogenous opioid with a high affnity for the m receptor. Indeed, evidence suggests that this hypothalamic β-endorphin system plays a central role in mediating the pain-relieving effect of acupuncture.

Furthermore, it has been shown that intense stimulation results in the activation of supraspinal pain inhibitory centres, and this mechanism is denoted diffuse noxious inhibitory controls (DNIC) or counterirritation.

In conclusion, the preoperative eletroacupuncture may be a useful adjunct for postoperative analgesia. Further large, well-designed studies are required to confirm those findings and to answer questions regarding the most efficacious type of acupuncture and optimal timing of administration.and the mechanism of acupuncture analgesia

4. Pain relief by acupuncture

Normal knee is freedom in flexion and extextension, which is limited now, just because of pain due to obstruction of Qi and blood in meridians, even there'stagnation. Where meridians pass, there is available to be treated. Accordingly, we should take local or remote acupoints in meridians where the disease is. Prescription: Yinlingquan (SP9), Yanglingquan (GB34), Neixiyan (EX-LE4), Taichong (LR3), Dachangshu (BL25), Quchi (LI11), Fengchi (GB20), both bilateral acupoints. If the course is long, we can add Zusanli (ST36), Sanyinjiao (SP6). Select 5 to 6 points each, after the arrival 0f Qi, we take reinforcing and reducing movement, needle retention 15min.2 to 3 times per week, 2 weeks as a course of treatment. Acupuncture treatment can be adjusted locally by tendon thinning the blood, promoting blood circulation, eliminating wind, removing obstrution from the meridians and relieving pain. Effective stimulation of acupuncture points receptors, so that pain signals are inhibited, anti-pain, enhance its ability to achieve the balance restored both inside and outside the state of the local meridian, and promote early recovery after surgery.

5. Application and effect of auricular acupoint pressing for analgesia in perioperative period of total knee arthroplasty

The role of Total knee arthroplasty has been widely recognized in the reconstruction of knee joint function and the remission the patient's pain. Effective postoperative analgesia is not just to alleviate the pain of patients, but also to help to do early ambulation, to do active physical therapy, to restore the knee's Range of motion as possible, to prevent deep vein thrombosis or other complications, to shorter hospital stay Time. In addition, effective postoperative analgesia reduces stress response, so that patients with stable internal environment, and can reduce patient anxiety and help patients sleep and rest, to improve the quality of life in patients with short-term.

Acupuncture has been used for more than 2, 000 years in traditional Chinese medicine to treat pain and other ailments. This technique was traditionally thought to work by channeling energy or Qi through body 'meridians' with acupuncture needles.And modern medicine has been trying to figure out the mechanism of acupuncture analgesia. And now various hypotheses about the mechanism of acupuncture analgesia are currently being discussed, e.g., the endogenous opioid system, gate-control mechanism, longterm depression, and diffuse noxious inhibitory controls (DNIC), as well as involvement of different neurotransmitters such as serotonin and norepinephrine, But none of them can explain it completely. Hence, acupuncture-induced analgesia seems to be a complex, multimodal interaction of neuronal and humoral pathways. On the other hand, large randomized controlled trials have proven a clinically relevant effect of acupuncture on pain conditions in the past years.

Auricular acupuncture is defined as 'a form of acupuncture in which needles are placed in various positions of the ear to affect the person. It postulates body correlates on the ear, so a treatment performed upon the ear will have effects reflected on the body part'. The Silk Book, China's earliest medical treatise written approximately 500 B.C, and Nei Jing, the Classic of Medicine, written around 200 B.C, both documented the theory Auricular acupuncture for analgesia.In Traditional Chinese Medical, it was concluded that all meridians converge at the ear.and the relationships of the Auricle, the Meridians, and the Zangfu Organs were very closely. Auricular acupuncture was first introduced into clinical western medicine by Nogier (1972)(Nogier PFM, 1972)., who empirically identified Auricular acupuncture points. The generally accepted view on auricular acupuncture is based on the conjecture that the human body is represented on the auricle in the form of an inverted fetus. It is claimed that this representation is constant, and can be detected by measuring the electrical resistance of the auricular skin and used for diagnostic purposes and/or treatment. Although the morphological structures connecting the specific auricular zones (acupuncture points) with corresponding parts of the body have not yet been identified, the effects of various stimulations applied to these regions have been verified in experimental and clinical studies.

Although no anatomical pathways exist to directly connect inner organs with the ear, a lot of nerve fiber distribution In the ear. The innervation of the central part of auricle (triangular fossa and concha) comes from trigeminal, geniculate and superior vagal ganglions, whereas the peripheral regions receive their innervation mainly by spinal nerves. The central parts of the neurons constituting the auricular branch of the vagal nerve are situated in the superior ganglion of the vagal nerve and nucleus tractus solitarii. Functionally, the stimulation of the inferior concha induced a significant increase in parasympathetic activity. In another study, the stimulation of the sympathetic AA point significantly decreased the stimulus-evoked electrodermal response compared with an AA stimulation to a non-specific point of the helix.. This resembles the design of studies performed by (Usichenko et al, 2005, 2007)where stimulation of the points in the central regions of the auricle was better than sham acupuncture at the non-specific points of the helix for reduction of postoperative analgesic requirement.

Early studies of Auricular acupuncture have demonstrated beneficial effects on both pain and anxiety including pain associated with cancer, knee arthroscopy, and hip fracture and hip arthroplasty. Several recent small studies have suggested that auricular acupuncture alone can relieve pain and anxiety in the prehospital transport phase of hip fracture and reduce acute pain due to a variety of causes in the emergency department setting.. Auricular acupuncture may be effective for the treatment of a variety of types of pain, especially postoperative pain

Auricular acupoint pressing(AAP), Vaccaria seeds be used to press in auricular acupoint, is the most commonly clinically Auricular acupuncture, In our hosptial we observe the effect of AAP for analgesia during perioperative period of total knee joint replacement, Methods: Sixty patients with osteoarthritis of ASA grade I to III scheduled to receive unilateral total knee joint replacement were equally randomized into the AAP group and the control group, 30 in each group. The general anesthesia on all patients was implemented by physicians of an identical group through endotracheal intubation. To the patients in the AAP group, AAP with Vaccaria seed was applied before operation, and the local analgesia on affected limb with acupoint pasting was used after operation. Besides, adm inistering of celecoxib 400 mg on the day before operation, and celecoxib 200 mg twice daily postoperation was given to all patients. When the visual analogue scales(VAS)reached more than 7 points, 0.1 g of bucinnazine hydrochloride was given for supplement Meantime same post-operative training methods were adopted in both groups. The resting VAS pain scores, contentment of sedation, incidence of adverse event, postoperative range of motion (ROM)Of knee joint and Hospital for Special Surgery(HSS) score were recorded Results: The resting VAS pain scores at 6 h and 24 h after operation was 5. 99±0. 67 scores and 4. 26±0. 59 scores in the AAP group respectively, which was significantly lower than that in the control group at the corresponding time (7. 02±0. 85 scores and 4. 92±0. 43 scores, P<0. 01), Through clinical observation we found that the resting VAS pain scores at 6 h and 24 h after operation reach its peak; but it showed insignificant difference between the two groups at 1 h and 48 h after operation (P>0. 05), which regard as the effect of Narcotic for analgesia at 1 h after operation is not eliminate Thoroughly, and Patients has tolerated the pain gradually at 48 h after operation so threshold of pain tolerance Increased, The result is the acute pain of the knee after surgery relieve gradually, After 48 hours after operation, patient's Acute pain was replaced by Chronic Pain that can be relieved by drugs for inflammation and pain, so the intergroup difference of the resting VAS pain scores at 1 h and 48 h after operation was statistically insignificant; sedation contentment in the two groups was similar: incidence of adverse event in the AAP groups seemed lower (4 cases VS. 1 1 cases), but the intergroup difference was statistically insignificant (P>0. 05). The application of postoperative narcotic analgesics and analgesic effects related to the occurrence of adverse reactions is the use of narcotic analgesics was positively correlated ROM before surgery were 75. 630±5. 74 and 75. 43±5. 63 in the two groups respectively, showing no significant difference (P>0. 05), two weeks after operation, the initiative ROM raised to 96. 500±3. 790 and 93. 500±3. 50 and the passive ROM reached 1 07. 80±3. 370 and 1 05. 27±3 250 in the two groups respectively, with statistical significance between them (P<0. 05) HSS score was similar between groups before operation (60. 23±3. 44 scores VS. 61. 70±2. 83 scores, p>0. 05); while it became 86. 97±2. 33 scores and 85. 37±2. 30 scores after operation. showing significant difference between groups(P<0. 05) so we draw the conclusion that Applying auricular acupoint pressing in perioperative period Of knee joint replacement is favorable for alleviating postoperative pain, decreasing narcotic consumption, and promoting early rehabilitation, and it has the advantages of low cost, less complication, simple manipulation and high safety.

After analysis the resting VAS pain scores at each time point, we must consider long enough analgesia for patient and additional analgesia aimed to the Peak pain point when we Select analgesic method. the satisfaction with analgesia in two groups of patients is about 50%, This shows that we must improved our Analgesia in the future, So in the next task we can combined many methods for better Analgesia in Perioperative Period of total knee arthroplasty, such as Auricular Acupoint Pressing, nerve block, intra-articular infusion reserved and so on, as far as Auricular Acupoint Pressing was considered, we prepare to Increase the intensity of the stimulus for better Analgesia through needle-embedding therapy and electric acupuncture in Auricle.

6. References

Albrecht S, le Blond R, Kohler V et al. Cryotherapy as analgesic technique in direct, postoperative treatment following elective joint replacement [J] z Orthop Ihre Grenzgeb, 1997, 135(1): 45-51

Alimi D, Rubino C, Pichard-Leandri E, et al. Analgesic effect of auricular acupuncture for cancer pain: A randomized, blinded, controlled trial. J Clin Oncol 2003;21:4120 - 4126

Bonica JJ. Postoperative pain/Bonica JJ, editor. The management of pain. 2nd ed. Philadelphia: Lea and Febiger, 1990: 461-480.

Bing Z, Villanueva L, Le Bars D. Acupuncture and diffuse noxious inhibitory controls: Naloxone-reversible depression of activities of trigeminal convergent neurons. Neuroscience 1990;37:809-18.

Bo Huijuan, Wang Haiyan, Xu Jianyang, etc. RA rats for experimental electrical pain explain and brainstem NO / NOS changes of [J]. Shanghai Journal of Acupuncture and Moxibustion, 2002, 21 (5): 48-50.

Barker R, Kober A, Hoerauf K, et al. Out-of-hospital auricular acupressure in elder patients with hip fracture: A randomized double-blinded trial. Acad Emerg Med 2006; 13: 19-23.

Brander V, Gondek S, Martin E, et a1. Pain and depression influence outcome 5 years after knee replacement surgery [J]. Clin Orthop Relat Res, 2007, 464: 21-26.

Chen Jin, Liu Guangpu, Zhou Chunyang. Pieces of the hypothalamus and POMC mRNA expression of EP in the role of after-effects of acupuncture analgesia [J]. Acupuncture Research, 2004, 29 (1): 5-9.

Chen J, Sandkuhler J. Induction of homosynaptic long-term depression at spinal synapses of sensory a delta-fibers requires activation of metabotropic glutamate receptors. Neuroscience 2000; 98: 141 - 8.

Dorr L D, Chao L. The emotional state of the patient after total hip and knee arthroplasty [J] Clin Orthop Relat Res, 2007, 463: 7-12.

Endres HG, Bowing G, Diener HC, et al. Acupuncture for tension-type headache: A multicentre, shamcontrolled, patient- and observer-blinded, randomized trial. J Headache Pain 2007;8:306 - 14.

Fang Zongren, Yu Qin, Li Yanhua. Transmission of peripheral C fibers in acupuncture analgesia in the observation of the effects [J]. Acupuncture Research, 1992, 17(1): 48-53.

GiuffreM, Asci J, Arnstein P, et al. Postoperative joint replacement pain: description and op ioid requirement[J]. Post Anesth Nurs, 1991, 6 (4) : 239-245.

Goertz CM, Niemtzow R, Burns SM, et al. Auricular acupuncture in the treatment of acute pain syndromes: A pilot study. Mil Med 2006;171:1010 - 1014.

Gao Chengshun, Xiong Junyu, Analgesic strategy after total knee arthroplasty [J]. Medicine & Philosophy, 2009, 30(1):49-50.

Gary N. Asher, Daniel E. Jonas, Remy R. et al. Auriculotherapy for Pain Management: A Systematic Review and Meta-Analysis of Randomized Controlled Trials. The Journal of Alternative and Complementary Medicine. October 2010, 16(10): 1097-1108

He Xiaoling, Liu Xiang, Zhu Bing, etc. Strong electro-acupuncture points on the dorsal horn neurons in the central mechanism of the analgesic effect of extensive [J]. Acta Physiologica Sinica, 1995, 47 (6): 605-609.

Huang Yong. Najia acupuncture on adjuvant arthritis in rabbits leucine effects of brain endorphins [J]. Chinese Clinical Rehabilitation, 2004, 8 (30): 6676-6677.

Han JS, Terenius L. Neurochemical basis of acupuncture analgesia. Annu Rev Pharmacol Toxicol 1982; 22: 193-220.

Hebl JR, Dilger JA, Byer DE et al. A pre-emptive multi-modal pathway featuring peripheral nerve block improves perioperative outcomes after major orthopedic surgery [J]. Reg Anesth Pain Med, 2008, 33(6): 510-517.

Haake M, Muller HH, Schade-Brittinger C, et al. German Acupuncture Trials (GERAC) for chronic low back pain: Randomized, multicenter, blinded, parallelgroup trial with 3 groups. Arch Intern Med 2007; 167:1892 – 8.

Jiang Li, Zhao Canghuan. From a psychological point of view of acupuncture analgesia [J]. Liaoning Journal of Traditional Chinese Medicine, 2007, 34 (9): 1240-1241.

Jonas WB. Mosby's Dictionary of Complementary and Alternative Medicine. St Louis US: Elsevier Mosby, 2005.

Liu Xiang. Cerebral cortex and subcortical nuclei of the raphe nucleus of control and their role in acupuncture analgesia [J] Acupuncture Research, 1986, 21(2):4-10.

Lu Fang, Tang Jinshi, Yuan Bin, etc. Bilateral damage to the ventrolateral orbital cortex on the rat tail flick reflex inhibition of EA's influence [J]. Acupuncture Research, 1996, 21 (2): 39-42.

Liu Xiang, Huang Pingbo, Jiang Wuchun. Capsaicin blocked nerve C fiber ranked overall effect and its impact on EA "Zusanli" analgesic effect [J]. Acupuncture Research, 1997, 22(4): 295-303.

Liang Fanrong, Luo Rong, Liu Yuxing, etc. The experimental study of Effect of electroacupuncture analgesia and inflammation after partial 5-HT, NE, DA content [J]. Chinese Journal of Basic Medicine in Traditional Chinese Medicine, 2001, 7 (1): 52-55.

Nogier PFM. Traite´ d' auriculotherapie. Moulinle´s-Metz: Maisonneuve; 1972.

NaliniVadivelu, ;SukanyaMitra, DeepakNarayan, RecentAdvances in Postoperative

Pain Management, YALE JOURNALOF BIOLOGYAND MEDICINE, 2010, 83, pp.11-25.

Peuker ET, Filler TJ. The nerve supply of the human auricle. Clinical Anatomy 2002; 15: 35-7.

Skinner HB. Multimodal acute pain management[J]. Am J Orthop, 2004, 33 (5 Supp l) : 5-9.

Saito N, Horiuchi H, Kobayashi S, et al.. Continuous local cooling for pain relief following total hip arthroplasty[J] J Arthroplasty, 2004, 19 (3): 334-337.

Scharf HP, Mansmann U, Streitberger K, et al. Acupuncture and knee osteoarthritis: A three-armed randomized trial. Ann Intern Med 2006;145

Tang Jinshi, Yuan Bin. A new discovery of pain modulation pathway[J]. Journal of Xi'an Jiaotong University(Medical Sciences), 2002, 23(4):329-332.

Tian Jinhua, Wang Xiaomin, Han Jisheng. Nitric oxide and pain modulation [J]. Progress in Physiological Sciences, 1996, 27(2):161-164.

Usichenko TI, Hermsen M, Witstruck T, et al. Auricular acupuncture for pain relief after ambulatory knee arthroscopy. Evidence Based Complementary and Alternative Medicine 2005; 2: 185 – 9.

Usichenko TI, Kuchling S, Witstruck T, et al. Auricular acupuncture for pain relief after ambulatory knee surgery: a randomized trial. Canadian Medical Association Journal 2007; 176: 179 – 83.

White R H, Henderson M C. Risk factors for venous thromboembolism after total hip and knee replacement surgery [J] Curr Opin Pulm Med, 2002, 8(5): 365-37L

Wu c L, Naqibuddin M, Rowlingson A J et al. The effect of pain on health-related quality of life in the immediate postoperative period [J] Anesth Analg, 2003, 97 (4): 1078-1085

Wang Yuexiu, Yuan Bin, Tang Jinshi. Central thalamic nucleus and under the front cover before the district were involved in mediating the nuclear strong and weak electroacupuncture analgesic effect of acupuncture [J]. Chinese Journal of Neuroscience, 1999, 15 (2): 125-130.

Wang Hongbei, Dong Xiaotong, Wang Shuangkun, etc. Different frequencies of electroacupuncture adjuvant arthritis in rats with acute pain and tissue reaction of P-endorphin content of the belly [J]. Chinese Acupuncture & Moxibustion, 1998, 18 (3): 163-166.

Wang Shengxu, Lai Xinsheng, He Haitang, etc. EA Jiaji on adjuvant arthritis in rats before spinal cord dynorphin mRNA expression in the belly yuan [J]. Chinese Journal of Traditional Medical Science and Technology, 1999, 6(10): 1-4.

Wang Shengxu, Hong Jun, Zhou Yilin, etc. EA Jiaji on adjuvant arthritis in rat peripheral blood monoamine content of the material[J]. Chinese Journal of Traditional Medical Science and Technology, 2000, 7(5):273-275.

Wang Shengxu, Hong Jun, Lai Xinsheng, etc. EA Jiaji on adjuvant arthritis in rats with spinal cord effects of substance P immunohistochemical study [J]. Chinese Journal of Traditional Medical Science and Technology, 2000, 7(3): 131-132.

Wang Shengxu, Hong Jun, Lai Xinsheng. EA Jiaji on adjuvant arthritis in rats with spinal cord content of monoamine neurotransmitters [J]. Chinese Journal of Traditional Medical Science and Technology, 2001, 80:1-3.

Wu CL, Naqibuddin M, Rowlingson AJ, et al. The effect of pain on health-related quality of life in the immediate postoperative period [J]. Anesth Analg, 2003, 97 (4): 1078-1085

Xun Rong, Guan Xinmin, Wang Caiyuan. Capsaicin treatment on rat sciatic nerve pain off and analgesic effect of EA[J]. Acupuncture Research, 1993, 18(4):280-284

Yin Xiaolei, Li Dan, Advances in postoperative analgesia [J]. People's Military Surgeon, 2004, 47 (4): 243-245.

Yang Jie, Tang Jinshi, Yuan Bin, etc. Rat hypothalamic neurons under the center's response to acupuncture [J]. Chinese Journal of Pain Medicine, 1997, 3(4): 223-227.

Yang Jiebin, Song Kaiyuan, Liang Fanrong, etc. Different acupuncture therapy on rat adjuvant arthritis of peripheral mechanism of analgesia[J]. Chinese Acupuncture & Moxibustion, 1999, 18(6):362-366.

Y. Sun, T. J. Gan, J. W. Dubose and A. S. Habib Acupuncture and related techniques for postoperative pain: asystematic review of randomized controlled trials British Journal of Anaesthesia 2008, 101 (2): 151 - 60

ZhangY Q, Tang J S, Yuan B, et al. Effect of the alamicnucleussubme diu sle sionso nt heta ilfli ckr eflexin hibitione vokedb yh indli mbelec trical st imulationi nt her at [J].NeuroR eport, 1995, 6(9): 1237-1240.

Zhao Canghuan. Electricity for local inflammation in adjuvant arthritis in rats the effects of opioid peptide gene expression[J]. Journal of Jinan University（Natural Science & Medicine Edition）, 1997, 18(5): 158-161.

Zhao Canghuan, Zhou Jun. Inflammation of the EP and LEK local injection of anti-serum components on the effect of electroacupuncture analgesia [J]. Shaanxi Journal of Traditional Chinese Medicine, 2002, 23(6): 569-570.

8

Research on Medication Rules of Chronic Gastritis and Allergic Rhinitis Based on the Complex System Entropy Clustering Method

Renquan Liu[1], Yuhao Zhao[2], Chenghe Shi[3] and Guoyong Chen[1]
[1]*Beijing University of Chinese Medicine, Beijing,*
[2]*School of Traditional Chinese, Medicine, Capital Medical University, Beijing,*
[3]*Department of TCM,Peking University Third Hospital, Beijing,*
P.R. China

1. Introduction

1.1 Mining principle of herbal combinations

The highlight of this research is providing a appropriate statistical method to find out medication rules of chronic gastritis and allergic rhinitis, which will help us to guarantee clinical effects for this two diseases.

Five Viscera Tonifying Method (FVTM) was established by Prof. Gao Zhongying, a national prestigious and experienced practitioner of Traditional Chinese Medicine (TCM). This method extends the implication of tonfiying method while making a break-through in traditional TCM theory. With this featured method in pattern identification and herbal prescription, Prof. Gao is famed for his significant clinical effects by using well-prescribed formula. Modified Lung Tonifying Decoction (LTD), a representative formula of five viscera tonifying method, is indicated and effective for various lung diseases. We employed complex system entropy cluster technique to mine the data of prescriptions by this prestigious and experienced TCM practitioner. It is clinically significant to explore prescription rules of herbal medicine in the treatment of lung diseases to guarantee clinical effects.

According to statistics from World Health Organization (WHO), lung diseases have been one of the four leading diseases that pose great threatens to human health. Conventional treatment using western drugs proves to be advantageous yet its side-effects are hindering patient compliances and thus the clinical effects. There are over 1000 formula indicated for lung diseases, which have been developed in the 2000-year history of Traditional Chinese Medicine (TCM). Modern prestigious and experience TCM practitioners also have developed numerous their own effective formula based on inheriting the essence of prescription rules by ancient practitioners. To study the rules of these formulas is of great significance to facilitate the prescription rules of effective herbal treatment and to explore new formula for lung diseases.

There have been very few studies on prescription rules of herbal medicine for lung diseases by prestigious and experienced TCM practitioners. This study employed complex system entropy cluster technique to mine the data of prescriptions of the prestigious and experienced TCM practitioner and to explore prescription rules of herbal medicine in the treatment of lung diseases to guarantee clinical effects.

1.2 Data mining methods based symptoms clustering

The syndrome is the basic pathological unit and the key concept in traditional Chinese medicine (TCM), and the herbal remedy is prescribed according to the syndrome a patient catches. Nevertheless, few studies are dedicated to investigate the number of syndromes in chronic heart failure (CHF) patients and what these syndromes are. In this paper, we carry out a clinical epidemiology survey and obtain 317 CHF cases, including 62 symptoms in each report. Based on association delineated by mutual information, we employed a pattern discovery algorithm to discover syndromes, which probably have overlapped symptoms in TCM. A revised version of mutual information is presented here to discriminate positive and negative association. The algorithm self-organizedly discovers 15 effective patterns, each of which is verified manually by TCM physicians to recognize the syndrome it belongs to. Therefore, we conclude that the algorithm provides an excellent solution to chronic heart failure problem in the context of traditional Chinese medicine.

Heart failure (CHF) is the most terminal stages of cardiovascular disease to the clinical development of overall performance, with the improvement of living standards and the popularity of interventional cardiology techniques, the proportion of heart failure was increased gradually become a cause of coronary heart disease The main basis for heart failure (Lu&Zhong,2010). Activities by the degree of heart failure symptoms of impaired heart function status was assessed clinically NYHA classification is more commonly used by the patients cardiac function contribute to determine the extent of the disease Qing Qian and treatment options. At present, this area on TCM Syndrome research is still small. In this study, clinical epidemiology, collected coronary heart disease signs and symptoms of heart failure patients, through the heap of entropy together to compare the cardiac function in different situations and syndromes four diagnostic elements of the evolution of features, designed to further grasp the law of the disease syndromes, diagnosis and treatment for the disease to provide a basis for Chinese medicine.

Data mining is a systematic approach used not only to identify biomarkers for a disease but also to investigate the cellular interaction in the context of a disease to construct biological networks.

Data mining also has a crucial role to play in TCM-related research activities. By text mining, a branch of data mining approaches, the biological networks underlying cold and hot syndromes phenotypes are constructed by NEI specifications (Li et al.,2007).Similarly, through a combination of Chinese literatures on TCM and related English counterparts on most diseases on PubMed database, biological networks for a syndrome in TCM in the context of a disease can be automatically generated through text mining approaches (Zhou et al.,2007).In addition, several novel data mining approaches were presented to deal with various kinds of clinical or in vivo animal data. An unsupervised cluster algorithm called pattern discovery algorithm was developed to discover syndromes in TCM in the context of a disease,which provides the targets for formulae or prescriptions since they are prescribed based on syndromes diagnosed (Chen et al.,2007). Furthermore, animal models for syndrome in TCM in the context of diseases were built by using supervised data mining approach to'clone' diagnosis criterion from clinics to animals, which paves a way for in vivo experimental validation of a prescription.8 However, when applying data mining approach in TCM, few research efforts are made in research activities of TCM, it is important to investigate the role of data mining approaches in them.

In information theory, mutual information (MI) of two random variables is a measure that scales mutual dependence of the two variables. It has been applied in many fields, in which researchers treat as divergence or distance between two distributions.

2. Materials and methods

2.1 Mining principle of herbal combinations

2.1.1 Formula source

All the formula comes from clinical prescriptions by Prof. Gao Zhongying. Prof. Gao Zhongying is a national prestigious and experienced TCM practitioner. He was born in a TCM family of generations and has been working in the fields of TCM clinics, teaching and research for 55 years. He has worked as the director of TCM internal medicine department and herbs & formula department. He has studied TCM theories and applied them in clinic with care before establishing Five Viscera Tonifying Method (FVTM). This method is a breakthrough in traditional TCM theory. It extends the implication of tonifying method and represents featured pattern identification and herbal administration. His formulas are well-prescribed with significant clinical effects. LTD has proven to be effective as a representative of FVTM. To mine the data of formula by Prof. Gao is mainly to collect and categorize LTD prescriptions in this study.

2.1.2 Establishment of formula database

To meet the requirements of data mining and analysis, processing and categorizing the data is a perquisite. Standardized terms were used as 'Final Term' to code the symptoms, signs, tests in the case records. Independent 'Pattern Elements' were summarized or extracted from the cases after standardizing the diagnosis, patterns and treatment according to international and textbook criteria. Phrase databases of patterns and treatments were thus finally established. A database of the medicinal used in the formulas was categorized by their classes, functions, prosperities and meridian entry. The names of medicinals are consistent with those used in the current 21 century textbook.

A module of structured case records based on Access platform was established to collect the clinical data of Prof. Gao Zhongying. All the information about the patients were included using a national standard case record format and access database platform. Clinical data of the 389 cases were carefully recorded in details based on Systemic and Structured Data Entry Criteria in Collecting Clinical Information of Prestigious and Experienced TCM Practitioners. The structured clinical information and other data was included into the system and a Prof. Gao's clinical database was thus formed.

2.1.3 Data analysis method

Before introducing the algorithm, we give a rigorous definition to mutual information

The definition of mutual information

Suppose system $X=(X_1,X_2,\cdots,X_a,\cdots,X_p)^T$ is consisted of p variables, $p\in N$ (N set of natural number), where $X_a=(X_{a_i})$, $a=1,2,\cdots,p$; $i=1,2,\cdots,q$. Here our objective is to obtain some subsets which have some close properties from set X. Let $C_a(a=1,\cdots,p)$ be set of classification of X_a, $C_{a_i}=i$ be i-th element of C_a, then we have $C_a=\{1,2,\cdots,i\cdots,k\}$, $k\le q$, and let n_i be quantity for X_a belong to i-th class, then entropy of X_a is defined as

$$H(X_a)=-\sum_{i=1}^{k} n_i/q\log n_i/q \tag{1}$$

The joint entropy of X_a,X_b is similarly defined as

$$H(X_a \cup X_b) = -\sum_i \sum_j n_{ij} / q \log n_{ij} / q \tag{2}$$

where n_{ij} is quantity for X_a belong to i -th class of C_a simultaneously X_b belong to j -th class of C_b . For the convenience of application, expressions (1) and (2) can respectively be represented as

$$H(X_a) = \log q - \frac{1}{q}\sum_{i=1}^{k} n_i \log n_i \tag{3}$$

$$H(X_a \cup X_b) = \log q - \frac{1}{q}\sum_i \sum_j n_{ij} \log n_{ij} \tag{4}$$

Having had above-mentioned definition of entropy, in what follows, correlative measure by which statistical dependence between X_a and X_b is denoted is defined by their mutual information.

Definition 1. Correlative measure between two variables

For arbitrary $X_a \in X$, $X_b \in X$, suppose $X_a \cap X_b = \phi$, then entropy

$$H(X_a, X_b) = H(X_a) + H(X_b) - H(X_a \cup X_b) \tag{5}$$

is called correlative measure $\mu(X_a, X_b)$ between X_a and X_b .

Definition 2. Correlative measure among multi-variables

Suppose $X_a \cap X_b = \phi$ for arbitrary $a, b (a \neq b)$, $p \in N$ then

$$\mu(X_1, X_2, \cdots, X_p) \overset{\Delta}{=} \sum_{a=1}^{p} H(X_a) - H\left(\sum_{a=1}^{p} X_a\right) \tag{6}$$

is called correlative measure among X_1, X_2,...and X_p.

We can also extend the definitions of correlative measure among variables to that of subsets of complex system. In fact, the variable itself is also one particular subset.

Definition 3. Correlative measure among multi-subsystems

Suppose system X be partitioned into m subsystems $s_1, s_2, \cdots, s_m$, for arbitrary i, j $(i \neq j)$, $s_i \cap s_j = \phi$, $X = \sum_{i=1}^{m} s_i$, then

$$\mu(s_1, s_2, \cdots, s_m) \overset{\Delta}{=} \sum_{i=1}^{m} H(s_i) - H\left(\sum_{i=1}^{m} s_i\right) \tag{7}$$

is called correlative measure among $s_1, s_2, \cdots, s_m$.

Let us consider nonempty finite set X and set-family $E(X)$ consisted of its subsets, P is a set-function defined on $E(X)$ with properties:

i. $P(A) \geq 0$, $\forall A \in E(X)$,

ii. $P(\varnothing) = 0$

The complex entropy cluster algorithm

The algorithm is detailedly presented in (Chen et al.,2007), we also present it here.

Once association for each pair (every two variables) is acquired, we propose a self-organized algorithm to automatically discovery the patterns. The algorithm can not only cluster, but also realize some variables appear in some different patterns. In this section, we use three subsections to introduce the algorithm. The first introduce the concept of "Relative" set. Based on this, the pattern discovery algorithm is proposed in second subsection. The last subsection is devoted to presenting an n-class association concept to back up the idea of the algorithm.

For a specific variable X, a set, which is collected by mean of gathering N variables whose associations with X are larger than others with regard to X, is attached to it and is denoted as $R(X)$. Each variable in the set can be regarded as a "Relative" of X while other variables that not belong to the set are considered as irrelative to X, so we name $R(X)$ "Relative" set of X. The "Relative" sets of all 20 variables can be denoted by a $20 \times N$ matrix. Based on the matrix, the pattern discovery algorithm is proposed.

A pair (variable X and Y) is defined to be significantly associated if and only if X belongs to the "Relative" set of Y ($X \in R(Y)$) and vice versa ($Y \in R(X)$). It is convenient to extend this definition to a set with multiple variables. If and only if each pair of these variables is significantly associated, then we can call that the set is significant associated. A pattern is defined as a significantly associated set with maximal number of variables. All these kinds of sets constitute the hidden patterns in the data. Therefore, a pattern should follow three main criteria: (1) the number of variables within a set is no less than 2. (2) Each pair of the variables belong to a set is significantly associated. (3) Any variable outside a set can not make the set significantly associated. This means the number of variables within the set reaches maximum.

We defined that two variables X and Y are correlated if and only if they are inter-relative, i.e., X is a 'relative' of Y and vice versa. It is convenient to extend this definition to the case with multi-variables, if each pair between these variables is correlated, then we called that they are correlated. A set that is comprised of maximal variables in which each pair is correlated is defined as a pattern and all sets constitute the hidden patterns in the data acquired above.

2.2 Data mining methods based symptoms clustering

2.2.1 Clinical epidemiology

317 patients with coronary heart disease patients with heart failure were collected from May 2009 to March 2010 Dongzhimen Hospital, Beijing University of Chinese Medicine, Dongfang Hospital, Beijing University of Chinese Medicine, Department of Cardiology of the patients.

2.2.2 Diagnosis criteria

(1) coronary artery disease with reference to the International Society of Cardiology and the Society, named after the World Health Organization standardized clinical report of the Joint Task Team, "named after ischemic heart disease and diagnostic criteria"; (2) diagnosis of heart failure based on diagnosis of chronic heart failure in China in 2007 treatment guidelines; cardiac function with reference to the New York Heart Association (NYHA) 1928 annual standard.

2.2.3 Inclusion criteria

Coronary heart disease and chronic heart failure meet the above diagnostic criteria, older than 18 years of age and less than or equal to 80 years of age and informed consent, patients participated in this study.

2.2.4 Exclusion criteria

Exclusion criteria isBy the expansion of heart disease, pulmonary heart disease, rheumatic heart disease, cardiomyopathy, congenital heart disease and other heart disease due to heart failure patients; with acute myocardial infarction, cardiogenic shock, severe arrhythmias associated with hemodynamic changes in persons; concurrent infection : ① fever; ② blood increased, white blood cell count> 10 × 109 / L, neutrophils> 85%; ③ chest X-ray shadows suggestive of sheet; with severe hepatic insufficiency (liver function values> normal 2 times), renal insufficiency (Ccr> 20%, Scr> 3mg/dl or> 265μmol / L), blood system, the primary disease, malignant tumor; pregnancy or breast-feeding women; mental illness, infectious diseases

2.2.5 Survey methods

Survey methods of clinical epidemiology, screening results in the literature and two rounds of preliminary questionnaire was developed based on expert clinical four diagnostic information collection form, in patients with heart failure collect demographic data, present illness, symptoms and signs, and tongue, veins and other information.

2.2.6 Quality control

Clinical Hospital, prior to the survey of the designated person responsible for, the research group to develop the work of the researchers involved in the study manual for the doctor and unified training. Establish Epidate3.1 database, all cases investigated by double data entry.

3. Conclusion

3.1 Mining principle of herbal combinations

By using the following data analysis methods, the corresponding results are given in Table 1 to Table 3 as well as Figure 1.

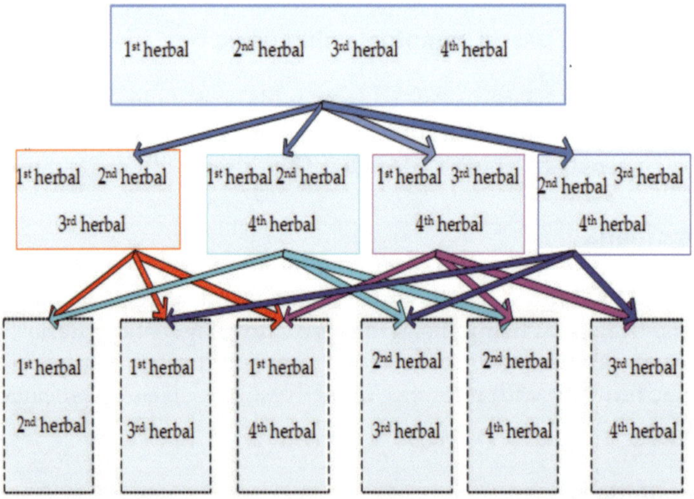

Fig. 1. The illustration of cluster process. Where 1st, 2nd ,3rd and 4th herbal represents milk-vetch root, rehmannia, heterophylly false satarwort root and Chinese magnolivine fruit respectively.

Herbal	Frequency	Usage	Herbal	Frequency	Usage
heterophylly false satarwort root	284	0.73008	scutellaria root	54	0.13882
milk-vetch root	270	0.69409	dwarf lilyturf tuber	52	0.13368
prepared rehmannia root	269	0.69152	common coltsfoot flower	46	0.11825
Chinese magnolivine fruit	265	0.68123	psoralea fruit	45	0.11568
tatarian aster root	222	0.57069	ephedra herb	43	0.11054
white mulberry root-bark	178	0.45758	Stir-baking bupleurum with vinegar	41	0.1054
pepperweed seed	136	0.34961	dried ginger rhizome	39	0.10026
snakegourd fruit; trichosanthes fruit	131	0.33676	Cassia twig	34	0.087404
pinellia rhizome	91	0.23393	great burdock achene	33	0.084833
platycodon root	91	0.23393	liquorice root	32	0.082262
rehmannia root	76	0.19537	heartleaf houttuynia herb	32	0.082262
tendrilled fritillaria bulb	64	0.16452	Chinese waxgourd seed	31	0.079692
stemona root	56	0.14396	smoked plum	31	0.079692
blackberry lily rhizome	55	0.14139	magnolia bark	30	0.077121
almond	55	0.14139			

Table 1. Commonly-used medicinal in the prescriptions of modified LTD for lung diseases

Herbal combination		Mutual information	Herbal combination		Mutual information
cockleburr fruit	blond magnolia flower	0.20823	euryale seed	pepperweed seed	0.07403
psoralea fruit	euryale seed	0.1568	perilla-seed	tatarian aster root	0.071148
blackberry lily rhizome	pepperwe ed seed	0.14528	snakegourd fruit	immature orange fruit	0.070149
ephedra herb	almond	0.1384	Stir-baking bupleurum with vinegar	blond magnolia flower	0.067455
platycodon root	pepperwe ed seed	0.13568	white atractylodes rhizome	ledebouriella root	0.064919
Indian bread	cassia twig	0.12965	common coltsfoot flower	pepperweed seed	0.063739
pinellia rhizome	red tangerine peel	0.1181	amur cork-tree bark	light yellow sophora root	0.06262
psoralea fruit	pepperwe ed seed	0.11559	stemona root	tatarian aster root	0.062125
prepared rehmannia root	Chinese magnolivi ne fruit	0.10894	Safflower	turmeric root tuber	0.061022
platycodon root	oroxylum seed	0.10519	atractylodes rhizome	light yellow sophora root	0.059596
platycodon root	great burdock achene	0.10188	tree peony bark	light yellow sophora root	0.059596
ephedra herb	great burdock achene	0.096925	donkey-hide gelatin pellets	dwarf lilyturf tuber	0.059468
bile arisaema	glabrous greenbrier rhizome	0.095717	pepperweed seed	tatarian aster root	0.05726
magnolia bark	almond	0.094751	light yellow sophora root	glabrous greenbrier rhizome	0.055996
platycodon root	white mulberry root-bark	0.088538	cassia twig	Safflower	0.055512
psoralea fruit	white mulberry root-bark	0.08771	kudzuvine root	Euonymi twig	0.055454

Herbal combination		Mutual information	Herbal combination		Mutual information
oldenlandia	bearded scutellaria	0.083543	snakegourd fruit	milk-vetch root	0.053697
suberect spatholobus stem	centipede	0.083543	common coltsfoot flower	blackberry lily rhizome	0.052638
rehmannia root	scutellaria root	0.083134	heterophylly false satarwort root	Chinese magnolivine fruit	0.052357
perilla-seed	pepperwe ed seed	0.082173	donkey-hide gelatin pellets	turmeric root tuber	0.052208
snakegourd fruit	scutellaria root	0.08126	great burdock achene	pepperweed seed	0.052098
cockleburr fruit	Stir-baking bupleuru m with vinegar	0.079804	Indian bread	Euonymi twig	0.050529
curcumae rhizome	cassia twig	0.077009	cockleburr fruit	ledebouriella root	0.050329
cnidium fruit	glabrous greenbrier rhizome	0.076576			

Table 2. Commonly-used medicinal combinations and combining values in the prescriptions of modified LTD for lung diseases

pinellia rhizome	**tendrilled fritillaria bulb**	**common coltsfoot flower**	**blackberry lily rhizome**
cockleburr fruit	Stir-baking bupleurum with vinegar	Chinese magnolivine fruit	blond magnolia flower
common coltsfoot flower	blackberry lily rhizome	perilla-seed	pepperweed seed
blackberry lily rhizome	perilla-seed	pepperweed seed	tatarian aster root
donkey-hide gelatin pellets	white peony root	atractylodes rhizome	
donkey-hide gelatin pellets	atractylodes rhizome	light yellow sophora root	

pinellia rhizome	**tendrilled fritillaria bulb**	**common coltsfoot flower**	**blackberry lily rhizome**
donkey-hide gelatin pellets	atractylodes rhizome	dwarf lilyturf tuber	
donkey-hide gelatin pellets	liquorice root	turmeric root tuber	
donkey-hide gelatin pellets	Safflower	turmeric root tuber	
donkey-hide gelatin pellets	dwarf lilyturf tuber	turmeric root tuber	
white peony root; peony	suberect spatholobus stem	centipede	
white atractylodes rhizome	aged tangerine peel	liquorice root	
white atractylodes rhizome	prepared rehmannia root	Chinese magnolivine fruit	
stemona root	platycodon root	oroxylum seed	
stemona root	cassia bark	oroxylum seed	
pinellia rhizome	common coltsfoot flower	white mulberry root-bark	
thunberg fritillary bulb	liquorice root	hogfennel root	
thunberg fritillary bulb	great burdock achene	hogfennel root	
psoralea fruit	common coltsfoot flower	white mulberry root-bark	
psoralea fruit	common coltsfoot flower	pepperweed seed	
psoralea fruit	euryale seed	pepperweed seed	
cockleburr fruit	ephedra herb	blond magnolia flower	

Table 3. Core medicinal combinations in the prescriptions of modified LTD for lung diseases

The name of Lung Tonifying Decocction (LTD) has been found in several ancient literatures. The ingredients recorded in Yun QI Zi Bao Ming Ji (Yun Qi Zi's Collections of Life-saving Formula) are different from those in Bei Ji Qian Jin Yao Fang (Essential Prescriptions Worth a Thousand Gold for Emergiences) and San Yin Ji Yi Bing Zheng Fang Lun (Treatise on Three Categories of Pathogenic Factors and Prescriptions). Prof. Gao used the ingredients of former source. Some Scholars says this formula was originated from Yong Lei Qian Fang written by Li Zhongnan in 1331 and Jing Yue Quan Shu (Complete Works of Jingyue). Sang Bai Pi (Cortex Mori), Di Huang (Radix Rehmanniae), Ren Shen (Radix et Rhizoma Ginseng),

Zi Wan (Radix et Rhizoma Asteris), Huang Qi (Radix Astragali), Wu Wei Zi (Fructus Schisandrae Chinensis) formulates a representative formula for tonifying lung qi. It was originally indicated for Lao Sou (consumptive cough) due to five viscera deficiency pattern manifested as afternoon tidal fever, spontaneous sweating or nigh sweating, cough with sputum, dyspnea with panting. In the formula, Ren Shen and Huang Qi are sweet and warm in nature. They are used to tonify qi, supplement the defense aspect and secure the exterior. The two medicinals are targeted at deficiency of spleen and lung. Di Huang is to supplement kidney essence to supply qi, tonify the lower to supplement the upper part of the body. It is also used to supply water to moisten the lungs and remove the deficiency dryness in the upper source. Wu Wei Zi and Zi Wan can astringe the lungs and moisten the dryness to relieve dryness and coughing. Sang Bai Pi clears the heat and calms down the reverse qi to resolve phlegm and stop coughing. These medicinals used together are to tonify the spleen and kidneys, moisten the dryness and stop coughing. That's how it works in most cases in the clinic.

In terms of the number of medicinal, Prof.Gao tends to use a few medicinals with specific targets. On average there are around 12 medicinals in each of his formula. Table 1 shows that Prof. Gao sticks to the original ingredients of the formula. The commonly-used medicinals ranked in the first 6 places are originally used in the formula. Modification is often used for specific symptoms. For example Ban Xia (Rhizoma Pinelliae) and Gua Lou (Fructus Trichosanthis) are combined to strengthen the effects of phlegm resolving. Table 2 shows that Prof. Gao tends to use Xin Yi (Flos Magnoliae) combined with Cang Er (Fructus Xanthii) to open the nasal orifice, Wu Wei Zi (Fructus Schisandrae Chinensis) combined with vinegar processed Chai Hu (Radix Bupleuri) to antagonize allergy. The results indicate that it is significant to mine data of prescriptions by prestigious and experienced TCM practitioners by using complex system entropy cluster technique.

Modified LTD is effective for various lung diseases, yet it has not been included by the current formula textbook. There has been few literature and clinical studies on this formula as well. According to incomplete statistics, Prof. Gao has used the modified LTD to treat Chronic Obstructive Pulmonary Diseases (COPD), Idiopathic Pulmonary Fibrosis (IPF), anthrasilicosis, bronchiectasis, allergic asthma and rhinitis besides coughing and panting in the clinic. Most attention should be drawn to this formula by the clinicians to improve clinical effects.

3.2 Data mining methods based symptoms clustering

Information collection form will be provided by the signs and symptoms of each patient were statistically and found 317 cases of heart failure in patients with systemic symptoms Shenpi fatigue (100%), shortness of breath (93%), less gas lazy words (71 %), spontaneous (39%), chills (39%), five upset hot (27%) majority; head, face the common symptoms of dizziness (73%), lips cyanosis (58%), dark complexion (22%); mind and flank the chest symptoms (88%), palpitations (76%), wheezing (57%), chest pain (37%), expectoration (30%) were more; stomach and abdominal symptoms of bloating (48 %) was the most common; waist and limbs Yaoxisuanruan common symptoms (73%), limb trapped weight (51%), and edema (55%), hand, foot and not warm (39%); restaurants and taste of symptoms to loss of appetite (59%), dry mouth (48%), sticky mouth (27%) were more symptoms of sleep and the two will be to insomnia (65%), nocturia (38%) most common; tongue in order to sublingual vein abnormalities (61%), tongue dark (55%), crack the tongue (34%), tongue pink (24%),

less or no moss moss (20%), fat large indentation tongue (19%) is more common; pulse late in the common pulse (49%), pulse astringent (21%), promoting Pulse (17%), pulse knot generation (10%).
By using pattern discovery algorithm, the 15 patterns were given in Table 4.

No.	Combination of symptoms	Syndrome diagnosed
1	Shortness of breath, asthma, fatigue, side limb edema	Qi Deficiency
2	Abdominal distention, gurgling, nausea, vomiting, mouth light thirsty	
3	Abdominal threatening pain, backache, headache, nausea expansion Xiong Xie	Qi stagnation
4	Subject to colds, cough, Long cough, sputum	
5	Shortness of breath, Shenpi, fatigue	Qi Deficiency
6	Shortness of breath, wheezing, sputum	
7	Shenpi, cough, bad air	
8	Fatigue, loss of appetite, shortness of breath	
9	Top-heavy, such as wrap, dizziness, limb paralysis Ma	
10	Ringing in the ears, knees soft, backache	
11	Tinnitus, backache, nausea expansion Xiong Xie	
12	Five upset hot, dry mouth, hot flushes and night sweats	Yin Deficiency
13	Five upset hot, constipation, hot flushes and night sweats	
14	Headache, nausea expansion Xiong Xie, channeling pain away	
15	Cough, Cough, the evil wind	

Table 4. 15 patterns for CHF

In heart failure have been recorded, including early, carved in Chinese medicine is a "heart palpitations", "Tan Yin" and "asthma card", "edema", "accumulation" and other areas. On the characteristics of the basic pathogenesis of heart failure, there are different points of view, Wong (Li et al.,2007) that the disease is mainly responsible for deficiency in the heart failure, falling seedlings lung, spleen, kidney all dirty and wet phlegm from each breeding Results from the heart Qi-oriented, blood stasis, water to drink as standard; Wang (Wang,2005) that the deficiency and yang-oriented virtual, blood stasis, water resistance, phlegm as the standard implementation of the levy; Chen (Li&Chen,2006) will be virtual, stasis, water summarized as the basic pathogenesis of the disease. 200 patients from four diagnostic methods of frequency analysis results, the heart failure patients often show the signs and False or True, false to qi deficiency, yang deficiency, yin deficiency is a common, real to stasis, water, sputum-based, I believe that deficiency may be associated with their hypertension, diabetes and other primary diseases related to each other based on the root theory of yin and yang, yang deficiency and yin, yang to a certain extent patients can occur when the signs of deficiency, it also Coronary Heart Yin decline in the basic pathogenesis of the important part.

Entropy algorithm for the clustering together of the heap in one, with the traditional method compared to non-supervised clustering, which is characterized by improved correlation between two variables method, effectively avoid the interference of negative data, through the calculate the two bivariate correlation coefficients between each variable designated the "friends group", after convergence, go to "friends group" within the limited number of variables, leaving the variables must be close to each other with higher levels of combination, this data extraction process and we are in the clinical symptoms and signs by a certain type of information gathering to designate property Panduan a similar card, therefore, become the method to explore between the clinical symptoms and Syndrome internal laws of the more common and objective mathematical method. In this study, patients with different cardiac function four diagnostic variables together elements of the heap after the analysis of the syndrome of basic and clinical match, but the law also has some defects, such as better together to make the variable into a class, we screened the raw data, which may lose some useful information. In conclusion, this study together after the data, while the heap is not fully reflect the clinical, but at least clinical symptoms of the disease trends in the evolution provide some reference.

4. References

Chen J, Xi G, Chen J et al., An unsupervised pattern (syndrome in traditional Chinese medicine) discovery algorithm based on association delineated by revised mutual information in chronic renal failure data, *J Biol Syst* 15(4):435–451, 2007.

LI Li-zhi. Chen Kej i'S Experience on the treatment of congestive heart failure. *Chinese Journal of Integrative Medicine on Cardio-/Cerebrovascular Disease*, 2006, 4(2): 136-138.

Li S, Zhang X, Wang Y et al., Understanding Zheng in traditional Chinese medicine in the context of neuro-endocrine immune network, *IET Syst Biol* 1(1):51–60, 2007.

LU Zai-ying, ZHONG Nan-shan. Internal Medicine. 7th ed. Beijing: People' s Medical Publishing House. 2010：170.

WANG Zhen-tao. Experience of syndrome differentiation and treatment on congestive heart failure. *Journal of Sichuan of Traditional Chinese Medicine* , 2005, 23(6): 9-10.

Zhou X, Liu B, Wu Z et al., Integrative mining of traditional Chinese medicine literature and MEDLINE for functional gene networks, *Artif Intell Med* 41(2):87–104,2007.

9

Effectiveness of Traditional Chinese Medicine in Primary Care

Wendy Wong[1], Cindy Lam Lo Kuen[1],
Jonathan Sham Shun Tong[2] and Daniel Fong Yee Tak[3]
[1]*Department of Family Medicine and Primary Care, LKS Faculty of Medicine,*
[2]*Department of Clinical Oncology, LKS Faculty of Medicine,*
[3]*Department of Nursing Studies, LKS Faculty of Medicine,*
The University of Hong Kong
Hong Kong

1. Introduction

This chapter first describes the role of Traditional Chinese Medicine (TCM) in health care. It then reviews the literature on the effectiveness of TCM with a special focus on primary care. An appraisal of the outcome measures in the context of TCM is made. The relationship between TCM and the concept of health-related quality of life (HRQOL) is discussed. The current applications and limitations of the HRQOL measures derived from Western culture to TCM are identified. The chapter ends with an overview of Chinese culture specific measures for evaluating the effectiveness of TCM in primary care.

2. The role of Traditional Chinese Medicine (TCM) in health services

In China, it was estimated that there were 3.1 billion TCM outpatient visits per year for the 1.3 billion population [1]. Currently, TCM accounts for 40% of all health services delivered in China, and it has been part of the formal Chinese healthcare system since 1950 under the political directives of Mao Tse Tung [2]. However, the development of TCM in Hong Kong followed a different path as it was not recognized by the Government as part of the formal healthcare system until 1997 when Hong Kong was reunited with China. The Hong Kong Special Administrative Region (SAR) government tried to re-integrate TCM into the health care system in the past decade by the establishment of the Chinese Medicine Council of Hong Kong (CMCHK) as a statutory body under the Chinese Medicine Ordinance to regulate and register Chinese Medicine Practitioners (CMP) in 1999 [3]. Although TCM in Hong Kong is still mostly a private service, piloting outpatient TCM clinics and limited inpatient services have started in public hospitals. Subsidized TCM primary care outpatient services have been provided by the Tung Wah Group Hospitals for nearly half a century in Hong Kong [4].

Even though Western Medicine consultation is the most commonly used type of primary care, 50 to 60% of people have consulted TCM in Hong Kong and 13.5% of the people have consulted TCM frequently or occasionally [5, 6]. There are 5604 registered CMP serving a population of 6.8 million in Hong Kong [3] and most of them provide primary care. A recent survey found that 19% of all private outpatient services were provided by Chinese Medicine Practitioners (CMP) [7] suggesting that many people find TCM helpful enough to be willing to pay for the service. Users of TCM were found to be more likely to be women, older persons, chronic disease patients with lower quality of life, and the lower socioeconomic group [8]. With its whole person approach, TCM may have a role in primary care to enhance the quality of life and health of people especially the elderly and those with chronic diseases.

TCM is regarded as a form of complementary and alternative medicines (CAM) in most countries other than China. CAM refers to a broad set of health practices that are not part of the country's own tradition and are not integrated into the dominant health care system [9]. The number of CAM visits exceeded the number of visits to all primary care physicians, and the estimated total out-of-pocket expenditure on CAM was US$27 billions in 1997 which was comparable to that for all primary care physician services for the same year [10]. TCM, especially acupuncture and bone-setting, is one of the most popular CAM globally being practiced widely in Asia, the United States (US), Canada, Europe and Australia [10]. TCM makes up a major proportion of the CAM services in the US [10] increasing from 34% in 1989 to 42% in 1997 [11]. Many of these patients reported improvement with their illnesses that Western Medicine failed to help [12]. In Denmark, the proportion of patients who had used TCM at least once annually increased from 23% in 1987 to 43.7% in 2007 [13]. TCM consultations accounts for a total expenditure of £580 million in the United Kingdom (UK) [14].

The increasing use of TCM has caused a profound impact on the global health care services. The National Centre of Complementary and Alternative Medicine (NCCAM) and the National Health Service (NHS) have been established in the US and the UK respectively, to allocate national budget for TCM services in primary care. Other European countries also have provided public financing for TCM [10]. The global increase use of TCM has called for more information on its function and outcomes to guide medical resource allocation.

3. Effectiveness of Traditional Chinese Medicine

The effectiveness of acupuncture in pain control was first demonstrated by an expert panel systematic review in the NIH conference in 1997 [15], which attracted the world's attention to TCM. This has established the place of TCM in health care. Artemisia annua was proved to be effective in against resistant malaria and gave hope of preventing more than 800 thousand deaths from malaria among children each year [16, 17]. In Geriatrics, TCM has been shown to not only improve health-related quality of life (HRQOL) in the treatment of illnesses, but also to promote healthy aging [18]. Wesnes and Ward et al. found Panax ginseng significantly improved an index of memory quality by 7.5% and this effect persisted for the whole treatment period until 2 weeks after washout [19]. TCM has also been studied for the prevention of acute severe respiratory syndrome (SARS) in hospital workers [20]. None of the health workers who took the supplement had contracted SARS compared to 0.4% of health care workers who did not ($p=0.014$). Improvement in influenza-like symptoms and quality of life were also observed among herbal supplement users. A remarkable effectiveness of TCM was found in patients with irritable bowel syndrome in a randomized controlled trial that showed an improvement measured by the total bowel symptoms scale and global improvement scores assessed by both patients and gastroenterologists [21]. Many studies in Europe were carried out in recent years to evaluate TCM treatments for specific conditions with variable results. In the UK, a daily decoction containing 10 herbs was found to be more effective than placebo in improving patients with chronic atopic dermatitis in erythema, surface damage, patients' subjective feeling on itching and sleep in a randomized, double-blind placebo-controlled trial [22, 23]. In Nerthlands, the effectiveness of Chinese herbal medicine (CHM) integrated with TCM diagnosis was confirmed for the treatment of postmenopausal symptoms when compared with hormone replacement therapy (HRT) or placebo in a randomized placebo-controlled trial [24]. It was found that CHM could significantly improve the amount of hot flushes than placebo. In addition, quality of care research in a TCM hospital in German found that TCM care could reduce the intensity of complaints, improve quality of life (in terms of both mental and physical-related HRQOL scores of SF-36) and subjective and objective global rating of conditions of inpatients subjects [25]. However, there were few research data on the effectiveness of TCM in primary care even though it is most commonly used for this purpose.

The National Health Service (NHS) of the UK conducted 4 large-scale population studies on the impact of CAM in reorganization of primary care services in 1999 [14, 26, 27]. Results showed that patients not only had their health outcomes significantly improved or expectation met after the consultation but also had significantly decreased in the use of medication and general practitioner time. A limitation of these surveys was that they did not differentiate between the different types of CAM.

A study by the Swiss Federal Department of Home Affairs evaluated and compared the health status and health care utilization rates of users of complementary and alternative medicine (CAM) clinics found that patients attending CAM clinics had higher consultation rates and more severe illnesses than patients in conventional primary care clinics [28]. This study gave evidence on poorer self-perced health status of CAM patients which need for a more physician-based medical services provided by CAM practitioners in primary care. The need for evaluating Chinese medicine and assure the quality of care was revealed by a population survey in Beijing [29] and a qualitative study in the UK [30]. Before this study, there were no data available on the effectiveness of TCM in primary care yet. The effectiveness of TCM primary care service as a whole remained unknown and that for the treatment of common problems were limited. Such information is needed to inform policy makers and the public how TCM is best utilized in our health care system [31, 32].

3.1 Evaluating the effectiveness of Traditional Chinese Medicine (TCM)

Despite the fact that TCM is popular globally and national institutes have been established for the integration of TCM into their health care systems, scientific evidence to support its use is not sufficient. The effectiveness of a highly individualized treatment made by a Chinese Medicine Practitioner (CMP) is usually subject to only the CMP's assessment and patients' subjective perception. The lack of a standardized outcome measurement method limits its scientific evaluation and generalizability of the results. The requirement of the paradigm of evidence based practice in using randomized controlled trials (RCT) as the 'gold standard' for the evaluation of treatment effectiveness has led to the denigration of non-experimental studies. A major conference held in 1993 concluded that only RCT was capable to confirm the benefit brought by TCM, and recommendation should not be made from evidence gathered in observational or case-control studies. However, only a few

Chinese herbal remedies and acupuncture have been proven by RCT [15]. Most claims on the effectiveness of TCM were based on empirical experience, leading to some people concluding that TCM was mostly not effective or even harmful [33]. Nevertheless, the debate on the most appropriate study designs for evaluating the effectiveness of TCM continues.

Unfortunately, most randomized controlled trials (RCT) conducted on TCM were rated to be poor in quality [34, 35] but RCT is not the only research study design and has its limitation. Classical RCT enforced the evaluation of TCM by the conventional Western medicine model, which can be impractical and inappropriate [36]. Black pointed out that not every intervention can be evaluated by a randomized trial and most importantly the rigorous random allocation may reduce the effectivenss of the intervention by not considering the subject's active participation, beliefs and preference [37]. We need observational or cohort studies to evaluate some interventions while others should be tested by RCT. Studies conducted by Thomas and Fitter showed the impossibilities of blinding Chinese Medicine Practitioners or patients during acupuncture interventions or giving individualized TCM treatments according to patients preference [38]. The realization of the inappropriateness of classical RCT to evaluate TCM led to the development of two alternative clinical trial methods: (1) the partial randomization design; and (2) the pragmatic design with prior randomization by Fitter [39] to evaluate the effectiveness of TCM. The partial randomization design takes patients' preference into account before they are randomized into treatment or placebo groups. Upon recruitment, patients are asked whether they have a preference for certain treatments, and if they do, they are assigned to the preferred treatment. If not, they are randomly assigned into either the study or the control treatments. The pragmatic design with prior randomization classifies eligible patients into syndrome groups by TCM practitioners before they are randomized to receive the appropriate treatment or placebo.

The study by Zaslawshi showed the pragmatic design with the integration of the CMP's syndrome differentiation based on TCM theory into a randomizd controlled trial was feasible in an acupuncture clinical trial [40]. This model was also used successfully in a RCT on the treatment of Irritable bowel syndrome (IBS) with Chinese herbal medicine showing better improvement in patients treated with individualized Chinese herbal formulae than standard TCM treatment and placebo groups [21].

The Medical Research Council in the UK [41], the NIH in the US [42] and WHO [43] have established guidelines on the research methodology for evaluating the effectiveness of CAM. All these recognize that conventional research methodology may not be applicable and recommended syndrome differenitaion in clinical trials. The pragmatic design of applying TCM syndrome differentiation to guide the formulation of the treatment before randomization is recommended to be a clinical trial model for attainining evidence-based TCM [44, 45].

4. Health outcome measures in the context of Traditional Chinese Medicine

Clinical outcomes can be categorized into four types (1) clinician-reported outcomes; (2) physiological outcomes; (3) caregiver-reported outcomes and (4) patient-reported outcomes (PROs) [46]. Clinician-reported outcomes are the observation, global impression or functional assessment made by professionals including doctors and nurses. Physiological outcomes include results from different laboratory tests (e.g. blood test, ultrasonic examination, X-ray etc). Caregiver-reported outcomes include the patient's behavior dependency and functional status observed by the caregiver. Patient reported outcomes (PROs) represent the patients' own perception of the changes in their own health condition, response to treatment and feelings, which include but not limited to general health status, symptoms, functional status and health-related quality of life (HRQOL). The first two types of outcomes used to be the main measures of efficacy or effectiveness of treatments but they are no longer adequate or sensitive enough for modern health care that aims at improving quality of life [47]. PROs started to gain popularity especially in the field of oncology. WHO defined the concept of 'health' as 'a state of complete physical, mental and social well-being and not merely the absence of disease or infirmity.'[48]. This definition has changed the conventional use of morbidity and mortality to measure health outcomes. Health care has become more concerned with the impact of health on social behavior and psychological well-being. In 1970s, quality of life began to be applied as an outcome to the medical field [49-53]. In 1975, the word 'quality of life' started to be used as a keyword in medical journals such as Annals of Surgery or Health Educaiton [54]. In 1977, 'quality of life' became indexed in the Index Medicus (Medline) database. In 1966, only four quality of life related articles published in Medline, 511 articles were published in 1998 and 4872 were published in 2008. The number of articles increased to a total of 72989 from 1966 to 2008 reflecting the increasing applications of QOL in medicine. The Oncologic Drugs Advisory Committee of the Food and Drug Administration (FDA) announced the beneficial effects on quality of life (QOL) as an endpoint and it could serve as the basis for approval of new oncology drugs [55]. Health-related quality of life (HRQOL) has become a standard outcome indicator in many clinical trials, population studies and health services in Western Medicine. There is potential for it to be used as a primary outcome measure for TCM.

5. The philosophy and conceptual base of Traditional Chinese Medicine

To evaluate the effectiveness of Traditional Chinese Medicine (TCM) its underlying philosophy and concepts of health must be defined. Dating back to the 8th century BC, Chinese defined the health by the concepts of the Yin and Yang which formed the theoretical base of TCM. Chinese Medicine practitioners (CMP) consider patients' symptoms in the context of an imbalance between Yin and Yang, In TCM, the equilibrium of Yin and Yang is best described in the earliest book on TCM, Internal Classic of Medicine [56].

"If the Yin and Yang energies of a man are kept in a state of equilibrium, his body will be strong and his spirit sound, if his Yin and Yang energies are dissociated, his vital energy will be declined and finally exhausted." and "A healthy man is one whose physique, muscle, blood and Qi are harmonious and appropriate with each other."

A perfect equilibrium between Yin and Yang indicates a perfect health state and implies good life quality. Disease is the result of a break down of the equilibrium between Yin and Yang with an excess or deficiency of either Yin or Yang. Symptoms develop as a result of the imbalance between Yin and Yang, which can be assessed by Chinese Medicine Practitioners (CMP) with the four diagnostic methods which are "Inspection", "auscultation-olfaction", "inquiry" and "palpation". A TCM treatment regimen aims at regulating and re-establishing the balance between Yin and Yang within the individual. This may involve reducing the redundancy of Yin or Yang or reinforcing the deficiency of Yin or Yang through the process of "planning treatment according to the individualized diagnosis called Bianzheng and lunzhi". By this principle, even though two patients presenting different symptoms/

illnesses, if the underlying TCM syndrome differentiation is the same, the treatments are still the same. This is known as different illnesses same treatment. On the other hand, two patients with the same presentation of symptoms/illness, if the underlying TCM syndrome differentiations are different, the treatments should be different. The main TCM treatments modalities include herbal medicines, acupuncture, moxibustion, exercises, breathing techniques and diets.

The health concept in TCM also emphasizes the importance of diet, daily activities, physical functioning and emotion, which conincides with that defined by the World Health Organization. In promoting health, Internal Classic of Medicine [56] described that:

"Those who knew the way of keeping good health in ancient times lived in accordance with nature, followed the principle of Yin and Yang, conformed with the art of prophecy, modulated their food and drinks, worked and rested in regular times and avoided overwork; therefore, they could maintain both the body and spirit to live to the natural old age of more than one hundred years."

6. Outcome indicators of TCM

As mentioned above, Traditional Chinese Medicine (TCM) has long been criticized for the lack of standardized outcome measures. The individualized prescription made by the Chinese Medicine Practitioner (CMP) is usually based on the CMP's subjective assessment. Particularly, the assessments between different CMP for the same patient can be greatly different, a lack of consistency in the assessment methods and outcome limits the generalizability of TCM and makes its evaluation difficult. Some researchers have tried to develop measures to standardize TCM syndrome differentiation diagnosis but it has been criticized that this method is limiting the strength of TCM in individualized treatment [57] and forcing TCM to adopt the classification of Western Medicine. In fact, the evaluation of TCM has little about measuring outcomes [58]. To evaluate the effectiveness of TCM, conventional outcome indicators such as laboratory or physical examination developed from Western Medicine have been applied in TCM research but there are great doubts on their appropriateness in the context of TCM. Some aspects such as complexion, spirit and vitality improvement cannot be captured by these indicators but they are very important indicators of health in TCM.

7. Traditional Chinese Medicine (TCM) and Health-related Quality of Life (HRQOL)

Health-related quality of life shares the same concepts and objectives as TCM. It should theoretically be the most appropriate outcome measure of the effectiveness of TCM. A paper by Lai et al [59] published in 2000 discussed and established the relationship between TCM and HRQOL. They pointed out that Chinese Medicine Practitioners (CMP) mainly rely on patients' reported symptoms and daily activities in their diagnostic process. The assessment of disease progression greatly depends on patients' feedback. Patients' subjective perception of the effect of their illness and treatment could be captured more scientifically by standardized HRQOL measures. To evaluate the effectiveness of TCM more scientifically, they suggested three directions: (1) Applying international generic HRQOL measures to evaluate the clinical effect of TCM; (2) Using standard methods to develop generic HRQOL measures for TCM, and (3) Developing TCM-condition specific HRQOL measures. Many other practitioners and researchers also agreed that HRQOL should be used as an important outcome of TCM because it can capture the latter's emphasis on the balance in physical, social and psychological well being [60, 61]. This outcome measure should complement conventional methods such as CMP assessment or laboratory results in the evaluation of TCM.

7.1 The concepts of health-related quality of life

The term Quality of life (QOL) is difficult to be defined. It summarizes a wide range of life events [62] and is a subjective appraisal of an individual of his/her life as a whole in various aspects. These aspects may range from the perception of well-being, satisfaction with one's life, achievement of personal goal, social usefulness, normalcy to duration of life, impairment, functional status (social, psychological, and physical), health perceptions, and opportunity. The definition of quality of life in fact depends on subjective perception which is greatly influenced by the environment, social, political and economic situations and cultures. Cummins had identified more than 100 definitions of QOL in the literature [63]. In general, QOL refers to a global state of satisfaction with life as a whole and the presence of positive feelings and the absence of negative ones. The broad and inclusive definitions of QOL go far beyond the medical model and only those aspects related to health are relevant to Medicine.

The term Health-related quality of life (HRQOL) is an attempt to quantify the net consequence of a disease and its treatment on the patients' perception of his ability to live a useful and fulfilling life [64]. It aims at measuring the effect of health by using a defined number of dimensions that are relevant to the person. These dimensions are structured firstly according to the WHO definitions of health to include the physical, psychological and social well-being [48]. Some authors extended the dimensions by adding spirituality. The purpose of HRQOL assessment is not only on measuring the presence and severity of illnesses but also on showing how an illness or treatment is experienced by an individual [65]. It has been used extensively in clinical trials [66-68], health economic research [69-72] and quality of care evaluations [73-76].

Although HRQOL has been criticized as too 'soft' or less reliable than conventional physiologic indicators, HRQOL can detect important clinical changes in many chronic conditions that other clinical outcome measures cannot. HRQOL differentiated patient adherence between three anti-hypertensive agents (captopril, methyldopa, and propranolol) that had similar efficacy in lowering blood pressure but different effects on quality of life [77]. Brown et al. found that a SF-36 physical functioning socre and role limitation score lower than the UK norm by 20 and 23, respectively, predicted a need for coronary revascularisation, the use of anxiolytics and the need for two or more angina drugs in patients who had acute myocardial infarctions [78]. Spertus et al. was able to show the benefit of a special angina clinic in that patients had greater improvements in quality of life measured by the Seattle Angina Questionnaire (SAQ) than those receiving usual care from a general medicine clinic [79]. Goodwin et al's systematic review concluded that HRQOL targeting specific symptoms could guide treatment decisions and was often the only significant outcome measure in breast cancer drug trials [80]. HRQOL is now regarded as the most important outcome indicator to guide medical decisions on the optimal treatment for breast cancer in the US [80].

7.2 HRQOL in measuring effectiveness of primary care

If HRQOL is to be used as an outcome measure of the effectiveness of TCM in primary care, it has to be valid and applicable to this setting. Primary care practitioners have always relied very much on patients' subjective symptoms in making diagnoses and evaluating treatment outcomes. A recent review on outcome measures for primary care showed the evolution and recognition of the importance of function and health-related quality of life as indicators of subjective health [81]. The accumulating evidence that HRQOL measures are valid and reliable has facilitated its increasing use in clinical service and research in primary care [82-84]. Before a HRQOL measure can be considered as applicable to primary care, it should [85],

- *Measure the aspects and effects of the illness that the patient decides are most important (relevant)*
- *Enable the patient to score the chosen variables (subjective)*
- *Be a sensitive measure of within person change over time (responsive)*
- *Be applicable to the whole spectrum of illness seen in primary care (generic)*
- *Be capable of measuring the effects of a wide variety of care (generic)*
- *Be brief and simple enough to complete in a 7-10 minute consultation.*

The first HRQOL that was applied to primary care was the COOP Charts, which was later adopted by the World Organization of Family Doctors (WONCA) and modified into the COOP/WONCA Charts for internatinal application in primary care [86]. It was translated and validated for the Chinese population in Hong Kong in 1994 [87, 88]. It demonstrated the negative impacts on the life of patients from common chronic diseases such as depression, diabetes mellitus, osteoarthritis and asthma in primary care (Lam and Lauder 2000). The MOS Short-form 36-item (SF-36) Health Survey has become a popular HRQOL measure worldwide since its first publication in 1992. Studies have shown that SF-36 can predict the utilization of primary care services [89], and low HRQOL in community-dwelling elderly had higher mortality rates [90]. Patients with gouts were found to have poorer HRQOL (lower functional limitation scores of the SF-36 Health Survey) and higher rates of inpatient utilization and mortality among all US veterans [91]. The Chinese (HK) version of the SF-36 Health Survey was validated and normed on the Hong Kong population in 1998. It was found to be a sensitive measure of the impact of chronic disease and determinant of primary care service utilization in the Chinese adult population in Hong Kong [88, 89, 92].

7.3 Application of health-related quality of life measures in Traditional Chinese Medicine

Since health-related quality of life (HRQOL) measures were recommended as an important outcome measures in clinical research by the World Health Organization and China Department of Health [93, 94], there has been a surge of HRQOL studies in TCM in the last two decades. Most of the applications were in the fields of cancer, cardiovascular diseases, pain management, geriatrics and respiratory diseases, but very few in primary care.

7.4 Application of HRQOL measures in TCM for the treatment of cancer

The first paper applying HRQOL measurement to TCM was published in 1986 on liver cancer patients [95]. The Karnofsky Performance Scale Index (KPSI) [96] was used as a pre-treatment assessment tool to predict the prognosis of liver cancer patients treated by Chinese herbs and radio-therapy. After this publication, HRQOL measures were used more often to assess the effectiveness of TCM after chemo- or radio therapy in liver and lung cancer patients [97-100]. The KPSI was the most commonly used in these early studies.

The KPSI was found to be responsive to improvement after TCM interventions. It was reported that 67.7% of stage II or III liver cancer patients [98] and 32 liver cancer patients who did not respond to chemo-therapy [99] had improved KPSI scores after TCM treatment. The KPSI scores was able to show in a cohort study on gastric, liver and esophagus cancer patients that the combination of Chinese herbs with chemotherapy was better than chemo-therapy alone [101]. Ma et al's meta-analysis further confirmed the sensitivity of KPSI in 7 randomized controlled clinical trials in showing TCM integrated with chemo-therapy was better than chemotherapy alone (OR = 3.4; 95% CI = 2.5 - 4.6, $p<0.05$) in the treatment of non-small cell lung cancer [102].

In recent years, more HRQOL measures have become available and being used in clinical trials on TCM. The European Organization for Research and Treatment of Cancer (EORTC QLQ-C30) questionnaire [103] was applied to evaluate the effect of medical qigong in cancer patients with or without chemotherapy [104]. It was found that EORTC QLQ-C 30 scores were significantly improved in both groups and medical qigong could also reduce the side effects of patients who underwent chemotherapy. Other HRQOL measures specific for cancer like Functional Assessment of Cancer Therapy-Prostate (FACT) have also been used. FACT-Prostate (FACT-P) [105] was used in assessing the effect of a dietary supplement containing eight herbal extracts (PC-SPES) on prostate cancer patients and reported a significant improvement in functional, emotional and physical well-being in the treatment group [106]. The FACT-Lung (FACT-L) [107] was used to asses the benefit of Chinese herbal medicine treatment on non-small cell lung cancer patient showing that integration of TCM with Western Medicine (WM) or TCM treatment alone were associated with better improvement in terms of total, physical and emotional status than WM alone [108].

7.5 Applications of HRQOL measures in TCM treatments of other conditions

Other than oncology, HRQOL measures have been applied to many studies on cardiovascular disease, pain management, geriatrics and respiratory diseases. A number of widely used international generic and disease-specific HRQOL measures have been used to assess the effectiveness of TCM treatment of cardiovascular diseases. The quality of life index (QLI) [109] and the Activities Daily Living Scale (ADL) [110] had been applied to cerebral hemorrhage patients to show that TCM was more beneficial than Western medicine in improving the cognitive function and the activities of daily living [111]. Wang et al. and Siu et al. found that TCM was equally effective as an antihypertensive drug, Norvasc, in improving all domains of SF-36 Health Survey in patients with hypertension [61, 112]. The Seattle Angina Questionnaire (SAQ) [113] was used in coronary artery bypass grafting patients and found that combining TCM with conventional Western care can significantly improve the domains of angina stability, angina frequency, treatment satisfaction and disease perception measured by the SAQ when compared with conventional Western care [114].

In evaluating the effectiveness of TCM treatment on patients with osteoarthritis, the SF-36 Health Survey, SF-12 Health Survey, Visual Analog Scale (VAS), Western Ontario and McMaster University osteoarthritis index (WOMAC), Lequesne Index and Global Satisfaction Scale have all been used [115-117]. The effectiveness of Complementary and Alternative Medicine (CAM) clinic in relieving pain of OA patients by the combination usage of herbs, chiropractice and acupuncture was detected by the SF-12v2 Health Survey [117]. Another study using the SF-36 v2 Health Survey showed that TCM could enhance social functioning and mental health in the elderly population [118]. The efficacy of willow bark extract was confirmed by a statistically significant difference of 14% in the WOMAC pain dimension between the treatment and placebo groups [116]. Ginger extracts were associated with a reduction of pain on a VAS and the Lequesne Index in a randomized placebo-controlled clinical trial [115, 119].

In evaluating the effectiveness of TCM in respiratory diseases [120], Xue et al. used a combination of symptoms scores diaries, the Rhinoconjunctvitis and Rhinitis Quality of Life Questionnaire (RQLQ), patient's global evaluations of improvement and physician's objective evaluation in a multi-center randomized double-blind, placebo-controlled clinical trials on allergic rhinitis. The RQLQ indicated significant beneficial effects of TCM treatment with an improvement in categorical items by 60.7% against an improvement by 29.6% from placebo. Their study also cross-validated improvement in quality of life by patients' global evaluation and practitioners' objective assessments.

HRQOL assessment of the effectiveness and efficacy of TCM have also been applied to studies on HIV[121] , hepatitis C virus [122, 123], vomiting and nausea in pregnant women [124], chronic alcoholism [125] and somatoform disorders [126].

7.6 Limitation of existing health-related quality of life measures in evaluation of Traditional Chinese Medicine

Despite the increasing applications of HRQOL measures developed from Western culture to the evaluation of TCM, their validity has been questioned. Song et al. stressed out that such applications should be only a transitional state [127] since the cultural context of Western HRQOL measures may not fully match the health concepts in the Chinese culture. Wu et al. pointed out that health concept from the Western culture may neglect the important Chinese concepts of the relationship between health and the seasonal changes or the importance of syndrome differentiation in TCM, which may hinder the development of TCM [128, 129].

Outcome measures of TCM should be coherent with its underlying philosophy and theory so that they could be sensitive and responsive to the changes brought about by TCM treatments [45, 130, 131]. For example, the commonly used Karnofsky Performance Scale Index (KPSI) [96] only focuses on objective assessment of the patient's ability to perform daily activities, work or self-care, it is not sufficient in describing other changes brought by TCM intervention such as the abilities to adapat to climatic changes or dinunal changes [132]. The domains measured by Western HRQOL measures may not be valid to TCM. Therefore it is uncertain whether the results truly reflect those related to TCM. This had called for the development of HRQOL measures specific for TCM.

7.7 Development of Chinese culture specific HRQOL measure for TCM

To develop HRQOL measures applicable to TCM, the Chinese health concepts must be first explored [133]. Cheung et al conducted a qualitative survey on TCM experts in their study on the content validity of a liver syndrome measure commented that the importance of meaning of health from the Chinese culture is unique and need further investigation [134].

Several TCM condition-specific HRQOL measures have been developed. The Emotion scale for Ganzangxiang of TCM was developed to measure HRQOL specific to the anxiety and depression syndrome that are classified under the liver-syndrome by the TCM theory [135,

136]. PiWei-syndrome differentiation measure [137] and the Liver-Fire Ascending Syndrome Scale [138, 139] were developed with similar principles to capture specific physical symptoms, psychological states changes related to specific TCM diagnosis. TCM syndrome differentiation indicators were included in the IBS-TCM differentiation measure for patients with irritable bowel syndrome [140].

While TCM-syndrome specific measures may be relevant and sensitive for a particular condition, there is doubt on the rationale and feasibility of developing a measure for each of the thousands TCM syndromes [141]. Others have urged the need for a generic TCM measure that should include the basic principles of TCM such as the balance of Yin and Yang or cold and heat, deficiency and excess. A generic HRQOL measure not only can evaluate the clinical effectiveness of different TCM treatments, it can also allow evaluation of health of the general population and comparison of patients with different illnesses [142]. A generic HRQOL measure applicable to TCM could also provide a common standard tool for the validation of the TCM syndromes specific measures to enhance research of TCM in clinical practice [143].

The Yin and Yang Scale was the first generic TCM measure developed based on the Yin and Yang principles. Although it was originally intended only for research purpose and not for clinical assessment, it was found that yin and yang scores could be used to differentiate groups of patients effectively in clinical practice. The Yin and Yang scale was also found to be easier to endorse than the detailed syndrome evaluation making it more useful in the research setting [144]. The Yin and Yang Scales served as a preliminary model of generic TCM measures, but it does not really measure HRQOL.

8. The Chinese Quality of Life instrument (ChQOL)

Leung et al. developed the first and probably the only generic TCM HRQOL measure, the Chinese Quality of Life (ChQOL) instrument in Mainland China in 2005 [145]. The initial model was developed from a review of the literature on TCM, which included the equilibrium of Yin Yang in four dimensions: (1) Physical form and Vitality & Spirit, (2) harmonization of man and society and (3) harmonization of man and nature and (4) Seven emotions. Based on these 4 dimensions, four TCM scholars generated 13 facets that were grouped into two domains: 1. Physical form and Vitatlity & Spirit, and 2. emotion. No facet could be identified for the dimensions on harmonization of man and society or the harmonization of man and nature because CMP rarely ask patients about these two dimensions, which were then excluded from the final Chinese Quality of Life instrument.

Items were then generated for the 13 identified facets and drafted in wordings that were used in the communication between Chinese Medicine Practitioners (CMP) and patients. Response options on intensity, frequency or capacity appropriate to the items were adopted from previously validated response options of the WHOQOL-100, The initial draft Chinese Quality of Life Instrument (ChQOL) had a 3-domain structure with 69 items. Each item was rated on a 5-point Likert scale and the scale scores were transformed to a range of 100, with higher scores indicating better HRQOL. The draft was reviewed by 100 CMP who added more items resulting in an 80-item instrument. The second draft was evaluated by a convenient sample of 15 subjects including both healthy and patients consulting a TCM clinic by cognitive debriefing interviews to confirm the linguistic and semantic clarity of the items. Two items were dropped and revisions were made to 78 items. These 78 items were then field tested on 273 subjects including in-patients and out-patients of a TCM hospital and healthy subjects conveniently recruited from the community of Southern Mainland China. Psychometric testing and factor analyses eliminated items that were below the standards of the respective psychometric properties resulting in the final ChQOL with a 3-domain structure and 50 items. The domains are namely physical form (20 items), vitality and spirit (12 items) and emotion (18 items). The three domain scores can be summarized into an overall score. The conceptual structure and the ChQOL are described in other published journal [146].

8.1 Validity and psychometric properties of the ChQOL

Construct validity of the 50-item ChQOL was confirmed by factor analysis and item-scale correlations. The facet-domain correlations ranged from 0.71-0.89 and domain-overall score correlations ranged from 0.56-0.78, supporting the scaling structure. Factor analysis also confirmed the 3-domain structure. The reliability of the ChQOL was supported by internal consistency with Cronbach's alpha ranging from 0.71-0.90 at the facet level and 0.80-0.89 at the domain level. Test-retest reliability was tested on 56 healthy subjects at 2-day interval, giving an intra-class correlations (ICC) ranging from 0.68-0.84 at the facet level and 0.83-0.87 at the domain level. Convergent construct validity was confirmed by moderate correlations between ChQOL scores and SF-36 or WHOQOL-100 scores. Responsiveness of the ChQOL had been examined on 32 subjects with congenital heart diseases showing effect size changes in the three ChQOL domain scores ranging from 0.25 to 0.93.

The ChQOL was adapted into a HK version and pilot tested on 122 Cantonese speaking people (69 patients with chronic diseases who consulted TCM clinic and 53 healthy subjects conveniently recruited in the community) in Hong Kong [132]. The ChQOL (HK version) scales showed good construct validity with the facet-domain correlations ranging from 0.64-0.89 and domain-overall score correlations ranging from 0.79-0.81. Internal consistency was supported by Cronbach's alpha ranged from 0.73-0.90 at the facet level and 0.73-0.83 at the domain level. Test-retest reliability tested in a 2-day interval was good with intra-class correlations (ICC) ranging from 0.77-0.88 at the facet level and 0.89-0.90 at the domain level. Convergent construct validity was confirmed by moderate correlations between the ChQOL (HK version) and the Hong Kong WHOQOL-100. In addition, the ChQOL (HK version) scores were able to discriminate between patients and healthy subjects.

Results from these pilot studies of the ChQOL and its HK version are encouraging. It can become a standard HRQOL measure for the evaluation of the effectiveness of TCM if further studies can confirm its acceptability, feasibility, validity, reliability, sensitivity and responsiveness in different Chinese populations and clinical settings.

8.2 Potential applications of the ChQOL

Over the past 50 years, molecular, cellular and pharmacological research have dominated the research in TCM, but clinical trials on effectiveness have been largely neglected [147]. The few TCM clinical studies evaluated effectiveness of TCM by conventional physical examination or laboratory tests [148] often showed only modest benefits. The use of a validated HRQOL measure can expand the scientific evidence on the effectiveness of TCM by capturing the improvement in HRQOL of patients. The Chinese Quality of Life instrument (ChQOL), if further proven to be responsive to changes related to TCM, can help to solve a major deficiency in evidence-based TCM practice. The ChQOL is generic so that it can be applied to people with different health status or illnesses. This is most suitable for evaluating the effectiveness of primary care that manages a wide spectrum of patients and conditions. Evidence on the effectiveness of TCM in primary care is important to establish its role in our health care system and to inform the public in their choice of service.

9. Summary

There is evidence supporting the role of Traditional Chinese Medicine (TCM) in primary care with increasing use, resources allocation, regulations, research and education. This trend is not only limited to China but also occurring in Western countries. Health-related quality of life (HRQOL) shares the same concepts and objectives as TCM, which should be a most appropriate outcome measure for assessing the effectiveness of TCM. As HRQOL has already been established as a standard outcome measure in Western medical care, it could be used for scientific evaluation of the effectiveness of TCM in primary care. HRQOL measures developed in the Western culture have been applied to oncology and other areas such as cardiovascular disease, pain management, and geriatrics with variable success. However, these Western measures cannot capture all the health benefits of TCM, which hinders further development and clinical research of TCM. The Chinese quality of life instrument (ChQOL), based on the Chinese cultural concepts of health, is a promising HRQOL measure that can become a scientific outcome measurement tool for TCM. The ChQOL is generic making it applicable to all types of patients and particularly suitable for primary care that manages a wide spectrum of illnesses.

10. References

[1] Dong, H. and X. Zhang, *An overview of traditional Chinese medicine. In: Traditional Medicine in Asia.*, World Health Organization Regional Office for South-East Asia, Editor. 2002, SEARO Regional Publication No. 39: New Delhi. p. 17-29.

[2] Xu, J. and Y. Yang, *Traditional Chinese medicine in the Chinese health care system.* Health Policy, 2008.

[3] CMCHK. *Chinese Medicine Council of Hong Kong*. 2008; Available from: http://www.cmchk.org.hk.

[4] Tung Wah Group of Hospitals. *Chinese Medicine Services.* 2008.

[5] Lau, J.T.F., E.M.F. Leung, and H.Y. Tsui, *Predicting traditional Chinese medicine's use and the marginalization of medical care in Hong Kong.* American Journal of Chinese Medicine, 2001. 29: p. 547-558.

[6] Lau, J.T.F. and A. Yu, *The choice between Chinese Medicine and Western Medicine practitioners by Hong Kong adolescents.* American Journal of Chinese Medicine, 2000. 28: p. 131-139.

[7] Leung, G.M., I.O.L. Wong, W.S. Chan, S. Choi, and S.V. Lo, *The ecology of health care in Hong Kong.* Social Science & Medicine, 2005. 61: p. 577-590.

[8] Chung, V., E. Wong, J. Woo, S.V. Lo, and S. Griffiths, *Use of Traditional Chinese medicine in the Hong Kong Special Administrative Region of China.* The Journal of Alternative and Complementary Medicine, 2007. 3: p. 361-367.

[9] WHO. *Traditional Medicine - Growing needs and potential.* in *WHO Policy Perspectives on Medicine.* 2002. Geneva.

[10] WHO, *WHO global atlas of traditional, complementary and alternative medicine,* WHO Centre for Health Development, Editor. 2005: Kobe, Japan.

[11] Eisenberg, D.M., *Trends in alternative medicine use in the United States, 1990 -1997: results of a follow-up national survey.* Journal of the American Medical Association, 1998. 280: p. 1569-1575.

[12] Fisher, P. and R. van Haselen, *Effectiveness gaps: a new concept for evaluating health service and research needs applied to complementary and alternative medicine.* Journal of Alternative and Complementary Medicine, 2004. 10(4): p. 627-632.

[13] Dateshidze, L. and N.K. Rasmussen, *Health and morbidity in Denmark 2000 - and the development since 1987,* National Institute of Public Health, Editor. 1987: Cophenhagen.

[14] Thomas, K.J., J.P. Nicholl, and P. Coleman, *Use and expenditure on complementary medicine in England: a population based survey.* Complementary Therapies in Medicine, 2001. 9: p. 2-11.

[15] National Institute of Health, *Acupuncture,* in *National Institute of Health Consensus Development Conference Statement.* 1997.

[16] Mueller, M.S., N. Runyambo, I. Wagner, S. Borrmann, K. Dietz, and L. Heide, *Randomized controlled trial of a traditional preparation of Artemisia annua L. (Annual Wormwood) in the treatment of malaria.* Transactions of the Royal Society of Tropical Medicine and Hygiene, 2004. 98: p. 318-321.

[17] WHO, *Assessment of therapeutic effect of antimalarial drugs for uncomplicated falciparum malaria in areas with intense trasmission,* in *World Health Orgaization.* 1996: Geneva.

[18] Bent, S., L. Xu, L.-Y. Lui, M. Nevitt, E. Schneider, G. Tian, s. Guo, and S. Cummings, *A randomized controlled trial of a Chinese herbal remedy to increase energy, memory, sexual function, and quality of life in elderly adults in Beijing, China.* The American Journal of Medicine, 2003. 115: p. 441-446.

[19] Wesnes, K.A., T. Ward, A. McGinty, and O. Petrini, *The memory enhancing effects of a Ginkgo biloba/Panax ginseng combination in healthy middle-aged volunteers.* Psychopharmacology, 2000. 152: p. 353-361.

[20] Lau, J.T.F., P.C. Leung, E.L.Y. Wong, C. Fong, K.F. Cheng, S.C. Zhang, C.W.K. Lam, V. Wong, K.M. Choy, and W.M. Ko, *The use of herbal formula by hospital care workers during the Severe Acute Respiratory Syndrome Epidemic in Hong Kong to prevent Severe Acute Respiratory Syndrome transmission, relieve Influenza-related symptoms, and improve quality of life: a prospective cohort study.* The Journal of Alternative and Complementary Medicine, 2005. 11: p. 49-55.

[21] Bensoussan, A., N.J. Talley, M. Hing, R. Menzies, A. Guo, and M. Ngu, *Treatment of irritable bowel syndrome with Chinese herbal medicine.* JAMA, 1998. 280: p. 1585-1589.

[22] Sheehan, M.P., M.H. Rustin, D.J. Atherton, C. Buckley, D.W. Harris, J. Brostoff, L. Ostlere, and A. Dawson, *Efficacy of traditional Chinese herbal therapy in Adult Atopic Dermatitis.* Lancet, 1992. 340: p. 13-17.

[23] Latchman, Y., B. Whittle, M. Rustin, D.J. Atherton, and J. Brostoff, *The efficacy of traditional Chinese herbal therapy in atopic eczema.* International Archives of Allergy and Immunology, 1994. 104(3): p. 222-226.

[24] Kwee, S.H., H.H. Tan, A. Marsman, and C. Wauters, *The effect of Chinese herbal medicines (CHM) on menopausal symptoms compared to horomone replacement therapy (HRT) and placebo.* Maturitas - The European Menopause Journal, 2007. 58: p. 83-90.

[25] Melchart, D., W. Weidenhammer, K. Linde, and R. Saller, *"Quality profiling" for complementary medicine: the example of a hospital for Traditional Chinese Medicine* The Journal of Alternative and Complementary Medicine, 2003. 9: p. 193-206.

[26] Ong, C.K., *Health status of people using complementary and alternative medical practitioner services in four English counties.* American Journal of Public Health, 2002. 92: p. 1653-1656.

[27] Ernst, E. and A. White, *The BBC survey of complementary medicine use in the UK.* Complementary Therapies in Medicine, 2000. 8: p. 32-36.

[28] Busato, A., A. Donges, S. Herren, M. Widmer, and F. Marian, *Health status and health care utilisation of patients in complementary and conventional primary care in Switzerland - an observational study.* Family Practice, 2006. 23: p. 116-124.

[29] Xie, Y.G., *The research on the needs and utilization of Chinese Medicine Service in Beijing.* Beijing Journal of Traditional Chinese Medicine, 2004. 3: p. 135-138.

[30] Frenkel, M.A. and J.M. Borkan, *An approach for integrating complemnetary alternative medicine into primary care.* Family Practice, 2003. 20(3): p. 324-332.

[31] Tang, J.L. and T.W. Wong, *The need to evaluate the clinical effectiveness of traditional Chinese medicine.* HKMJ, 1998. 4: p. 208-210.

[32] Kelner, M.J., H. Boon, B. Wellman, and S. Welsh, *Complementary and alternative groups contemplate the need for effectiveness, safety and cost-effectiveness research.* Complementary Therapies in Medicine, 2002. 10: p. 235-239.

[33] Ernst, E., *Complementary medicine - doing more good than harm?* British Journal of General Prcatice, 1996. 46: p. 60-61.

[34] Tang, J.L., S.-Y. Zhan, and E. Ernst, *Review of randomized controlled trials of traditional Chinese medicine.* British Medical Journal, 1999. 319: p. 160-161.

[35] Leung, P.C. and M.W.N. Wong, *A critical analysis of professional and academic publications on traditional Chinese medicine in China.* The American Journal of Chinese Medicine, 2001. 30: p. 177-181.

[36] Kaptchuk, T.J., *The double-blind, randomized, placebo-controlled trial: gold standard or golden calf?* Journal of Clinical Epidemiology, 2001. 54: p. 541-549.

[37] Black, N., *Why we need observational studies to evaluate the effectiveness of health care.* BMJ, 1996. 312: p. 1215-1218.

[38] Thomas, K.J. and M.J. Fitter, *Evaluating complementary therapies for use in the national health service: 'horses for courses'. part 2: alternative research strategies.* Complementary Therapies in Medicine, 1997. 5: p. 94-98.

[39] Fitter, M.J. and K.J. Thomas, *Evaluating complementary therapies for use in the national health service: 'horses for courses'. part 1: the design challenge.* Complementary Therapies in Medicine, 1997. 5: p. 90-93.

[40] Zaslawski, C., *Clinical reasoning in traditional Chinese medicine: implications for clinical research.* Clinical Acupuncture and Oriental Medicine, 2003. 4: p. 94-101.

[41] Medical Research Council. *A framework for development and evaluation of RCTs for complex interventions to improve health.* 2000 [cited 2005 8-8-2005]; Available from: http://www.mrc.ac.uk/pdf-mrc_cpr.pdf.

[42] Levin, J.S., T.A. Glass, L.H. Kushi, J.R. Schuck, L. Steele, and W.B. Jonas, *Quantitative methods in research on complementary and alternative medicine: a methodological manifesto.* Medical Care, 1997. 35: p. 1079-1094.

[43] WHO, *General guidelines for methodologies on research and evaluation of traditional medicine.* 2000. p. 1-74.

[44] Critchley, J.A.J.H., Y. Zhang, C.C. Suthisisang, T.Y.K. Chan, and B. Tomlinson, *Alternative therapies and medical science: designing clinical trials of alternative/complementary*

medicines - is evidence-based traditional Chinese medicine attainable? Journal of Clinical Pharmacology, 2000. 40: p. 462-467.

[45] Tonelli, M.R. and T.C. Callahan, *Why alternative medicine cannot be evidence-based.* Academic Medicine, 2001. 76: p. 1213-1220.

[46] Acquadro, C., R. Berzon, D. Dubois, N. Leidy, P. Marquis, D. Revicki, M. Rothman, and PRO Harmonization Group, *Incoporating the patient's perspective into drug development and communication: an ad hoc task force report of the Patient-Reported Outcomes (PRO) Harmonization Group meeting at the Food and Drug Administration, February 16, 2001.* Value in Health, 2003. 6(5): p. 503-504.

[47] Donald, L.P., *Patients-Reported Outcomes (PROs): An Organizing Tool for Concepts, Measures, and Applications.* Quality of Life Newsletter, 2003. 31: p. 1-5.

[48] WHO, *The first ten years of the World Health Organization, WHO.* 1985: Genevq.

[49] Crowne, D.P., *A new scale of social desirability independent of psychopathology.* J Consult Psychol, 1960. 24: p. 349-354.

[50] Seiler, L.H., *The 22-item scale used in field studies of mental illness: a question of method, a question of substance and a question of theory.* J Health Soc Behav, 1973. 14: p. 252-264.

[51] Chapman, C.R., *Measurement of pain: problems and issues.* , in *Advanced in pain research and therapy,* Bonica JJ and A. DG, Editors. 1976, Raven Press. p. 345-353.

[52] Clark, W.C., *Pain sensitivity and the report of pain: an introduction to sensory decision theory,* in *Pain new perspectives in therapy and research,* Weisenberg M and Tursky B, Editors. 1976, Plenum Press: New York. p. 195-222.

[53] Rosser, R.M., *Recent studies using a global approach to measuring illness.* Med Care, 1976. 14 (suppl): p. 138-147.

[54] Hu, X.J., B.L. Zhang, and G.X. Cai, *The application and research of health-related quality of life instruments in Chinese Medicine.* Gianjin Journal of Traditional Chinese Medicine, 2002. 19: p. 72-74.

[55] Johnson, J. and R. Temple, *Food and drug administration requirements for approval of new anticancer drugs.* Cancer Treatment Reports, 1985. 69(10): p. 1155-1159.

[56] Wu, L.N. and Q.A. Wu, *Yellow Empeor's canon of internal medicine.* 1997, Beijing: Zhongguo ke xue ji shu chu ban she.

[57] Yang, W.Y., *Chinese Medicine: Macroscopical coordination of functional Medicine.* 2001. 416.

[58] Lai, S.L., *The clinical efficacy of Traditional Chinese Medicine.* Chinese Journal of Information on TCM, 2000. 7: p. 88-89.

[59] Lai, S.L., J.Q. Hu, and X.F. Guo, *Evidence-based Medicine and clinical studies of Traditional Chinese Medicine.* Journal of Guangzhou University of Traditional Chinese Medicine, 2000. 17: p. 1-8.

[60] Liu, F.B., J.H. Wang, and W.W. Chen, *Investigation of application of health-related quality of life instruments in Traditional Chinese Medicine.* Traditional Chinese Drug Research and Clinical Pharmacology, 1997. 8: p. 179-181.

[61] Xiao, J.F. and J.Z. Cai, *Impact of the health-related quality of life of type-II hypertension elderly by treatment of integration of Chinese and Western Medicine* Fujian Journal of Traditional Chinese Medicine, 2002. 33(1): p. 10-11.

[62] Fayers, P.M. and D. Machin, *Quality of life: assessment, analysis, and interpretation.* 2000.

[63] Cummins, R.A. *Quality of life definition and terminology: a discussion document from the International Society for Quality of Life studies.* 1998. Virginia: Blackburg.

[64] Schipper, H., J.J. Clinch, and C.L.M. Olweny, *Quality of life studies. Definition and conceptual issues*, in *Quality of life and Pharmaeconomics in Clinical Trials*, B. Spiker, Editor. 1996, Lippincott-Raven: Philadelphia. p. 11-24.

[65] Bullinger, M., *Assessing health related quality of life in medicine. An overview over concepts, methods and applications in international research.* Restorative Neurology and Neuroscience, 2003. 20: p. 93-101.

[66] Lourander, L., I. Ruikka, and J. Rautakorpi, *Psychological methods applied to evaluate symptomatic geratric treatment.* Geriatrics, 1970. 25(8): p. 124.

[67] Morgan, W.P. and D.H. Horstman, *Psychometric correlates of pain perception.* Perceptual & Motor Skills, 1978. 47(1): p. 27-39.

[68] Edelstyn, G.A., K.D. MacRae, and F.M. MacDonald, *Improvement of life quality in cancer patients undergoing chemotherapy.* Clinical Oncology, 1979. 43-49.

[69] Weinstein, M.C. and W.B. Stason, *Foundations of cost-effectiveness analysis for health and medical practices.* New England Journal of Medicine, 1977. 296(13): p. 716-21.

[70] Jean, G.L., *Day care: cost effectiveness vs. quality of life.* Aging & Leisure Living, 1978. 1(1): p. 8-10.

[71] Mathias, C.M.J., *Improving the quality of life for the elderly.* Journal of the American Geriatrics Society, 1979. 27(9): p. 385-388.

[72] Kriedel, T., *Cost-benefit analysis of epilepsy clinics.* Social Science & Medicine - Medical Economics, 1980. 14(1): p. 35-39.

[73] Cattell, R.B., *Evaluating therapy as total personality change: theory and available instruments.* American Journal of Psychotherapy, 1966. 20(1): p. 69-88.

[74] Salzberg, H.C. and D.R. Bidus, *Development of a group psychotherapy screening scale: an attempt to select suitable candidates and predict successful outcome.* Journal of Clinical Psychology, 1966. 22(4): p. 478-481.

[75] Barrett, G.V., T.R. Williamson, and C.L. Thornton, *Perception of depth as measured by magnitude estimation.* Perceptual & Motor Skills, 1967. 25(3): p. 905-908.

[76] Cattell, R.B. and L.R. Killian, *The pattern of objective test personality factor differences in schizophrenia and the character disorders.* Journal of Clinical Psychology, 1967. 23(3): p. 342-348.

[77] Croog, S.H., S. Levine, and M.A. Testa, *The effects of antihypertensive therapy on the quality of life.* New England Journal of Medicine, 1986. 314: p. 1657-1664.

[78] Brown, N., M. Melville, D. Gray, T. Young, J. Munro, A.M. Skene, and J.R. Hampton, *Quality of life four years after acute acute myocardial infarction: shor form 36 scores compared with a normal population.* Heart, 1999. 1999(81): p. 352-358.

[79] Spertus, J.A., T.A. Dewhurst, C.M. Dougherty, P. Nichol, M. McDonell, B. Bliven, and S.D. Fihn, *Benefits of an "angina clinic" for patients with coronary artery disease: A demostration of health status measures as markers of health care quality.* American Heart Journal, 2002. 143: p. 145-150.

[80] Goodwin, P.J., J.T. Black, L.J. Bordeleau, and P.A. Ganz, *Health-related quality-of-life measurement in randomized clinical trials in breast cancer--taking stock.* Journal of the National Cancer Institute, 2003. 95: p. 263-281.

[81] Wilkin, D., I. Hallan, and M. Doggett, eds. *Measures of need and outcome for primary health care.* 1992, Oxford University Press: Oxford.

[82] Mossey, J.M. and E. Shapiro, *Self-rated health: a predictor of mortality among the elderly.* American Journal of Public Health, 1982. 72: p. 800-808.

[83] McDowell, I. and C. Newell, eds. *Measuring health: a guide to rating scales and questionnaires*. 2nd ed. ed. 1996, Oxford University Press.

[84] Spertus, J.A., P. Jones, M. McDonell, V. Fan, and S.D. Fihn, *Health status predicts long-term outcome in outpatients with coronary disease.* Circulation, 2002. 106: p. 43-49.

[85] Ruta, D.A., A.M. Garratt, M. Leng, and I.T. Russell, *A new approach to quality of life: the patient-generated index.* Medical Care, 1994. 32: p. 1109-1126.

[86] Landgraf, J.M.N., E C, *Summary of the WONCA/COOP International health assessment field trial. The Dartmouth COOP primary care network.* Australian Family Physicians, 1992. 21(3): p. 255-257, 260-262, 266-269.

[87] Lam, C.L.K., C. Van Weel, and I.J. Lauder, *Can the Dartmouth COOP/WONCA charts be used to assess the functional status of Chinese patients?* Family Practice, 1994. 11: p. 85-94.

[88] Lam, C.L.K. and I.J. Lauder, *The impact of chronic diseases on the health-related quality of life (HRQOL) of Chinese patients in primary care.* Family Practice, 2000. 17(2): p. 159-66.

[89] Lam, C.L.K., D.Y.T. Fong, I.J. Launder, and T.P. Lam, *The effect of health-related quality of life (HRQOL) on health service utilisation of a Chinese population.* Social Science & Medicine, 2002. 55(9): p. 1635-1646.

[90] Tsai, S.Y., L.Y. Chi, L.C. Hsen, and P. Chou, *Health-related quality ofe life as a predictor of mortality among community-dwelling older persons.* European Journal of Epidemiology, 2007. 19-26.

[91] Singh, J.A. and V. Strand, *Gout is associated with more comorbidities, poorer health-related quality of life and higher healthcare utilisation in US veterans.* Annals of the Rheumatic Diseases, 2008. 67(9): p. 1310-1316.

[92] Lam, C.L.K., I.J. Launder, T.P. Lam, and B. Gandek, *Population based norming of the Chinese (HK) version of the SF-36 health survey.* The Hong Kong Practitioner, 1999. 21: p. 460-470.

[93] Ministry of Health of the People's Republic of China, *Guidelines of the Prevention and Treatment of Cancers,* Ministry of Health of the People's Republic of China, Editor. 1986-2000.

[94] WHO, *The development of the WHO quality of life assessment instrument.* WHO, 1993.

[95] Yu, E.X., *Radiotherapy of hepatic carcinoma.* Chinese Journal of Practical Surgery, 1986. 3: p. 157-158.

[96] Grieco, A. and C.J. Long, *Investigation of the Karnofsky Performance Status as a measure of quality of life.* Health Psychology, 1984. 3: p. 129-142.

[97] Pu, B.K., W.X. Tang, Z.Q. Zhang, and H.S. Lin, *The clinical observation of Fei Liu Ping Gao in treating late stage primary lung cancer.* Journal of Traditional Chinese Medicine, 1991. 4: p. 21-23.

[98] Huang, L.Z., S.L. Ceng, Y.L. Jian, Y.H. Wu, Y.B. Sun, and M.Q. Pan, *Clinical obversation of 31 cases of primary liver cancer treated by Gan Fu Lei Pian.* Hunan Journal of Traditional Chinese Medicine, 1997. 13: p. 4-5, 12.

[99] Zhou, L.M., J.J. Zhu, J.Y. Hong, X.C. Fu, G.M. Cheng, and L. Wu, *Injection of Kang Lai Te in treating post-radiotherapy failure of non small cell pulmonary carcinoma.* Journal of Practical Oncology, 1999. 14: p. 313-314.

[100] Cai, Z.R., *The impact of Yan Su on the quality of life of late stage liver cancer patients.* Heilongjiang Journal of Traditional Chinese Medicine, 1999. 6: p. 62.

[101] Tan, L.X. and J.F. Ji, *Clinical efficacy of new cancer drugs of Lan Xiang Xi Ru in treating late stage carcinoma.* Chinese Journal of Information on TCM, 1997. 4: p. 11-12.

[102] Ma, L., Y.N. Weng, and X. Xiao, *Intergration of Traditional Chinese Medicine and chemotherapy for the treatment of non-small cell lung cancer - meta analysis of the impact on clinical efficacy and health-related quality of life.* Chinese Journal of Practical Chinese with Modern Medicine, 2004. 4: p. 709-712.

[103] King, M.T., *The interpretation of scores from the EORTC quality of life questionnaire QLQ-C30.* Quality of Life Research, 1996. 5(6): p. 555-567.

[104] Oh, B., P. Butow, and B. Mullan, *Medical qigong for cancer patients: pilot study of impact on quality of life, side effects of treatment and inflammation.* The American Journal of Chinese Medicine, 2006. 36(3): p. 459-472.

[105] Esper, P., F. Mo, G. Chodak, M. Sinner, D. Cella, and K.J. Pienta, *Measuring Quality of life in men with prostate cancer using the Functional Assessment of Cancer Therapy-Prostate (FACT-P) instrument.* Urology, 1997. 50(6): p. 920-928.

[106] Pfeifer, B.L., J.F. Pirani, S.R. Hamann, and K.F. Klippel, *PC-SPES, a dietary supplement for the treatment of horomone-refractory prostate cancer.* BJU International, 2000. 85: p. 481-485.

[107] Cella, D.F., A.E. Bonomi, S.R. Lloyd, D.S. Tulsky, E. Kaplan, and P. Bonomi, *Reliability and validity of the Functional Assessment of Cancer Therapy - Lung (FACT-L) quality of life instrument.* Lung Cancer, 1995. 12: p. 199-220.

[108] Li, L.N., W.S. Liu, K. Xu, W.Y. Wu, Y.L. Liu, D.Y. Zhu, H.Y. Luo, and C.Y. Chen, *Clinical efficacy and health-related quality of life of Chinese Medicine Syndrome differentiation for the treatment of stage III and IV non-small cell lung carcinoma.* Chinese Journal of Lung Cancer, 2003. 6: p. 216-219.

[109] Spitzer, W.O., *Measuring the quality of life of cancer patients. A concise QL-index for use by physicians.* Journal of Chronic Diseases, 1981. 34(12): p. 585-597.

[110] Mahoney, F.I. and D.W. Baarthel, *Functional evaluation: The Barthel index.* Maryland State Medical Journal, 1965. 14: p. 61-65.

[111] Liang, Q., X. Li, and G. He, *The observation of the quality of life on cerebral hemorrhage treated with decotion of Ping Gan Xi Feng.* Bulletin of Hunan Medical University, 1996. 21(5): p. 403-406.

[112] Wang, Y., R.B. Zhang, and B.R. He, *The impact of health-related quality of life of Chinese and Western medication on hypertension patients.* Zhejiang Journal of Integrated Traditional Chinese and Western Medicine, 1999. 9: p. 86-88.

[113] Spertus, J.A., J.A. Winder, T.A. Dewhurst, R.A. Deyo, J. Prodzinski, M. McDonnell, and S.D. Fihn, *Development and evaluation of the Seattle Angina Questionnaire: A new functional status measure for coronary artery disease.* Journal of the American College of Cardiology, 1995. 25(2): p. 333-341.

[114] Ruan, X.M., Y. Lin, W. Jiang, J.X. Hu, Q.X. Chen, H.L. Wu, Z.J. Chen, H.C. Zhou, and C.L. Huang, *Clinical observation on quality of life in coronary artery bypass grafting patients treated according to syndrom differentiation of TCM.* Chinese Journal of Integrated Traditional and Western Medicine, 2003. 23(11): p. P. 804-807.

[115] Bliddal, H., A. Rosetzsky, P. Schlichting, M.S. Weidnet, L.A. Andersen, H.-H. lbfelt, K. Christensen, O.N. Jensen, and J. Barslev, *A randomized, placebo-controlled, cross-over study of ginger extracts and lbuprofen in osteoarthritis.* Osteoarthritis and Cartilage, 2000. 8: p. 9-12.

[116] Schmid, B., R. Ludtke, H.-K. Selbmann, I. Kotter, B. Tshidewahn, W. Schaffner, and L. Heide, *Efficacy and tolerability of a standardized Willow Bark Extract in patients with Osteoarthritis: randomized Placebo-controlled, double blind clinical trial.* Phytotherapy Research, 2001. 15: p. 344-350.

[117] Secor, E.R.J., J.H. Blumberg, M.J. Markow, J. MacKenzie, and R.S. Thrall, *Implementation of outcome measure in a complementary and alternative medicine clinic: evidence of decreased pain and improved quality of life.* The Journal of Alternative and Complementary Medicine, 2004. 10: p. 506-513.

[118] Cicero, A.F.G., G. Derosa, R. Brillante, R. Bernardi, S. Nascetti, and A. Gaddi, *Effects of Siberian Ginseng (Eleutherococcus senticosus maxim.) on elderly quality of life: a randomized clinical trial.* Arch. Gerontol. Geriatr. Suppl., 2004. 9: p. 69-73.

[119] Altman, R.D. and K.C. Marcussen, *Effects of a Ginger extract on knee pain in patients with osteoarthritis.* Arthritis and Rheumatism, 2001. 44: p. 2531-2538.

[120] Xue, C., F. Thien, J. Zhang, W. Yang, C.D. Costa, and C. Li, *Effects of adding a Chinese herbal preparartion to acupuncture for seasonal allergic rhinitis: randomised double-blind controlled trial.* Hong Kong Medical Journal, 2003. 9: p. 427-434.

[121] Weber, R., L. Christen, M. Loy, S. Schaller, S. Christen, R.B. Joyce, U. Ledermann, B. Ledergerber, R. Cone, R. Luthy, and M.R. Cohen, *Randomized, placebo-controlled trial of Chinese herb therapy for HIV-1-infected individuals.* Journal of Acquired Immune Deficiency Syndromes, 1999. 22(1): p. 56.

[122] Kainuma, M., J. Hayashi, S. Sakai, K. Imai, N. Mantani, K. Kohta, T. Mitsuma, Y. Shimada, S. Kashiwagi, and K. Terasawa, *The efficacy of herbal medicine (Kampo) in reducing the adverse effects of IFN-B in Chronic Hepatitis C.* The American Journal of Chinese Medicine, 2002. 30: p. 355-367.

[123] Jakkula, M., T.A. Boucher, U. Beyendorff, S.M. Conn, J.E. Johnson, C.J. Nolan, J.p. Craig, and J.H. Albrech, *A randomized trial of Chinese herbal medicines for the treatment of symptomatic hepatitis C.* Archives of Internal Medicine, 2004. 164: p. 1341-1346.

[124] Vutyavanich, T., T. Kraisarin, and R. Ruangsri, *Ginger for nausea and vomiting in pregnancy: randomized, double-masked, placebo-controlled trial.* Obstetrics and Gynecology, 2001. 97: p. 577-582.

[125] Shebek, J. and J.P. Rindone, *A pilot study exploring the effect of Kudzu Root on the drinking habits of patients with Chronic Alcoholism.* The Journal of Alternative and Complementary Medicine, 2000. 6: p. 45-48.

[126] Yamada, K., R. Den, K. Ohnishi, and S. Kanba, *Effectiveness of herbal medicine (Kampo) and changes of quality of life in patients with Somatoform Disorders.* Journal of Clinical Psychopharmacology, 2005. 25: p. 199-201.

[127] Song, J. and K.J. Chen, *Several critical questions needed to be asked for clinical observation of Traditional Chinese Medicine.* Chinese Journal of Integrated Traditional and Western Medicine, 2003. 23: p. 564-565.

[128] Hu, S.Y., Z. Wang, T.S. Cai, J.S. You, and Q. Yao, *Preliminary Development of Emotion rating scale for Ganzangxiang of Traditional Chinese Medicine.* Chinese Journal of Clinical Psychology, 2001. 9: p. 84-89.

[129] Hu, S.Y., Z. Wang, C.Y. Yu, and J.S. You, *Researching thoughts and methods of emotion scale for Gangzangxiang of Traditional Chinese Medicine.* China Journal of Basic Medicine in Traditional Chinese Medicine, 2001. 7: p. 9-11.

[130] Edwards, R.A., *Our research approaches must meet the goal of improving patient care.* Alternative Therapies in Health and Medicine, 1997. 3: p. 99.

[131] Matko, M., "*Complementary and alternative*" *medicine - a measure of crisis in academic medicine* Croatian Medical Journal, 2004. 45: p. 684-688.

[132] Zhao, L., K.F. Leung, and K. Chan, *The Chinese Quality of Life instrument: reliability and validity of the Hong Kong Chinese version (ChQOL-HK).* The Hong Kong Practitioner, 2007. 29: p. 220-232.

[133] Yang, X.B., J.Q. Hu, and S.L. Lai, *Thoughts on the Standardization of Syndrome differentiation of Chinese Medicine.* Chinese Journal of Information on TCM, 2001. 8: p. 10-11.

[134] Zhang, H.N., S.Y. Hu, Z.Q. Chen, and J.Q. Luo, *An analysis on the first questionnaires for the syndrome standard of hepatic stagnation causing phlegm retention among cases with depression.* Journal of Hunan College of Traditional Chinese Medicine, 2002. 27: p. 519-521.

[135] Wang, Z., S.Y. Hu, T.S. Cai, and D.S. Xia, *Development of emotion rating scale for Ganzangxiang of Traditional Chinese Medicine (ERSG).* Chinese Journal of Behavioral Medical Science, 2004. 13: p. 104-106.

[136] Wang, Z., S.Y. Hu, and T.S. Cai, *Factor analysis of emotion rating scale for ganzangxiang of Traditional Chinese Medicine.* Chinese Mental Health Journal, 2003. 17: p. 306-308.

[137] Liu, F.B., J.Q. Fang, Z.H. Pan, Q. Li, X.L. Liu, and Y.T. Hao, *The development of syndrom differential scale of the spleen-stomach disease used for computer aided expert diagnosis system.* Academic Journal of Sun Yat-Sen University of Medical Sciences, 2000. 21(4S): p. 112-116.

[138] Liu, Z.Z., Z.Q. Chen, and Q. Guo, *Study on syndrome scale for Liver-qi stagnation syndrome.* Journal of Traditional Chinese Medicine University of Hunan, 2007. 27: p. 48-51.

[139] Liu, X.Z., Z.Q. Chen, and Q. Guo, *Primary compilation of a scale for Liver-fire ascending syndrome.* Chinese Journal of Clinical Rehabilitation, 2006. 10: p. 1-3.

[140] Quan, K.X. and W.J. Wu, *Establishment and evaluation of irritable bowel syndrome instruments for TCM.* Journal of Traditional Chinese Medicine and Chinese Materia Medica of Jilin, 2004. 24: p. 6-8.

[141] Zhao, L., K.T. Chan, K.F. Leung, and F.B. Liu. *Quality of Life and Chinese Medicine - The development of health status measures for Chinese Medicine.* in *The 2nd World Integrative Medicine Congress.* 2004. Beijing.

[142] Li, F.L. and R. Liang, *Application and thoughts of TCM syndrome differentiation in questionnaire development.* Journal of Beijing Univeristy of Traditional Chinese Medicine, 2006. 29: p. 162-164.

[143] Li, G.C., W.K. Chen, X.Y. Mei, C.X. Peng, and L. Zou, *Discussion on quantitative analysis method about variable of macroscopical differentiation of syndromes of TCM.* China Journal of Basic Medicine in Traditional Chinese Medicine, 2005. 11: p. 650-652.

[144] Langevin, H.M., G.J. Badger, B.K. Povolny, R.T. Davis, A.C. Johnston, K.J. Sherman, J.R. Kahn, and T.J. Kaptchuk, *Yin scores and Yang scores: a new method for quantitative diagnostic evaluation in traditional Chinese medicine research.* The Journal of Alternative and Complementary Medicine, 2004. 10: p. 389-395.

[145] Leung, K.F., F.B. Liu, L. Zhao, J.Q. Fang, K. Chan, and L.Z. Lin, *Development and validation of the Chinese quality of life instrument* Health and quality of life Outcomes, 2005. 3: p. 26.

[146] Wong, W., C.L.K. Lam, K.F. Leung, and L. Zhao, *Is the Content of the Chinese Quality of Life Instrument (ChQOL) Really Valid in the Context of Traditional Chinese Medicine in Hong Kong?* Complementary Therapies in Medicine, 2009. 17(1): p. 29-36.

[147] Tang, J.L. and P.C. Leung, *An efficacy-driven approach to the research and development of traditional Chinese medicine.* Hong Kong Medical Journal, 2001. 7: p. 375-380.

[148] Guo, X.F., S.L. Lai, and W.X. Liang, *Choice and application of the outcome indexes for clinical effectivenesss assessment of Traditional Chinese Medicine.* Journal of Guangzhou University of Traditional Chinese Medicine, 2002. 19: p. 251-255.

10

A Comparison Study on Arterial Blood Pressure and Pulse Data of Condenser Microphone*

Yin-Yi Han[1], Yih-Nen Jeng[2], Si-Chen Lee[3] and Hao-Jian Hung[4]
[1]Department of Trauma, National Taiwan University Hospital,
Graduate institute of Electrical Engineering, National Taiwan University,
[2]Department of Aeronautics and Astronautics, National Cheng-Kung University,
[3]Department of Electrical Engineering, National Taiwan University,
[4]Department of Aeronautics and Astronautics, National Cheng-Kung University,
Taiwan

1. Introduction

Recently, [Wang et al. 1989; Young et al. 1989, 1992; Jan et al, 2003; Wang Lin et al, 2004; Kuo et al, 2004; and Hsu et al. 2006] developed the resonance theory that each arterial bed in the vascular system is oscillated by the pressure waves at its own resonant frequency. They reported that ligating the renal, gastric, splenic or superior mesenteric artery of Wistar rats for a short duration could cause specific changes to the individual harmonics. They also showed that the ligation effects of different systems were linearly additive: as the renal artery and the superior mesenteric artery were simultaneously ligated, the change in the pulse spectrum was similar to the direct addition of two spectra resulting from the two individual ligations. They came to two important conclusions: First, the organ spectra can be used as parameters to elucidate the physical status of the specific vascular beds. Specifically, the magnitude of a harmonic mode reflects the amount of blood spent by the corresponding organ. Second, as the physical properties of a specific arterial bed change, the amplitude of the corresponding resonant mode changes more than that of the others. However, the corresponding resonant frequency will be approximately maintained by the heart rate control system to minimize the energy loss [Jan et al. 2003]. Most of their experimental data used pressure transducers to collect tail arteries of Wistar rats.
Based on this theory, Yu and Wang developed an artery blood pressure pulse acquisition system to take the wrist arterial blood pulse pressure data via a commercial microphone [Yu & Wang, 2006]. Unlike the experimental data of Wang et al., the sensor of the sonocardiography system of Yu and Wang are non-invasive and were more convenient to collect data than most existing systems. However, the interested frequency range of the wrist pulse data of the traditional Chinese medicine is lower than the announced range of most commercial microphone, say 20-20kHz. In [Jeng & Lee, 2008; Jeng, et al., 2011], it was proven that, if the acoustic signal source, pressure waves and small air cell containing the diaphragm of the electret condenser microphone are properly confined to a small air

* Project 2009101017D under the regulation of National Taiwan University Hospital, Research Ethics Committee A.

chamber, the lower bound of the effectively frequency response can be as low as 0.5Hz. The environment of signal confinement is equivalent to the situation that one firmly presses the microphone to the measured skin. In other words, the system using an electret condenser microphone is a potential tool to re-study the human organ-meridians which had achieved great achievement in the traditional Chinese medicine.

The above discussions confirm the fact that the arterial signals picked up by the sonocardiography system are closely related to the human organ-meridians. An interested problem is whether the microphone arterial pulse data also closely relates to the modern medicine data such as the well known invasive ABP and ECG. The ECG and ABP are the two commonly employed physiological parameters to monitor patients in the setting of critical illness [Civetta et al. 1992 & Marino 2007]. They offer the basic information of how the circulatory system performs in complex clinical conditions.

In order to look into complicated information embedded in signals of microphone's arterial pressure, ABP and ECG, both the FFT [Brigham, 1998] and time-frequency transform should be simultaneously used [Jeng & Lee, 2008; Jeng, et al., 2011]. The FFT provides a spectral parameter representation and the time frequency transform even give us the possibility of revolving the temporal varied amplitude and frequency of a wave component. In this study the Gabor transform will be employed.

In some sense, the ECG data reflects the input command, whereas the ABP signal reflects the corresponding vascular response. In case of homeostasis, the circulatory system should behave as a linear transfer function in the spectral band of the heart beat mode that the variation of ABP should be highly correlated with that of ECG. When the system is not properly functioning, the correlation may be violated such that the person may have healthy problem. From this view point, the correlation between variation of ECG and ABP can be a potential biomarker of human health assessment. However, continuous ABP data is usually only conveyed in critically ill patient with invasive intra-arterial measurement. Being non-invasive and more easily applicable, microphone pressure sensor is an alternative choice to get the continuous pulse signals. If we can prove that the microphone arterial signal's heart rate mode can be used to provide the index, the preventive medicine would become a practical issue for the general population. Moreover, the connection between the ancient Chinese and modern medicines will become more solid in near future.

2. Data and method

2.1 Theoretical development

Because the time series picked up by the microphone system, ECG or ABP may involve drift and/or trend, it frequently involves a monotonic non-periodic part. Therefore, a time series data string, $y_j = y(t_j), j = 0,1,2...,J$, can be written in the following form [Jeng et al. 2009]:

$$y_j = \sum_{l=0}^{J-1}[c_l \cos\frac{2\pi t_j}{\lambda_l} + d_l \sin\frac{2\pi t_j}{\lambda_l}] + \sum_{n=0}^{N} a_n t_j^n, \quad 0 < j < J-1 \tag{1}$$

where $t_{j+1} - t_j = \Delta t$ = constant, l is the mode index, and $\lambda_l = J\Delta t \,/\, l$ is the wavelength of the l-th mode, the second summation represents the non-sinusoidal drift and/or trend and N represents the largest power for which $a_n \to 0$ for all $n > N$. For most engineering applications, N = 250 is a reasonable value. The non-sinusoidal trend is interpreted as the sum of monotonic parts and all the Fourier modes whose wavelengths are longer than the data span $T = J\Delta t$. This study uses the iterative Gaussian smoothing method in the spectral domain to serve as a high-passed filter. It can be proven the resulting response takes the following form [Jeng et al. 2008, 2009, 2011]:

$$y'_{j,m} \approx \sum_{l=0}^{J}[1-\exp[-2\pi^2\sigma^2/\lambda^2]^m\left[c_l\cos\frac{2\pi t_j}{\lambda_l}+d_l\sin\frac{2\pi t_j}{\lambda_l}\right]+O(\Delta t^2)$$
$$\bar{y}_j^m = y_j - y'_{j,m} \tag{2}$$

where $y'_{j,m}$ and $\bar{y}_j^m$ represent smooth and high frequency responses after applying the iterative Gaussian smoothing method for m cycles and $[1\text{-}\exp[-2\pi^2\sigma^2/\lambda_l^2]^m$ represents the attenuation factor, in which σ is the smoothing factor of the Gaussian smoothing method and $m>N/2$. In this study, the iteration parameter m and smoothing factor σ use the value of 127 and 0.8seconds, respectively. These parameters means that the filter's transition zone is $\lambda_2/\lambda_1=2$ and $\lambda_1 \approx \sigma/0.772 \approx 1.036$seconds. More specifically, all wave modes of y'_m with wavelength $\lambda \leq 1.036$seconds are almost the same as that of original data and those wave modes with wavelength $\lambda \leq 2.072$seconds are removed. Now the trend is ultimately removed. Because this result is principally derived by assuming the data span running from $-\infty$ to ∞, small errors are thus induced by the missing data beyond the two ends. Next, the zero crossing points around the two ends can be located by a search procedure and interpolation formula. After dropping the data segments beyond the two zeros, a monotonic cubic interpolation [Huynh, 1993;Jeng et al. 2009, 2011] is used to redistribute the data into uniform spacing whose points equal an integer power of 2. Subsequently, the odd function mapping is used to double the data span. Finally, the FFT [Brigham, 1998] will generate a Fourier sine spectrum. This spectrum reflects many details in the low frequency region because the trend has already been removed and all the required periodic conditions are ensured by the odd function mapping.

In this study, the following Gabor wavelet transform using the Gaussian window (with a given window width a on the time domain) is used for the sinusoidal data y'_m:

$$G(f,\tau) = \frac{1}{\sqrt{a}}\int_0^T y'_m(t)e^{-2i\pi f(t-\tau)}e^{-(t-\tau)^2/(2a^2)}dt \tag{3}$$

in which τ denotes the central time instant of the Gaussian window and f is the central frequency index on spectral domain. By scanning both f and τ over the desired range of time-frequency domain, the desired two-dimensional Gabor wavelet coefficient plot or the spectrogram can be obtained. It can be proven it is about equal to the following form [Jeng et al. 2009, 2011]:

$$G(f,\tau) \approx \sqrt{\frac{a\pi}{2}}\sum_{l=1}^{J-1}\{[d_l - ie_l]e^{i2\pi f_l\tau}\exp[-2a^2\pi^2(f_l-f)^2]\} \tag{4}$$

where $d_l \approx (1-2\pi^2\sigma^2/\lambda_l^2)^m b_l$ and $e_l \approx (1-2\pi^2\sigma^2/\lambda_l^2)^m c_l$ are Fourier spectrum of y'_m. These relations indicate the wavelet coefficient is just an inverse FFT of a finite spectrum band specified by an associated Gaussian window whose window width is $1/(2a\pi)$ and is centered at the frequency of *f*. For the sake of completeness, the procedures are summarized below [Jeng et al. 2009, 2011].

1. Use the iterative Gaussian smoothing method to remove the non-sinusoidal part and a fraction of several lowest modes whose wavelengths are ranged from λ_L to T, where $T=J\Delta t$ is the data length.
2. Find the Fourier sine spectrum : find the zero around the two ends; discard data segments beyond the zeros; redistribute the data via a proper interpolation method so that the data point is an integer power of 2 (= 2**k > 2L, where L denotes the original data size); make an odd function mapping with respect to one end; employ in an FFT.
3. Choose the frequency resolution $f_i = f_0 + i\Delta f$ and $a = 2c / \Delta f$ to evaluate the band-pass limited spectrum via the Gaussian window with window width c, where f_0 is the lowest frequency employed to plot the spectrogram and c is an user specified parameter (e.g. c =1.5).
4. Find the inverse FFT of the band-pass limited spectrum, which is the real part of the spectrogram coefficient corresponding to the f_i mode. The corresponding amplitude distribution with respect to time is then evaluated by applying the Hilbert transform.
5. Scan all f_i s and plot the spectrogram.

Note that the resulting wavelet coefficients (spectrograms) are subject to the blur effect of the uncertainty principle [Goswami & Chan, 1999; Mallat, 1999; Jeng et al. 2009, 2011]. At most one obtains the best resolution with certain compromise between the temporal and spectral scales. In practical application, an approximate optimal resolution can be achieved via a few trial and error procedures by varying the parameter c in the third step.

A careful inspection upon Eq.(2) reveals that one can simultaneously remove the trend and obtain the high frequency spectrum by merely calculating in the spectral domain. Moreover, one can further obtain a single mode or a band-pass-limited spectrum by imposing a suitable window upon the spectrum of the high frequency part.

In this study, the relation between the microphone pulse data, ECG, and ABP is assumed to be determined by the cross-correlation of two wave components of the heart rate mode. The following familiar method directly calculates the cross-correlation coefficient [Bendat & Piersol 2000] between two wave components $y_1(t)$ and $y_2(t)$ is employed.

$$c = \frac{\int_{t_0}^{t_f} y_1(t)y_2(t)dt}{\left[\int_{t_0}^{t_f} y_1^{\,2}(t)dt \int_{t_0}^{t_f} y_2^{\,2}dt\right]^{1/2}} \tag{5}$$

where t_0 and t_f are the initial and final instances of the two wave components. The associated time series wave component, say $y_1(t)$ or $y_2(t)$, is obtained by the inverse FFT algorithm of the spectral band. For convenience, only two Fourier modes are considered here.

In order to eliminate the phase lag induced by the pressure wave propagation along the artery wall, one of the two wave components will be shifted, say $y_1(t \pm \tau)$ or $y_2(t \pm \tau)$. The parameter τ is the amount of time shift which achieves the maximum absolute value of c in Eq.(5). For a person not in critical state, his heart beat modes of ECG and ABP should be highly correlated in this sense.

For a patient in an intensive care unit, the modern medicine provides many effective supports and treatments. He may still survive even if his heart beat modes of ECG and ABP are not correlated. The reason is Eq.(5) principally depends on the phase lag between these modes. With the strong support of the intensive care unit, it seems that the correlation between the envelopes of these ECG and ABP modes is also an important index for such a patient. The envelopes, which represent the energy or amplitude of these modes, are believed to be roughly reflected by the shapes of corresponding wave components in spectrograms of amplitude [Jeng & Cheng, 2007].

According to the above discussions, in addition to Eq.(5), a partial information of the cross-correlation between two sinusoidal data strings is roughly considered to be the similarity of wave components in the spectrograms of amplitude. It is clearly that, as two wave components are partially correlated, the phase lag may or may not occur. If the phase lag is insignificant, it is certain that $|c| \geq 0.6$. If a large phase lag exists between two wave components with partial energy correlation, their correlation coefficient calculated by Eq.(5) may be low, say $|c| < 0.5$. To explain this state, consider the correlation between the heart rate modes of ECG and ABP of a patient as an example. Suppose their temporal amplitude and frequency distributions are similar so that energies of their corresponding wave components are correlated. The command of the heart (ECG) is transferred to the point of measuring the wrist pulse (ABP) via the pressure wave propagation through a series of vascular tubes. Due the some reasons, however, the wave propagation speed is not homogeneous and not invariant from one location to another. Thus, the periodicity of the heart rate is distorted at the ABP measuring point and the phase lag occurs. Although this stage is not perfect, the entire circulation system still partially functioned.

2.2 Data acquisition

In this study, the ECG signals were obtained from the three-lead ECG recording device. The ABP signals were conveyed from an invasive arterial-line system which involves an insertion of an arterial catheter connecting to a conducting tube filled with properly pressured fluid (see Fig.1). The mechanical signals were then transformed to the electrical ones with a midway pressure transducer. Both ECG and ABP data were transferred back to the Philips MP60 module which was the physiological signal monitoring system used in our study. The analog signals were output to the data acquisition card where they would be converted to the digital signals with a sampling rate of 500Hz and then forwarded to the portable computer for further analysis.

In order to achieve a stable sensitivity in response to the tiny wrist arterial pressure data, a commercial electret condenser microphone is employed, whose instructions are 20-20,000 Hz, 100mw, 32 Ω 105db sound pressure level sensitivity at 1kZ ±2 %. The experimental facilities include a digital audio board (Onkyo Inc. SE-150 PCI, SN ratio 100dB, 0.3-44KHz, sampling rate 32-192KHz). Before the wrist artery with a sampling rate of 500Hz was acquired, the measuring point should be carefully located by human finger so as to make sure that the pulse signal is prominent. The schematic diagram is shown in Fig.2a where the front face with the actuating diaphragm of microphone (Figs.2b and 2c) was firmly attached to the measuring point.

The data of six different patients in the intensive care unit of a hospital in Taiwan were included in our study. The ECG, ABP, and microphone data were in all cases successfully and simultaneously recorded in the same sampling rate. During the period of acquiring data, the ABP data was taken from the left wrist while the microphone data from the right wrist.

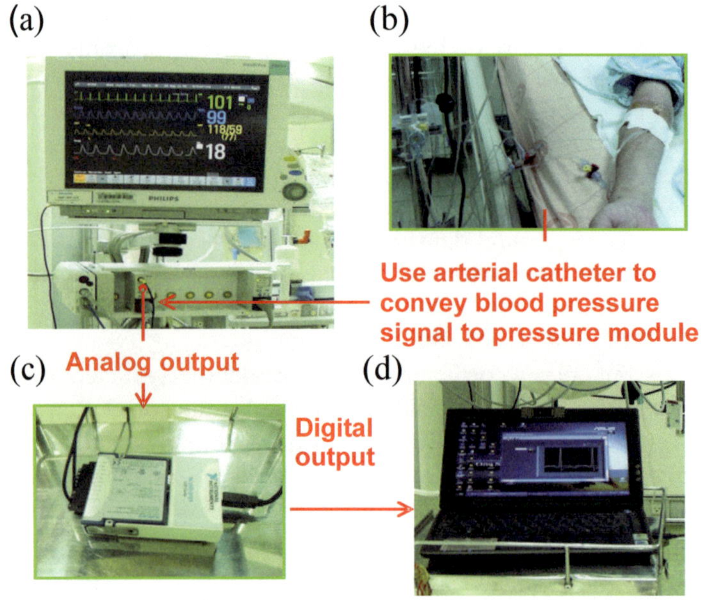

Fig. 1. Experimental instruments for the signal acquisition. (a) physiological signal monitoring system, Philips MP60, and pressure module; (b) invasive ABP monitoring system including an arterial catheter connecting to a conducting tube filled with fluid; (c) data acquisition card; (d) portable computer for displaying and storing the vital signs.

Although the direct invasive arterial-line system applied here provides the advantage of continuous and real-time monitoring, it may introduce additional signal damping, especially when the pressure conducting tube is long [Marino, 2007]. The inertia of the medium within the tube would inevitably remove most high frequency Fourier modes. Nevertheless, it is the currently available method to collect a continuous ABP signal during surgery.

Principally speaking, an electret condenser microphone uses the rate change of capacity to collect pressure signal so that it picks up the motion signal of the pulse. In other words, the microphone data reflect variations of pulse pressure rather than the pressure itself. In Ref.[Yu and Wang, 2006; Jeng & Lee, 2008], this signal had been successfully linked to the Wang pulse spectrum theory. However, in order to study the relation between ABP and microphone signal, the latter will be integrated once so that they have the same base.

3. Results and discussions

Consider the case of Fig. 7 of [Jeng & Lee, 2008] that the person had slight spleen disease as an example. Figure 3.1a plots the data before and after performing the integration once and their corresponding spectra are shown in Fig.3b. These figures indicate that the integration significantly smears the irregularity and rendering the fast attenuation of mode amplitude as the mode index increases. For the sake of clarity, their corresponding spectrograms of amplitudes are plotted in Fig.4a and 4b, respectively, in which the amplitude is transformed to be $\log_{10}(1+\text{amp})$ to reveal the detailed information. According to the arterial wave theory [Wang et al. 1989; Young et al. 1989, 1992; Jan et al, 2003; Wang Lin et al, 2004; Kuo et al, 2004; and Hsu et al. 2006] the fourth mode reflects the healthy condition of the spleen. The significant amplitude and frequency variations of the spleen mode of both figures provided by microphone system indicate that the person had better to see a doctor. In other words, the integration of the microphone arterial signal does not much alter its capability of resolving the detailed information.

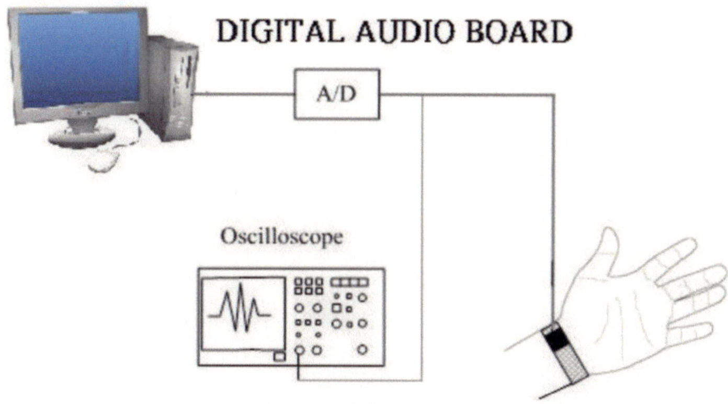

(a)

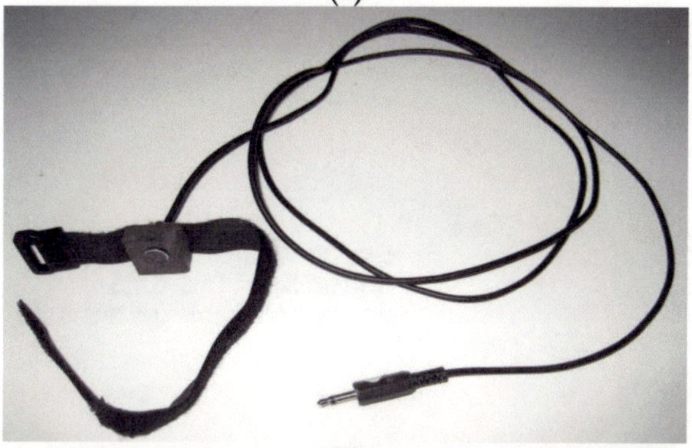

(b)

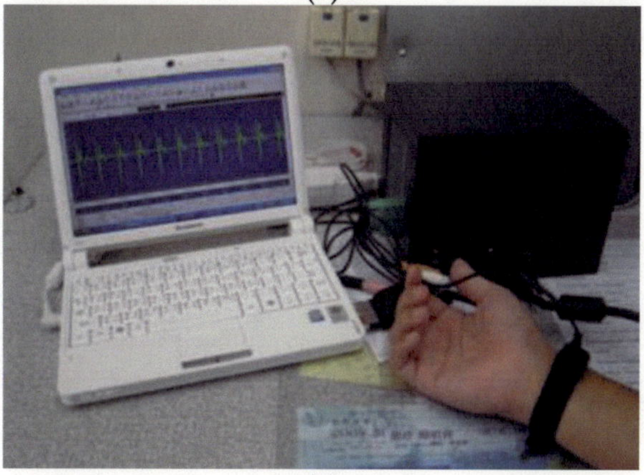

(c)

Fig. 2. An example of the sonocardiography system: (a) schematic diagram; (b) the microphone; and (c) an example of acquiring pulse data.

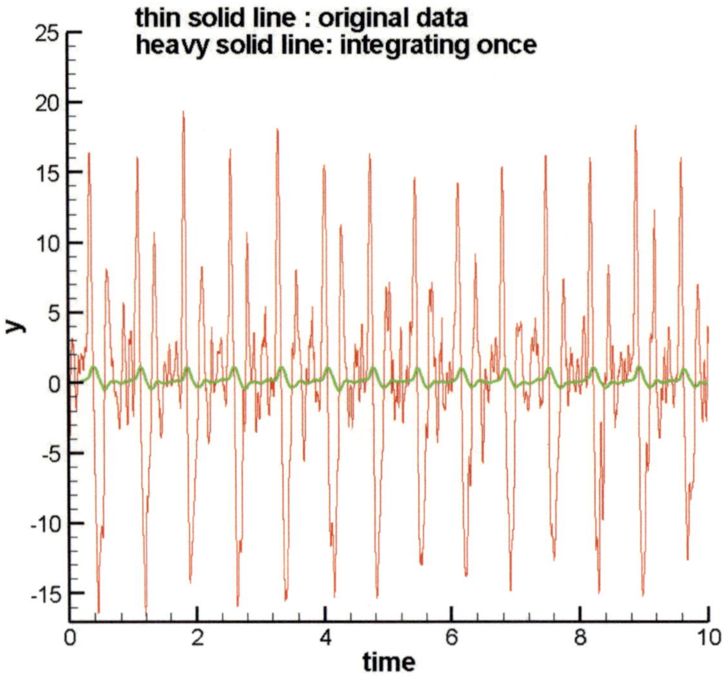

(a)

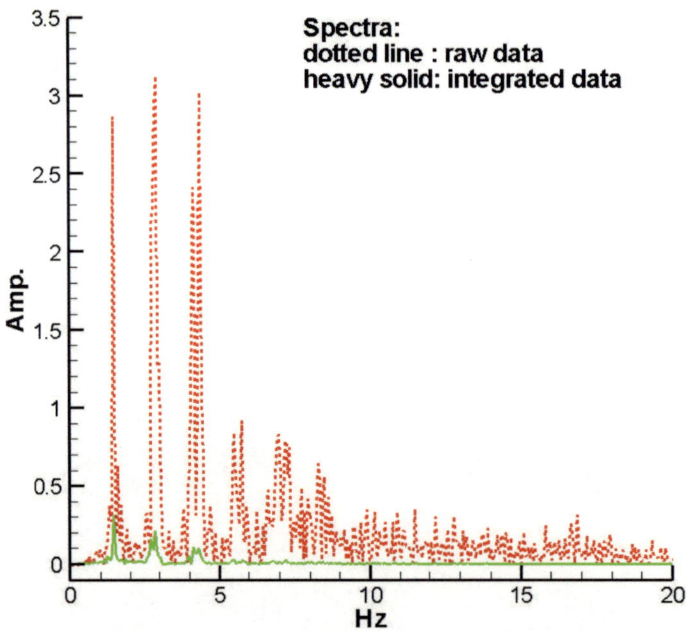

(b)

Fig. 3. Data and spectrum of a people with slight spleen disease: (a) raw (thin solid line) and integrated (heavy solid line) data; (b) spectrum of the raw and integrated data.

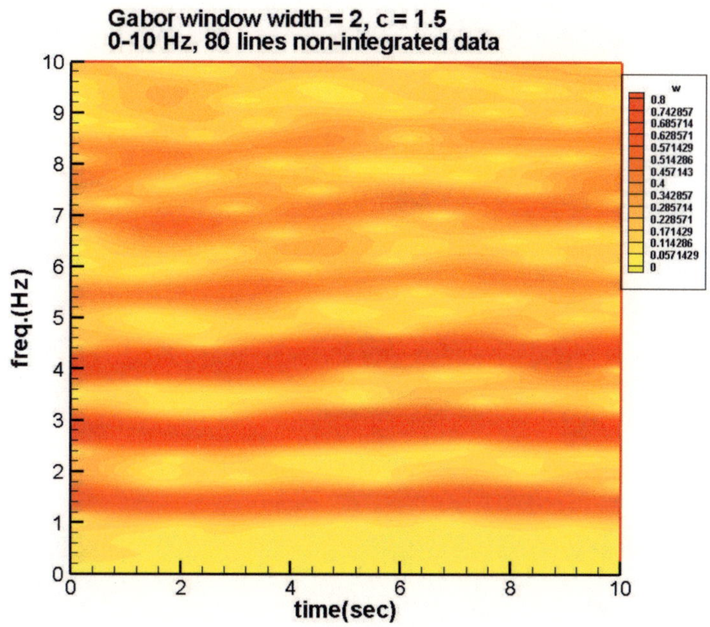

(a)

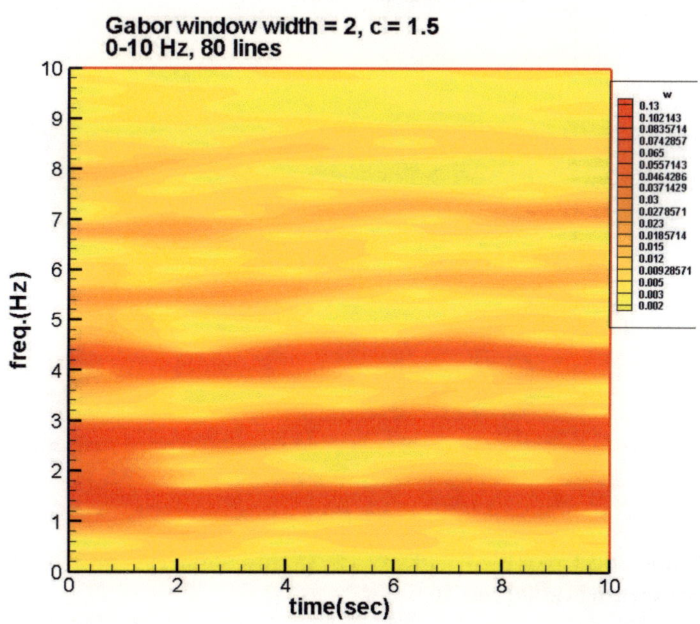

(b)

Fig. 4. Three-dimensional spectrograms: (a) raw data; and (b) integrated data.

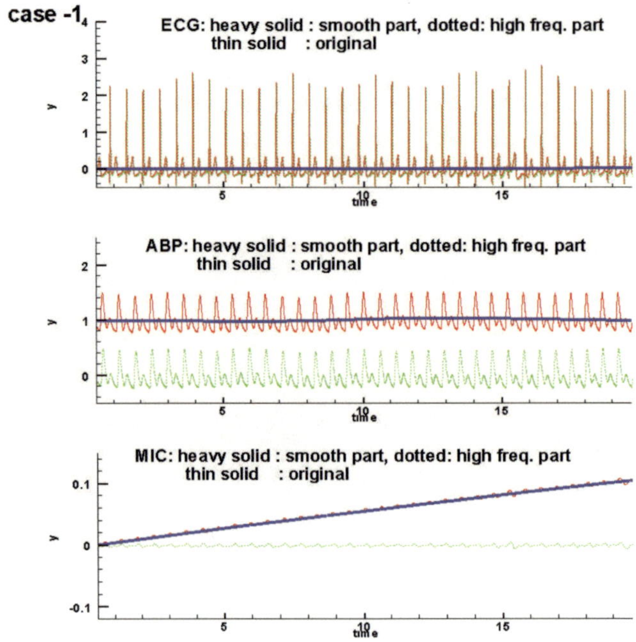

(a)

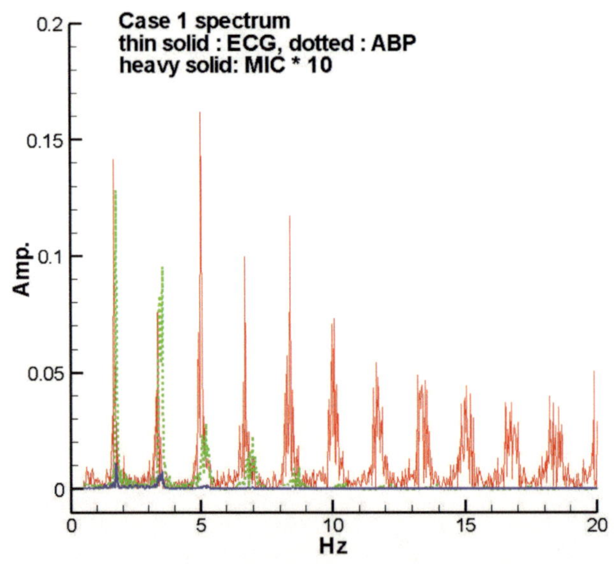

(b)

Fig. 5. The data and spectra of the first test case: (a) raw data; (b) spectrum in which the microphone's spectrum is enlarged 10 times.

In this study, data of six test cases are examined. All of them survived. However, the third case stayed in the hospital for one year after data collection. They are separately discussed below.

The first one is a case of head injury with epidural hematoma resulted from a car accident. His raw data are shown in Fig.5a, in which the ECG, ABP and microphone data are plotted from top to bottom, respectively. He was in comatose state with ventilator use while the data was collected. As the governing center had some problems, the output command of the heart rate control system, say the envelope of his ECG, is obviously variable so as to keep a highly adaptive state as shown in Fig.5a. According to the wave theory [Wang et al. 1989; Young et al. 1989, 1992; Jan et al, 2003; Wang Lin et al, 2004; Kuo et al, 2004; and Hsu et al. 2006] and ancient Chinese medicine, the fourth (lung mode) and sixth harmonic (gall mode) are closely related to the circulatory homeostasis of lung and brain, respectively. The spectrograms of Figs.6b and 6c show that the amplitude and frequency of the sixth mode are variable. However, since the steady mechanical ventilator use under sedation provides a smooth breathing pattern, the fourth mode is slightly more stable than the sixth mode.

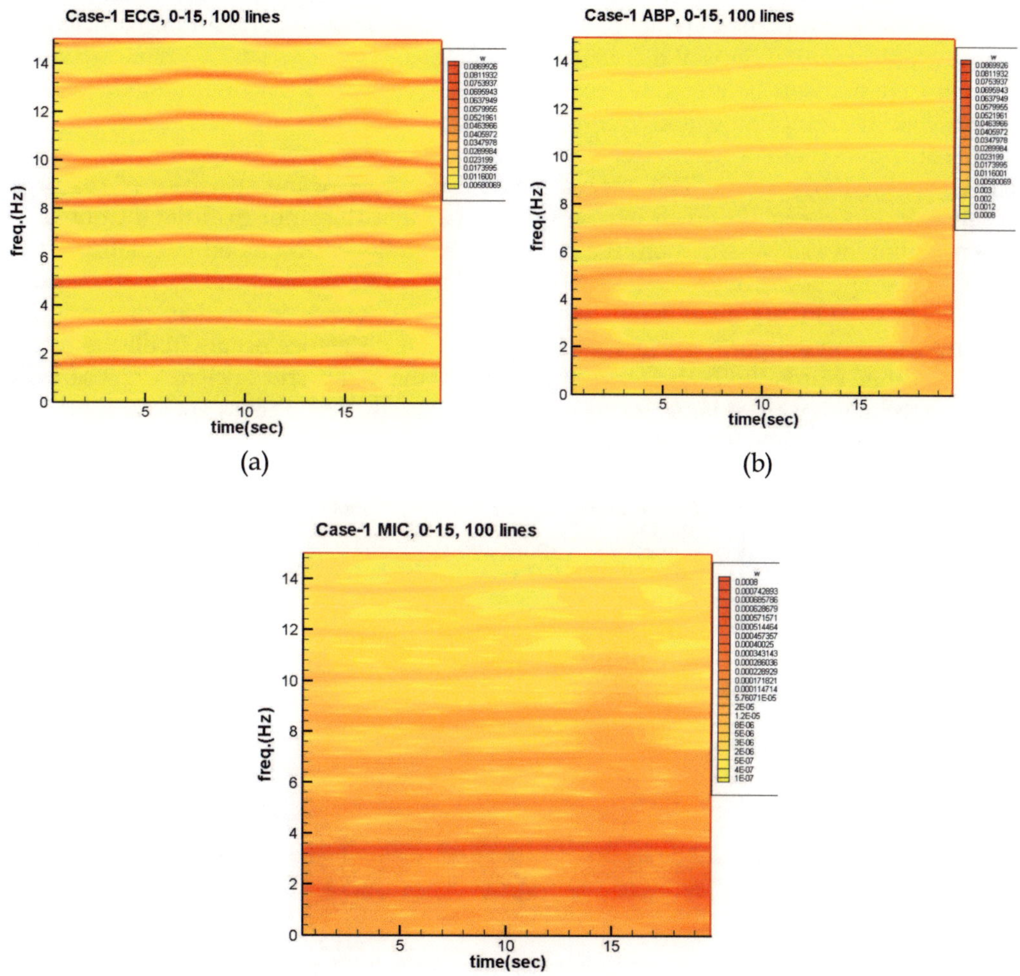

Fig. 6. The spectrograms of the first case: (a) ECG; (b) ABP; and (c) microphone wrist arterial signal.

The cross-correlations between three signals are plotted in Fig.7a through 7c, which are ECG, ABP, and microphone from top to bottom. Note that the time series of the three signals are measured at different points. Therefore, they should have certain phase differences between one another. Because the wave propagation speed distribution through the circulation system is not known, we shift the time scale of one of the wave components so as to attain a maximum absolute value of cross correlation coefficients. The shifted amounts are marked on the figures as shown. It seems that, around the heart rate mode of 1.7Hz, the ECG and ABP are almost totally correlated. In fact, the patient finally recovered after one month. It is interested to see that the correlations of both ECG and ABP with respect to the microphone signal are very high too.

It is interesting to see that the color distributions (represent the amplitude distribution) and wavy shapes (represent the frequency variation) of the fundamental and harmonics of Fig.7a are not similar to those of Fig.7b and 7c, respectively. Nevertheless, their differences of the heart beat wave component are not significant so that their cross-correlation coefficients are still very high and vital signs of the patient are stable.

A careful comparison between the sixth mode of Fig.6c and the fourth mode of Fig.5b reveals that the amplitude and frequency variations of the latter are obviously more complicated than those of the former. The former is corresponding to the signal of emergent case while the latter is not. This means that the behavior of the spectrum of the organ-meridian in emergency is much less sensitive than that does not in serious trouble. The reason is that, in critical situation, the adaptive capability of the blood circulation system concentrates on how to survive so that it takes care of the entire organ-meridians simultaneously. On the other hand, when only one organ is in trouble, the circulation system focuses on supporting this specific target. This difference occurs in all the rest test cases. In other words, both the wave theory of Wang et al. and ancient Chinese organ-meridian technology are suitable for most people before they face emergent health problems and are closely related to the preventive medicine.

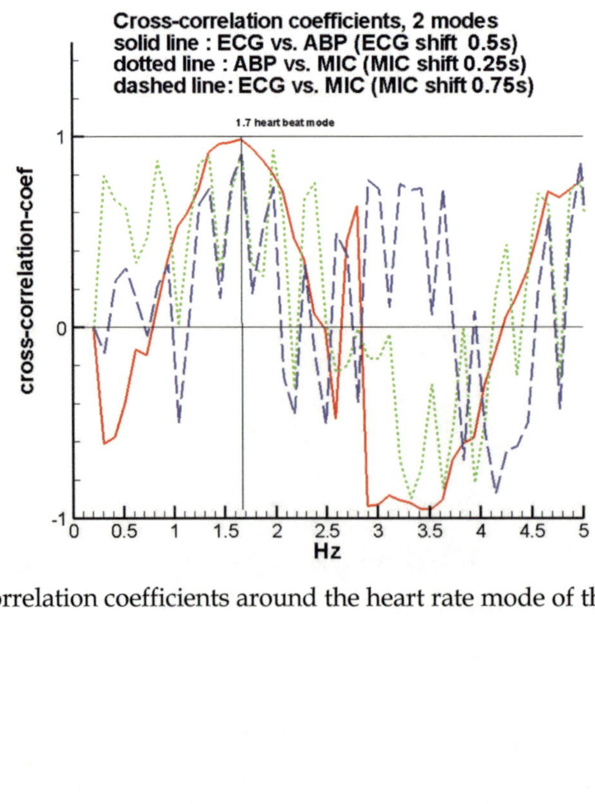

Fig. 7. The cross-correlation coefficients around the heart rate mode of the first test case.

The second one is a case of liver laceration resulted from a car accident. When the data was collected, the patient was in a stable hemodynamic state and non-operative management was applied. The corresponding raw data and spectra are shown in Figs.8a and 8b, respectively. It is seen that the spectral band around the fundamental (heart) and harmonics

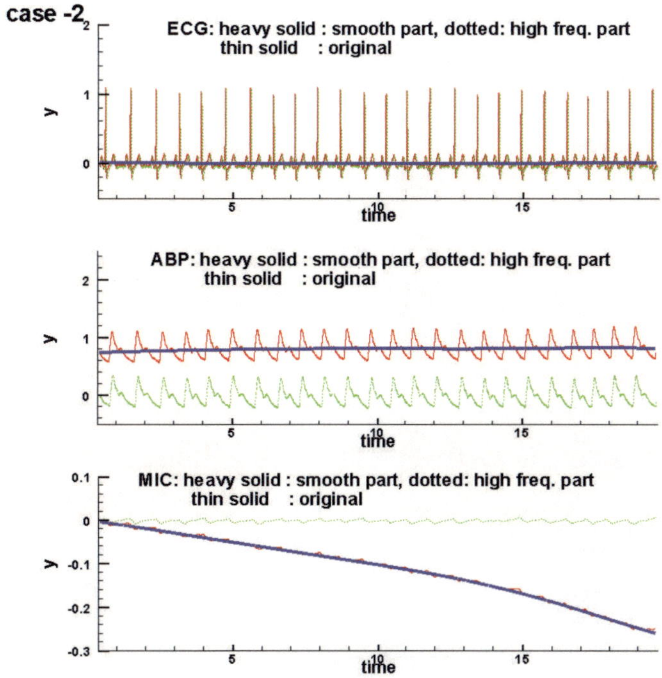

(a)

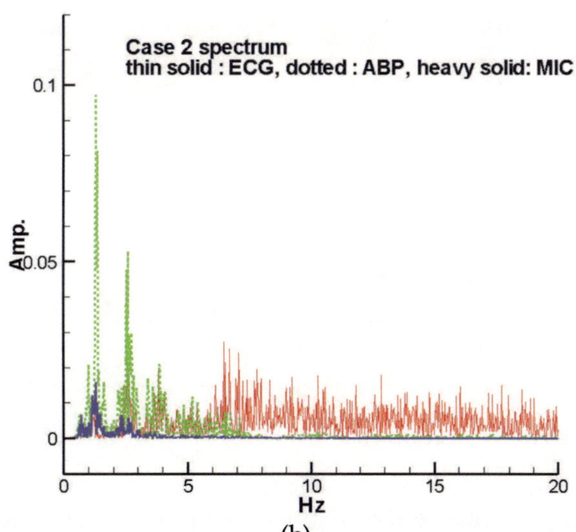

(b)

Fig. 8. The data and spectra of the second test case: (a) raw data; (b) spectrum in which the microphone's spectrum is enlarged 10 times.

seriously scattered. All the corresponding spectrograms of ECG, ABP and microphone signals exhibit significant variations of both amplitude and frequencies. It seems that the spectral scattering of a wave component is corresponding to the variation of one or two of the amplitude and frequency. The degrees of these dominant modes' variations are not less than the first harmonic (live mode). It seems that the injury of the major organ, liver, brought great impact on the operation of other systems, and the adaptation of the entire system was switched on. Fortunately, the situation is not serious enough to become chaos so that we can still trace every mode.

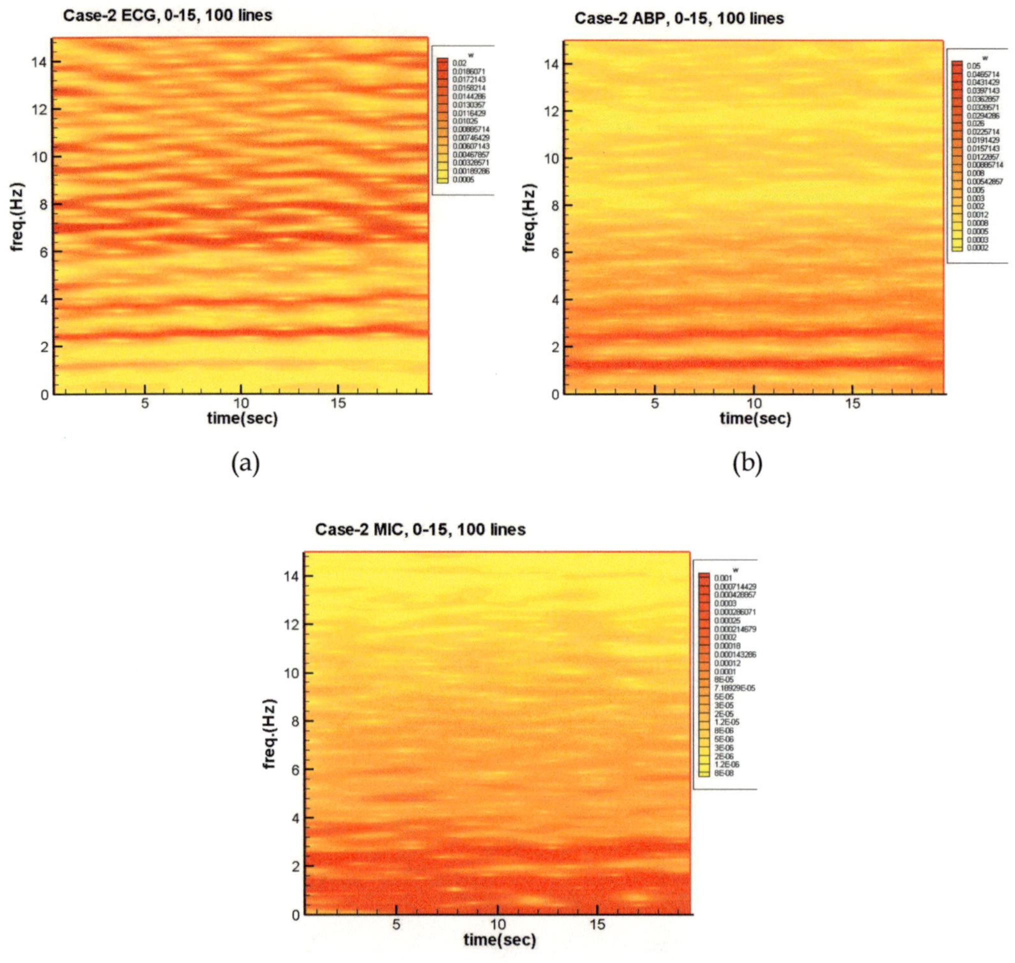

(c)

Fig. 9. The spectrograms of the second case: (a) ECG; (b) ABP; and (c) microphone wrist arterial signal.

The cross correlation coefficients are shown in Fig.10. The correlations of ECG-ABP and ABP-microphone are moderately high (about 0.7 and 0.6 respectively). The ECG and microphone signal is in highly negative correlation (-0.9). Now the color distributions and wavy shapes of most organ meridians shown in the three spectrograms are similar to each other such that they are also partially correlated. Therefore, the patient's circulation system is healthy. This explanation was confirmed by the record that the patient had recovered after one month.

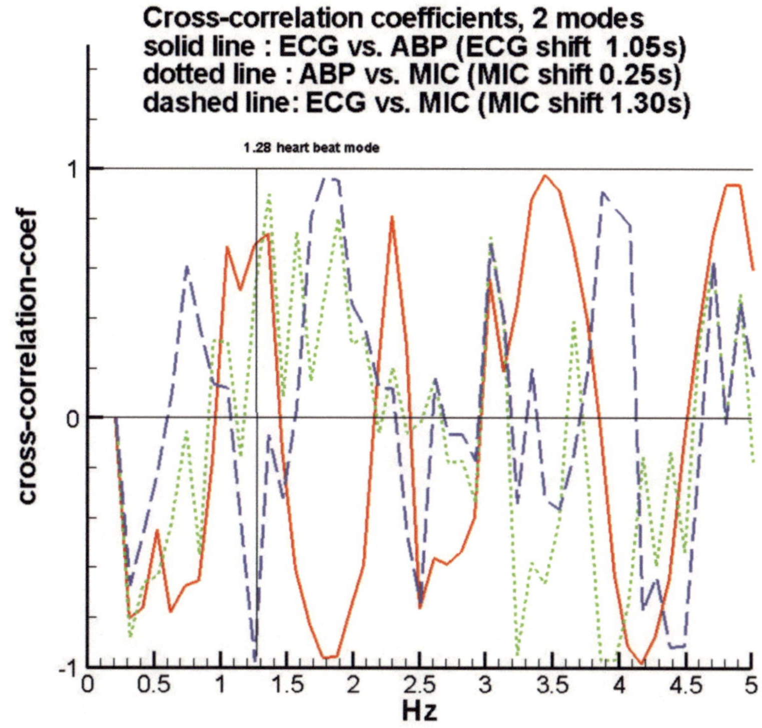

Fig. 10. The cross-correlation coefficients around the heart rate mode of the second test case.

The third test case suffered from serious electric shock and had cardiopulmonary resuscitation right before onto the ambulance. Though the vital signs resumed, he remained in comatose state with ventilator support while the data was collected. Unfortunately, the case had prolonged hospitalization for one year after that. The raw data and spectra are shown in Figs.11. Like the spectra shown in Fig.11b, spectrograms of Figs.12a through 12c are regular and do not have much amplitude variation. It seems that the coma had suppressed the system adaptation. Moreover, the similarity of color distribution and wavy shape of every organ meridian indicates that the three data are partially correlated too. Moreover, Fig.13 shows that all the correlation coefficients of the heart rate mode are very high as shown. In spite of the fact that the patient can not completely recover for a long time, the highly correlated state indicates that vital signs are stable.

The next case got right frontal parietal and temporal subdural hematoma after falling down. She also had the history of old stroke. The corresponding raw data and spectra are plotted in Figs.14a and 14b, respectively. From these signal we can not have much information. From the resulting spectrograms, it is obviously that the gall mode (related to brain organ-meridian) has obvious variations of both amplitude and frequency. Consequently, the second and still higher harmonics are all affected too.

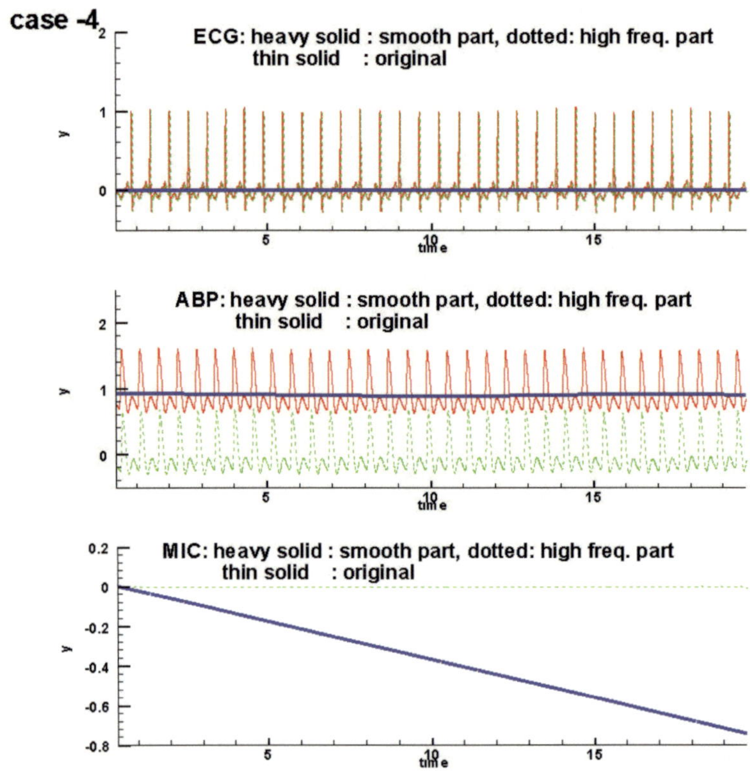

(a)

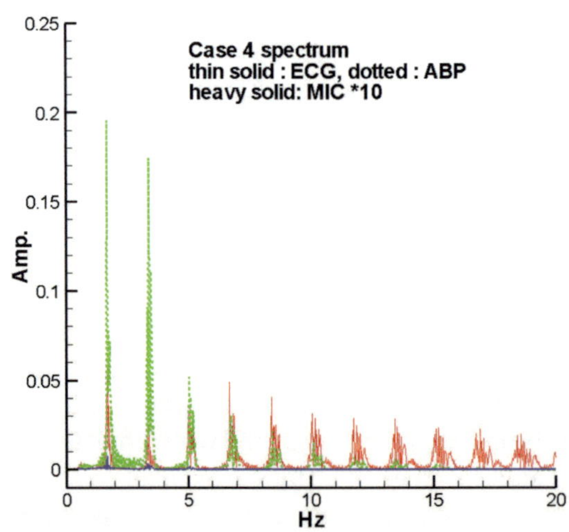

(b)

Fig. 11. The data and spectra of the third test case: (a) raw data; (b) spectrum in which the microphone's spectrum is enlarged 10 times.

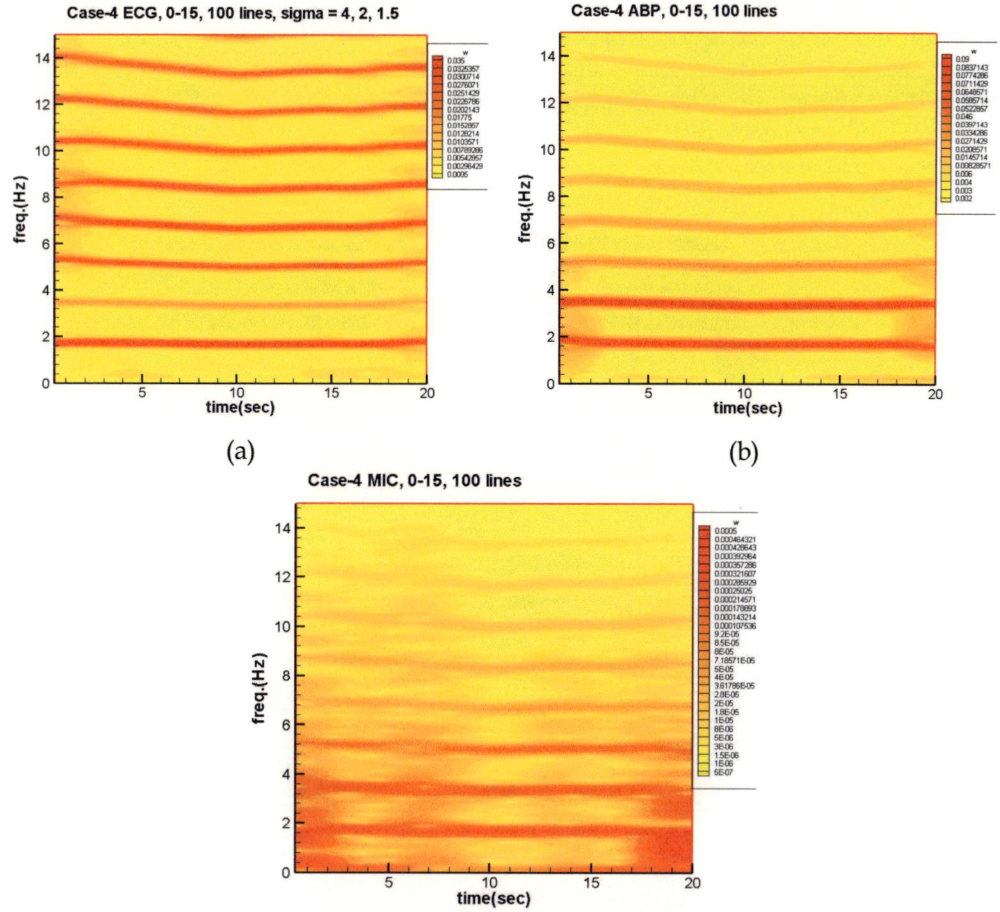

(c)

Fig. 12. The spectrograms of the third case: (a) ECG; (b) ABP; and (c) microphone wrist arterial signal.

The cross correlation between the ECG and ABP are very high (about 0.9 as shown in Fig.15). On the other hand, signals of ABP-microphone and ECG-microphone have negative correlations of about -0.6. The reason may be cause by the weak wrist pulse signal of the patient. Nevertheless, it seems that the system adaptation of the patient worked very well so that mode wave components gradually fluctuated as shown. These fluctuations are similarly existed in the three spectrograms of Figs.14a-14c which show that their energies are partially correlated. These correlations reflect the high possibility of recover which is verified by the fact that the patient had recovered after one month.

The fifth test case was suffered from a cervical vertebra injury after falling down and received the support of the endotracheal intubation. At the instant of measuring data, the patient lost consciousness and was quadriplegia. His raw data and spectra are shown in Figs.17a and 17b, respectively. The resulting spectrograms (Figs.18a-18c) show that both fundamental mode and harmonics have obvious amplitude and frequency fluctuations. His gall modes even have jumps at the instances of the tenth and fifteenth second as shown. It indicates his self-protection system was in the adaptive state and tried to recover his health. In Fig.19, it is seen the ECG, ABP, and microphone signal have very high correlation between one another such that his circulation worked very well. The partial correlations among their energy are also reflected by the similarity between their organ meridians' amplitude and frequency distributions. These conclusions have the strong evident that he finally recovered after six months.

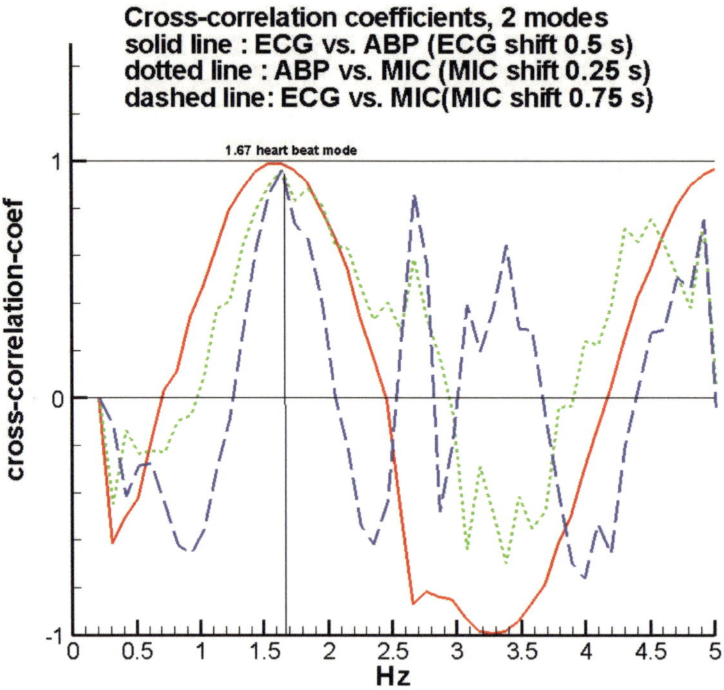

Fig. 13. The cross-correlation coefficients around the heart rate mode of the third test case.

The last test case got severe head injury with intracranial hemorrhage, subdural hematoma and subarachnoid hemorrhage. The raw data and spectra are shown in Figs.20a and 20b, respectively. Envelopes of the ECG and APP raw data have obvious oscillations as shown. The corresponding spectrograms of Figs.21a through 21b show that his circulation system tried to adapt itself. The three gall modes has abnormal jump in the interval of 5-7 second as shown. In this case, the heart rate modes of ABP and microphone signal are highly correlated (correlation coefficient is about 0.9 in Fig.22). Figure 22 shows that his cross-correlation coefficients of ECG-ABP and ECG-microphone are about 0.3 and 0.1, respectively. Obviously, the phase lags are serious between these two signals. That indicates he was in a life-threatening situation at that time. Fortunately, the patient has partial correlation between three data because his amplitude and frequency fluctuations of all the organ meridian modes of three spectrograms are similar to one another. He recovered gradually and was transferred to the general ward within one month. Recently, he returned to the clinic for the treatment of epilepsy, a neurological sequel of the previous head injury. That means his neural control system is impaired. Although his circulation system has phase lag problems, the overall response is not too bad so that he finally recovered under the proper supports and treatments in the intensive care unit. These messages indicate that he effectively struggled for his life during the period in the intensity care unit.

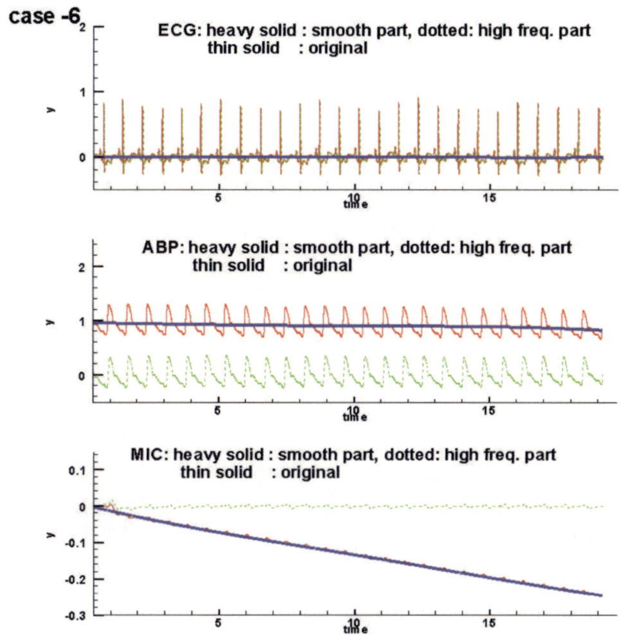

(a)

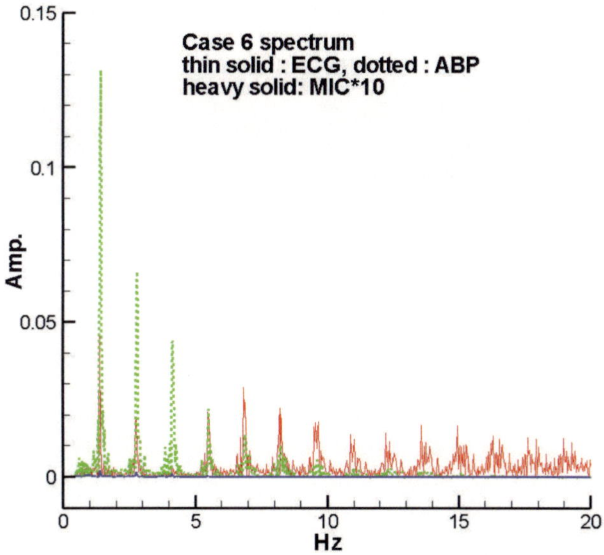

(b)

Fig. 14. The data and spectra of the fourth test case: (a) raw data; (b) spectrum in which the microphone's spectrum is enlarged 10 times.

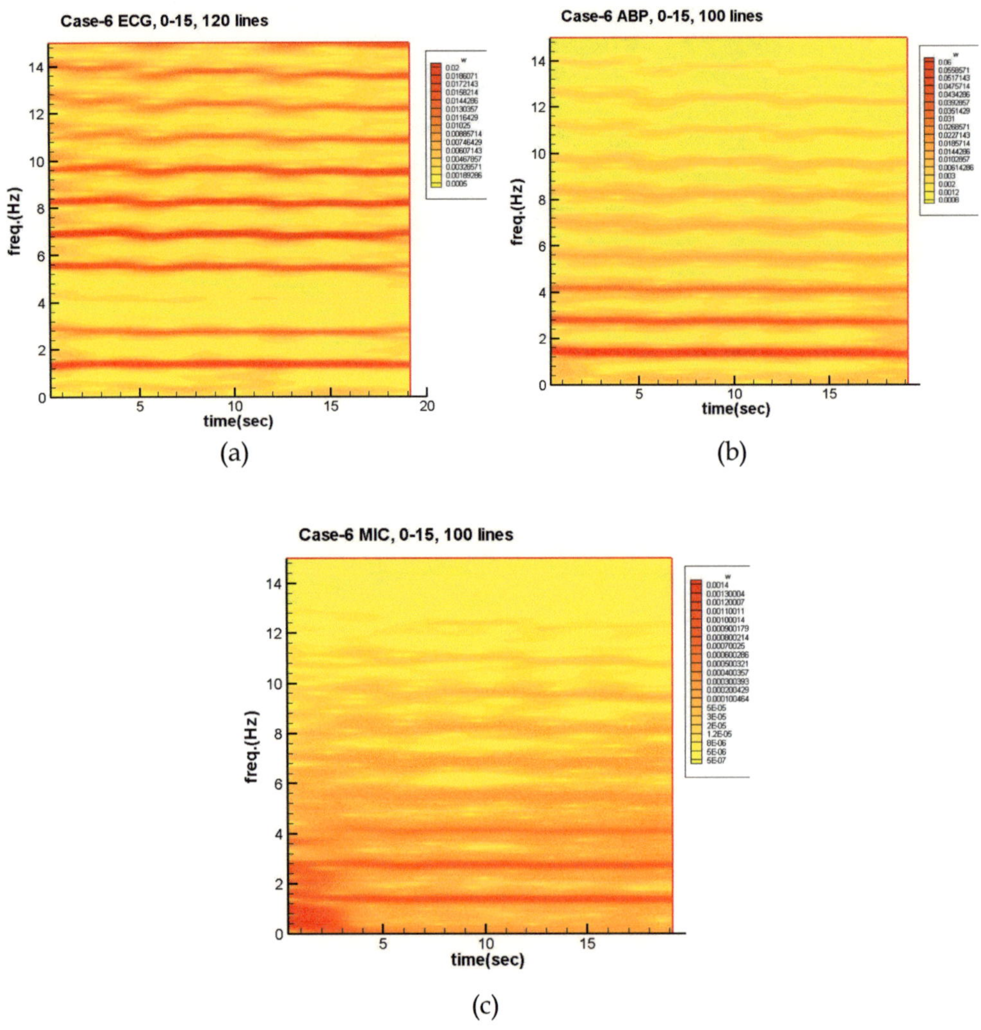

Fig. 15. The spectrograms of the fourth case: (a) ECG; (b) ABP; and (c) microphone wrist arterial signal.

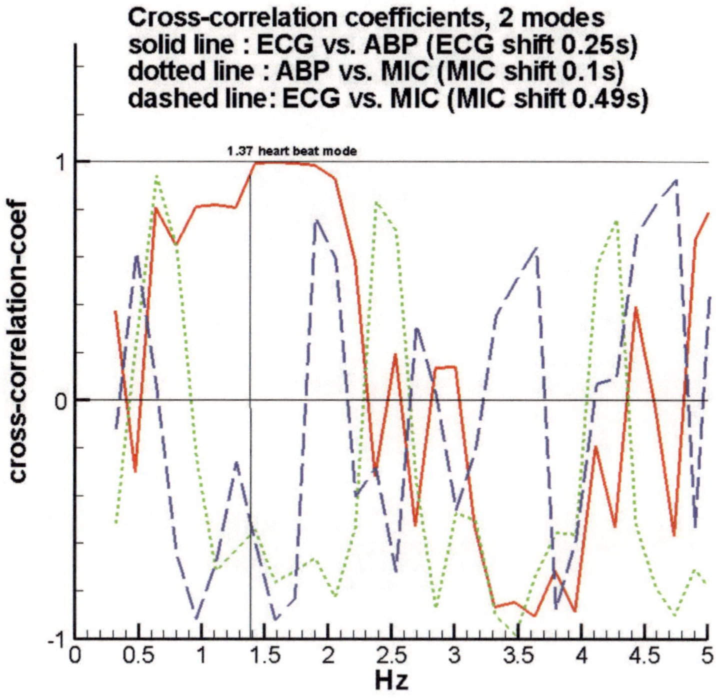

Fig. 16. The cross-correlation coefficients around the heart rate mode of the fourth test case.

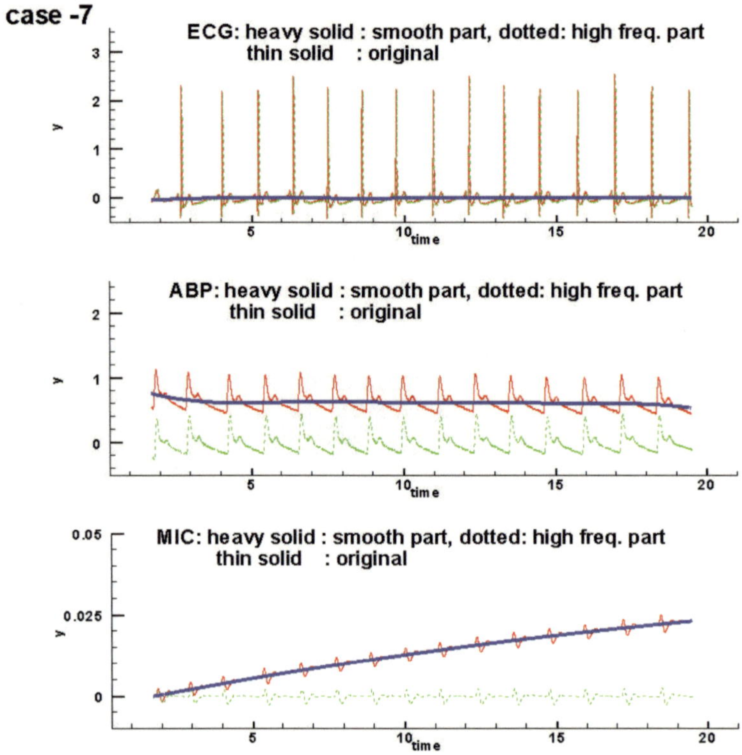

(a)

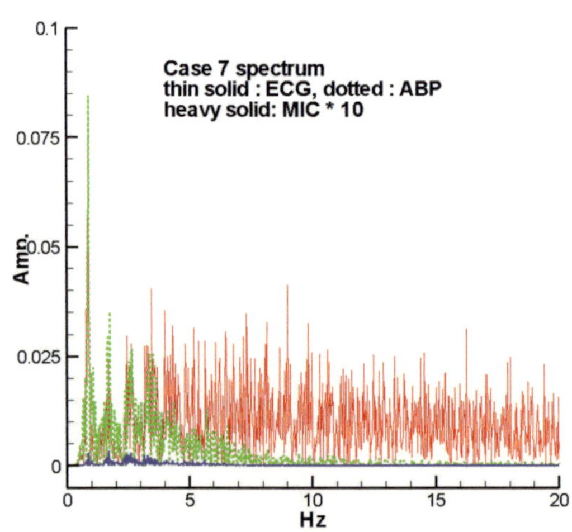

(b)

Fig. 17. The data and spectra of the fifth test case: (a) raw data; (b) spectrum in which the microphone's spectrum is enlarged 10 times.

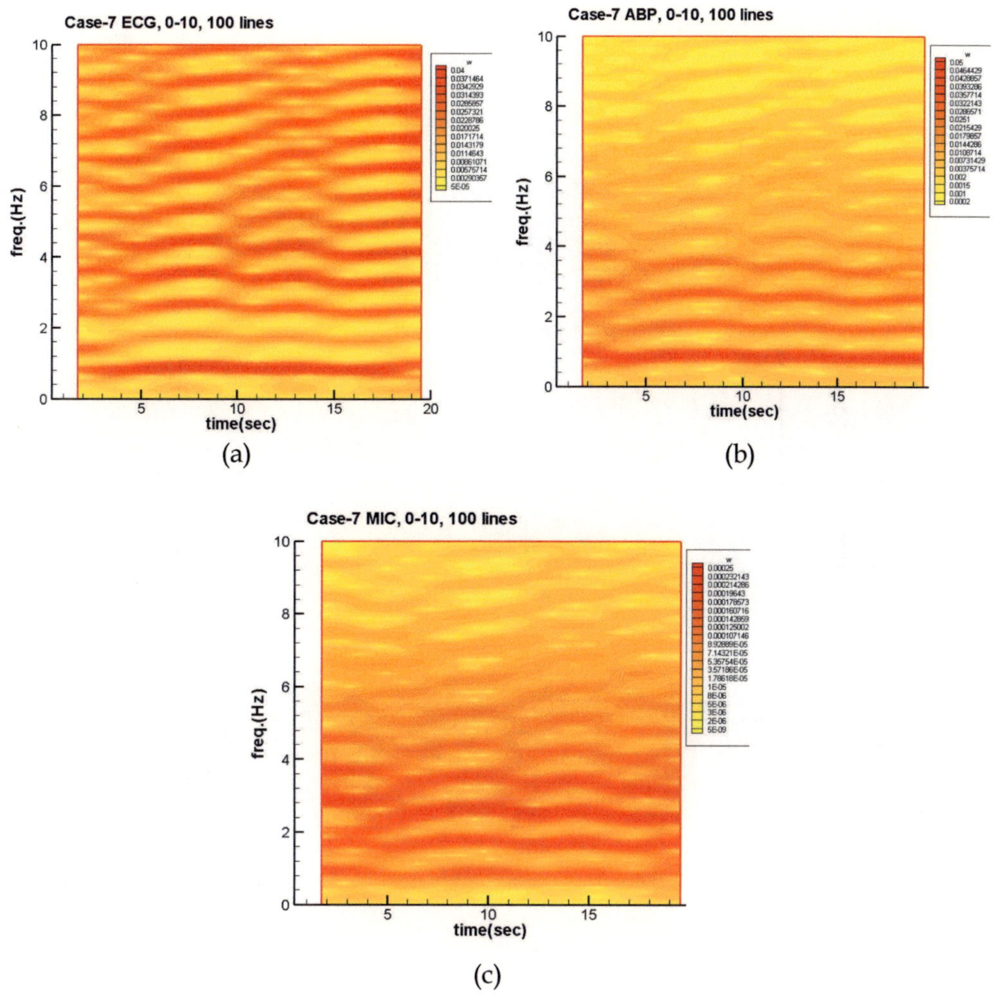

Fig. 18. The spectrograms of the fifth case: (a) ECG; (b) ABP; and (c) microphone wrist arterial signal.

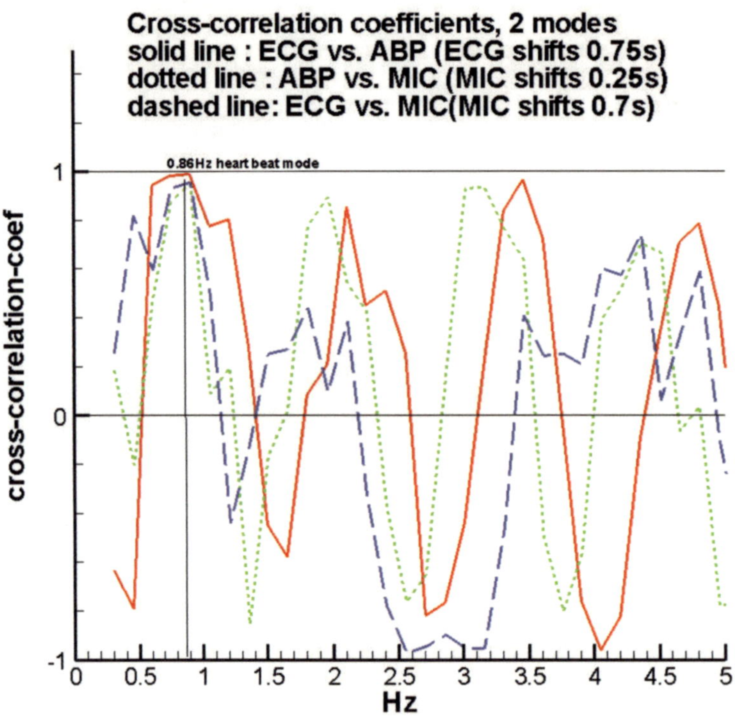

Fig. 19. The cross-correlation coefficients around the heart rate mode of the fifth test case.

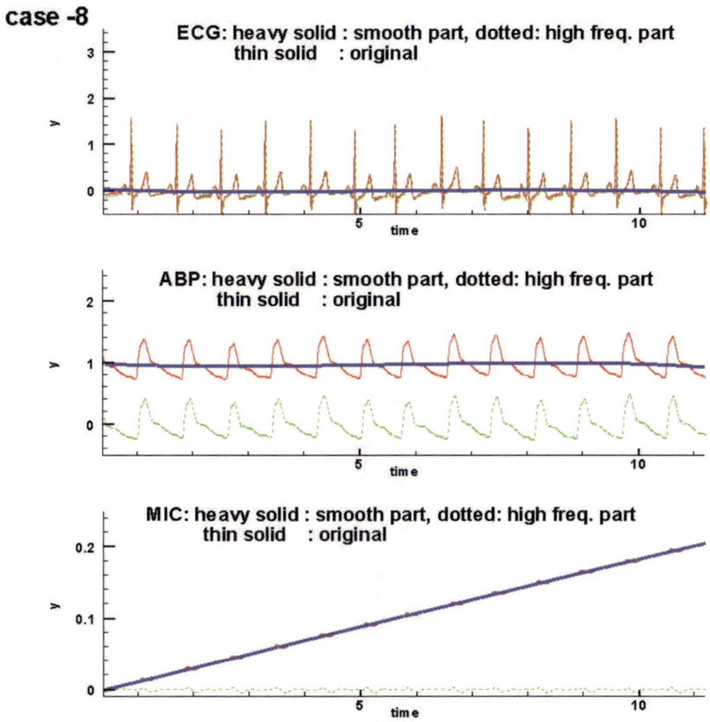

(a)

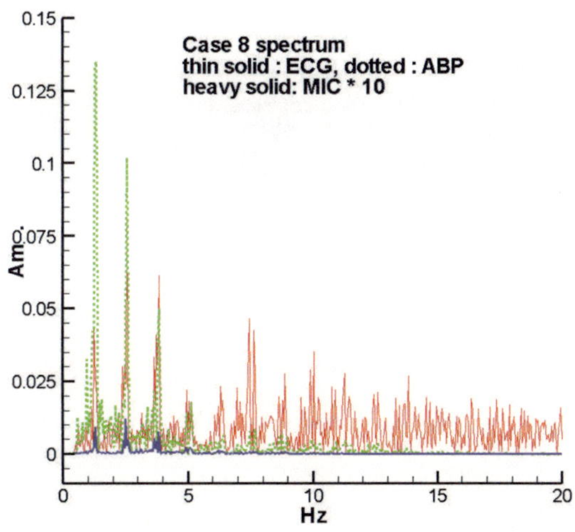

(b)

Fig. 20. The data of the sixth test case, fell down, bilateral temporal bone fractures extends into the right middle ear cavity: (a) raw data; (b) spectrum in which the microphone's spectrum is enlarged 10 times.

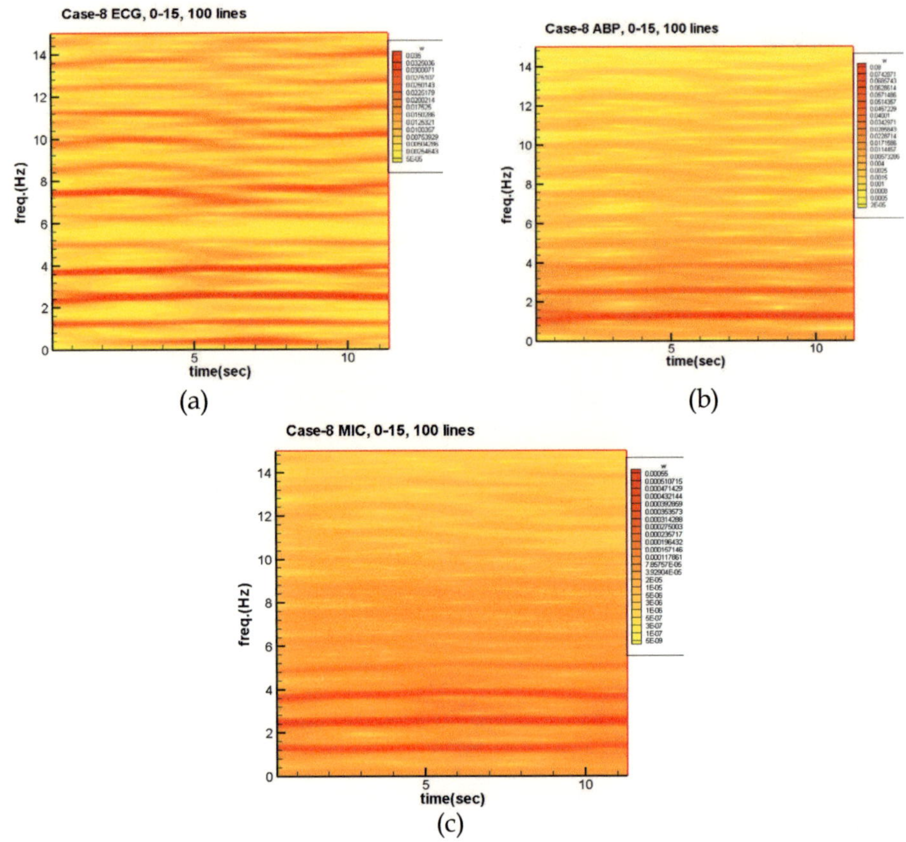

Fig. 21. The spectrograms of the sixth case: (a) ECG; (b) ABP; and (c) microphone wrist arterial signal.

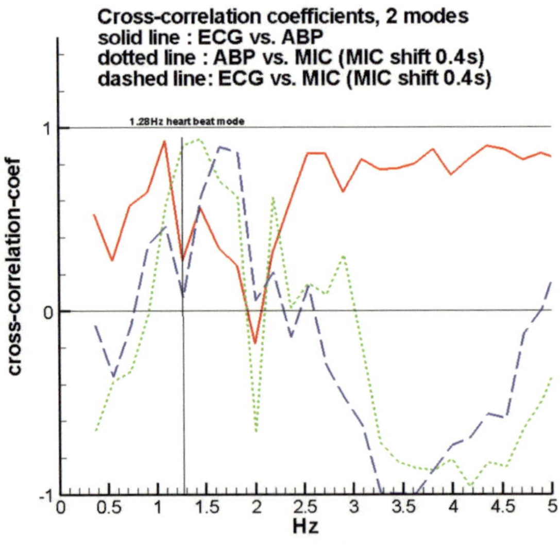

Fig. 22. The cross-correlation coefficients around the heart rate mode of the sixth test case.

In summary, several consistent points of the above discussions are listed below.

1. The heart modes of microphone signal and ABP are correlated. It indicates the possibility that the electret condenser microphone system is a potential tool to be an alternative of ABP system. Since the microphone is a non-invasive sensor and closely related to the ancient Chinese medicine, it can be equipped with simple ECG system to become a valuable tool of clinic and preventive medicine.
2. The cross-correlations between ECG, ABP and microphone can be examined either by the directly calculating the coefficient among time domain heart rate components or by checking the similarity of every organ meridian's shape and color variations with respect to time in their spectrograms. All the test cases show that the heart rate modes of ECG and ABP are correlated. The followed up records show that all these patients remain alive under the effective treatments of the intensive care unit.
3. In critical cases, the wave theory of Wang et al. about single organ meridian still works but is not prominent as in the less emergent situations.
4. When the state is not critical, all the organ-meridians fluctuate which reflect the adaptation of the blood circulation system to struggle for survive.

Since the sample size is too small to achieve a statistical level, further studies will be done to enrich the data base so as to make these facts become useful.

4. Conclusions

The precise post processing algorithm combining the trend removal, Fourier transform and modified Gabor transform provides a tool to look into details of ECG, ABP, and microphone data of wrist arterial signal. The heart modes of all the microphone signals are correlated with ABP. In other words, the non-invasive acoustic sensor can also be a potential tool to monitor human healthy state. The cross correlation coefficient between heart beat modes of ECG and ABP seems to be a possible index of human vital sign. In summary, the microphone system is a potential tool to effectively construct a bridge among ancient and modern medicine and modern technologies.

5. References

Bendat, J. S. & Piersol, A. G.. (2000). *Random Data Analysis and Measurement Procedures*, 3rd ed., John Wiley & Sons, New York, Chapters 10 & 11, pp.349-456.

Brigham, E.O. (1998). *The Fast Fourier Transform and Its Applications;* Prentice Hall: Englewood Cliffs, NJ, USA.

Civetta, J. M.; Taylor, R. W. & Kirby, R. R. (1996). *Critical Care.* 3rd ed., Lippincott-Raven, Ch. 16 & 26, pp. 227-245, 368-372

Goswami, J. C., & Chan, A. K. (1999). *Fundamentals of Wavelets, Theory, Algorithms, and Applications,* John Wiley & Sons, New York.

Hsu, T. L.; Chao, P. T., Hsiu, H., Wang, W. K., Li, S. P. & Lin Wang Y. Y. (2006). Organ-Specific Ligation-Induced Changes in Harmonic Components of the Pulse Spectrum and Regional Vasoconstrictor Selectivity in Wistar Rats, *Experimental Physiology*, vol. 91, no.1, pp.163-170, 2006.

Huynh, H.T. (1993). Accurate monotone cubic interpolation. *SIAM. J. Numer. Anal.* Vol.*30*, pp.57-100

Jan, M. Y.; Hsiu, H., Hsu, T. L., Wang, W. K., & Wang, Y. Y. (2003). The Physical Conditions of Different Organs Are Reflected Specifically in the Pressure Pulse Spectrum of the Peripheral Arterial, *Cardiovascular Engineering: An Int. J.*, vol. 3. no.1, pp.21-29.

Jeng, Y. N. & Lee, S. Y.. (2008). Qualitative Frequency Response Calibration of Sonocardiography System to Sense Wrist Pulse, *The 7th Asian-Pacific Conference on Medical and Biological Engineering,* APCMBE 2008 March 21-26, 2008, Beijing, China, paper no. T22. No.5-15.

Jeng, Y. N. and Cheng, Y. C. (2007). A First Study of Speech Processing via a Novel Mode Decomposition Basing on the Fourier Sine Spectrum and Spectrogram, *Proc. IEEE 2007 TENCON,* 10/30~11/2 Taipei, Taiwan, WeSP-01 section, paper no.00079.

Jeng, Y. N.; Yang, T. M. & Lee, S. Y. (2011). Response Identification in the Extremely Low Frequency Region of an Electret Condenser Microphone, *Sensors,* vol.11, pp.623-637; doi:10.3390/s110100623.

Jeng, Y.N.; Huang, P.G. & Cheng, Y.C. (2008). Decomposition of one-dimensional waveform using iterative Gaussian diffusive filtering methods. *Proc. R. Soc. Lond. A* 2008, *464,* 1673-1695.

Jeng, Y.N.; Yang, T.M. & Wu, C.H. (2009) Low Frequency Analysis of Acoustic and Vibration Data of a Remote Control Electronic Helicopter. *Proceeding of 47th AIAA Aerospace Sciences Meeting.* Orlando, FL, USA, January 2009; pp. 5-8.

Kuo, Y. C. Kuo; Chiu, T. Y., Jan, M. Y., Bau, J. G., Li, S. P., Wang, W. K. & Wang, Y. Y. (2004). Losing Harmonic Stability of Arterial Pulse in Terminally Ill Patients, Clinical Methods and Pharmachology, *Blood Pressure Monitoring,* vol. 9. no. 5, pp.255-258, Oct. 2004.

Mallat, S. G. (1999). *A Wavelet Tour of Signal Processing*. Academic Press, New York.

Marino, P. L. (2007). *The ICU book.* 3rd ed., Lippincott Willian & Wilkins, Ch 8 & 12, pp.151-159, 211-230.

Wang Lin, Y. Y.; Jan, M. Y., Shyu, C. S., Jiang, C. A. & Wang, W. K. (2004). The Natural Frequencies of the Arterial System and Their Relation to the Heart Rate," *IEEE Trans. Biomed. Eng.*, vol. 51. no.1, Jan. 2004, pp. 193-195.

Wang, W. K.; Lo, Y. Y., Chiang, Y., Hsu, T. L. & Wang Lin Y. Y (1989). Resonance of Organs with the Heart, *Biomedical Engineering – An International Symposium,* ed. Young, W. J., Hemisphere, Washington, DC. USA, pp.259-268.

Young, S. T.; Wang, W. K., Chang, L. S. & Kuo, T. S. (1992). The Filter properties of the Arterial Beds of Organs in Rats, *Acta Physiol Scand.*, vol. 145, pp.401-406.

Young, S. T.; Wang, W. K., Chang, L. S., & Kuo, T. S. (1989). Specific Frequency Properties of the Renal and the Superior Mesenteric Arterial Beds in Rats, *Cardiovas Res.* Vol. 23, pp.265-467.

Yu, F. M. & Wang, S. C. (2006). Design of a Sonocardiography System and Its Application in the Diagnostic of the Cardiovascular Disease, *Proceedings of 2006 TSB conference,* Taiwan, Paper No. TSB2006-O-205, pp.16, Dec. 2006.

Part 3

Pharmacological Experimental Research

11

Traditional Chinese Herbal Medicine – East Meets West in Validation and Therapeutic Application

John W.M. Yuen, Sonny H.M. Tse
and Jolene Y.K. Yung
School of Nursing, The Hong Kong Polytechnic University, Hong Kong SAR, China

1. Introduction

Chinese herbal medicine has been practiced for thousands of years, and is used increasingly in western countries in conjunction with or in place of allopathic medicine. The earliest extant book of material medica, known as *Shen Nong Bencaojing* (The divine farmer's material medica), appeared in the third century AD. At that time, the Father of Chinese herbal medicine Shen Nong, had classified 365 entities of herbs and drugs (Yang, 2005). The herbal tradition reached its peak some thousand years later, in 1552-1578 AD, of when Li Shi-zhen compiled his Great Herbal *Bencao Gangmu* (Compendium of Materia Medica) of 52 volumes which described 1,892 herbal entities in details (Li, 2003). The World health Organization (WHO) estimates that at least 75% of the world's population utilizes traditional medicines for healing and curing diseases (Robinson & Zhang, 2011). However, the holistic concepts of traditional Chinese medicine (TCM) are far removed from the reductionist principles of the modern day Western approach, and are difficult to express and comprehend in western terms. Western medicine is evidence-based and disease-focused, and relies on the double blinded, randomized, controlled clinical trial as the gold standard to assess clinical utility and safety of treatment, which is usually a pure chemical with a defined pharmacological action. Conversely, TCM is based on history, experience, culture and belief, and most herbal medicines are complex mixtures of largely unknown chemical composition. In western terms, the health benefits of most herbal remedies remain unsubstantiated by scientific evidence in well-designed human studies, and this limits their acceptance by western trained health professionals. In addition to efficacy, the issues of toxicity and of herb-herb and herb-drug interaction that might be additive, synergistic or antagonistic need comprehensive scientific study. In this chapter, we overview the divergence and convergence between the two systems, and explore into nowadays methods used in herbal case-studies representing different stages of herbal use and evaluation. More importantly, the need for and feasibility of performing controlled trials for scientific validation of herbal medicine are discussed, thus repositioning the herbal research, and helping to decide the most favorable direction for East meets West.

2. The conceptual divergence between Western and Eastern perspectives

Looking into the world history, modern medicine is known to be originated from the ancient Egyptian medicine, and largely influenced by the Greek medical ideas about anatomy, physiology and practical medicine. Different cultures, from their very beginning, have established their own special ways in the care of the sick (Longrigg, 1997). The earliest written evidences (10,000-2000 BC) have mentioned the practice of Chinese medicine and imhotep in Egypt, which both commonly used medicinal herbs as the treatment modality (Bynum, 2008). Such ancient medical approaches, were largely influence by the cultural and religious beliefs, have later on transformed into scientific disciplines to its own effective and safe practice. The beginnings of true medical science in the West were laid when the reliance on superstition that underpinned tribal medicine was replaced by civilized and rational curiosity about the cause of illness. Modern medicine, at first glance, especially in the past century, is moving from triumph to triumph with the growing number of survivors, it has gained the prevailing acceptance. However, Chinese medicine, holding the key traditional beliefs of healing – holism, is divided into special disciplines e.g. herbalism and acupuncture in the alternative and complementary medicine. Scientific and alternative medical approaches have followed different paths at different speeds. Rational treatment ultimately depends upon properly understanding the true nature of disease. Orthodox and unorthodox practitioners have relied for centuries on 'tried-and-tested' methods to ensure the efficacy of empirical remedies. Empiricism has become the general principle to explain the purpose and rationale of therapy (Tong, 2010). The conundrum of east meets west - let's first look into the theory and thinking of the two perspectives.

2.1 The Western perspective

During the last two centuries, western medicine has developed and been practiced both generally and officially in those industrial nations that are collectively known as 'the West'. The modernization of medicine begun with the taxonomy and classification by grouping of signs and symptoms into disease entities (Bliss, 2011). The anatomic concept has formed the basis of disease identification, explaining and visualizing the cause of illness in the patient's internal anatomical organs (Duffin, 2010). Later on, disease and environment were bonded upon the discovery of small living organisms, i.e. microorganisms like bacteria and fungi, using microscope (Duffin, 2010). Thus, illnesses are diagnosed based on something so called the "demonstrable pathology". For cures, chemical drugs and surgery are the main therapeutic lines used to remove specifically the notable causes of the illness (e.g. antibiotics killing pathogenic bacteria, tumor removal in malignant diseases) or at least alleviation of symptoms and distress (Lock, 1997). In simple words, western medicine has a single-minded, materialistic approach that, basically, reduces all bodily function and dysfunction to material causes, mechanical mechanisms and structural flaws that can be thought of and studied in isolation from those who suffer from them – the so called 'science', which relies on objective, demonstrable, measurable, and self-evident observations. Western practitioners, at least many of them, are in fact treating the diseases rather than the patients. Empirical beliefs and tried remedies often persist beyond the actual needs of the patients and consequently affect quality-of-life, for example life-term hormone supplementation (with possible side-effects) is needed after the surgical removal of thyroid. Scientific medicine rejects all concepts of 'vitalism', the belief on immaterial spiritual or vital forces to explain natural phenomena (Lock, 1997). It has no place for 'life forces' or vital principles distinct from physical and chemical processes, and thus differs from the Eastern medical systems, particularly TCM.

2.2 The Eastern perspective

Traditional Chinese Medicine is originated from the culture and lives of the ancient orient, who considered life and death as the meaning of life forces. The underlying philosophy was established based on methods non-differentiable from the western one, namely objective observation, clinical practice, comparison, categorization, production, analysis, integration, and advancement. In other words, TCM is a subject of science specialty. The main difference between Chinese medicine and other medicine lies on "The sages in ancient times who knew the *Dao* (the tenets for cultivating health) who followed the rules of *yin* and *yang* and adjusted *Shushu* (the way to cultivate health)". According to the earliest text of Chinese medicine (206 BC-220 AD) *Huangdi neijing* (Yellow Emperor's Inner Canon), the doctrine of *Dao* is drawn from speculations of the two central theories, the creation of the universe (cosmology) and from direct observation of the natural world (Beinfield & Korngold, 2003). It postulated that all states of being, characteristics and physical phenomena could be categorized as either Yang, which was formless and existed conceptually in an association with heaven, light, heat and masculinity, or Yin, which corresponded to earth, darkness, cold and femininity. The principals of yin-yang suggest that each of these opposites produce the other, however, these verses draw lines of correspondence or association between sets of opposing states (Kaptchuk, 2000; van Wijk et al., 2010). The production of yin from yang and yang from yin occurs cyclically and constantly, so that no one principle continually dominates the other or determines the other (Mann, 2001; Unschuld, 2003). The *Tai Chi* (infinite void) symbol of yin yang (Figure 1) is emblematic of the continual change and renewal (Kaptchuk, 2000). Chinese people believe what the existence of human being is an organic whole which is integrated with the external environment. This idea is known as holism, dispute from the demonstrable anatomy in western medicine, concerning the functional rather than the physical body (Kaptchuk, 2000). Thus, the visceral organs in Chinese anatomy are actually groups of closely related physiological functions, which composed of *jing* (body essence), *qi* (energy), *shen* (spirit) - collectively known as the *San Bao* or 'three gems' and allowed the transportation of qi within the meridians for health maintenance (Kaptchuk, 2000; Unschuld, 2003). The essential qi of the five viscera, further divided into *Zang* (yin organs) and *Fu* (yang organs) are supplied by five corresponding tastes of foods, of each has its corresponding phase (known as five phases theory) (Table 1). The ingestion and storage of the five tastes nourish the five kinds of *qi* (*visceral qi*), however, the harmony of qi is essential for the production of jing and shen in the healthy body (Unschuld, 2003). The concept of five tastes of medicinal foods, derived from the long history of living and clinical experiences, has the direct linkage to the basic theories of yin-yang, five phases, viscera, meridian and collateral, in order to explain the cause of disease and therapeutic principle in TCM. Therefore, medicinal foods including large entities of herbs are commonly used for life nurturing and healing.

Disease diagnose in TCM is based on the pattern identification and syndrome differentiation. Rooting from the doctrine of yin and yang, the 'eight principles' were developed as the guiding principle to categorize illnesses into yin and yang, exterior and interior, cold and heat, deficiency and excess (Shiang & Li, 1971; Unschuld, 2003). Signs and symptoms of illness were comprehensively analyzed through the four examinations known as inspection, listening and smelling, inquiry, and palpation. With then, Chinese practitioners can determine the cause, nature and location of the pathogens, consider the disharmony between the disease and healthy qi, and conclude to identify the pattern of a certain nature following the rules of the eight principles. Upon identifying the disease pattern, a treatment plan, normally using herbal medicine and/or acupuncture, can be determined to rebalance the patient's inner yin and yang energy, and thus treating the root of the illness. Herbs may be prescribed individually or as part of a formula, of which formula are polyherbals including four typical components (Table 2) that promote the effective use of herbs (Covington, 2001). The ultimate aim of Chinese healing is to preserve or restore the healthy equilibrium of the body to adapt to the living environment. Chinese also believed that changing states either of body or of mind could affect the healthy balanced state, and therefore, an excessive emotion might cause a bodily illness or vice versa. Asian healers and practitioners treat consciousness as an organ of the body rather than a separate entity residing within it.

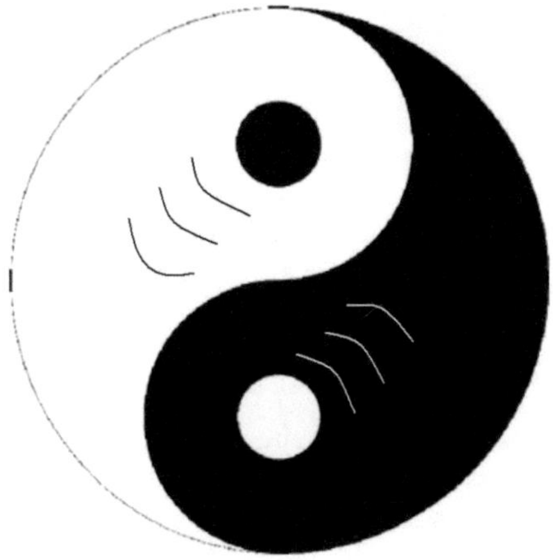

Fig. 1. Taijitu in motion. The forces of yin and yang are expressed in dark and white, respectively, are interdependent and interact constantly to form the integrated whole. Furthermore, the small circles of opposite shading illustrate that within the yin there is yang and vice versa, whereas the dynamic curve dividing them indicates that yin and yang are continuously merging, overall representing yin and yang's ability to create, control, and transform into each other (Yuen & Gohel, 2008).

Phases (Elements)	Tastes	Zang (yin organs)	Fu (yang organs)	Tissues	Sense organs
Wood	Sour	Liver	Gallbladder	Tendons	Eye
Fire	Bitter	Heart	Small intestine	Vessels	Tongue
Earth	Sweet	Spleen	Stomach	Muscles	Mouth
Metal	Pungent	Lung	Large intestine	Skin/hair	Nose
Water	Salty	Kidney	Bladder	Bones	Ear

Table 1. The Five phase theory. The five elements control the corresponding tissues and organs that are also correspondent with the five tastes of foods.

Components	Purpose
Principal	Use to treat the principal pattern of disease.
Associate	Use to assist the principal ingredient(s) in treating the major syndrome or serve as the main ingredient against a coexisting syndrome.
Adjutant	To enhance the effect of the principal ingredient, moderate or eliminate the toxicity of the principal or associate ingredients, or can have the opposite function of the principal ingredient(s) to produce supplementing effects.
Guide	To focus the actions of the formula on a certain meridian or area of the body or harmolize and integrate the actions of the other ingredients.

Table 2. The composition of typical herbal formula in TCM. Each component may consist of more than one herb, and a formula may not consist of all four components.

3. Junctions between the two systems of medicine – The dynamic equilibrium of the body as yin-yang interplay

While the maintenance of health and the treatment of disease are expressed in very different terms in the two cultures, the physiological processes and pathological changes that define human health are common in many aspects on each side of the East-West divide. Yet despite how difficult it is being illustrated in the language of modern medicine, the yin-yang theory governs the underlying principle of occurrence and development of diseases in TCM (Kaptchuk, 2000). An algorithmic scoring system is now available to group human subjects quantitatively into broad categories of yin and yang, in accordance to their health conditions expressed in the western terms (Langevin et al., 2004). More recently, a mathematical reasoning model using steady multilateral systems was successfully applied to guide the treatment of diseases based on the "*yin yang wu xing*" principle of TCM (Zhang, 2011). This is an important milestone, in East meets West, expressing the yin and yang entities numerically, which permits the mathematical manipulation and provides quantitative parameters for statistical analysis, which eventually make acceptance of TCM diagnosis to modern medicine with a standardized method and scientific validity. Maintaining yin and yang in harmony is akin to attaining the homeostatic state in modern medicine. However, the logic of yin-yang is often misunderstood as a matter of two complementary opposite qualities only, whereas the compensatory, synthetic and dialectical natures are entirely omitted. On the other hand, researchers have attempted to align the yin-yang concept with different physiological mechanisms of the body.

3.1 Oxidation and antioxidation

Reactive oxygen species (ROS), by-products of mitochondrial combustion, are generated alongside the adenosine triphosphate (ATP) during the process of oxidative phosphorylation in metabolism (Halliwell, 2009). ROS are known to be detrimental leading to oxidative damage of DNA, protein and lipid molecules, while the accumulation of such damage has been regarded as an endogenous cause of ageing as well as age-related disorders inclduing cancers (Finkel & Holbrook, 2000; Halliwell, 2009). Fortunately, our body has an antioxidant defense mechanism, in forms of endogenous enzymatic and dietary non-enzymatic molecules, to counteract the harmful activities of ROS *in vivo* (Gutteridge, 1994). Therefore, the balance between antioxidation and oxidation play an important role in health maintenance. The analogy of yin-yang balance with that of antioxidation-oxidation has been suggested by different researchers (Ko et al., 2004, 2006; Ou et al., 2003; Szeto & Benzie, 2006), who come up with a general agreement that yin corresponds to antioxidation and Yang corresponds to oxidation involved in energy metabolism. Researchers (Ou et al., 2003) proposed that, inside the body, yang represents the driving force for energy-generating oxidation processes, while yin exhibits the protective role of antioxidation. Pharmacologically, the 'yang-invigorating' herbs were found to promote ATP-generation capacity through stimulating the mitochondrial electron transport, in rat heart homogenates *ex vivo* (Ko et al., 2004, 2006) and cultured cardiomyocytes *in vitro* (Wong et al., 2011). In TCM, the heart plays a pivotal role in fueling the vital activities in all organs, hence promoting the body function in terms of 'Qi' (Kaptchuk, 2000;Ko et al., 2004). Experimental analysis has demonstrated that yang-herbs processed protective effects on DNA *ex vivo* from hydrogen peroxide challenge (Szeto & Benzie, 2006). Authors of the work then argued that the antioxidation-oxidation relationships are not necessarily obeyed to the opposite nature of yin and yang. In fact, apart from the antioxidant activities derived from the phytochemicals, ROS such as superoxides and nitric oxide, are also present in herbs (Achike & Kwan, 2003; Lin et al., 1995). In general, yin-herbs were found to have higher free-radical scavenging activities than yang-herbs (Ko & Leung, 2007; Szeto & Benzie, 2006). Herbs by themselves are not explicitly absolutely antioxidant or oxidant in nature. Antioxidant and ATP generation (oxidation) actions could be coexisted amongst yang-promoting herbs, while the ATP generation capacity was absence in yin-tonic herbs (Ko et al., 2004). Therefore, it is not surprising that yang-invigorating herbs are able to enhance the antioxidant status of human red cells after ingestion (Mak et al., 2004) and simultaneously protect DNA (Szeto & Benzie, 2006), further supporting the important role of the yin nature of yang-herbs being played in safeguarding the ATP generation process with ROS production. According to the Chinese Materia Medica (Bensky et al., 2004), some single herbs such as *Ganoderma lucidum* (Lingzi), are neutral in nature as they presumably contain complex chemical constituents and so have both yin and yang properties. The differential biochemical analysis of Lingzhi indicated that the water-soluble extract containing higher antioxidant capacities than its ethanol counterpart, were designated as the yin and yang, respectively (Yuen & Gohel, 2008). Functionally, in this study, the former (yin) reduced the carcinogen-induced oxidative DNA damage, while the later (yang) induced the formation of ROS and oxidative DNA damage resulting in apoptosis, in a pre-cancerous cell line (Yuen & Gohel, 2008). The authors anticipated that, even in a single herb, phytochemicals are interacting as yin and yang interplay that may be responsible for its multiple functions-bearing characteristic.

3.2 Immune balance

Given that many antioxidants are immunomodulating. The herb Cordyceps (*Cordyceps sinensis)* enhanced the concanavalin A (Con A)-stimulated splenocytes proliferation and the myocardial ATP generation capacity, which were disseminated in terms of TCM as 'yin-nourishment' and 'yang-invigoration', respectively (Siu et al., 2004). This is consistent with the notion of Ko and Leung (Ko & Leung, 2007) that yin-herbs, in addition to their significant antioxidant capcities, also possess immunomodulatory properties, including mitogen-stimulated proliferation of mouse splenocytes, cytokines secretion, leukocyte migration, and antibody production. In TCM, "Fu-zheng" therapy is one of the basic principles, literally equivalent to the promotion of the natural host defense mechanism, following the immunological balance of yin and yang (Macek, 1984). The Chinese believe that the herbal regimens may not only stimulate host defense but also enhance the vitality of their patients, hence the immune system resembles the yin aspect to support such vital yang aspects as the heart force and energy generation (Ko & Leung, 2007). The immunological yin-yang is considered as the cross-talk between the innate and adaptive arms of the immune system: the former serving to initiate a response of the latter, and the latter amplifying the former, defending the body from pathogens but sometimes exaggerating it certain immunological disorders (Lafaille & Mathis, 2002). The intricate immune network is composed of uncountable pairs of cells with activating/suppressive activities and stimulatory/inhibitory molecules, analogous regulatory interplay (Lafaille & Mathis, 2002; Macek, 1984). No doubt, T-suppressor and T-helper cells are in opposition but are totally interdependent, and an imbalance of either cell population can result in disease (Macek, 1984). Proinflammatory and antiinflammatory processes formed another interplaying pair that must be balanced to maintain health (Mann, 2001; Mills & Bhatt, 2004; Zhang, 2007). The interplay of interferon-gamma (IFN-γ) with other immune components was crucial to the development of autoimmune disease (Zhang, 2007). Hence, the inside views of yin-yang in the system denoted inflammatory process as yang, while its regulation as yin. Once an inflammatory process (yang) is initiated, IFN-γ is produced to promote inflammation until reaching the peak level, the inflammation then intensifies and compresses its opposite to activate a regulatory process (yin), and finally resulting in the reduction of inflammation. The differential immunological study of Lingzhi demonstrated that the ethanol extract in yang nature induced the secretion of proinflammatory interleukins (IL)-2, -6, and -8 via nuclear factor-kappaB (NF-κB) pathway in the apoptotic pre-cancer cells, but such effects were not exhibited by the water extract in yin nature (Yuen et al., 2011). This is explained that "yang initiates the expression of yin. Yang controls the origination and enjoys the completion of a process while yin follows the effects produced by yang and completes the work of yang" (Chan, 1969). In viral myocarditis, interleukin 6 (IL-6) played the paradoxical roles in promoting and suppressing the inflammation, to avert deleterious viral effects and to increase tissue destruction, respectively (Mann, 2001). Given that C-reactive protein (CRP) plays critical roles in atherosclerosis central to plaque progression and plaque rupture, the interplay of proinflammation and antiinflammation, that affecting the CRP levels is considered as a determinant for vascular health or illness (Mills & Bhatt, 2004). Such arterial inflammatory process is closely regulated by the local T-helper 1 (Th1)-type and Th2-type responses, with the principal inducers IL-12 and IL-10, respectively (Yang et al., 2010). Previous researches have demonstrated the presence of both IL-12 and IL-10 in atherosclerotic lesions, and the increase of IL-10 secretion led to the reduction in lesion size, that suggesting IL-10 is a counterbalancing factor that exerts its effect on Th1-Th2 cooperation by downregulating IL-12 and IL-18 production and inhibiting the Th1-based immune response, altogether to fully illustrate the yin-yang picture (Yang et al., 2010). The Th1/Th2 imbalance, an expression of yin-yang disharmony, causing the dichotomy between the humoral and cellular arms is related to pathological changes, such that cancerous tumor with Th2 dominant (Witz, 2008) and spontaneous abortion when Th1 reaction is in excess during pregnancy (Wilczynski, 2005).

3.3 Hormonal harmony

The biochemical meaning of yin-yang is extendable to the interaction between the immune system and other systems, involving a variety of hormones as key mediators. The endocrine system is known as one of the regulatory machineries to the immune response. Established literatures have documented that high levels of stress elevate the concentration of hormones such as glucocorticoids (cortisol or corticosterone) and catecholamines (epinephrine or norepinephrine), which exert immunosuppressive activities by binding the receptors on lymphocytes and impairing the immune defense, so that overall health will be altered (Kaye & Lightman, 2005; Vegiopoulos & Herzig, 2007). Consequently, certain soluble factors of the immune system, i.e. cytokines and interleukins, are altered to act on the brain and variety of endocrine pathways, to trigger feedback reactions in the Hypothalamic-pituitary-adrenal (HPA) axis (Dunn, 1996). The bidirectional interaction between the immune and the endocrine system is also reflected by its influence on the reproductive system, probably via the hypothamus-gonadal axis. Gonadal hormone like estrogen involves in the development of the thymus (an important lymphoid organ for lymphocyte differentiation), while the removal of thymus can induce pathologies in ovaries, testes and thyroid endocrine tissues, hence changes in one system will likely influence the other (Ahmed, 2000). The gender differences in brain development and immune response, possibly also in other non-gonadal organs, were explained as the compensatory yin-yang effects between sex chromosome and sex hormone status (Palaszynski et al., 2005). Furthermore, the functions of endocrine glands are explicitly controlled by the antagonizing sympathetic and parasympathetic activities of the autonomic nervous system in response to stimulation. In a recent human psychophysiological study, the decreases of parasympathetic and sympathetic activity were associated with the deficiency of yin and yang, respectively (Taitano et al., 2003). This is exemplified by the cardiac autonomic control that the activation of parasympathetic and sympathetic inputs to the heart in tandem results in greater cardiac output, demonstrating the synergistic and complementary properties of yin-yang interplay (Paton et al., 2005). In patients with hypothyroidism they are classified as having a deficiency of yang in terms of the TCM diagnosis, and the usage of yang tonifying herbs was shown to help in alleviating the symptoms (Kuang et al., 1988). As previously mentioned, yang-herbs actively promote the ATP-generation capacity and cardiac activity, and in hypothyroid rabbits, serum levels of thyroxine (T_3) and triiodothyronine (T_4) were elevated by intake of selected yang tonifying herbs, following the enhancement of myocardial β-adrenoceptor density and affinity (Min et al., 1998).

4. Feasibility of validating Eastern medicine by Western methods

The theory of yin-yang is explanatory to the biochemical activities of various biological phenomena, which supporting the feasibility of using western methods for TCM validation.

Regardless of what treatment principle behind, science and technology provide objective, accurate and reliable platforms for examining the effectiveness and efficacy of traditional therapeutic modalities. Herbal remedies are often marketed as dietary supplements, where they are not required to meet with the stringent clinical testing of pharmaceuticals, even though their usage may be for the same purpose, i.e. treatment of disease. Most herbal-derived medicines are complex mixtures of largely unknown chemical composition. They may be decoctions, infusions or extracts of one or many herbs, the quality and identity of which may vary widely, whose active ingredients are not well defined and whose molecular action is unknown. In light of the increasing globalization of herbal medicines, the WHO-leading authorities have put plenty of efforts to setup guidelines and regulations for the herbal identification and quality control (World Health Organization Special Programme for Research and Training in Tropical Diseases (WHO-TDR, 2005).

4.1 Authentication of herbal identity and quality control of ingredients

In TCM, herbs are traditionally authenticated by smell, taste and appearance that are totally dependent on the prescriber's experience. Even a famous herb such as ginseng, cases of misidentification have caused adverse reactions after use have been reported (Yap et al., 2008). Right herb possessing the right properties must be given to a right person for the right purpose. Therefore, reliable authentication becomes an important issue to safeguard the efficacy and safety about the usage of herbal medicine. Fingerprint analysis is accepted as the standard methodology for the assessment of natural products (WHO-TDR, 2005). Each herbal species has its unique fringerprint chemical profile containing an array of individual compounds separated and developed by chromatographic technique coupled with suitable detection methods (Schaneberg et al., 2003; Tistaert et al., 2011). There are several chromatographic techniques that can be used for the fingerprint profiling, including *Thin layer chromatography* for fast screening of samples, *High performance liquid chromatography* (*HPLC*) for high resolution, selectivity and sensitivity, *Ultra-High performance liquid chromatography* for superior sensitivity and resolution to HPLC, *Hydrophilic interaction chromatography* for retention and separation of hydrophilic compounds, and *Gas chromatography* for characterization and identification for volatile compounds (Tistaert et al., 2011). Additionally, there are some pattern recognition methods (some sort of statistical methods), which enable the visualization and further exploratory data analysis on information that is included in the chromatographic profile, are available for addressing the difficult differentiation of some closely related species (Lu et al., 2005; Tistaert et al., 2011; Zhao et al., 2009). The quality of herbs may vary due to the cultivation conditions, breeds and places of origin, for examples, liquid chromatographic coupled with multistage mass spectrometry (HPLC-MS) technique has revealed there to be non-stable and inconsistence of chemical constituents amongst different batches of Lingzhi samples (Chen et al., 2008a). In this regard, the research team (Chen et al., 2008b) has demonstrated the feasibility of employing multiple statistical analyses of HPLC fingerprints of Lingzhi to discriminate samples in accordance of origin of cultivation (Chen et al., 2008b). For fingerprinting the complicated decoctions, multi-herb botanical drug products, multiple chromatographic fingerprinting was suggested, in order to capture the complete picture of chemical profile (Fan et al., 2006). By employing such chromatographic technology, herbs of different species that share the identical bioactive ingredients, or at least a particular chemical fraction, can be merged and classified to facilitate the standardization of herbal products (Xie et al., 2010). In the past decade, the rapid growth of molecular techniques has also benefited the herbal authentication. Numerous polymerase chain reaction (PCR)-based and sequencing methods using specific probes have shown to be applicable for validating the herbal identities (Chang et al., 2009; Herrero et al., 2010; Law et al., 2011). Particularly, random amplified polymorphic DNA (RAPD) profiling, a newly developed cost-effective PCR-based technique, has extensively used to differentiate large number of medicinal species from their close relatives or adulterants (Khan et al., 2011; Kiran et al., 2010). Not surprising, encouraging outcomes support the development of DNA barcoding technique, which enables the fast screen of botanical identities just like we checking out at the supermarkets (Song et al., 2009).

4.2 Extraction and fractionation of herbs – recovery of the active ingredients

For pharmaceutical preparation, the technique of HPLC-MS is still promising the characterization and isolation of chemical constituents from medicinal plants (Han et al., 2009; Yang et al., 2009). In addition to polysaccharides and flavanoids which have been commonly identified in many herbs, phytochemical analyses revealed 'marker components' that could be used for quality evaluation and standardization of specific herbs, for example, triterpenoids and β-glucans in *Ganoderma* (Wang et al., 2006), cordycepin and ergosterol in Cordyceps (Paterson, 2008), ginsenoside in *Ginseng* (Chen et al., 2009). The complexity of TCM samples, particularly multiple active constituents and low concentration levels of active compounds, poses a big challenge to analytical chemistry for active ingredients recovery (Tang et al., 2009). To solve this problem, researchers have devoted to develop and optimize a wide variety of sample preparation methods for herbs, such as shaking, ultrasonic, soxhlet, boiling, distilling, high/ultrahigh pressure, heat reflux, supercritical-fluid (CO_2), microwave, etc (Chen et al., 2009, 2007; Shouqin et al., 2004). Usually, traditional techniques for extraction are time consuming and with low efficiency in recovery and purification of active ingredients. The technique of high pressure extraction coupled with selective solvents have been suggested in providing cost-effective and time-saving methods for obtaining single components of high purity (Shouqin et al., 2004). With the ultrahigh pressure extraction, not only the yielding of ginsenosides extracted from ginseng roots was increased, but the extract was shown to have enhanced free radical scavenging activity, when compared with other extraction methods (Chen et al, 2009). However, the extraction conditions and solvents being used need to be carefully decided based on the chemical characteristics and physical natures of the target molecules. For Lingzhi as an example it was found that the fraction of polysaccharides and triterpenes, each contains more than 100 molecules, can be simply extracted by water and ethanol (Yuen & Gohel, 2005). The most abundant polysaccharides type found in Lingzhi was β-glucans (Askin et al., 2010; Yuen & Gohel, 2005). The problems with β-glucan are low extraction yielding and poor purity, although various extraction methods using organic solvents have been applied (Askin et al, 2010). Recently, Askin and co-workers (Askin et al., 2010) have used a hydrothermal extraction method with 'subcritical water', conditioned at 473 K temperature at 10 MPa atmospheric pressure, and successfully obtained the maximum total amount (57.4% yielding) of β-glucans from Lingzhi. Besides, extraction of total triterpenes with organic solvents and water have long been practiced, however, isolation of the acidic triterpenes, mainly highly oxygenated triterpenoids which responsible for the bitter taste of the Lingzhi, from the total triterpenes fraction can be achieved with 95% aqueous ethanol under reflux and evaporation under reduced pressure, followed by chloroform extraction under acidic condition (Huie & Di, 2004). Silica gel column chromatography has also been described as an additional purification procedure for such acidic triterpenes (Huie & Di, 2004). To extract the specific triterpenoid saponins from another *Ganoderma species*, microwave-assisted extraction was demonstrated to be superior over other techniques, in terms of high yielding and short extraction time (Chen et al., 2007). Because of its gentle extraction conditions of supercritical CO_2 used with relatively low viscosity, high diffusivity, low extraction temperature, rapid and minimal use of halogenated solvents, supercritical fluid extraction (SFE) is a widely accepted extraction technique, however, its application is largely limited by the non-polar nature of CO_2 (Chen et al., 2011; Tang et al., 2009). Nonetheless, the dissolving and penetrating powers of SFE were employed to aid the breaking of extremely hard and resilient sporoderm of *Ganoderma lucidum* spores, in order to obtain the spore components and easy the subsequent extraction (Fu et al., 2009; Liu et al., 2002). Furthermore, activity-guided fractionation of herbal remedies has remained a hot field in the separation science. Constituents sharing similar chemical structures or physical properties can be isolated together into fraction during the chromatographic separation. Hence, the time-specific fraction can be tested for certain desired bioactivities such as anti-tumor (Li et al. 2010), antimicrobial (Kitzberger et al., 2007), antioxidant (Chen et al., 2009; Kitzberger et al., 2007), and many other activities by using any *in vitro* platforms and animal models. Results will then guide to identify the potent fractions and the effective bioactive ingredients. For example, in the study of Wang et al (Wang et al., 2005), four fractions namely R, F1, F2 and F3 were produced by the SFE of Cordyceps sinensis with CO_2, followed by bioassays that indicated that fraction R was the most active fraction to scavenge free radicals and induce apoptosis on human colorectal and liver cancer cells, while the remaining fractions exhibited only low to moderate levels of scavenging activities but no antitumor effect.

4.3 *In vitro* experiments and animal studies

In translational research, tissue culture and animal models serve as convenient tools for drug screening and mechanistic investigation. As presented in a scientific review (Yuen & Gohel, 2005), huge numbers of cancer cell lines and tumor-bearing animal models were used to address the antitumor properties of Lingzhi, its extracts or isolated compounds. By employing a well-established tumorigenic transformation model of uroepthelial cells, a series of chemopreventive properties were demonstrated by the ethanol extract of *Ganoderma lucidum* (GLe) to inhibit the carcinogen-induced tumorigenesis of bladder cancer through the inhibition of growth and cell migration (Lu et al., 2004; Yuen et al., 2008), telomerase-associated apoptosis (Yuen et al., 2008), oxidative DNA damage (Yuen & Gohel, 2008), and stimulation of selected cytokines and neutrophilic migration (Yuen et al., 2011). Meanwhile, an *ex vivo* orthotopic organ culture model is being used to establish the synergistic effects between GLe and other conventional chemotherapeutics. Anticancer effects of Lingzhi were also supported by the induction of cell cycle arrest and apoptosis amongst human and rodent tumor cells of various origins through signaling pathway controlling cell death, inhibition of cell adhesion, invasion and migration in foci formation assays, and stimulation of anti-angiogenesis, anti-metastasis and tumor regression in tumor-bearing rat/mice models (Wachtel-Galor et al., 2011). To delineate the cause-and-effect mechanism of particular genes and/or proteins, sometimes techniques of cell transfection and transgenic mice will be applied to create overexpression or suppression of certain gene(s), and used to test the herbal products. These experimental models are excellent to study the mechanism of action under the well-controlled microenvironments; however, they also limit on a focused pathway, ignoring the holism, and might not reflect the actual response inside the human bodies, especially issues about bioavailability and drug distribution. On the other hand, animal studies allow the determination of therapeutic and toxic dosage ranges, which are crucial before human trials can be admitted. Furthermore, animal models enable the whole body physiological examination and individual organ tissues can be isolated to study the drug effects as well as toxicities. Some pathological conditions, for example diabetic rats can be induced by intraperitoneal injection of streptozotocin, and was used to establish the mechanism underlying the antioxidant enzyme activity of Lingzhi polysaccharides to diminish pancreatic damage through the bax/bcl-2 modulation (Yang et al., 2010). In another experiment conducted by Tam et al. (Tam et al., 2011), a two-herb formula (with Radix Astragali and Radix Rehmanniae) was designed according to the classical theory of Chinese medicine, that was shown to elicit the actions of fibroblast proliferation, angiogenesis and anti-inflammation which favored the wound healing, in a chemically induced diabetic foot ulcer rat model. Nowadays, advanced molecular technology such as DNA micro-arrays also allowed the rapid high-throughput gene expression screening to conclude the outcomes of herbal remedies when tested on animal and cell culture studies (Hudson & Altamirano, 2006).

4.4 Safety and efficacy issues

For anything being applied inside the human body, regardless it is for treatment or health maintenance purpose, safety and efficacy are the first concerned. Despite the general public perceived herbal products as low risk because of the long history of usage, the current body of scientific evidence is seldom conveyed. In fact, herbal medicines may carry potential harms due to contamination, adulteration, misidentification, as well as unknown interactions with other herbal products, pharmaceutical drugs or even diets (Jordan et al., 2010). Unlike conventional drugs which are single chemical compounds, the complex composition of whole herbs or their extracts contain a myriad of phytochemicals, making the toxicological evaluation difficult, especially the therapeutic effects are also possibly based on the interaction of these different components could hardly be separated (Jordan et al., 2010). In terms of quality control, it is suggested that markers used for Chinese herbal medicine should be strongly correlated with their safety and efficacy, and thus 'marker components' of specific herb should be the 'effective components' which consisting both the active (bioactivity for therapeutic effects) and relative (no specific action but affect the therapeutic effects of active components) components, rather than just the most abundant chemical constituents mentioned in 4.1 as convenient (Li et al., 2011). One more challenge is that, the *in vivo* target sites for herbal remedies are usually unknown because of their complicated natures, and thus antidotes are unavailable in case of adverse reactions occur (Li et al., 2011). Therefore, scientifically, not so much can be done regarding the safety and efficacy concerns of traditional herbal medicine, but only taking the passive role in waiting for the case reports of adverse reaction are inadequate, demanding proper designed randomized controlled trails to conduct.

4.5 *In vivo* human trails – randomized controlled trails

Human controlled trails that use randomized allocation are the gold standard to restrain bias and confounding in trials evaluating pharmaceuticals. So as for TCM, randomized controlled trials (RCTs) of herbal medicine were not uncommon, at least in China. During 1999-2004, a total of 7,422 RCTs has been identified from 13 randomly selected journals published in Mainland China, and the number is kept increasing (Wang et al., 2007). However, by reviewing these RCTs, outcomes were discouraging, not because of the treatment outcomes themselves, but the poor qualities as assessed by using international standards, i.e. the Jadad score scare and the Consolidated Standards of Reporting Trials (CONSORT) checklist, more than 90% of these studies were poorly designed or reported with poor scientific rigor (Gagnier et al., 2011; Wang et al., 2007; Wolsko et al., 2005; Zhong et al., 2010). Some essential RCT components, such as sample size calculation, randomization sequence, allocation concealment, implementation of the random-allocation sequence, analysis of intention-to-treat (ITT), lacking syndrome differentiation of TCM, and the use of placebo was not justified and was ethically contradictory, were not sufficiently described in the methodologies of the studies (Gagnier et al., 2011; Wang et al., 2007; Zhong et al., 2010). Even limiting to the RCTs published in English, many investigators have failed to provide proper characterization to the study herbs such as identity, purity, quality, strength, and composition in their articles (Wolsko et al., 2005). A systemic review has conducted to assess 49 trials which included 3992 cancer patients who have given Chinese medicinal herbs concurrently with conventional cancer treatments (Molassiotis et al., 2009). Majority of the studies has shown positive herbal drug effects in terms of treatment toxicity, quality of life, survival, and tumor regression, however, no clinical recommendation could be concluded because of the poor intervention qualities (Molassiotis et al., 2009). Up to 2005, there were at least 127 Chinese RCTs identified of studying a single compound β-Elemene isolated from the Chinese herb *Curcuma wenyujin*, in order to characterize its efficacy on antitumorgenecity (Peng et al., 2006). Since the middle 1990s, although this chemical component has already been widely used in clinical practice for cancer treatment in China, there were less than two percents of trials performed with the double-blinding in the subject allocation, just four percents have carried out statistical analysis on baseline data, and none have used the intention-to-treat analysis (Peng et al., 2006). On the other hand, an international research team has conducted a series of well-designed RCTs (at phase I/II) on advanced cancer patients, which supported the efficacy of use of Lingzhi as an adjunct cancer therapy where it enhanced the conventional treatment outcome, by improving the immune response, increasing quality of life and survival, and decreasing side effects from conventional treatments (Gao et al., 2002, 2003a, 2003b, 2005). More recently, a perspective, multiple-center, randomized, double-blind, placebo-controlled trial was conducted to study the efficacy and safety of Antiwei granule (with ma huang and Baimaogen as the principals) on infected adults of influenza (Wang et al., 2010). The report provided sufficient evidence to recommend antiwei as an effective influenza treatment based on the positive outcomes, of which increased the patients' recovery by 17% and reduced the severity of illness by 50%. The study was considered as perfectly designed since there was a well characterized herbal prescription, the use of visually indistinguishable starch coupled with a bitter agent as a placebo, fulfillment of all items listed in the CONSORT checklist as an objective outcome measurement using median symptom scores was used, and objective side effects monitored using ECG and vital signs.

5. The spectrum of East meets West: The transition from traditional cure to conventional drug really necessary?

Many folk remedies have maintained their reputation for effectiveness, to be handed on from generation to generation, on the word of the village elders. Faith in the efficacy of a treatment plays a large part in feeling better. Confidence in a remedy is reinforced by word-of-mouth repetition, when everyone tells everyone else in everyday conversation that they simply know it works. Their over-the-counter availability and reputation as natural, 'safe' and effective alternatives to drug treatment makes herbal products attractive to consumers. The great increase in consumption of herbal products is a cause for concern, however, because, in addition to their efficacy, the issues of toxicity and of herb-herb and herb-drug interactions that might be additive, synergistic or antagonistic will require comprehensive scientific study. Scientists all over the world consider herbal species as a rich source for new chemical entities and used them successfully to isolate compounds, such as ephedrine, digoxin, morphine, taxol, atropine and vinblastine, are nowadays conventional drugs in allopathic medicine (Tistaert et al., 2011). To develop a new drug from herbs, the WHO has setup guidelines related on chemical drug development and traditional experience of using herbs. The paradigm of chemical drug development: drug discovery, drug design, pre-clinical studies, and clinical studies. A chemical drug always requires 10-12 years for optimization and evaluation to allow in prescription. Herbal medicine starts with human use and finally become an isolated purified form of chemical(s) for approval to be marketed. Considering the unique features of herbal products are multiple component mixtures and that substantial prior human use precedes their formal investigation, the WHO has issued a set of clear and concise recommendations for preparing well supported clinical trials to evaluate the actual benefits and risks of traditional herbal products being used for clinical purpose (WHO-TDR, 2005). Such operational guidance was built according to the principles of modern clinical sciences with four sets of issues: chemical manufacturing-control (CMC) issues, non-clinical issues, clinical issues, and ethical issues, and considerations have to translate into terms appropriate to support the justification for a clinical trial of a traditional herbal remedy, as summarized in a flowchart (Figure 2). Looking into the recommendations, the WHO has acted supportively in preserving the traditions of herbal medicine, i.e. candidate herbal substance or product should be prepared in accordance with the traditionally-used formulation, where purified chemicals are not required WHO-TDR, 2005).

6. The current positioning: Right or wrong direction of research in traditional Chinese herbal medicine

In western terms, the health benefits of most herbal remedies remain unsubstantiated by scientific evidence in well-designed human studies, and this limits their acceptance by western trained health professionals. Nonetheless, herbal medicine offers an enormous potential for health promotion and treatment of disease, and several commonly used western drugs have their origins in herbal medicine. On the other hands, the traditional essence of TCM is reconsidered by other investigators, who have used western criteria to validate scientifically the traditional theories and their usage. Based on what are the personal beliefs, the applications of herbal medicine are splitting into either one of the two paths: transition into pure chemicals or holding the traditional way of practice. Right or wrong is always up your decision, or actually there is no answer. However, whatever it is decided will lead the future research direction of herbal medicine very differently.

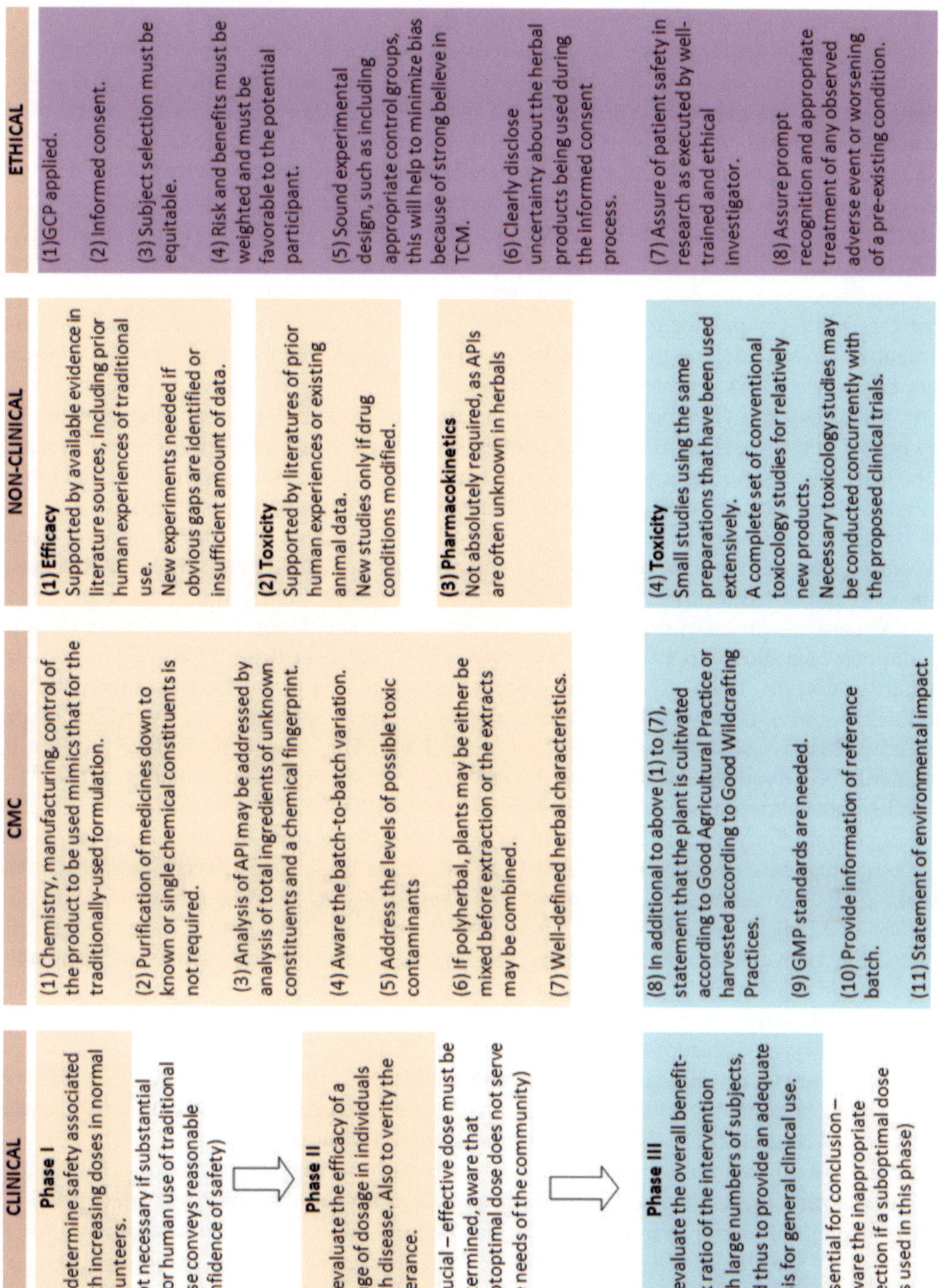
CLINICAL
Phase I
To determine safety associated with increasing doses in normal volunteers.
(not necessary if substantial prior human use of traditional dose conveys reasonable confidence of safety)
Phase II
To evaluate the efficacy of a range of dosage in individuals with disease. Also to verity the tolerance.
(Crucial – effective dose must be determined, aware that subtoptimal dose does not serve the needs of the community)
Phase III
To evaluate the overall benefit-risk ratio of the intervention with large numbers of subjects, and thus to provide an adequate basis for general clinical use.
(Essential for conclusion – beware the inappropriate rejection if a suboptimal dose was used in this phase)
CMC
(1) Chemistry, manufacturing, control of the product to be used mimics that for the traditionally-used formulation.
(2) Purification of medicines down to known or single chemical constituents is not required.
(3) Analysis of API may be addressed by analysis of total ingredients of unknown constituents and a chemical fingerprint.
(4) Aware the batch-to-batch variation.
(5) Address the levels of possible toxic contaminants
(6) If polyherbal, plants may be either be mixed before extraction or the extracts may be combined.
(7) Well-defined herbal characteristics.
(8) In additional to above (1) to (7), statement that the plant is cultivated according to Good Agricultural Practice or harvested according to Good Wildcrafting Practices.
(9) GMP standards are needed.
(10) Provide information of reference batch.
(11) Statement of environmental impact.
NON-CLINICAL
(1) Efficacy
Supported by available evidence in literature sources, including prior human experiences of traditional use.
New experiments needed if obvious gaps are identified or insufficient amount of data.
(2) Toxicity
Supported by literatures of prior human experiences or existing animal data.
New studies only if drug conditions modified.
(3) Pharmacokinetics
Not absolutely required, as APIs are often unknown in herbals
(4) Toxicity
Small studies using the same preparations that have been used extensively.
A complete set of conventional toxicology studies for relatively new products.
Necessary toxicology studies may be conducted concurrently with the proposed clinical trials.
ETHICAL
(1)GCP applied.
(2) Informed consent.
(3) Subject selection must be equitable.
(4) Risk and benefits must be weighted and must be favorable to the potential participant.
(5) Sound experimental design, such as including appropriate control groups, this will help to minimize bias because of strong believe in TCM.
(6) Clearly disclose uncertainty about the herbal products being used during the informed consent process.
(7) Assure of patient safety in research as executed by well-trained and ethical investigator.
(8) Assure prompt recognition and appropriate treatment of any observed adverse event or worsening of a pre-existing condition.

Fig. 2. Recommended information needed to support a clinical trial for an herbal medicine (WHO-TDR, 2005). CMC: chemical-manufacturing-control; API: Active pharmaceutical ingredient; GMP: Good Manufacturing Practices; GCP: Good Clinical Practice.

6.1 The transition of herbs into pure chemicals

Referring to the development of plant-derived medicines, the Western approach with clinically effective plant extracts was to ask "what is the active principle?", and then to isolate, purify, determine its structure and produce a standardized dosage form. Herbal medicine has made many contributions to commercial drug preparations manufactured today including ephedrine from ma huang (*Ephedra sinica*) (Gaddum & Kwiatkowski, 1938). Ephedra, which is being used for weight loss, antiasthmatic, or as stimulant for athletic performance, and clinical trials recognized common side effects as increased risk of psychiatric, autonomic or gastrointestinal symptoms, and heart palpitations (Schaneberg et al., 2003; Shekelle et al., 2003). Serious adverse reactions, including death, have occurred; in most cases, the people were abusingly taking two or four times the recommended dose (Samenuk et al., 2002). In this relation, one should realize the fact that definite phytopharmaceuticals are highly concentrated that no longer represent the whole herb. In many cases they are vast more effective than the whole herb, but some effects of the herb may be lost and the potential for adverse effects and herb/drug interactions may increase.

In the last 30 years, no plant compounds discovered have generated as much public interest and excitement as has taxol (paclitaxel). Pure taxol, a complex polyoxygenated diterpene, was isolated in 1969 in 0.01% yield from the bark of *Taxus brevifolia Nutt*, following a series of screening experiments for anticancer activity (Kingston, 2007). Later on, taxol was known to be extractable from other *Taxus* species of Yew trees including the Chinese yew Hong Dou Shan (*Taxus chinensis*) grows in china (Siow et al., 2005). Upon the selection of taxol as a development candidate in 1977 and the approval as anticancer drug by U.S. Food and Drug Administration in 1992, efforts were non-stopped to explore methods to enhance its production and synthesis, although the current yielding has achieved over 90% of pure paclitaxel (Khosroushahi et al., 2006; Pyo et al., 2007). The drug is nowadays the first-line treatment for advanced ovarian and breast cancer, the second-line treatment for AIDS-related Kaposi's sarcoma, and used in combination with cisplatin for treating nonsmall-cell lung carcinoma (Siow et al., 2005), however, intensive studies are still underway for its anti-cancer mechanisms (Varbiro et al., 2001) as well as its toxic side effects (Atas et al., 2006; Rabah, 2010). Nonetheless, according to the *Dongbei Yaozhi zhi* (Records of Plant Herb in Northeast China), TCM used *Hong Dou Shan* to detoxify the body and releases cough (Siow et al., 2005) Perhaps, the traditional use of *Hong Dou Shan* has long been forgotten which attract no more attention at the rear of the successful toxal (Figure 3). Of course, taxol is not the only TCM-derived anticancer drug, but many others such as homoharringtonine from *Cephalotaxus species*, camptothecin from *Camptotheca acuminate*, and vincristine from *Catharanthus roseus*, are all used for cancer chemotherapy in Western medicine (Efferth et al., 2007). This is not East-meets-West, by just turning herbal species into conventional chemical drugs, which contradict the theory and application of traditional medicine.

At edge, Lingzhi is standing at the middle point waiting for you to decide which way to go. Not mentioning it is named to be a superior tonic in the very first pharmacopeia - The divine farmer's material medica, Lingzhi has been used over two thousand years for the promotion of health and longevity. Thousands of studies have been performed with large proportion was focused on its anticancer effects, ranging from experiments *in vitro* and animals to humans' *in vivo*, merely supported its applicability for cancer treatment and prevention (Yuen & Gohel, 2005). Effective and toxic dosages have long been established by animal studies (Kim et al., 1986) in addition to the substantial prior human use. Toxicities were rarely reported, and the safe usage has been convinced by scientific evidence and history (Mizuno et al., 1995). Several Lingzhi products have already been well characterized by fingerprinting and genotyping techniques for authentication and quality control (Chen et al., 2008a, 2008b). The above conditions explicitly supported the clinical trials at phase I and II. In fact, A New Zealand-based research team (Gao et al., 2002, 2003a, 2003b, 2005) has conducted several phase II trials with advanced cancer patients as mentioned; however, the study aims were just placing Lingzhi as an adjunct therapy, where the outcome measurements were not really the valid disease endpoint. Besides, several isolated compounds, such as ganoderic acids and lucialdehydes, and their efficacy and safety have already characterized by using tissue culture and animal models (Yuen & Gohel, 2005). According to the WHO recommendations (WHO-TDR, 2005), both the crude mushrooms and isolated compounds are justified proceeding to large-scale phase III clinical trials, at least for their anticancer properties. Therefore, the choices are up to your decision, for traditional or conventional? Remember, your determination will lead the future research.

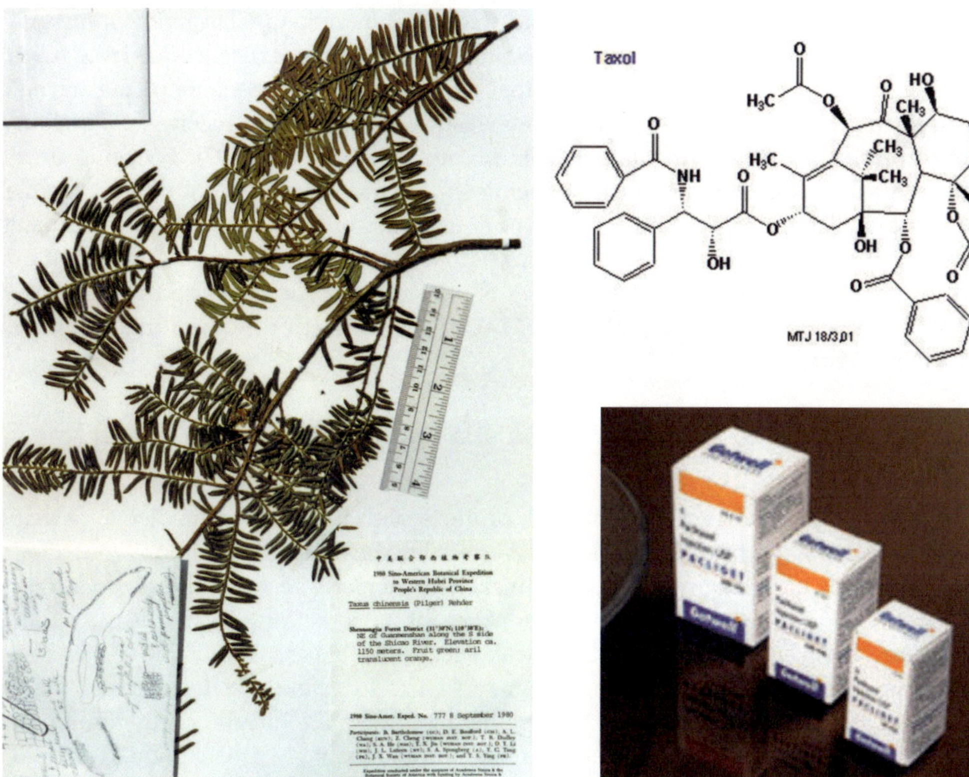

Fig. 3. The chemical structure of taxol in the package of Paclitaxel ®, reminding *Hong Dou Shan (Taxus chinensis)* available in Hubei China (diagram adopted from © The world Botanical Associates Web page) is one of the herbal sources of taxol.

6.2 The validation of holistic application of herbal formulations

We have seen for ourselves herbal medicine's ability both to heal those disorders that often fail to respond to the best of Western medicine, and treat major diseases with methods that are more sympathetic to the human system and have fewer harmful side effects. The WHO has published a list of ailments and conditions for which treatment or alleviation with Chinese medicine is considered appropriate which include diabetes. In Western medicine, diabetes is deemed as an incurable disease that patients have persistent hyperglycemia associated with high morbidity and mortality due to complications if blood glucose levels are not controlled. In view of TCM, diabetes is referred as *Xiao Ke* which is a syndrome of "wasting and thirsting" (Duan, 2008). The disease is described as the constitutional deficiency of yin of the kidney and lung and associated with the internal heat that consumes fluids, and thus causes wasting and thirst (Covington, 2001; Duan, 2008). There were 13 traditional herbal formulations for treating Xiao Ke according to the Yellow Emperor's Inner Canon, and later on derived into hundreds of prescriptions to aim at different symptoms of diabetes (Duan, 2008; Li et al., 2004). Whilst 33 most frequently used Chinese herbs for clinical treatment of diabetes and its complications were listed (Li et al., 2004). The "Herbal drink to strengthen muscle and control swelling", which is a six-component formula using Radix Astragali (*Astragalus membranaceus*) and Radix Rehmanniae (*Rehmannia glutinosa*) as principals, have been shown to promote the healing of diabetic foot ulcers effectively (Chan et al., 2007). Experimental studies revealed that all individual components of the formula were active in modifying tissue glucose homeostasis *in vitro* but inactive to improve glycaemic control of diabetes in diabetic rats *in vivo* (Chan et al., 2007). Focusing on its mechanism for the ulcer healing effects, a chemically induced diabetic foot ulcer rat model was used to establish the *in vivo* anti-inflammatory activities of the two principal ingredients (Tam et al., 2011). This is a typical example of herbal case demonstrating the feasibility of examining the traditionally used cures using of Western approach. More of this caliber should be conducted to eventually place TCM onto the context of modern medicine, and thus East meets West.

7. Conclusion – A need for compromise and agreement – A new model for investigation

The holistic views of TCM generally have no conflicts with the western medicine, perhaps they were just expressed in different terms. Western medicine is usually more concrete in diagnosis and judgment. Treatment is often quicker, particularly in acute cases, and surgery is its strength. Its weak points are that it sees disease as something to be measured and quantified and often ignores the psychological, social and behavioral factors involved in illness. Chinese medicine, on the other hand, can be too flexible and too general where diagnosis and judgment are concerned, and sometimes relies too heavily on the individual practitioner's experiences. Its strong points are its highly flexible approach, which enabling treatments to be changed as the patient improve, and its emphasis on prevention. The Chinese way tends to treat the whole body rather than to try to isolate a particular infected area. And, finally, the herbs themselves, compared with chemically produced medicines, are relatively cheap and easy to use. They have minimal side-effects, and most have been tried and tested for over many thousand years. Western medicine focuses more on symptomatic management, whereas TCM focuses more on cause and effect. Western medicine is more useful for first-aid and surgical interventions, whereas TCM is more useful in treating internal and chronic illnesses. An ideal health care system should be established to concern people's physical and mental health, to deal with all personal problems, and to improve people's quality of life. A new model of health care should be composed by a different medical system to provide a holistic approach. TCM, today as an alternative and complementary medicine should be included into the conventional medicine to form the new modern medicine. This is in line with the aim of the WHO to promote recognition of traditional medicine and to support its integration into the mainstream health service. There is space of integration for TCM and modern medicine. A new paradigm for developing medicine is needed, and Chinese medicine could make a significant contribution in this field. To achieve such integration, modern science and technology had to be used to study the action, efficacy and toxicity of Chinese medicines. Although, there are many issues to concern, especially safe and effectiveness, some compromise and agreement are needed. Thus botanicals should be defined, authenticated and documented as to their source and conditions of cultivation using modern methodology. Manufacturing and preparation processes of Chinese medicine should be carefully monitored and standardized. Claims for Chinese medicine should be verified from rigorous controlled trials. Interaction between Western and Chinese medicines should be better studied and information obtained centralized into accessible databases. This would be an enormous undertaking requiring international collaboration and participation of governments worldwide. In fact, the feasibility of herbal validation by using Western methods is well-illustrated. In particular, concerns about identity authentication, quality control, evidences of efficacy and safety of herbal remedies, are being addressed with the modern science and technology, and ultimately allow the gathering of information necessarily to support clinical trials. Along with this route, efforts being played will return with the transition of TCM into a recognized science specialty to fill up the gaps between Eastern and Western medical approaches. In this perspective, it may not be necessary to isolate the active ingredients from herbal remedies or purity them to finally become chemical drugs. To promote the effectiveness, Chinese herbal medicine can remain in formulae but standardizations are needed. Meanwhile, both Chinese and western practitioners should come together and sort out the best treatment they can offer to patients, which very often may be the combination of the modern and Chinese medicine, instead of favoring one over the other. Conventional Western medicine and Chinese medicine should be seen as complementary to each other, rather than as alternatives. Both types of medicine have their advantages and drawbacks, which is why they need to work hand in hand for optimal results. Together, Chinese and Western medicine could form the most effective disease treatment the world has ever known.

8. Acknowledgement

The authors are grateful to be supported the research by the Hong Kong Polytechnic University Grants G-997 and G-U979.

9. References

Achike, F.I. & Kwan, C.Y. (2003). Nitric oxide, human diseases and the herbal products that affect the nitric oxide signalling pathway. *Clinical and Experimental Pharmacology and Physiology*, Vol.30, No.9, (September 2003), pp. 605-615, ISSN 0305-1870

Ahmed, S.A. (2000). The immune system as a potential target for environmental estrogens (endocrine disrupters): a new emerging field. *Toxicology*, Vol.150, No.1-3, (September 2000), pp. 191-206, ISSN 0300-483X

Askin, R., Sasaki, M., & Goto, M. (2010). Recovery of water-soluble compounds from Ganoderma lucidum by hydrothermal treatment. *Food and Bioproducts Processing*, Vol.88, No.C2-3, (July 2009), pp. 291-297, ISSN 0960-3085

Atas, A., Agca, O., Sarac, S., Poyraz, A., & Akyol, M.U. (2006). Investigation of ototoxic effects of Taxol on a mice model. *International Journal of Pediatric Otorhinolaryngology*, Vol.70, No.5, (May 2006) pp. 779-784, ISSN 0165-5876

Beinfield, H. & Korngold, E. (2003). Dao and the doctor: The thought and practice of Chinese medicine. *Seminars in Integrative medicine*, Vol.1, No.3, (September 2003), pp. 136-144, ISSN 1543-1150

Bensky, D., Clavery, S., & Stoger, E. (2004). Substances that clam the spirit, In: *Chinese Herbal Medicine: Materia Medica*, A. Gamble, (Ed.), pp. 933-935, Eastland Press, ISBN 0939616424, Seattle

Bliss, M. (2011). *The marking of modern medicine: Turning points in the treatment of disease* (1st edition), The University of Chicago Press, ISBN 9780226059013, Chicago, London

Bynum, W.F. (2008). *History of medicine* (1st edition), Oxford University Press, ISBN 9780199215430, Oxford

Chan, C.M., Chan, Y.W., Lau, C.H., Lau, T.W., Lau, K.M., Lam, F.C., Che, C.T., Leung, P.C., Fung, K.P., Lau, C.B., & Ho, Y.Y. (2007). Influence of an anti-diabetic foot ulcer formula and its component herbs on tissue and systemic glucose homeostasis. *Journal of Ethnopharmacology*, Vol.109, No.1, (January 2007), pp. 10-20, ISSN 0378-8741

Chan, W.T. (1969). *A source book in Chinese philosophy* (1st edition), Princeton University Press , ISBN 1400811228, Princeton, New Jersey

Chang, H., Huang, W., Tsao, D., Huang, K., Lee, S., Lin, S., Yang, S., & Yeh, C. (2009). Identification and Authentication of Burdock (Arctium lappa Linn) Using PCR Sequencing. *Fooyin Journal of Health Science*, Vol.1, No.1, (August 2009), pp. 28-32, ISSN 1877-8607

Chen, R.Z., Meng, F.L., Zhang, S.Q., & Liu, Z.Q. (2009). Effects of ultrahigh pressure extraction conditions on yields and antioxidant activity of ginsenoside from ginseng. *Separation and Purification Technology*, Vol.66, No.2, (April 2009), pp. 340-346, ISSN 1383-5806

Chen, T., Zhao, X., Wu, J., Yu, D., & Wu, Y. (2011). Supercritical fluid CO2 extraction, simultaneous determination of components in ultra-fine powder of Ganoderma sinense by HPLC-ESI-MS method. *Journal of the Taiwan Institute of chemical Engineers*, Vol.42, No.3., (May 2011), pp. 428-434, ISSN 1876-1070

Chen, Y., Xie, M.Y., & Gong, X.F. (2007). Microwave-assisted extraction used for the isolation of total triterpenoid saponins from Ganoderma atrum. *Journal of Food Engineering*, Vol.81, No.1, (July 2007), pp. 162-170, ISSN 0260-8774

Chen, Y., Yan, Y., Xie, M.Y., Nie, S.P., Liu, W., Gong, X.F., & Wang, Y.X. (2008a). Development of a chromatographic fingerprint for the chloroform extracts of Ganoderma lucidum by HPLC and LC-MS. *Journal of Pharmaceutical and Biomedical Analysis*,Vol.47, No.3, (July 2008), pp. 469-477, ISSN 0731-7085

Chen, Y., Zhu, S.B., Xie, M.Y., Nie, S.P., Liu, W., Li, C., Gong, X.F., & Wang, Y.X. (2008b.) Quality control and original discrimination of Ganoderma lucidum based on high-performance liquid chromatographic fingerprints and combined chemometrics methods. *Analytica Chimica Acta*, Vol.623, No.2, (August 2008), pp. 146-156, ISSN 0003-2670

Covington, M. B. (2001). Traditional Chinese medicine in the treatment of diabetes. *Diabetes Spectrum*, Vol.14, No.3, (November 2001), pp. 154-159, ISSN 1944-7353

Duan, Q.F. (2008). *Huangdi nei jing* (2nd edition), Chong wen shu ju, ISBN 9787540312350, Wuhan Shi

Duffin, J. (2010). *history of medicine: A scandalously short introduction* (2nd edition), University of Toronto Press, ISBN 9780802098252, Toronto

Dunn, A. J. (1996). Psychneuroimmunology, stress and infection, In: *Psychoneuimmunology, stress, and infection*, H.K.T.W. Friedman & A.L. Friedman (Eds.), pp. 25-78, CRC Press , ISBN 0849376386, Boca Raton, New York, London, tokyo

Efferth, T., Li, P.C., Konkimalla, V.S., & Kaina, B. (2007). From traditional Chinese medicine to rational cancer therapy. *Trends in Molecular Medicine*, Vol.13, No.8, (August 2007), pp. 353-361, ISSN 1471-4914

Fan, X.H., Cheng, Y.Y., Ye, Z.L., Lin, R.C., & Qian, Z.Z. (2006). Multiple chromatographic fingerprinting and its application to the quality control of herbal medicines. *Analytica Chimica Acta*, Vol.555, No.2, (January 2006), pp. 217-224, ISSN 0003-2670

Finkel, T. & Holbrook, N.J. (2000). Oxidants, oxidative stress and the biology of ageing. *Nature*, Vol.408, No.6809, (November 2000), pp. 239-247, ISSN 0028-0836

Fu, Y.J., Liu, W., Zu, Y.G., Shi, X.G., Liu, Z.G., Schwarz, G., & Efferth, T. (2009). Breaking the spores of the fungus Ganoderma lucidum by supercritical CO_2. *Food Chemistry*, Vol.112, No.1, (January 2009), pp. 71-76, ISSN 0308-8146

Gaddum, J.H. & Kwiatkowski, H. (1938). The action of ephedrine. *Journal of Physiology*, Vol.94, No.1, (October 1938), pp. 87-100, ISSN 0022-3751

Gagnier, J.J., Moher, D., Boon, H., Beyene, J., & Bombardier, C. (2011). Randomized controlled trials of herbal interventions underreport important details of the intervention. *Journal of Clinical Epidemiology*, Vol.64, No.7, (July 2011), pp. 760-769, ISSN 1179-1349

Gao, Y., Tang, W., Dai, X., Gao, H., Chen, G., Ye, J., Chan, E., Koh, H.L., Li, X., & Zhou, S. (2005). Effects of water-soluble Ganoderma lucidum polysaccharides on the immune functions of patients with advanced lung cancer. *Journal of Medicinal Food*, Vol.8, No.2, (Summer 2005), pp. 159-168, ISSN 1096-620X

Gao, Y., Zhou, S., Jiang, W., Huang, M., & Dai, X. (2003a). Effects of ganopoly (a Ganoderma lucidum polysaccharide extract) on the immune functions in advanced-stage cancer patients. *Immunological Investigatioms*, Vol.32, No.3, (August 2003), pp. 201-215, ISSN 1532-4311

Gao, Y. H., Dai, X. H., Chen, G. L., Ye, J. X., & Zhou, S. F. (2003b). A randomized, placebo-controlled, multicenter study of Ganoderma lucidum (W.Curt.: Fr.) Lloyd (Aphyllophoromycetideae) polysaccharides (Ganoploy (R)) in patients with advanced lung cancer. *International Journal of Medicinal Mushrooms*, Vol.5, No.4, (December 2003), pp. 369-381, ISSN 1521-9437

Gao, Y. H., Zhou, S. F., Chen, G. L., Dai, X. H., & Ye, J. X. (2002). A phaseI/II study of a Ganoderma lucidum (Curt.: Fr.) P. Karst extract (Ganopoly) in patients with advanced cancer. *International Journal of Medicinal Mushrooms,* Vol.4, No.3, (September 2002), pp. 207-214., ISSN 1521-9437

Gutteridge, J.M. (1994). Biological origin of free radicals, and mechanisms of antioxidant protection. *Chemico Biological Interactions,* Vol.91, No.2-3, (June 1994), pp. 133-140, ISSN 0009-2797

Halliwell, B. (2009). The wanderings of a free radical. *Free Radical Biolology and Medicine,* Vol.46, No.5, (March 2009), pp. 531-542, ISSN 0891-5849

Han, T., Zhang, Q.Y., Zhang, H., Wen, J., Wang, Y., Huang, B.K., Rahman, K., Zheng, H.C., & Qin, L.P. (2009). Authentication and quantitative analysis on the chemical profile of Xanthium fruit (Cang-Er-Zi) by high-performance liquid chromatography-diode-array detection tandem mass spectrometry method. *Analytica Chimica Acta,* Vol.634, No.2, (Feburary 2009), pp. 272-278, ISSN 0003-2670

Herrero, B., Madrinan, M., Vieites, J.M., & Espineira, M. (2010). Authentication of Atlantic cod (Gadus morhua) using real time PCR. *Journal of Agricultural and Food Chemistry,* Vol.58, No.8, (April 2010), pp. 4794-4799, ISSN 0021-8561

Hudson, J. & Altamirano, M. (2006). The application of DNA micro-arrays (gene arrays) to the study of herbal medicines. *Journal of Ethnopharmacology,* Vol.108, No.1, (November 2006), pp. 2-15, ISSN 0378-8741

Huie, C.W. & Di, X. (2004). Chromatographic and electrophoretic methods for Lingzhi pharmacologically active components. *Journal of Chromatography B Analytical Technologies in the Biomedical and Life Science,* Vol.812, No.1-2, (December 2004), pp. 241-257, ISSN 1570-0232

Jordan, S.A., Cunningham, D.G., & Marles, R.J. (2010). Assessment of herbal medicinal products: challenges, and opportunities to increase the knowledge base for safety assessment. *Toxicology and Applied Pharmacology,* Vol.243, No.2, (March 2010), pp. 198-216, ISSN 0041-008X

Kaptchuk, T.J. (2000). *Chinese medicine: The web that has no weaver* (1st edition), Rider, ISBN 071260281X, London, Sydney, Auckland, johannesburg

Kaye, J. M. & Lightman, S. L. (2005). Psychologucak stress and endrine axes, In: *Human psychoneuroimmunology,* K. Vedhara & M. Irwin, (Eds.), pp. 25-52, Oxford University Press , ISBN 019852840X, New York

Khan, S., Mirza, K.J., Al-Qurainy, F., & Abdin, M.Z. (2011). Authentication of the medicinal plant Senna angustifolia by RAPD profiling. *Saudi Journal of Biological Sciences,* Vol.18, No.3, (March 2011), pp. 287-292, ISSN 1319-562X

Khosroushahi, A.Y., Valizadeh, M., Ghasempour, A., Khosrowshahli, M., Naghdibadi, H., Dadpour, M.R., & Omidi, Y. (2006). Improved Taxol production by combination of inducing factors in suspension cell culture of Taxus baccata. *Cell Biology International,* Vol.30, No.3, (March 2006), pp. 262-269, ISSN 1065-6995

Kim, M. J., Kim, H. W., Lee, Y. S., Shim, M. J., Choi, E. C., & Kim, B. K. (1986). Stduies on safety of ganoderma lucidum. *Korean Journal of Mycology,* Vol.14, (March 1986), pp. 49-60, ISSN 1226-4709

Kingston, D.G. (2007). The shape of things to come: structural and synthetic studies of taxol and related compounds. *Phytochemistry,* Vol.68, No.14, (July 2007), pp. 1844-1854, ISSN 0031-9422

Kiran, U., Khan, S., Mirza, K.J., Ram, M., & Abdin, M.Z. (2010). SCAR markers: a potential tool for authentication of herbal drugs. *Fitoterapia*, Vol.81, No.8, (December 2010), pp. 969-976, ISSN 0367-326X

Kitzberger, C.S.G., Smania, A., Pedrosa, R.C., & Ferreira, S.R.S. (2007). Antioxidant and antimicrobial activities of shiitake (Lentinula edodes) extracts obtained by organic solvents and supercritical fluids. *Journal of Food Engineering*, Vol.80, No.2, (May 2007), pp. 631-638, ISSN 0260-8774

Ko, K.M., Leon, T.Y., Mak, D.H., Chiu, P.Y., Du, Y., & Poon, M.K. (2006). A characteristic pharmacological action of 'Yang-invigorating' Chinese tonifying herbs: enhancement of myocardial ATP-generation capacity. *Phytomedicine*, Vol.13, No.9-10, (November 2006), pp. 636-642, ISSN 0944-7113

Ko, K.M. & Leung, H.Y. (2007). Enhancement of ATP generation capacity, antioxidant activity and immunomodulatory activities by Chinese Yang and Yin tonifying herbs. *Chinese Medicine*, Vol.2, No.3, (March 2007), available from: http://www.cmjournal.org/content/2/1/3

Ko, K.M., Mak, D.H., Chiu, P.Y., & Poon, M.K. (2004). Pharmacological basis of 'Yang-invigoration' in Chinese medicine. *Trends in Pharmacoogical Science*, Vol. 25, No.1, (January 2004), pp. 3-6, ISSN 0165-6147

Kuang, A. K., Ding, T., Chen, G. L., Xu, M. Y., Zhang, D. Q., Chi, Y. S., Lo, S. Z., Chen, M. Y., Wang, X. L., & Wang, Q. Q. (1988). Study on clinical effect of treatment of myxedema with TCM alone and TCM supplemented with thyroid tablets. *Chinese Journal of Integrated Traditional and Western Medicine*, Vol.8, No.2, (Feburary 1988), pp. 74-76, ISSN 1003-5370

Lafaille, J.J. & Mathis, D. (2002). Immunological Yin-Yang. *Current Opinion in Immunology*, Vol.14, No.6, (December 2002), pp. 741-743, ISSN 0952-7915

Langevin, H.M., Badger, G.J., Povolny, B.K., Davis, R.T., Johnston, A.C., Sherman, K.J., Kahn, J.R., & Kaptchuk, T.J. (2004). Yin scores and yang scores: A new method for quantitative diagnostic evaluation in traditional Chinese medicine research. *Journal of Alternative and Complementary Medicine*, Vol.10, No.2, (April 2004), pp. 389-395, ISSN 1075-5535

Law, S.K., Simmons, M.P., Techen, N., Khan, I.A., He, M.F., Shaw, P.C., & But, P.P. (2011). Molecular analyses of the Chinese herb Leigongteng (Tripterygium wilfordii Hook.f.). *Phytochemistry*, Vol.72, No.1, (January 2011), pp. 21-26, ISSN 0031-9422

Li, M., Jiang, R.W., Hon, P.M., Cheng, L., Li, L.L., Zhou, J.R., Shaw, P.C., & But, P.P.H. (2010). Authentication of the anti-tumor herb Baihuasheshecao with bioactive marker compounds and molecular sequences. *Food Chemistry*, Vol.119, No.3, (April 2010), pp. 1239-1245, ISSN 0308-8146

Li, S.P., Zhao, J., & Yang, B. (2011). Strategies for quality control of Chinese medicines. *Journal of Pharmacutical and Biomedical Analysis.*, Vol.55, No.4, (June 2011), pp. 802-809, ISSN 0731-7085

Li, S.Z. (2003). *Compendium of materia medica (Bencao Gangmu)* (1st edition), Foreign Language Press, ISBN 9787119032603, Beijing

Li, W.L., Zheng, H.C., Bukuru, J., & De, K.N. (2004). Natural medicines used in the traditional Chinese medical system for therapy of diabetes mellitus. *Journal of Ethnopharmacology*, Vol.92, No.1, (May 2004), pp. 1-21, ISSN 0378-8741

Lin, W.S., Chan, W.C., & Hew, C.S. (1995). Superoxide and traditional Chinese medicines. *Journal of Ethnopharmacology*, Vol.48, No.3, (November 1995), pp. 165-171, ISSN 0378-8741

Liu, X., Yuan, J.P., Chung, C.K., & Chen, X.J. (2002). Antitumor activity of the sporoderm-broken germinating spores of Ganoderma lucidum. *Cancer Letters*, Vol.182, No.2, (Auguet 2002), pp. 155-161, ISSN 0304-3835

Lock, S. (1997). Medicine in the second half of the twentieth century, In: *Western Medicine: An Illustrated History*, I. Loudon, (Ed.), pp. 123-146, Oxford University Press, ISBN 0198205090, Oxford, New York

Longrigg, J. (1997). Medicine in the classical world, In: *Western Medicine: An Illustrated History*, I. Loudon, (Ed.), pp. 25-39, Oxford University Press, ISBN 0198205090, Oxford, New York

Lu, G.H., Chan, K., Liang, Y.Z., Leung, K., Chan, C.L., Jiang, Z.H., & Zhao, Z.Z. (2005). Development of high-performance liquid chromatographic fingerprints for distinguishing Chinese Angelica from related umbelliferae herbs. *Journal of Chromatography A*, Vol.1073, No.1-2, pp. 383-392, ISSN 0021-9673

Lu, Q.Y., Jin, Y.S., Zhang, Q., Zhang, Z., Heber, D., Go, V.L., Li, F.P., & Rao, J.Y. (2004). Ganoderma lucidum extracts inhibit growth and induce actin polymerization in bladder cancer cells in vitro. *Cancer Letters*, Vol.216, No.1, (December 2004), pp. 9-20, ISSN 0304-3835

Macek, C. (1984). East meets West to balance immunologic yin and yang. *Journal of American Medical Association*, Vol.251, No.4, (Januray 1984), pp. 433-439, ISSN 0098-7484

Mak, D.H., Chiu, P.Y., Poon, M.K., Ng, T.T., Chung, Y.K., Lam, B.Y., Du, Y., & Ko, K.M. (2004). A yang-promoting Chinese herbal suppository preparation enhances the antioxidant status of red cells in male human subjects. *Phytotherapy Research*, Vol.18, No.7, (July 2004), pp. 525-530, ISSN 0951-418X

Mann, D.L. (2001). Interleukin-6 and viral myocarditis: the Yin-Yang of cardiac innate immune responses. *Journal of Molecular and Cellular Cardiology*, Vol.33, No.9, (September 2001), pp. 1551-1553, ISSN 0022-2828

Mills, R. & Bhatt, D.L. (2004). The Yin and Yang of arterial inflammation. *Journal of American College of Cardiology*, Vol.44, No.1, (July 2004), pp. 50-52, ISSN 0735-1097

Min, X., Xiaohui, Z., Zhaixiang, D., & Ming, O. (1998). Effect of the Yang tonifying herbs on myocardial beta-adrenoceptors of hypothyroid rabbits. *Journal of Ethnopharmacology*, Vol.60, No.1, (February 1998), pp. 43-51, ISSN 0378-8741

Mizuno, T., Wang, G.Y., Zhang, J., Kawagishi, H., Nishitoba, T., & Li, J.X. (1995). Reishi, Ganoderma lucidum and Ganoderma tsugae - Bioactive Substances and Medicinal Effects. *Food Reviews International*, Vol.11, No.1, (November 2009), pp. 151-166, ISSN 8755-9129

Molassiotis, A., Potrata, B., & Cheng, K.K. (2009). A systematic review of the effectiveness of Chinese herbal medication in symptom management and improvement of quality of life in adult cancer patients. *Complementary Therapies Medicine*, Vol.17, No.2, (April 2009), pp. 92-120, ISSN 0965-2299

Ou, B., Huang, D., Hampsch-Woodill, M., & Flanagan, J.A. (2003). When east meets west: the relationship between yin-yang and antioxidation-oxidation. *The FASEB Journal*, Vol.17, No.2, (October 2002), pp. 127-129, ISSN 0892-6638

Palaszynski, K.M., Smith, D.L., Kamrava, S., Burgoyne, P.S., Arnold, A.P., & Voskuhl, R.R. (2005). A yin-yang effect between sex chromosome complement and sex hormones on the immune response. *Endocrinology*, Vol.146, No.8, (August 2005), pp. 3280-3285, ISSN 0013-7227

Paterson, R.R. (2008). Cordyceps: a traditional Chinese medicine and another fungal therapeutic biofactory? *Phytochemistry*, Vol.69, No.7, (May 2008), pp. 1469-1495, ISSN 0031-9422

Paton, J.F., Boscan, P., Pickering, A.E., & Nalivaiko, E. (2005). The yin and yang of cardiac autonomic control: vago-sympathetic interactions revisited.*Brain Research Reviews.*, Vol.49, No.3, (Novermber 2005), pp. 555-565, ISSN 0165-0173

Peng, X., Zhao, Y., Liang, X., Wu, L., Cui, S., Guo, A., & Wang, W. (2006). Assessing the quality of RCTs on the effect of beta-elemene, one ingredient of a Chinese herb, against malignant tumors. *Contemporary Clinical Trials*, Vol.27, No.1, (February 2006), pp. 70-82, ISSN 1551-7144

Pyo, S.H., Cho, J.S., Choi, H.J., & Han, B.H. (2007). Evaluation of paclitaxel rearrangement involving opening of the oxetane ring and migration of acetyl and benzoyl groups. *Journal of Pharmaceutical and Biomedical Analysis*, Vol.43, No.3, (February 2007), pp. 1141-1145, ISSN 0731-7085

Rabah, S. O. (2010). Acute taxol nephrotoxicity: Histological and ultrastructural studies of mice kidney parenchyma. *Saudi Journal of Biological Sciences, Vol.*17, No.2, (April 2010), pp. 105-114, ISSN 1319-562X

Robinson, M. M. & Zhang, X. 2011, *The World Medicine situation 2011: Traditional medicine: Global situation, issues and challenges*, WHO Press, Geneva, Retrived from http://www.who.int/medicines/areas/policy/world_medicines_situation/WMS_ch18_wTraditionalMed.pdf

Samenuk, D., Link, M.S., Homoud, M.K., Contreras, R., Theoharides, T.C., Wang, P.J., & Estes, N.A., III (2002). Adverse cardiovascular events temporally associated with ma huang, an herbal source of ephedrine. *Mayo Clinic Proceedings*, Vol.77, No.1, (January 2002), pp. 12-16, ISSN 0025-6196

Schaneberg, B.T., Crockett, S., Bedir, E., & Khan, I.A. (2003). The role of chemical fingerprinting: application to Ephedra. *Phytochemistry*, Vol.62, No.6, (March 2003), pp. 911-918, ISSN 0031-9422

Shekelle, P.G., Hardy, M.L., Morton, S.C., Maglione, M., Mojica, W.A., Suttorp, M.J., Rhodes, S.L., Jungvig, L., & Gagne, J. (2003). Efficacy and safety of ephedra and ephedrine for weight loss and athletic performance: a meta-analysis. *Journal of American Medical Association*, Vol.289, No.12, (March 2003), pp. 1537-1545, ISSN 0098-7484

Shiang, E. & Li, F.P. (1971). The Yin-Yang (cold-hot) theory of disease. *Journal of American Medical Association*, Vol.217, No.8, (August 1971), pp. 1108, ISSN 0098-7484

Shouqin, Z., Junjie, Z., & Changzhen, W. (2004). Novel high pressure extraction technology. *International Journal of Pharmaceuticals*, Vol.278, No.2, (July 2004), pp. 471-474, ISSN 1811-7775

Siow, Y.L., Gong, Y., Au-Yeung, K.K., Woo, C.W., Choy, P.C., & O K (2005). Emerging issues in traditional Chinese medicine. *Canadian Journal of Physiology and Pharmacology*, Vol.83, No.4, (April 2005), pp. 321-334, ISSN 0008-4212

Siu, K.M., Mak, D.H., Chiu, P.Y., Poon, M.K., Du, Y., & Ko, K.M. (2004). Pharmacological basis of 'Yin-nourishing' and 'Yang-invigorating' actions of Cordyceps, a Chinese tonifying herb. *Life Science*, Vol.76, No.4, (December 2004), pp. 385-395, ISSN 1730-413X

Song, J., Yao, H., Li, Y., Li, X., Lin, Y., Liu, C., Han, J., Xie, C., & Chen, S. (2009). Authentication of the family Polygonaceae in Chinese pharmacopoeia by DNA barcoding technique. *Journal of Ethnopharmacology*, Vol.124, No.3, (July 2009), pp. 434-439, ISSN 0378-8741

World Health Organization Special Programme for Research and Training in Tropical Diseases (WHO-TDR). 2005. *Operational guidance: Information needed to support clinical trials of herbal products*, WHO Press, Geneva, Switcerland, Retrived from http://whqlibdoc.who.int/hq/2005/TDR_GEN_Guidance_05.1_eng.pdf

Szeto, Y.T. & Benzie, I.F. (2006). Is the yin-yang nature of Chinese herbal medicine equivalent to antioxidation-oxidation? *Journal of Ethnopharmacology*, Vol.108, No.3, (December 2006), pp. 361-366, ISSN 0378-8741

Taitano, K., Schnyer, R., Allen, J. J. B., Manber, R., & Hitt, S. K. (2003). The psychophysiology of yin and yang. *Journal of Herbal Pharmacotherapy*, Vol.3, pp. 63 ISSN 1552-8940

Tam, J.C., Lau, K.M., Liu, C.L., To, M.H., Kwok, H.F., Lai, K.K., Lau, C.P., Ko, C.H., Leung, P.C., Fung, K.P., & Lau, C.B. (2011). The in vivo and in vitro diabetic wound healing effects of a 2-herb formula and its mechanisms of action. *Journal of Ethnopharmacology*, Vol.134, No.3, (April 2011), pp. 831-838, ISSN 0378-8741

Tang, F., Zhang, Q.L., Nie, Z., Chen, B., & Yao, S.Z. (2009). Sample preparation for analyzing traditional Chinese medicines. *Trends in Analytical Chemistry*, Vol.28, No.11, (December 2009), pp. 1253-1262, ISSN 0165-9936

Tistaert, C., Dejaegher, B., & Vander, H.Y. (2011). Chromatographic separation techniques and data handling methods for herbal fingerprints: a review. *Analytica Chimica Acta*, Vol.690, No.2, (April 2011), pp. 148-161, ISSN 0003-2670

Tong, W. (2010). Challenge from the Philosophy of Scientific Practice and New Empiricism. *Systems Research and Behavioral Science*, Vol.27, No.2, (February 2010), pp. 190-199, ISSN1712-851X

Unschuld, P.U. (2003). *Huangdi nei jing su wen: Nature, kowledge, imagery in an ancient Chinese medical text* (1st edition), University of California Press, ISBN 0585468583, Berkeley

van Wijk, R., van der Greef, J., & van Wijk, E. (2010). Human ultraweak photon emission and the yin yang concept of Chinese medicine. *Journal of Acupuncture and Meridian Studies*, Vol.3, No.4, (December 2010), pp. 221-231, ISSN 2005-2901

Varbiro, G., Veres, B., Gallyas, F., Jr., & Sumegi, B. (2001). Direct effect of Taxol on free radical formation and mitochondrial permeability transition. *Free Radical Biology and Medicie*, Vol.31, No.4, (August 2001), pp. 548-558, ISSN 0891-5849

Vegiopoulos, A. & Herzig, S. (2007). Glucocorticoids, metabolism and metabolic diseases. *Molecular and Cellular Endocrinology*, Vol.275, No.1-2, (September 2007), pp. 43-61, ISSN 0303-7207

Wachtel-Galor, S., Yuen, J., Buswell, J. A., & Benzie, I. F. F. (2011). Ganoderma lucidum (Lingzhi or Reishi): A medicinal mushroom, In: *Herbal medicine - Biomolecular and clinical aspects*, (2nd edition), I.F.F. Benzie & S. Wachtel-Galor, (Eds.), pp. 175-198, CRC Press, ISBN 978143980132, Boca Raton, London, New York

Wang, B.J., Won, S.J., Yu, Z.R., & Su, C.L. (2005). Free radical scavenging and apoptotic effects of Cordyceps sinensis fractionated by supercritical carbon dioxide. *Food and Chemical Toxicology*, Vol.43, No.4, (April 2005), pp. 543-552, ISSN 0278-6915

Wang, G., Mao, B., Xiong, Z.Y., Fan, T., Chen, X.D., Wang, L., Liu, G.J., Liu, J., Guo, J., Chang, J., Wu, T.X., & Li, T.Q. (2007). The quality of reporting of randomized controlled trials of traditional Chinese medicine: a survey of 13 randomly selected journals from mainland China. *Clinical Therapeutics*, Vol.29, No.7, (July 2007), pp. 1456-1467, ISSN 0149-2918

Wang, L., Zhang, R.M., Liu, G.Y., Wei, B.L., Wang, Y., Cai, H.Y., Li, F.S., Xu, Y.L., Zheng, S.P., & Wang, G. (2010). Chinese herbs in treatment of influenza: a randomized, double-blind, placebo-controlled trial. *Respiratory Medicine*, Vol.104, No.9, (September 2010), pp. 1362-1369, ISSN 0954-6111

Wang, X.M., Yang, M., Guan, S.H., Liu, R.X., Xia, J.M., Bi, K.S., & Guo, D.A. (2006). Quantitative determination of six major triterpenoids in Ganoderma lucidum and related species by high performance liquid chromatography. *Journal of Pharmaceutical and Biomedical Analysis*, Vol.41, No.3, (June 2006), pp. 838-844, ISSN 0731-7085

Wilczynski, J.R. (2005). Th1/Th2 cytokines balance-yin and yang of reproductive immunology. *European Journal of Obstetrics and Gynecology and Reproductive Biology*, Vol.122, No.2, (Oct 2005), pp. 136-143, ISSN 0301-2115

Witz, I.P. (2008). Yin-yang activities and vicious cycles in the tumor microenvironment. *Cancer Research*, Vol.68, No.1, (January 2008), pp. 9-13, ISSN 0008-5472

Wolsko, P.M., Solondz, D.K., Phillips, R.S., Schachter, S.C., & Eisenberg, D.M. (2005). Lack of herbal supplement characterization in published randomized controlled trials. The *American Journal of Medicine*, Vol.118, No.10, (October 2005), pp. 1087-1093, ISSN 0002-9343

Wong, H. S., Leung, H. Y., & Ko, K. M. (2011). 'Yang-invigorating' chinese tonic herbs enhance mitochondrial ATP generation in H9c2 cardiomyocytes. *Chinese Medicine*, Vol.2, No.1, (March 2011), pp. 1-5, ISSN 2151-1918

Xie, P.S., Yan, Y.Z., Guo, B.L., Lam, C.W., Chui, S.H., & Yu, Q.X. (2010). Chemical pattern-aided classification to simplify the intricacy of morphological taxonomy of Epimedium species using chromatographic fingerprinting. *Journal of Pharmaceutical and Biomedical Analysis*, Vol.52, No.4, (August 2010), pp. 452-460, ISSN 0731-7085

Yang, M., Sun, J., Lu, Z., Chen, G., Guan, S., Liu, X., Jiang, B., Ye, M., & Guo, D.A. (2009). Phytochemical analysis of traditional Chinese medicine using liquid chromatography coupled with mass spectrometry. *Journal of Chromatography A*, Vol.1216, No.11, (March 2009), pp. 2045-2062, ISSN 0021-9673

Yang, Q., Wang, S., Xie, Y., Sun, J., & Wang, J. (2010). HPLC analysis of Ganoderma lucidum polysaccharides and its effect on antioxidant enzymes activity and Bax, Bcl-2 expression. *International Journal of Biological Macromolecules*, Vol.46, No.2, March 2010, pp. 167-172, ISSN 0141-8130

Yang, S.Z. (2005). *The divine famer's materia; medica: a translation of the shen nong ben cao jing* (1st edition)., Blue Poppy Press, ISBN 0585105464, Boulder, Colorado

Yap, K.Y.L., Chan, S.Y., & Lim, C.S. (2008). The reliability of traditional authentication - A case of ginseng misfit. *Food Chemistry*, Vol.107, No.1, (March 2008), pp. 570-575, ISSN 0308-8146

Yuen, J.W. & Gohel, M.D. (2005). Anticancer effects of Ganoderma lucidum: a review of scientific evidence. *Nutrition and Cancer: An International Journal*, Vol.53, No.1, (November 2005), pp. 11-17, ISSN 0163-5581

Yuen, J.W. & Gohel, M.D. (2008). The dual roles of Ganoderma antioxidants on urothelial cell DNA under carcinogenic attack. *Journal of Ethnopharmacology*, Vol.118, No.2, (July 2008), pp. 324-330 ISSN 0378-8741

Yuen, J.W., Gohel, M.D., & Au, D.W. (2008). Telomerase-associated apoptotic events by mushroom ganoderma lucidum on premalignant human urothelial cells. *Nutrition and Cancer: An International Journal*, Vol.60, No.1, (January 2008), pp. 109-119, ISSN 0163-5581

Yuen, J.W., Gohel, M.D., & Ng, C.F. (2011). The differential immunological activities of Ganoderma lucidum on human pre-cancerous uroepithelial cells. *Journal of Ethnopharmacology*, Vol.135, No.3, (June 2011), pp. 711-718, ISSN 0378-8741

Zhang, J. (2007). Yin and yang interplay of IFN-gamma in inflammation and autoimmune disease. *The Journal of Clinical Investigations*, Vol.117, No.4, (April 2007), pp. 871-873, ISSN 0021-9738

Zhang, Y. S. (2011). Mathematical reasoning of treatment principle based on "yin yang wu xing" theory in traditional Chinese medicine. *Chinese Medicine*, Vol.2, (March 2011), pp. 6-15, ISSN 2151-1918

Zhao, Y.Y., Zhang, Y., Lin, R.C., & Sun, W.J. (2009). An expeditious HPLC method to distinguish Aconitum kusnezoffii from related species. *Fitoterapia*, Vol.80, No.6, (September 2009), pp. 333-338, ISSN 0367-326X

Zhong, Y., Fu, J., Liu, X., Diao, X., Mao, B., Fan, T., Yang, H., Liu, G., & Zhang, W. (2010). The Reporting Quality, Scientific Rigor and Ethics of Randomized Placebo-Controlled Trials of traditional Chinese Medicine Compound Formulations and the Differences Between Chinese and Non-Chinese Trials. *Current Therapeutic Research*, Vol.71, No.1, (February 2010), pp. 30-49, ISSN 0011-393X

12

Effects of Vasoactive Chinese Herbs on the Endothelial NO System

Huige Li
Department of Pharmacology, University Medical Center, Johannes Gutenberg University, Mainz, Germany

1. Introduction

In the vasculature, nitric oxide (NO) is produced from the endothelium mainly by endothelial NO synthase (eNOS), which is activated by agonists such as bradykinin and acetylcholine or by shear stress produced by the flowing blood. NO is a potent vasodilator and protects blood vessels from thrombosis by inhibiting platelet aggregation and adhesion. In addition, endothelial NO possesses multiple anti-atherosclerotic properties, which include (i) prevention of leukocyte adhesion to the vascular endothelium and leukocyte migration into the vascular wall; (ii) decreased endothelial permeability, reduced influx of lipoproteins into the vascular wall and inhibition of low density lipoprotein (LDL) oxidation; and (iii) inhibition of DNA synthesis, mitogenesis, and proliferation of vascular smooth muscle cells [1, 2]. Recent studies suggest that eNOS is also involved in mitochondrial biogenesis, anti-aging effects and extension of lifespan in mammals [3, 4].
Based on the abovementioned protective effects of eNOS-derived NO, a pharmacological enhancement of NO production is of therapeutic interest. Indeed, numerous Chinese medicinal plants, herbal preparations, or isolated compounds thereof have been shown to stimulate endothelial NO production, which is likely to be a contributing mechanism for their therapeutic effects.

2. Regulation of endothelial NO production

Endothelial NO production is regulated at different levels, including

- Regulation of eNOS expression: expression of the eNOS enzyme is regulated at both the transcriptional and post-transcriptional levels. Estrogens, for example, increase eNOS expression by stimulating eNOS promoter activity. TNFα, on the other hand, reduces eNOS expression by destabilizing eNOS mRNA [5, 6]. Several Chinese herbal products have been shown to enhance eNOS expression (Table 1).
- Regulation of eNOS activity by post-translational modifications: the enzymatic activity of eNOS is regulated by different cellular events such as increased intracellular Ca^{2+}, interactions with substrates, co-factors, adaptors and regulatory proteins, and through shuttling between distinct subcellular domains [7]. In addition, eNOS activity is also regulated by post-translational modification of the eNOS protein. For example, phosphorylation of serine 1177 enhances eNOS activity, whereas phosphorylation of

threonine 495 decreases eNOS activity [7]. Recent studies indicate that eNOS activity can be also enhanced by SIRT1-mediated deacetylation of lysine residues in the calmodulin-binding domain [8].

- Regulation of eNOS activity by changing the intracellular concentration of asymmetric dimethylarginine (ADMA): elevated plasma levels of ADMA have been shown to be associated with cardiovascular events and mortality. ADMA is believed to be an endogenous eNOS inhibitor, although NO-independent effects of ADMA have also been reported [9]. ADMA is formed during proteolysis and is degraded by the intracellular enzyme dimethylarginine dimethylaminohydrolase (DDAH). Decreased DDAH expression/activity is evident in disease states associated with endothelial dysfunction [10].
- Regulation of eNOS functionality: under a number of pathological conditions, the enzymatic reduction of molecular oxygen by eNOS is no longer coupled to L-arginine oxidation, resulting in production of superoxide rather than NO. This phenomenon is referred to as "eNOS uncoupling" [1, 5]. A number of potential mechanisms have been reported to contribute to eNOS uncoupling. Among all of these mechanisms, a deficiency of the NOS cofactor tetrahydrobiopterin (BH_4) seems to be the primary cause for eNOS uncoupling in pathophysiology. In BH_4 deficiency, the reduction of molecular oxygen still occurs at the heme site of eNOS, but oxidation of the guanidine nitrogen of L-arginine is prevented, so that the reduced oxygen comes off the enzyme as superoxide [11, 12]. eNOS-mediated superoxide production has been observed in animal models of atherosclerosis, hypertension, diabetes mellitus and nitroglycerin tolerance, and also in patients with endothelial dysfunction resulting from hypercholesterolemia, diabetes mellitus, or essential hypertension, in chronic smokers, and in nitroglycerin-treated patients [11, 12]. Thus, eNOS uncoupling turns eNOS from a NO-producing protective enzyme into a superoxide-generating deleterious molecule. It is therefore of therapeutic interest to reverse eNOS uncoupling and restore eNOS functionality. An elevation of endothelial BH_4 levels (by enhancing BH_4 biosynthesis and/or by preventing oxidative stress-mediated BH_4 oxidation) may reverse eNOS uncoupling [13]. Chinese herbs containing large amounts of polyphenolic compounds with antioxidant properties may have the potential to prevent BH_4 oxidation and eNOS uncoupling.
- Regulation of NO bioactivity by reducing the levels of reactive oxygen species (ROS): NO can be rapidly inactivated by superoxide. A reduction of oxidative stress (by downregulating ROS-producing enzymes, upregulating antioxidant enzymes, or by ROS scavenging activities) may enhance NO bioactivity by two means: prevention of eNOS uncoupling and reduction of superoxide-mediated NO inactivation [1].

3. Searching for eNOS-enhancing Chinese herbs

Numerous Chinese herbs have been shown to enhance endothelial NO production. These reports are summarized in Table 1. This chapter focuses on our own findings.

EA.hy 926 cells are an immortalized endothelial cell line derived from human umbilical vein endothelial cells (HUVEC). This cell line has been generated by fusing HUVEC with the permanent human alveolar epithelial cell line A549 [14]. We cloned the 5'-flanking region (3.5 kb in length) of the human eNOS gene into pGL_3-neo, which contains a promoterless luciferase reporter gene and a neomycin resistance gene [15]. Stable transfection of EA.hy 926 cells with this construct (selection using G418) resulted in an immortalized human endothelial cell line (termed "stable EA.hy cells" for simplicity) that expresses the luciferase gene driven by the human eNOS promoter. Luciferase activity in cell homogenates, which can be easily measured in a luminometer or on a chemiluminescence plate reader, is used as a determinant of promoter activity of the human eNOS gene.

To search for eNOS-regulating Chinese herbs, we generated aqueous extracts of 17 herbs possessing "circulation-improving" effects according to traditional Chinese medicine (TCM) [16]. These were:

- Angelicae sinensis radix
- Astragali radix
- Carthami flos
- Celosiae semen
- Chrysanthemi indici flos
- Eucommiae cortex
- Ligustici radix
- Metaphyreum roseum
- Moutan radicis cortex
- Paeoniae rubrae radix
- Panacis notoginseng radix
- Persicae semen
- Prunella vulgaris L.
- Puerariae radix
- Salviae miltiorrhizae radix
- Uncariae ramulus et unci
- Zizyphi spinosae semen

Human EA.hy 926 endothelial cells stably transfected with a 3.5 kb fragment of the human eNOS promoter (stable EA.hy cells) were treated with each extract (corresponding to 5 g of raw plant extract per ml) at dilutions of 1:100000 to 1:300 for 18 hours to study their effects on eNOS promoter activity. Ten herbal extracts increased eNOS promoter activity in a concentration-dependent manner with a maximal effect over 150%: *Carthami flos, Chrysanthemi indici flos, Eucommiae cortex, Ligustici radix, Paeoniae rubrae radix, Prunella vulgaris L., Puerariae radix, Uncariae ramulus et unci, Salviae miltiorrhizae radix* and *Zizyphi spinosae semen*.

These ten herbal extracts were further analyzed in a second screening (RNase protection assay) for their effect on eNOS mRNA levels in normal EA.hy 926 cells. In this experiment, only *Prunella vulgaris L., Salviae miltiorrhizae radix* and *Zizyphi spinosae semen* significantly increased eNOS mRNA expression [16].

Our screening procedure using stable EA.hy cells has some limitations: (i) it is based on eNOS promoter activity and the positive results must be verified by additional methods for analyses of mRNA expression to exclude false positive hits. (ii) Herbs/compounds that regulate NO production via mechanisms other than modulating eNOS expression will provide false negative results. For example, *Astragali radix* had no effect on eNOS expression and was negative in our screening. However, *Astragali radix* can stimulate NO production from eNOS by enhancing eNOS enzymatic activity [17]. Despite of its limitations, this screening procedure has the advantages of being a low-cost method of relatively high efficiency which is easy to perform. Because of these strengths, it has also been used by pharmaceutical companies in the screening for eNOS enhancers [18]. Based on this screening, we have identified *Prunella vulgaris L., Salviae miltiorrhizae radix* and *Zizyphi spinosae semen* as eNOS-regulating Chinese herbs.

Plant	Compounds / extracts	Cells / models	Effects on eNOS	Additional effects	References
Astragali radix	extract	HUVEC	eNOS activity↑	VEGF↑, PI3K-Akt↑, angiogenesis↑	[17]
Epimedii herba	icariin	coronary artery isolated from canine	eNOS activity↑	vasodilation	[74]
Ginseng	ginsenosides	I/R in Langendorff hearts; HAEC	eNOS-P↑	cardiac function↑, coronary perfusion flow↑, prostacyclin↑, PI3K-Akt↑	[75]
Ginseng (Korean red ginseng)	saponin fraction	Hypertensive rats	eNOS activity↑	blood pressure↓	[76]
Magnolia officinalis	honokiol	oxLDL-treated HUVEC	eNOS protein expression↑	adhesion molecules↓, EC-monocyte interaction↓, LDL-oxidation↓, ROS↓	[77]
Panax notoginseng	saponin extract	HUVEC / zebrafish	eNOS-P↑	angiogenesis↑, VEGF↑, PI3K-Akt↑	[78]
Polygonum multiflorum	TSG	aorta isolated from fat-fed rats	eNOS expression↑	endothelial function↑, intimal remodeling↓ , iNOS↓	[79]
Pueraria lobata	puerarin	fat-fed rats	eNOS expression↑	cholesterol↓	[80]
Prunella vulgaris	extract	EA.hy / HUVEC	eNOS expression↑	NO↑	[16]
Salvia miltiorrhiza (Danshen)	crypto-tanshinone	HUVEC	eNOS expression↑	ET-1↓, NF-κB↓	[81]
	magnesium lithospermate B	HUVEC (hyperglycemia) / OLETF rats	eNOS-P↑	Endothelial function↑ Akt↑, Nrf-2↑, HO-1↑	[82]
	tanshinone IIA	angiotensin II-treated rat cardiac fibroblasts	eNOS-P↑	ET-1↓, ROS↓, fibroblast proliferation ↓	[83]
	tanshinone IIA	renovascular hypertension model in hamsters	eNOS expression↑ eNOS -P↑	Vasodilation, blood pressure↓	[84]
	extract / ursolic acid	EA.hy 926 / HUVEC	eNOS expression↑	NADPH oxidase↓	[24]
	extract	rat hypoxic pulmonary hypertension	eNOS expression↑	media thickening↓, iNOS↓	[85]
Seabuckthorn	flavonoids	EA.hy 926	eNOS expression↑	LOX-1↓, cell death↓	[86]

Plant	Compounds / extracts	Cells / models	Effects on eNOS	Additional effects	References
Sophora flavescens roots	matrine	RIMEC	eNOS expression↑	IL-6, IL-8 & sICAM-1↓	[87]
Szechwan lovage rhizome	TMP	Cerebral vasospasm in rabbit	eNOS expression↑	cerebral vasospasm↓	[88]
Xanthoceras sorbifolia	ethanol extract	Rat aorta	eNOS activity↑	vasodilation	[89]
Zizyphi Spinosi semen	betulinic acid	EA.hy / HUVEC	eNOS expression↑	ROS↓	[62]
Combinations & compounds					
A&A	decoction	obstructed rat kidney	eNOS activity↑	renal fibrosis↓, ROS↓	[90]
ELCAS	extract	H_2O_2-treated ECV304	eNOS expression↑	SOD↑, CAT↑, GPx↑	[91]
Qing Huo Yi Hao	TMP	glucose-treated bEnd.3	eNOS-P↑	ROS↓, Akt↑, UCP2↑	[92]
Refined Qing Kai Ling	injection	MCAO in rats	eNOS expression↑	infarct size↓	[93]
Shen-fu	injection	myocardial I/R in diabetic rats	eNOS-P↑	infarct size↓, Akt↑	[94]
Tongxinluo	compound	HUVEC / aortic rings from rats on a methionine-rich diet	eNOS expression↑	Endothelial function↑, PI3K- Akt↑	[95]
		myocardial no-reflow and I/R in minipigs	eNOS-P↑	PKA↑, infarct size↓	[96]

A&A, a combination of roots Astragalus membranaceus var. mongholicus and Angelica sinensis; bEnd.3, mouse brain microvascular cells; CAT, catalase; EA.hy 926, an immortalized human endothelial cell line derived from HUVEC; ECV 304, a misidentified (as endothelial cells) human bladder cell line of epithelial origin; ELCAS, an extract of Ligusticum chuanxiong and Angelica sinensis; eNOS-P, eNOS phosphorylation at serine 1177; GPx, glutathione peroxidase; HAEC, human aortic endothelial cells; HO-1, heme oxygenase-1; H/R, hypoxia/reoxygenation; HUVEC, human umbilical vein endothelial cells; I/R, ischemia-reperfusion injury; MCAO, middle cerebral artery occlusion; Nrf-2, nuclear factor erythroid 2-related factor-2; OLETF, Otsuka Long-Evans Tokushima Fatty rats; RIMEC, rat intestinal microvascular endothelial cells; ROS, reactive oxygen species; SOD, superoxide dismutase; TMP, tetramethylpyrazine; TSG, 2,3,4',5-tetrahydroxystilbene 2-O-beta-D-glucoside; UCP2, uncoupling protein 2.

Table 1. Effects of Chinese herbs on endothelial NO production.

3.1 *Prunella vulgaris L.* (PVL)

PVL is used in TCM as well as in Western herbal medicine. In the West, the plant has been used primarily as a remedy to alleviate pains in the throat, to treat fevers and to accelerate wound healing. Modern pharmacological studies have revealed a wide array of biological effects and numerous therapeutic possibilities for the herb, including anti-viral and anti-bacterial effects, immunomodulatory, anti-allergy and anti-cancer potential, as well as antioxidant activity [16].

In TCM, PVL (fruiting spikes) is used as an anti-microbial, anti-inflammatory and anti-tumor drug [19], but it is also commonly used as a component in combination therapy for hypertension.

PVL extracts relax isolated epinephrine-precontracted rabbit aorta [20]. Intravenous injection of PVL saponins results in a reduction of both systolic and diastolic blood pressures in anesthetized rats [21]. A PVL-containing Chinese herb combination (consisting of *Crataegus pinnatifida Bge, Uncariae ramulus et uncis, Alisma orientalis radix* and PVL at 1:1:1:1, w/w) reduces blood pressure and lowers cholesterol and triglyceride in hypertensive and hypercholesterolemic patients [22].

Our study demonstrated that PVL is an effective eNOS-upregulating herb; it significantly increases eNOS promoter activity, eNOS mRNA and protein expression and NO production in human endothelial cells [16].

PVL extracts contain a variety of chemical constituents, including triterpenoids (such as ursolic acid, betulinic acid, oleanolic acid, vulgarsaponins), steroids (such as β-sitosterol, stigmasterol, α-spinasterol), flavonoids (such as rosmarinic acid, luteolin, cynaroside, homoorientin, quercetin), coumarins (such as umbelliferone, scopoletin, esculetin), organic acids (such as caffeic acid, palmitic acid, stearic acid, oleic acid, arachidic acid, lauric acid, myristic acid), sugars, as well as essential oils [23].

Importantly, our studies have demonstrated that ursolic acid (also present in *Salviae miltiorrhizae radix*) [24], betulinic acid (also a constituent of *Zizyphi spinosae semen*) [24], luteolin and cynaroside (also constituents of artichoke, *Cynara scolymus L.*) [25] are eNOS-upregulating compounds. Ursolic acid and betulinic acid are two of the main PVL triterpenoids; luteolin and cynaroside are two of the main PVL flavonoids [23]. Therefore, these four compounds, possibly in combination with other yet unidentified compounds, may be responsible for the observed eNOS-upregulating effect of PVL.

Our recent experience indicates that the effects of PVL on eNOS may vary significantly from batch to batch. With the last two batches of PVL products we bought recently, we could not find any eNOS-enhancing activities. This might be due to concentration variation of the active constituents in the PVL plant.

3.2 *Salviae miltiorrhizae radix* (Danshen)

Danshen, the dried root of *Salvia miltiorrhiza* Bunge (Lamiaceae), is one of the most commonly used TCM remedies. A Danshen-containing preparation was the first TCM product approved for phase II and III clinical trials by the Food and Drug Administration (FDA) [26]. Ancient TCM books describe Danshen as a drug "improving circulation" and "removing blood stasis". Today, Danshen is available in China, Japan, the United States, and also in many European countries and is used for the treatment of angina pectoris, hyperlipidemia, and acute ischemic stroke [26]. Clinical trials have indicated that Danshen preparations are superior to nitroglycerin or isosorbide dinitrate for the treatment of stable angina pectoris, with respect to efficacy and side effects [27, 28].

Various *in vitro* and *in vivo* studies have demonstrated that several constituents of Danshen can improve microcirculation, dilate coronary arteries, increase blood flow, and prevent myocardial ischemia. Aqueous Danshen extracts and purified active principles of Danshen (tanshinones) have been shown to cause vasodilation of coronary, renal, femoral, and mesenteric arteries, and suppress systemic blood pressure in rats and rabbits [29, 30]. In a rat acute myocardial infarction model, Danshen extracts increased the survival rate and reduced the infarct size to an extent comparable with that of the angiotensin converting enzyme inhibitor ramipril [31]. Tanshinone IIA, a pharmacologically active component isolated from Danshen, reduced myocardial infarct size by about 50% in a rabbit ischemia-reperfusion model [32].

Interestingly, the cardiovascular protective effects of Danshen resemble the action profile of endothelium-derived NO. Danshen extracts and constituents inhibit platelet aggregation [33] and attenuate neutrophil-endothelial adhesion [34]. Danshen also lowers plasma cholesterol levels, enhances smooth muscle apoptosis and attenuates neointimal hyperplasia in the balloon-injured abdominal aorta of hypercholesterolemic rabbits [35]. Danshen has also been shown to reduce lipid peroxidation, inhibit LDL oxidation, and reduce atherosclerosis in cholesterol-fed rabbits [36].

In stable EA.hy cells we have identified Danshen as an eNOS-enhancer. Danshen extracts increase eNOS promoter activity, eNOS mRNA and protein expression, as well as endothelial NO production [24]. Danshen extracts contain large amounts of polyphenolic compounds with antioxidant properties [26, 37]. This may prevent BH_4 oxidation and eNOS uncoupling.

So far, more than 100 compounds have been isolated and identified from Danshen. Most of the lipophilic compounds are diterpene chinone compounds of the tanshinone type, including tanshinone I, IIA, and IIB, cryptotanshinone, dihydrotanshinone, and other related compounds [26, 37]. Hydrophilic constituents include polyphenolic acids (such as various salvianolic acids) and related compounds (such as danshensu, i.e. salvianic acid A, protocatechuic aldehyde, and protocatechuic acid); but also rosmarinic acid and isoferulic acid. Baicalin and ursolic acid have been isolated from alcohol extracts of Danshen [26].

In EA.hy 926 cells, an aqueous extract of Danshen and a methanol extract of the plant increase eNOS promoter activity, eNOS mRNA and protein expression. On the contrary, a dichloromethane extract does not change eNOS gene expression [24]. Thus, hydrophilic and alcohol-soluble, but not lipophilic constituents of Danshen seem to be responsible for its eNOS-upregulating effect. Accordingly, the commercially available lipophilic compounds (tanshinone I, tanshinone IIA, cryptotanshinone and dihydrotanshinone) of Danshen have no effect on eNOS expression in EA.hy 926 cells [24]. We have also tested several commercially available hydrophilic compounds, including protocatechuic acid, protocatechuic aldehyde, rosmarinic acid, isoferulic acid, salvianic acid A, and salvianolic acid B. They show no significant effects on eNOS expression [24]. Therefore, the hydrophilic compounds that are responsible for the eNOS-upregulating effect of Danshen still remain to be identified. Among the alcohol-soluble compounds, we have found that ursolic acid, but not baicalin, significantly enhances eNOS mRNA and protein expression [24]. Therefore, ursolic acid is likely to represent one of the compounds responsible for enhanced eNOS expression in response to Danshen.

3.3 Ursolic acid

Ursolic acid is a secondary plant metabolite not only found in Danshen [38], but also widespread in some other plants including apple pomace, rosemary leaves, and sage leaves (*Salvia officinalis*) [39]. This pentacyclic triterpenoid has emerged as a multifunctional compound with diverse pharmacological properties, including anticancer, antioxidant, anti-inflammatory, anti-HIV, antimicrobial, and hepatoprotective activities. Currently, ursolic acid is in human clinical trials for treating cancer and skin wrinkles [40, 41]. In addition, ursolic acid possesses anti-obestic and anti-diabetic effects. It prevents abdominal adiposity

[42, 43], improves pancreatic beta-cell function [44], ameliorates glucose intolerance [45], inhibits hepatic glucose production in diabetic mice [46], and inhibits diabetic nephropathy [47, 48].

Also in the cardiovascular system, ursolic acid shows therapeutic effects. In rat models of hypertension, ursolic acid prevents the development of severe hypertension which may be attributed to a potent diuretic/saluretic activity and a negative chronotropic effect. In addition, ursolic acid shows antihyperlipidemic (reduction of LDL and triglycerides), antioxidant (upregulation of glutathione peroxidase, GPx, and superoxide dismutase, SOD), and hypoglycemic effects [49].

The reported effects of ursolic acid on atherogenesis are controversial. TNFα-induced E-selectin expression is shown to be suppressed by ursolic acid via the inhibition of NF-κB [50]. In the rat carotid artery injury model, ursolic acid has been demonstrated to inhibit neointima formation [51]. In contrast, a recent study has shown that oral treatment of apolipoprotein E-knockout mice with ursolic acid for 24 weeks accelerates atherosclerotic plaque formation in a dose-dependent manner [52]. In the latter study, ursolic acid inhibited endothelial proliferation and induced endothelial cell death. Ursolic acid caused DNA damage, followed by the activation of a p53-, BAK-, and caspase-dependent cell-death pathway [52]. Further studies are needed to clarify this controversy.

We have provided the first evidence that ursolic acid enhances eNOS mRNA and protein expression in human endothelial cells [24]. This leads to increased NO production and improved endothelial cell function. In a recent study by Lee et al., treatment of human coronary artery endothelial cells with ursolic acid increased tube formation, endothelial cell migration capacities and the expression of allograft inflammatory factor-1 (AIF-1, a mediator of vasculogenesis) through an NO-related mechanism [53]. In a mouse hind limb ischemia model, ursolic acid enhanced eNOS and AIF-1 expression, and increased collateral blood flow and capillary density through the induction of neovascularization [53].

In addition to this stimulatory effect on gene expression observed at concentrations of 1-10 μM, ursolic acid at higher concentrations also stimulated eNOS activity. In organ chamber experiments with isolated rat aorta, ursolic acid (and a methanolic extract of *Lepechinia caulescens*) induced an endothelium-dependent, NO-mediated vasodilation (EC_{50} for ursolic acid 44 μM) [54].

Ursolic acid also possesses anti-oxidative effects. It has been shown to reduce endothelial superoxide production by suppressing the expression of NOX4 [24], which is the predominant NADPH oxidase isoform in endothelial cells [55]. In addition, ursolic acid also enhances ROS inactivation by upregulating the expression/activity of antioxidant enzymes, e.g., GPx and SOD [49]. Thus, ursolic acid may also have the potential to prevent BH_4 oxidation and eNOS uncoupling.

3.4 *Zizyphi spinosae semen* (ZSS)

ZSS is a sedative and hypnotic drug with additional effects on the cardiovascular system [19]. ZSS protects cardiomyocytes from ischemic injury, and oxygen and glucose deprivation-induced damage of cultured neonatal rat myocardial cells can be markedly reduced by ZSS total saponins [56]. Anoxia/reoxygenation of cultured neonatal rat myocardial cells results in increased intracellular malondialdehyde and lipid peroxides, increased intercellular calcium concentration and decreased SOD activity. All of these parameters can be reversed by ZSS total saponins [56, 57].

ZSS has also antihypertensive effects. Intravenous injection of an aqueous solution of ZSS extract markedly decreases blood pressure in anesthetized rats, dogs, and cats without any significant effect on coronary blood flow, heart rate, or myocardial contractility [58]. Oral treatment of spontaneously hypertensive rats with ZSS jujubosides resultes in a reduction in blood pressure [59]. Blood pressure reduction can be observed as early as 30 min and lasted for at least 3.5 h; the effect declined after 7.5 h [59]. Moreover, treatment of hypercholesterolemic rabbits with ZSS for three months leads to a reduction in total cholesterol, LDL cholesterol and triglycerides, an increase in HDL and a decrease in atherosclerotic lesions [60].

The molecular mechanisms underlying these cardiovascular effects are poorly understood. Interestingly, treatment of rats with ZSS resulted in increased plasma levels of NO through unknown mechanisms [61]. We have found that ZSS increases eNOS promoter activity, eNOS mRNA and protein expression, as well as NO production in human endothelial cells [62].

The active constituents of ZSS include saponins, triterpenoids, flavonoids, alkaloids, and fatty acids [19, 63, 64]. The most important ZSS saponins are triterpenoid oligoglycosides, such as jujubosides A and B. Triterpenoids found in ZSS include betulin and betulinic acid [63, 65].

Jujuboside A, B and betulin show no effect on eNOS promoter activity or eNOS mRNA expression. Interestingly, treatment of human endothelial cells with betulinic acid results in a significant up-regulation of eNOS mRNA and protein expression [62]. The content of betulinic acid in ZSS is approximately 7 mg/kg [63]. When cells are treated with this ZSS extract (concentration of 5 g/ml) at a 1:100 dilution, the estimated final concentration of betulinic acid is in the low micromolar range. In our study, betulinic acid increases eNOS mRNA expression even at 1 μM. Thus, betulinic acid is likely to be one of the compounds responsible for the eNOS up-regulation induced by ZSS [62].

3.5 Betulinic acid

The pentacyclic triterpenoid betulinic acid is not only found in ZSS, but is also widespread in fruit peel, leaves and stem bark of several species of plants, including white birch bark (*Betula pubescens*), plane bark (*Plantanus acerifolia*), rosemary leaves (*Rosmarinus officinalis*), Ber tree (*Ziziphus mauritiana*) and selfheal (*Prunella vulgaris*) [39, 66]. The compound is mainly known for its anti-tumor, anti-viral and anti-inflammatory activities [66, 67]. Our study has identified betulinic acid as an eNOS-stimulating compound [62].

Interestingly, accumulating data in the recent years support a protective effect of betulinic acid in the cardiovascular system. In a rat renal ischemia/reperfusion (I/R) injury model, betulinic acid attenuates I/R-induced oxidant responses, inhibits microscopic damage, and improves renal function by regulating the apoptotic function of leukocytes and inhibiting neutrophil infiltration [68]. Recently, betulinic acid and ursolic acid have been identified as selective agonists of the G protein-coupled receptor TGR5, which plays an important role in the control of energy metabolism. This suggests the therapeutic potential of betulinic acid and ursolic acid for metabolic diseases [69].

In HUVEC, betulinic acid has been shown to inhibit TNFα-induced ROS production and NF-κB activation. The resulting inhibition of endothelial activation and leukocyte adhesion points to a protective role of the compound against vascular inflammation [70].

We have found that betulinic acid upregulates eNOS expression in endothelial cells [62]. As mentioned above, upregulation of eNOS does not necessarily result in an increase in bioactive NO. Under pathological conditions of oxidative stress, eNOS is often uncoupled and dysfunctional. The primary cause of eNOS uncoupling is a deficiency of its cofactor BH_4 due to oxidative stress-mediated oxidation (e.g. by peroxynitrite) [1, 12]. Importantly, betulinic acid also reduces the expression of NADPH oxidases (NOX4 and p22phox) [62], a major source of ROS in the vasculature [71]. We have demonstrated that betulic acid reduces the levels of peroxynitrite in the mouse *in vivo* [72]. These results suggest the potential of betulinic acid to reverse eNOS uncoupling. In a mouse stroke model, betulinic acid upregulates eNOS and downregulated NADPH oxidases, events which are associated with a reduction in infarct size [72].
Our recent results indicate that betulinic acid not only enhances eNOS expression but also enhances eNOS enzymatic activity. Treatment of human endothelial cells with betulinic acid leads to phosphorylation of eNOS at serine 1177 and dephosphorylation of eNOS at threonine 495, and an increase in NO production [Hohmann N, Xia N, Forstermann U and Li H, unpublished data]. This is consistent with a recent report demonstrating that betulinic acid induces an endothelium-dependent, NO-mediated relaxation of isolated rat aorta [73].

4. Conclusion

Numerous vasoactive Chinese herbs possess stimulating effects on endothelial NO production, e.g. by enhancing eNOS expression and/or by modulating eNOS phosphorylation status. Such molecular events are likely to be contributing mechanisms for the therapeutic effects of these herbs described in traditional Chinese medicine.

5. References

[1] Li H, Forstermann U. Prevention of atherosclerosis by interference with the vascular nitric oxide system. *Curr Pharm Des.* 2009; 15: 3133-3145.
[2] Li H, Forstermann U. Nitric oxide in the pathogenesis of vascular disease. *J Pathol.* 2000; 190: 244-254.
[3] Csiszar A, Labinskyy N, Pinto JT, Ballabh P, Zhang H, Losonczy G, Pearson K, de Cabo R, Pacher P, Zhang C, Ungvari Z. Resveratrol induces mitochondrial biogenesis in endothelial cells. *Am J Physiol Heart Circ Physiol.* 2009; 297: H13-20.
[4] Nisoli E, Tonello C, Cardile A, Cozzi V, Bracale R, Tedesco L, Falcone S, Valerio A, Cantoni O, Clementi E, Moncada S, Carruba MO. Calorie restriction promotes mitochondrial biogenesis by inducing the expression of eNOS. *Science.* 2005; 310: 314-317.
[5] Li H, Wallerath T, Munzel T, Forstermann U. Regulation of endothelial-type NO synthase expression in pathophysiology and in response to drugs. *Nitric Oxide.* 2002; 7: 149-164.
[6] Li H, Wallerath T, Forstermann U. Physiological mechanisms regulating the expression of endothelial-type NO synthase. *Nitric Oxide.* 2002; 7: 132-147.
[7] Fleming I. Molecular mechanisms underlying the activation of eNOS. *Pflugers Arch.* 2010; 459: 793-806.
[8] Mattagajasingh I, Kim CS, Naqvi A, Yamamori T, Hoffman TA, Jung SB, DeRicco J, Kasuno K, Irani K. SIRT1 promotes endothelium-dependent vascular relaxation by

activating endothelial nitric oxide synthase. *Proc Natl Acad Sci USA.* 2007; 104: 14855-14860.

[9] Maas R, Boger R, Luneburg N. ADMA and the role of the genes: lessons from genetically modified animals and human gene polymorphisms. *Pharmacol Res.* 2009; 60: 475-480.

[10] Pope AJ, Karuppiah K, Cardounel AJ. Role of the PRMT-DDAH-ADMA axis in the regulation of endothelial nitric oxide production. *Pharmacol Res.* 2009; 60: 461-465.

[11] Forstermann U, Li H. Therapeutic effect of enhancing endothelial nitric oxide synthase (eNOS) expression and preventing eNOS uncoupling. *Br J Pharmacol.* 2010: DOI: 10.1111/j.1476-5381.2010.01196.x.

[12] Forstermann U, Munzel T. Endothelial nitric oxide synthase in vascular disease: from marvel to menace. *Circulation.* 2006; 113: 1708-1714.

[13] Xia N, Daiber A, Habermeier A, Closs EI, Thum T, Spanier G, Lu Q, Oelze M, Torzewski M, Lackner KJ, Münzel T, Förstermann U, Li H. Resveratrol reverses endothelial nitric-oxide synthase uncoupling in apolipoprotein E knockout mice. *J Pharmacol Exp Ther.* 2010; 335: 149-154.

[14] Edgell CJ, McDonald CC, Graham JB. Permanent cell line expressing human factor VIII-related antigen established by hybridization. *Proc Natl Acad Sci USA.* 1983; 80: 3734-3737.

[15] Li H, Oehrlein SA, Wallerath T, Ihrig-Biedert I, Wohlfart P, Ulshofer T, Jessen T, Herget T, Forstermann U, Kleinert H. Activation of protein kinase C alpha and/or epsilon enhances transcription of the human endothelial nitric oxide synthase gene. *Mol Pharmacol.* 1998; 53: 630-637.

[16] Xia N, Bollinger L, Steinkamp-Fenske K, Forstermann U, Li H. Prunella vulgaris L. Upregulates eNOS expression in human endothelial cells. *Am J Chin Med.* 2010; 38: 599-611.

[17] Zhang Y, Hu G, Lin HC, Hong SJ, Deng YH, Tang JY, Seto SW, Kwan YW, Waye MM, Wang YT, Lee SM. Radix Astragali extract promotes angiogenesis involving vascular endothelial growth factor receptor-related phosphatidylinositol 3-kinase/Akt-dependent pathway in human endothelial cells. *Phytother Res.* 2009; 23: 1205-1213.

[18] Wohlfart P, Xu H, Endlich A, Habermeier A, Closs EI, Hubschle T, Mang C, Strobel H, Suzuki T, Kleinert H, Forstermann U, Ruetten H, Li H. Antiatherosclerotic effects of small-molecular-weight compounds enhancing endothelial nitric-oxide synthase (eNOS) expression and preventing eNOS uncoupling. *J Pharmacol Exp Ther.* 2008; 325: 370-379.

[19] Huang KC. *The pharmacology of Chinese herbs.* Second edition ed. Boca Raton: CRC Press; 1999.

[20] Sun H, Yuan B, Liu B, Zhang C. The effect of Prunella vulgaris L. extracts on isolated rabbit artery. *Xi'an Jiao Tong Da Xue Xue Bao.* 2005; 26: 19-21.

[21] Wang HB, Zhang ZY, Su ZW, Li CG. [The effect of total saponins from common selfheal (Prunella vulgaris) on experimental myocardial infarction and hypertension of anesthetized rats]. *Zhong Cao Yao.* 1994; 25: 264-266.

[22] Heart-Disease-Group. [Clinical observation with Jiangya-Jiangzhi-chongji]. *Zhonghua Xin Xue Guan Bing Za Zhi.* 1976; 16: 54-56.

[23] Liu Y, Song S-J, Xu S-X. [Advances in the study on the chemical constituents and biological activities of Prunella vulgaris L.]. *Journal of Shenyang Pharmaceutical University*. 2003; 20: 55-59.

[24] Steinkamp-Fenske K, Bollinger L, Voller N, Xu H, Yao Y, Bauer R, Forstermann U, Li H. Ursolic acid from the Chinese herb danshen (Salvia miltiorrhiza L.) upregulates eNOS and downregulates Nox4 expression in human endothelial cells. *Atherosclerosis*. 2007; 195: e104-111.

[25] Li H, Xia N, Brausch I, Yao Y, Forstermann U. Flavonoids from artichoke (Cynara scolymus L.) up-regulate endothelial-type nitric-oxide synthase gene expression in human endothelial cells. *J Pharmacol Exp Ther*. 2004; 310: 926-932.

[26] Zhou L, Zuo Z, Chow MS. Danshen: an overview of its chemistry, pharmacology, pharmacokinetics, and clinical use. *J Clin Pharmacol*. 2005; 45: 1345-1359.

[27] Wang G, Wang L, Xiong ZY, Mao B, Li TQ. Compound salvia pellet, a traditional Chinese medicine, for the treatment of chronic stable angina pectoris compared with nitrates: a meta-analysis. *Med Sci Monit*. 2006; 12: SR1-7.

[28] Zhang JH, Shang HC, Gao XM, Zhang BL, Xiang YZ, Cao HB, Ren M, Wang H. Compound Salvia droplet pill, a traditional Chinese medicine, for the treatment of unstable angina pectoris: a systematic review. *Med Sci Monit*. 2008; 14: RA1-7.

[29] Lam FF, Yeung JH, Cheung JH. Mechanisms of the dilator action of Danshen (Salvia miltiorrhiza) on rat isolated femoral artery. *J Cardiovasc Pharmacol*. 2005; 46: 361-368.

[30] Lei XL, Chiou GC. Studies on cardiovascular actions of Salvia miltiorrhiza. *Am J Chin Med*. 1986; 14: 26-32.

[31] Ji X, Tan BK, Zhu YC, Linz W, Zhu YZ. Comparison of cardioprotective effects using ramipril and DanShen for the treatment of acute myocardial infarction in rats. *Life Sci*. 2003; 73: 1413-1426.

[32] Wu TW, Zeng LH, Fung KP, Wu J, Pang H, Grey AA, Weisel RD, Wang JY. Effect of sodium tanshinone IIA sulfonate in the rabbit myocardium and on human cardiomyocytes and vascular endothelial cells. *Biochem Pharmacol*. 1993; 46: 2327-2332.

[33] Wang Z, Roberts JM, Grant PG, Colman RW, Schreiber AD. The effect of a medicinal Chinese herb on platelet function. *Thromb Haemost*. 1982; 48: 301-306.

[34] Chen YH, Lin SJ, Ku HH, Shiao MS, Lin FY, Chen JW, Chen YL. Salvianolic acid B attenuates VCAM-1 and ICAM-1 expression in TNF-alpha-treated human aortic endothelial cells. *J Cell Biochem*. 2001; 82: 512-521.

[35] Chen YL, Yang SP, Shiao MS, Chen JW, Lin SJ. Salvia miltiorrhiza inhibits intimal hyperplasia and monocyte chemotactic protein-1 expression after balloon injury in cholesterol-fed rabbits. *J Cell Biochem*. 2001; 83: 484-493.

[36] Wu YJ, Hong CY, Lin SJ, Wu P, Shiao MS. Increase of vitamin E content in LDL and reduction of atherosclerosis in cholesterol-fed rabbits by a water-soluble antioxidant-rich fraction of Salvia miltiorrhiza. *Arterioscler Thromb Vasc Biol*. 1998; 18: 481-486.

[37] Wang X, Morris-Natschke SL, Lee KH. New developments in the chemistry and biology of the bioactive constituents of Tanshen. *Med Res Rev*. 2007; 27: 133-148.

[38] Kong DY. Chemical constituents of Salvia miltiorrhiza. *Zhongguo Yiyao Gongye Zazhi*. 1989; 20: 279-285.

[39] Jager S, Trojan H, Kopp T, Laszczyk MN, Scheffler A. Pentacyclic triterpene distribution in various plants - rich sources for a new group of multi-potent plant extracts. *Molecules.* 2009; 14: 2016-2031.

[40] Sultana N. Clinically useful anticancer, antitumor, and antiwrinkle agent, ursolic acid and related derivatives as medicinally important natural product. *J Enzyme Inhib Med Chem.* 2011.

[41] Shao JW, Dai YC, Xue JP, Wang JC, Lin FP, Guo YH. In vitro and in vivo anticancer activity evaluation of ursolic acid derivatives. *Eur J Med Chem.* 2011; 46: 2652-2661.

[42] Kim J, Jang DS, Kim H, Kim JS. Anti-lipase and lipolytic activities of ursolic acid isolated from the roots of Actinidia arguta. *Arch Pharm Res.* 2009; 32: 983-987.

[43] Rao VS, Melo CL, Queiroz MG, Lemos TL, Menezes DB, Melo TS, Santos FA. Ursolic acid, a pentacyclic triterpene from Sambucus australis, prevents abdominal adiposity in mice fed a high-fat diet. *J Med Food.* 2011; in press. doi:10.1089/jmf.2010.0267.

[44] Jang SM, Yee ST, Choi J, Choi MS, Do GM, Jeon SM, Yeo J, Kim MJ, Seo KI, Lee MK. Ursolic acid enhances the cellular immune system and pancreatic beta-cell function in streptozotocin-induced diabetic mice fed a high-fat diet. *Int Immunopharmacol.* 2009; 9: 113-119.

[45] Jayaprakasam B, Olson LK, Schutzki RE, Tai MH, Nair MG. Amelioration of obesity and glucose intolerance in high-fat-fed C57BL/6 mice by anthocyanins and ursolic acid in Cornelian cherry (Cornus mas). *J Agric Food Chem.* 2006; 54: 243-248.

[46] Jang SM, Kim MJ, Choi MS, Kwon EY, Lee MK. Inhibitory effects of ursolic acid on hepatic polyol pathway and glucose production in streptozotocin-induced diabetic mice. *Metabolism.* 2010; 59: 512-519.

[47] Zhou Y, Li JS, Zhang X, Wu YJ, Huang K, Zheng L. Ursolic acid inhibits early lesions of diabetic nephropathy. *Int J Mol Med.* 2010; 26: 565-570.

[48] Wang ZH, Hsu CC, Huang CN, Yin MC. Anti-glycative effects of oleanolic acid and ursolic acid in kidney of diabetic mice. *Eur J Pharmacol.* 2010; 628: 255-260.

[49] Somova LO, Nadar A, Rammanan P, Shode FO. Cardiovascular, antihyperlipidemic and antioxidant effects of oleanolic and ursolic acids in experimental hypertension. *Phytomedicine.* 2003; 10: 115-121.

[50] Takada K, Nakane T, Masuda K, Ishii H. Ursolic acid and oleanolic acid, members of pentacyclic triterpenoid acids, suppress TNF-alpha-induced E-selectin expression by cultured umbilical vein endothelial cells. *Phytomedicine.* 2010; 17: 1114-1119.

[51] Pozo M, Castilla V, Gutierrez C, de Nicolas R, Egido J, Gonzalez-Cabrero J. Ursolic acid inhibits neointima formation in the rat carotid artery injury model. *Atherosclerosis.* 2006; 184: 53-62.

[52] Messner B, Zeller I, Ploner C, Frotschnig S, Ringer T, Steinacher-Nigisch A, Ritsch A, Laufer G, Huck C, Bernhard D. Ursolic acid causes DNA-damage, p53-mediated, mitochondria- and caspase-dependent human endothelial cell apoptosis, and accelerates atherosclerotic plaque formation in vivo. *Atherosclerosis.* 2011: doi:10.1016/j.atherosclerosis.2011.1005.1025.

[53] Lee AW, Chen TL, Shih CM, Huang CY, Tsao NW, Chang NC, Chen YH, Fong TH, Lin FY. Ursolic acid induces allograft inflammatory factor-1 expression via a nitric oxide-related mechanism and increases neovascularization. *J Agric Food Chem.* 2010; 58: 12941-12949.

[54] Aguirre-Crespo F, Vergara-Galicia J, Villalobos-Molina R, Javier Lopez-Guerrero J, Navarrete-Vazquez G, Estrada-Soto S. Ursolic acid mediates the vasorelaxant activity of Lepechinia caulescens via NO release in isolated rat thoracic aorta. *Life Sci.* 2006; 79: 1062-1068.

[55] Xu H, Goettsch C, Xia N, Horke S, Morawietz H, Forstermann U, Li H. Differential roles of PKCalpha and PKCepsilon in controlling the gene expression of Nox4 in human endothelial cells. *Free Radic Biol Med.* 2008; 44: 1656-1667.

[56] Chen XJ, Yu CL, Liu JF. [Protective effects of total saponins of semen Ziziphi spinosae on cultured rat myocardial cells]. *Zhongguo Yao Li Xue Bao.* 1990; 11: 153-155.

[57] Wan HY, Ding L, Kong XP, Liu SJ, Chen XJ. [Effect of total saponins of semen Ziziphi spinosae on hypoxia-reoxygenation injury in myocardial cells]. *Zhongguo Bingli Shengli Za Zhi.* 1997; 13: 522-526.

[58] Gu WX, Liu JF, Zhang JX, Liu XM, Liu JS, Chen YR. [Blood pressure-lowering effect and mechanism of total saponins from Ziziphus Mill seeds]. *Di Yi Jun Yi Da Xue Xue Bao.* 1987; 7: 8-10.

[59] Zhang D, Yuang BX, Sun H. [The effect of jujuboside on rats with spontaneous hypertension]. *Xi'an Jiao Tong Da Xue Xue Bao.* 2003; 24: 59-60.

[60] Wu SX, Lang XC, Jia BY, Zhao SX, Li MX, Lan MY. [Effects of Ziziphus spinosa Hu on serum lipoprotein and experimental atherosclerosis]. *Zhongguo Zhong Yao Za Zhi.* 1989; 14: 434-451, 448.

[61] Wang X, Xie M. [Effects of suanzaoren decoction on serum NO and the Level of cytokines in rats]. *Beijing Zhong Yi Yao Da Xue Xue Bao.* 2004; 11: 16-18.

[62] Steinkamp-Fenske K, Bollinger L, Xu H, Yao Y, Horke S, Forstermann U, Li H. Reciprocal regulation of endothelial nitric-oxide synthase and NADPH oxidase by betulinic acid in human endothelial cells. *J Pharmacol Exp Ther.* 2007; 322: 836-842.

[63] Li L-M, Liao X, Peng S-L, Ding L-S. Chemical constituents from the seeds of Ziziphus jujuba var. spinosa (Bunge) Hu. *Journal of Integrative Plant Biology.* 2005; 47: 494-498.

[64] Zhao J, Li SP, Yang FQ, Li P, Wang YT. Simultaneous determination of saponins and fatty acids in Ziziphus jujuba (Suanzaoren) by high performance liquid chromatography-evaporative light scattering detection and pressurized liquid extraction. *J Chromatogr A.* 2006; 1108: 188-194.

[65] Zhang M, Zhang Y, Xie J. Simultaneous determination of jujuboside A, B and betulinic acid in semen Ziziphi spinosae by high performance liquid chromatography-evaporative light scattering detection. *J Pharm Biomed Anal.* 2008; 48: 1467-1470.

[66] Mullauer FB, Kessler JH, Medema JP. Betulinic acid, a natural compound with potent anticancer effects. *Anticancer Drugs.* 2010; 21: 215-227.

[67] Fulda S. Betulinic acid: a natural product with anticancer activity. *Mol Nutr Food Res.* 2009; 53: 140-146.

[68] Eksioglu-Demiralp E, Kardas ER, Ozgul S, Yagci T, Bilgin H, Sehirli O, Ercan F, Sener G. Betulinic acid protects against ischemia/reperfusion-induced renal damage and inhibits leukocyte apoptosis. *Phytother Res.* 2010; 24: 325-332.

[69] Genet C, Strehle A, Schmidt C, Boudjelal G, Lobstein A, Schoonjans K, Souchet M, Auwerx J, Saladin R, Wagner A. Structure-activity relationship study of betulinic acid, a novel and selective TGR5 agonist, and its synthetic derivatives: potential impact in diabetes. *J Med Chem.* 2010; 53: 178-190.

[70] Yoon JJ, Lee YJ, Kim JS, Kang DG, Lee HS. Protective role of betulinic acid on TNF-alpha-induced cell adhesion molecules in vascular endothelial cells. *Biochem Biophys Res Commun.* 2010; 391: 96-101.

[71] Forstermann U. Oxidative stress in vascular disease: causes, defense mechanisms and potential therapies. *Nat Clin Pract Cardiovasc Med.* 2008; 5: 338-349.

[72] Lu Q, Xia N, Xu H, Guo L, Wenzel P, Daiber A, Munzel T, Forstermann U, Li H. Betulinic acid protects against cerebral ischemia-reperfusion injury in mice by reducing oxidative and nitrosative stress. *Nitric Oxide.* 2011; 24: 132-138.

[73] Fu JY, Xia ML, Lu JF, Liu Q, Cai X, Yang J, Wang HP, Xia Q. [Betulinic acid ameliorates impairment of endothelium-dependent relaxation induced by oxidative stress in rat aorta]. *Zhejiang Da Xue Xue Bao Yi Xue Ban.* 2010; 39: 523-529.

[74] Xu HB, Huang ZQ. Vasorelaxant effects of icariin on isolated canine coronary artery. *J Cardiovasc Pharmacol.* 2007; 49: 207-213.

[75] Yi XQ, Li T, Wang JR, Wong VK, Luo P, Wong IY, Jiang ZH, Liu L, Zhou H. Total ginsenosides increase coronary perfusion flow in isolated rat hearts through activation of PI3K/Akt-eNOS signaling. *Phytomedicine.* 2010; 17: 1006-1015.

[76] Jeon BH, Kim CS, Kim HS, Park JB, Nam KY, Chang SJ. Effect of Korean red ginseng on blood pressure and nitric oxide production. *Acta Pharmacol Sin.* 2000; 21: 1095-1100.

[77] Ou HC, Chou FP, Lin TM, Yang CH, Sheu WH. Protective effects of honokiol against oxidized LDL-induced cytotoxicity and adhesion molecule expression in endothelial cells. *Chem Biol Interact.* 2006; 161: 1-13.

[78] Hong SJ, Wan JB, Zhang Y, Hu G, Lin HC, Seto SW, Kwan YW, Lin ZX, Wang YT, Lee SM. Angiogenic effect of saponin extract from Panax notoginseng on HUVECs in vitro and zebrafish in vivo. *Phytother Res.* 2009; 23: 677-686.

[79] Zhang W, Xu XL, Wang YQ, Wang CH, Zhu WZ. Effects of 2,3,4',5-tetrahydroxystilbene 2-O-beta-D-glucoside on vascular endothelial dysfunction in atherogenic-diet rats. *Planta Med.* 2009; 75: 1209-1214.

[80] Yan LP, Chan SW, Chan AS, Chen SL, Ma XJ, Xu HX. Puerarin decreases serum total cholesterol and enhances thoracic aorta endothelial nitric oxide synthase expression in diet-induced hypercholesterolemic rats. *Life Sci.* 2006; 79: 324-330.

[81] Zhou Z, Wang SQ, Liu Y, Miao AD. Cryptotanshinone inhibits endothelin-1 expression and stimulates nitric oxide production in human vascular endothelial cells. *Biochim Biophys Acta.* 2006; 1760: 1-9.

[82] Kim SH, Choi M, Lee Y, Kim YO, Ahn DS, Kim YH, Kang ES, Lee EJ, Jung M, Cho JW, Williams DR, Lee HC. Natural therapeutic magnesium lithospermate B potently protects the endothelium from hyperglycaemia-induced dysfunction. *Cardiovasc Res.* 2010; 87: 713-722.

[83] Chan P, Liu JC, Lin LJ, Chen PY, Cheng TH, Lin JG, Hong HJ. Tanshinone IIA inhibits angiotensin II-induced cell proliferation in rat cardiac fibroblasts. *Am J Chin Med.* 2011; 39: 381-394.

[84] Kim DD, Sanchez FA, Duran RG, Kanetaka T, Duran WN. Endothelial nitric oxide synthase is a molecular vascular target for the Chinese herb Danshen in hypertension. *Am J Physiol Heart Circ Physiol.* 2007; 292: H2131-H2137.

[85] Chen Y, Ruan Y, Li L, Chu Y, Xu X, Wang Q, Zhou X. Effects of Salvia miltiorrhiza extracts on rat hypoxic pulmonary hypertension, heme oxygenase-1 and nitric oxide synthase. *Chin Med J (Engl).* 2003; 116: 757-760.

[86] Bao M, Lou Y. Flavonoids from seabuckthorn protect endothelial cells (EA.hy926) from oxidized low-density lipoprotein induced injuries via regulation of LOX-1 and eNOS expression. *J Cardiovasc Pharmacol.* 2006; 48: 834-841.

[87] Suo Z, Liu Y, Ferreri M, Zhang T, Liu Z, Mu X, Han B. Impact of matrine on inflammation related factors in rat intestinal microvascular endothelial cells. *J Ethnopharmacol.* 2009; 125: 404-409.

[88] Shao Z, Li J, Zhao Z, Gao C, Sun Z, Liu X. Effects of tetramethylpyrazine on nitric oxide/cGMP signaling after cerebral vasospasm in rabbits. *Brain Res.* 2010; 1361: 67-75.

[89] Jin SN, Wen JF, Kim HY, Kang DG, Lee HS, Cho KW. Vascular relaxation by ethanol extract of Xanthoceras sorbifolia via Akt- and SOCE-eNOS-cGMP pathways. *J Ethnopharmacol.* 2010; 132: 240-245.

[90] Meng L, Qu L, Tang J, Cai SQ, Wang H, Li X. A combination of Chinese herbs, Astragalus membranaceus var. mongholicus and Angelica sinensis, enhanced nitric oxide production in obstructed rat kidney. *Vascul Pharmacol.* 2007; 47: 174-183.

[91] Hou YZ, Zhao GR, Yang J, Yuan YJ, Zhu GG, Hiltunen R. Protective effect of Ligusticum chuanxiong and Angelica sinensis on endothelial cell damage induced by hydrogen peroxide. *Life Sci.* 2004; 75: 1775-1786.

[92] Kang Y, Hu M, Zhu Y, Gao X, Wang MW. Antioxidative effect of the herbal remedy Qin Huo Yi Hao and its active component tetramethylpyrazine on high glucose-treated endothelial cells. *Life Sci.* 2009; 84: 428-436.

[93] Hua Q, Zhu X, Li P, Tang H, Cai D, Xu Y, Jia X, Chen J, Shen Y. Refined Qing Kai Ling, traditional Chinese medicinal preparation, reduces ischemic stroke-induced infarct size and neurological deficits and increases expression of endothelial nitric oxide synthase. *Biol Pharm Bull.* 2008; 31: 633-637.

[94] Wu Y, Xia ZY, Meng QT, Zhu J, Lei S, Xu J, Dou J. Shen-Fu injection preconditioning inhibits myocardial ischemia-reperfusion injury in diabetic rats: activation of eNOS via the PI3K/Akt pathway. *J Biomed Biotechnol.* 2011; 2011: 384627.

[95] Liang JQ, Wu K, Jia ZH, Liu C, Ding J, Huang SN, Yin PP, Wu XC, Wei C, Wu YL, Wang HY. Chinese medicine Tongxinluo modulates vascular endothelial function by inducing eNOS expression via the PI-3K/Akt/HIF-dependent signaling pathway. *J Ethnopharmacol.* 2011; 133: 517-523.

[96] Li XD, Yang YJ, Geng YJ, Jin C, Hu FH, Zhao JL, Zhang HT, Cheng YT, Qian HY, Wang LL, Zhang BJ, Wu YL. Tongxinluo reduces myocardial no-reflow and ischemia-reperfusion injury by stimulating the phosphorylation of eNOS via the PKA pathway. *Am J Physiol Heart Circ Physiol.* 2010; 299: H1255-1261.

13

JIN Formula Inhibits Tumorigenesis Pathways in Human Lung Carcinoma Cells and Tumor Growth in Athymic Nude Mice

Yuhui Zhou et al.*
Nanjing University of Chinese Medicine,
Tianjing Medical University General Hospital,
Hongkong Baptist University, Hongkong,
China

1. Introduction

Lung cancer as the most common cancer in the world represents a major public health problem (1). Worldwide it has the highest rate of cancer mortality, exceeding the mortality rates of colorectal, breast and prostate cancers combined (2). Despite major advances in the treatment and management of lung cancer, most patients with lung cancer eventually die of this disease. Because conventional therapies have failed to make a major impact on survival, newer approaches are necessary in the battle against lung cancer. The poor lung cancer survival figures argue powerfully for new approaches to control this disease through chemoprevention, which has been defined as the use of agents that could reverse, suppress or completely halt tumor development. Developing novel mechanism-based chemopreventive approaches for lung cancer which humans can accept has become an important goal.

Many traditional Chinese medicine (TCM) formulas have been used in cancer therapy. JIN formula, an ancient herbal formula from classical book JIN KUI YAO LUE (Golden Chamber) for the treatment of lung cancer, which is composed of Ophiopogon japonicus 30g, Prepared Rhizoma Pinelliae15g, Ginseng radix 30g, Glycyrrhiza radix 12g, Peach Kernel 15g, Unprepared Coix lachryma jobi seed 30g, Chinese waxgourd seed 30g, and Phragmititis Caulis 30g. TCM theory regarded that lung cancer is related with both deficiency of Qi and Yin, or Qi insufficiency of the Spleen and Lung, as well as pathological changes of Qi stagnation, blood stasis, and accumulation of phlegm and toxin. Whereas, JIN formula could replenish both Qi and Yin, strengthen the Spleen and Lung, clear lung, resolve phlegm, activate blood circulation and remove stasis.

* Fei Xiong[1], Zhenzhou Huang[1], Luyu Zheng[1], Miao Jiang[1], Ming Jiang[3], Yuping Tang[1], Jian Ma[1], Zhen Zhan[1], Jinao Duan[1] and Xu Zhang[**,1],
[1]*Nanjing University of Chinese Medicine, China*
[2]*Tianjing Medical University General Hospital, China*
[3]*Hongkong Baptist University, Hongkong, China*
**Corresponding Author

We extracted JIN formula with different solvents, hereafter referred to as JIN formula extracts (JFE). It is hypothesized that JFE may afford chemopreventive as well as chemotherapeutic effects against lung cancer. In the present study, we first demonstrated the antiproliferative effects of JFE (including E1 to E8) in A549 cells. This involves the tumorigenesis network of cells. Next, we determined the chemopreventive potential of JFE on regulation of PI3K/Akt, MAPK, NF-kB pathways in A549 and H157 human lung carcinoma cells. Based on the results of our in vitro data, we next carried out in vivo study in mice. We found that oral administration of a human acceptable dose of JIN formula (3%, wt/vol) to athymic nude mice implanted with A549 and H157 cells resulted in significant inhibition of tumor growth.

2. Materials and methods

2.1 Materials

Akt, JNK, and p38 antibodies were obtained from Cell Signaling Technology. The polyclonal antibodies NF-kB/p65, ERK1/2 were procured from Santa Cruz Biotechnology Inc. Anti-mouse and anti-rabbit secondary antibody horseradish peroxidase (HRP) conjugate was obtained from Amersham Life Science Inc.

2.2 Methods

2.2.1 Preparation of JFE

Fresh JIN formula was decocted in distilled water. As shown in Figure 1, different solvents were applied to acquire the following eight extracts: Water extraction concentrate (E1), Ethanol precipitation (E2), Precipitates in ethanol recovery (E3), Ethanol concentration (E4), Cyclohexane extract (E5), Ethyl acetate extract (E6), N-butanol extract (E7) and Water solution (E8). The extracts were condensed and freeze dried. The freeze-dried extracts were stored at 4°C to be used for various treatments.

2.2.2 Cell culture and treatment

The human lung carcinoma A549 and H157 cells were obtained from American Type Culture Collection and cultured in DMEM medium, supplemented with 10% fetal bovine serum, 1% penicillin/streptomycin (P-S) in a 5% CO_2 atmosphere at 37°C. The extracts were dissolved in dimethyl sulfoxide (DMSO) and were used for the treatment of cells. A total of 50–60% confluent cells were treated with the extracts (1–100 μg/ml) for 72 h in complete growth medium.

2.2.3 Cell viability (MTT assay)

The effect of JFE on the viability of cells was determined by 3-[4,5-dimethylthiazol-2-yl]-2,5-diphenyl tetrazoliumbromide assay. The cells were plated at 1×10^4cells/well in 200 μl of complete culture medium containing 1–100 μg/ml concentrations of JFE in 96-well microtiter plates for 72 h. After incubation for specified times at 37°C in a humidified incubator, 3-[4,5-dimethylthiazol-2-yl]-2,5-diphenyl tetrazoliumbromide (5 mg/ml in PBS) was added to each well and incubated for 4 h, after which the plate was centrifuged at 1800g for 5 min at 4°C. The absorbance was recorded on a microplate reader at the wavelength of 540 nm. The effect of JFE on growth inhibition was assessed as percent cell viability where DMSO-treated cells were taken as 100% viable. DMSO at the concentrations used was without any effect on cell viability.

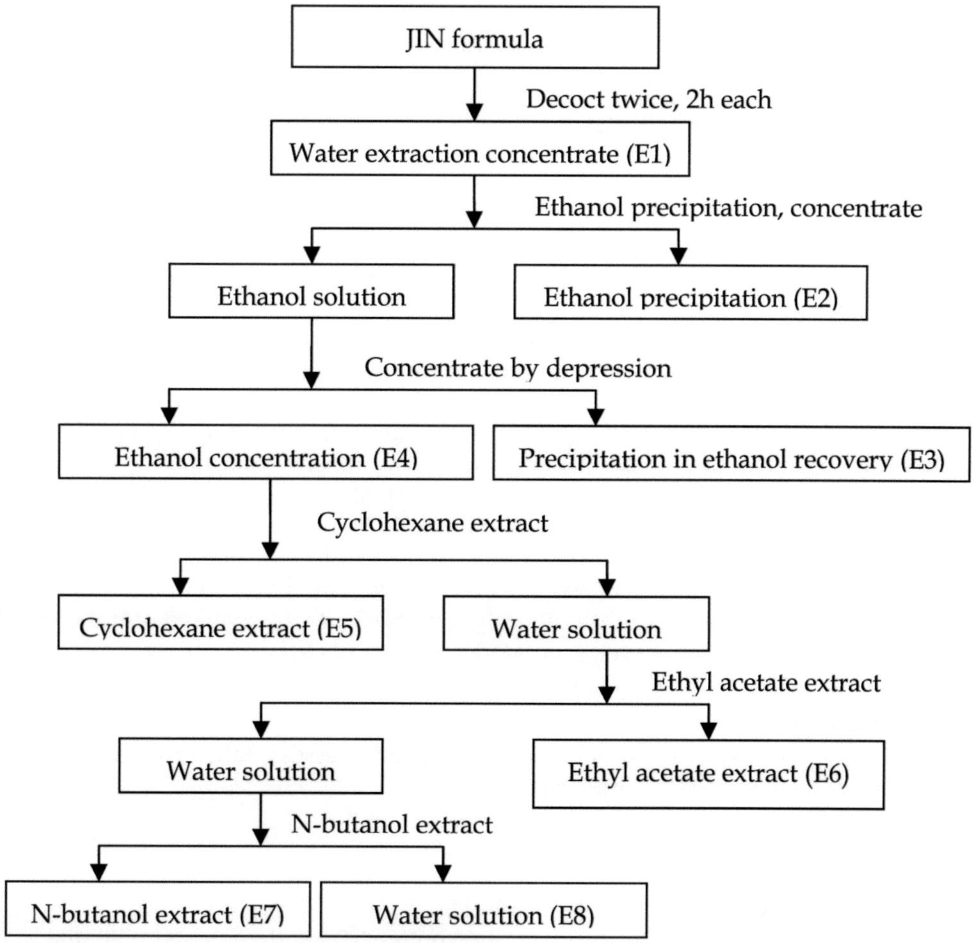

Fig. 1. The Extracting Procedure of JIN formula

2.2.4 Protein extraction and western blotting

Following the treatment of cells as described above, the media was aspirated, the cells were washed with cold PBS (pH 7.4), and ice-cold lysis buffer (50 mM Tris-HCl, 150 mM NaCl, 1 mM EGTA, 1 mM EDTA, 20 mM NaF, 100 mM Na_3VO_4, 0.5% NP-40, 1%Triton X-100, 1 mM PMSF (pH 7.4) with freshly added protease inhibitor cocktail (Protease Inhibitor Cocktail Set III; Calbiochem) over ice for 30 min. The cells were scraped and the lysate was collected in a microfuge tube and passed through needle to break up the cell aggregates. The lysate was cleared by centrifugation at 14 000g for 15 min at 4°C and the supernatant (whole cell lysate) was used or immediately stored at -80°C.

For western blotting, 30-50 mg protein was resolved over 8-12% polyacrylamide gels and transferred to a nitrocellulose membrane. The blot was blocked in blocking buffer (5% non-fat dry milk/1% Tween 20; in 20 mM TBS, pH 7.6) for 1 h at room temperature, incubated with appropriate monoclonal or polyclonal primary antibody in blocking buffer for 1.5 hours to overnight at 4 °C, followed by incubation with anti-mouse or anti-rabbit secondary antibody HRP conjugate obtained from Amersham Life Science Inc. Densitometric measurements of the band detected by chemiluminescence in western blot analysis were performed using digitalized scientific software program Quantity One.

2.2.5 In vivo tumor xenograft model

Balb/c athymic (nude) mice (male, 6–8 weeks) weighing 21–25 g were purchased from Animal Center, Academy of Military Medical Sciences, (Beijing, China) and were housed under specific pathogen-free conditions according to the guidelines of Animal Care, Nanjing University of Chinese Medicine. The animal room was controlled for temperature (22 ±2°C), light (12 hour light/dark cycle) and humidity (50±10%). All laboratory feed pellets and bedding was autoclaved.

The tumor regression model in nude mice has been successfully applied to evaluate antitumor activity. This model was therefore used to evaluate suppression of solid tumor growth in JIN Formula (JIN). A total of 1×10^7 A549, H157 cells in 0.2 ml culture medium were injected subcutaneously into the flank of each mouse using a 26-gauge needle. After 7 days observation, an apparently solid tumor mass was excised from mice inoculated with lung cancer cells. When the tumor volume reached about 50 mm^3 in the nude mice, xenografted tumor model were randomly distributed into normal group, model group, Jin group, after sacrifice of animals with oral administration of JIN formula (3%, wt/vol) for 16 days, tumor inhibiting rate was recorded to show the effects of drugs on tumor growth.

Tumor inhibiting rate= (average of tumor weight in model group-average of tumor weight in JIN group) /average of tumor weight in model group ×100%.

2.3 Statistical analysis

Results were analyzed using a two-tailed Student's t-test to assess statistical significance and P-values<0.05 were considered significant.

3. Result

3.1 Inhibition of cell growth by JFE in A549 cells

This study was designed to show the chemopreventive/chemotherapeutic potential of JIN formula against lung cancer. Initially in our study, we investigated the antiproliferative effects of JFE treatment on human lung carcinoma A549 cells. Therefore, using A549 cells, we first evaluated the effect of JFE on the growth of these cells by MTT assay. We compared the antiproliferative effects of JFE (including E1 to E8) on A549 cells. As shown in Figure 2, treatment of JFE (1–100 μg/ml) for 72 h was found that E6 and E7 could decrease the viability of A549 cells.

3.2 Inhibition of tumorigenesis pathways by JFE in A549 and H157 cells

To explore the mechanism of antiproliferative effects of JIN formula against lung cancer, we investigated the involvement of Akt, ERK1/2, JNK1/2, p38 and NF-κB machinery during the inhibition of tumorigenesis by JFE in A549 and H157 cells.

Akt, also known as protein kinase B, which is a serine or threonine kinase, has been identified as an important component of tumorigenesis signaling pathway. The PI3K/Akt promotes cell survival by activating the NF-kB signaling pathway (3). Studies have shown that Akt plays an important role in carcinogenesis. We first investigated the effect of JFE on Akt protein expression in human lung carcinoma cells. In our study, we have demonstrated that the treatment of A549 and H157 cells with JFE (E1–E8) resulted in different degree inhibition of Akt pathways on tumor promotion processes as shown in Figure 3.

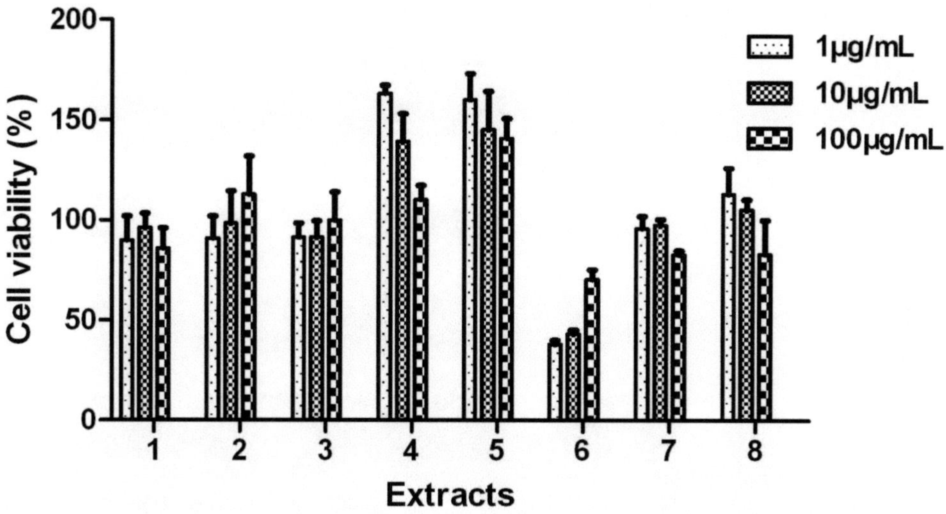

Fig. 2. The effects of JFE (including E1 to E8) on A549 cells growth

The MAP kinase superfamily (MAPKs) has been characterized into three groups which include extracellular signal-regulated kinase p44/42 (ERK), JNK/SAPK (c-jun N-terminal kinase/stress activated protein kinase) and p38 MAP kinase. MAPKs, a group of serine/threonine-specific, proline-directed protein kinases are known to modulate transcription factor activities. (4, 5). The involvement of the MAPK pathway in tumor proliferation is well documented. Transient activation of ERK is responsible for proliferation and differentiation and has also been shown to be involved in tumor promotion processes (3). Stimulation of JNK/SAPK and p38 can mediate differentiation, inflammatory responses and cell death (6). In the present study, we assessed the effect of JFE on MAPK pathway in A549 and H157 human lung carcinoma cells. The immunoblot analysis demonstrated that the treatment of cells with JFE inhibited ERKl/2, JNK1/2 and p38 proteins, and this inhibition of JNK1/2 and p38 in A549 cells was stronger than in H157 (Figure 3). Several studies have shown that JNK pathway plays a major role in cellular function, such as cell proliferation and transformation, whereas the ERK pathway suppresses apoptosis and enhances cell survival or tumorigenesis (4). ERK1/2 and p38 are also involved in the transcriptional activation of NF-kB (7, 8).

NF-kB is a sequence specific transcription factor that is known to be involved in the inflammatory and innate immune responses (9, 10). NF-kB is sequestered in the cytoplasm in an inactive form through interaction with IkB. Phosphorylation of IkB by IkB kinase (IKK) causes ubiquitination and degradation of IkB, thus releasing NF-kB which then translocates to the nucleus, where it binds to specific kB binding sites in the promoter regions of several genes (11). Studies have shown that NF-kB activation plays an important role in cell survival, by its ability to block or reduce apoptosis (12). In the present study, we further investigated the effect of JFE on the pattern of NF-kB activation and whether treatment with JFE inhibits nuclear translocation of NF-kB/p65 in A549 and H157 cells. As is evident from western blot analysis data and the relative density of bands, we found that JFE (E2, E3, E7) treatment of A549 cells resulted in inhibition of translocation of NF-kB/p65, meanwhile, we demonstrated that NF-kB is activated in H157 human lung carcinoma cells treated with JFE (E2, E3, E7) and is translocated to the nucleus when measured by western blot analysis (Figure 3).

(A)

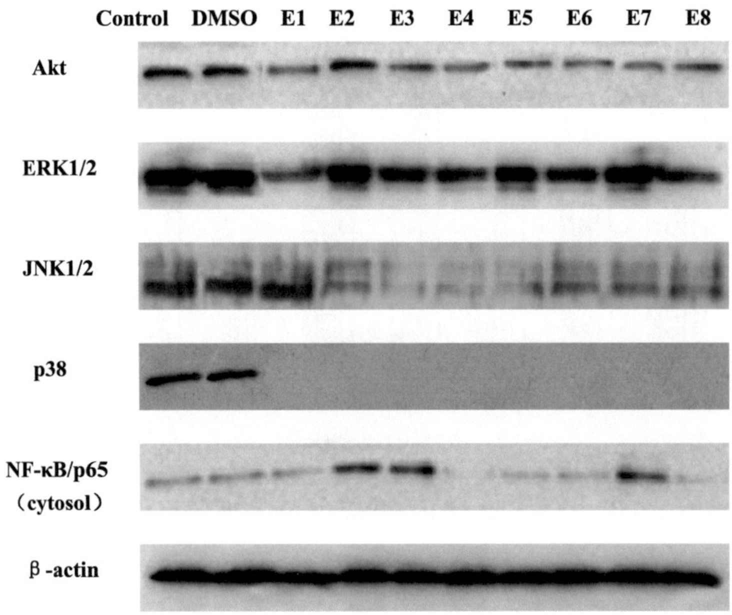

(B)

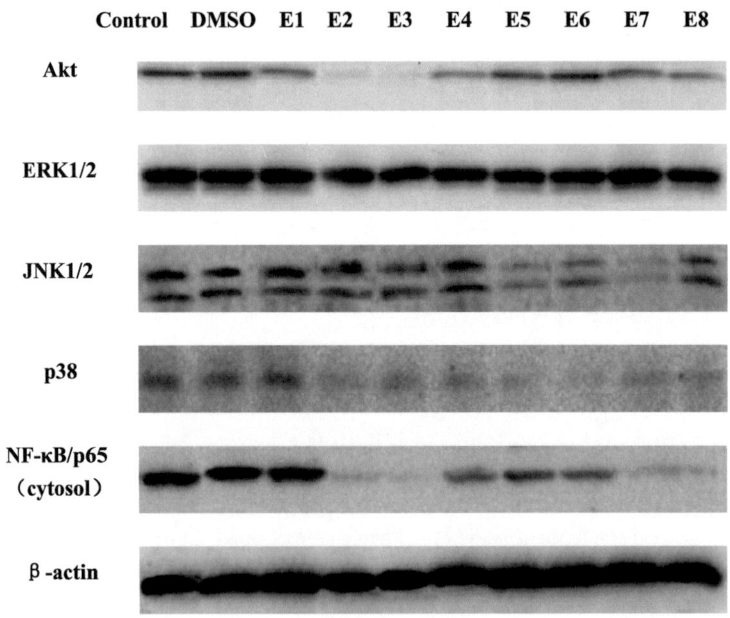

Fig. 3. (A) Inhibitory effects of JFE on tumorigenesis pathways in human lung carcinoma A549 cells (B) Inhibitory effects of JFE on tumorigenesis pathways in human lung carcinoma H157cells

The immunoblot analysis demonstrated that JFE (E1–E8) treatment could induce (i) inhibition of AKt, (ii) inhibition of ERK1/2 (p44 and p42), (iii) inhibition of JNK1/2 (p54 and p46), (iv) inhibition of p38 protein and (v) regulation of NF-kB.

3.3 Inhibition on the growth of human lung carcinoma A549 and H157 cells by JIN formula in nude mice

JFE inhibits the development of lung tumorigenesis by modulating and inhibiting PI3K/Akt, MAPK, and NF-kB signaling. To establish the relevance of these in vitro findings to in vivo situation, athymic nude mice were implanted with human lung carcinoma A549 and H157 cells. Compared with model group, Jin formula could significantly inhibit volume growth of A549 and H157 xenografted tumors. The inhibiting rate could reach to 28.5% and 25% in A549 and H157 tumor-bearing mice respectively ($p<0.05$). We found that the oral administration of JIN formula significantly slowed the progression of A549 and H157 tumor growth in nude mice.

4. Discussion

Lung cancer as the most common cancer in the world represents a major public health problem. Worldwide it accounts for 1.18 million cancer-related deaths and is the most common cause of cancer death in both men and women (13). Lung carcinogenesis is a chronic and multistep process resulting in malignant lung tumors. This progression from normal to neoplastic pulmonary cells or tissues could be arrested or reversed through pharmacological treatments. These therapeutic interventions should reduce or avoid the clinical consequences of lung cancer by treating early neoplastic lesions before the development of clinically evident signs or symptoms of malignancy. Preclinical, clinical and epidemiological findings relating to different classes of candidate chemopreventive agents provide strong support for lung cancer prevention as a therapeutic strategy (14). Cancer chemoprevention is an attractive approach to reduce lung cancers by treating early steps in lung carcinogenesis. There is a convergence of basic scientific and clinical findings in lung cancer chemoprevention. Pharmacological interventions also can be used to reverse or arrest the progression of lung carcinogenesis. For this reason, additional clinical trials are needed that emphasize a mechanistic approach in which mechanisms identified in vitro can be validated in vivo.

This study was designed to show the chemopreventive/chemotherapeutic potential of JIN formula against lung cancer. we assessed the efficacy of the JIN formula, which is an ancient herbal formula from classical book JIN KUI YAO LUE (Golden Chamber) for the treatment of lung cancer and explored its probable molecular mechanisms. Initially, employing human lung carcinoma A549 cells, we compared the growth inhibitory effects of JIN formula extracts (JFE, including E1 to E8). The results showed that E6 and E7 could decrease the viability of A549 cells by the MTT assays. To explore the mechanism of antiproliferative effects of JIN formula against lung cancer, we investigated the involvement of Akt, ERK1/2, JNK1/2, p38 and NF-κB pathway during the inhibition of tumorigenesis by JFE in A549 and H157 cells. The immunoblot analysis demonstrated that JFE treatment could result in different degree inhibition of above signaling pathways on tumor promotion processes. Oral administration of JIN formula (3%, wt/vol) to athymic nude mice implanted with A549 and H157 cells resulted in a significant inhibition in tumor growth.

In conclusion, the present study demonstrates that human non small cell lung cancer A549 and H157 cells are highly sensitive to JIN formula both in vitro and in vivo experimental models. JIN formula inhibits the development of lung tumorigenesis by modulating the imbalance of proliferative and apoptotic signaling network. Based on the present study it is tempting to suggest that JIN formula and its effective extracts have strong potential for development as a chemopreventive and possibly as a chemotherapeutic agent against lung cancer.

5. Acknowledgements

This study was supported by National Science & Technology Pillar Program in the 11th Five year Plan of China (2006BAI11B08－01) and the Priority Academic Program Development (PAPD) of Jiangsu Higher Education Institutions.

6. References

[1] Parkin, D.M., Bray,F., Ferlay,J. and Pisani,P. (2001) Estimating the world lung cancer burden: Globocan 2000. Int. J. Cancer, 94, 153–156.

[2] Parkin, D.M., Bray,F., Ferlay,J. and Pisani,P. (2005) Global cancer statistics, 2002. CA Cancer J. Clin., 55, 74–108.

[3] Adhami, V.M., Siddiqui,I.A., Ahmad,N., Gupta,S. and Mukhtar,H. (2004) Oral consumption of green tea polyphenols inhibits insulin-like growth factor-I-induced signaling in an autochthonous mouse model of prostate cancer. Cancer Res., 64, 8715–8722.

[4] Afaq, F., Ahmad,N. and Mukhtar,H. (2003) Suppression of UVB-induced phosphorylation of mitogen-activated protein kinases and nuclear factor kappa B by green tea polyphenol in SKH-1 hairless mice. Oncogene, 22, 9254–9264.

[5] Katiyar, S.K., Afaq, F., Azizuddin, K. and Mukhtar, H. (2001) Inhibition of UVB-induced oxidative stress-mediated phosphorylation of mitogen-activated protein kinase signaling pathways in cultured human epidermal keratinocytes by green tea polyphenol (-) -epigallocatechin-3-gallate. Toxicol. Appl. Pharmacol., 176, 110–117.

[6] Cobb, M.H. and Goldsmith, E.J. (1995) How MAP kinases are regulated. J. Biol. Chem., 270, 14843–14846.

[7] Adderley, S.R. and Fitzgerald, D.J. (1999) Oxidative damage of cardiomyocytes is limited by extracellular regulated kinases 1/2-mediated induction of cyclooxygenase-2. J. Biol. Chem., 274, 5038–5046.

[8] Carter, A.B., Knudtson, K.L., Monick, M.M. and Hunninghake,G.W. (1999) The p38 mitogen-activated protein kinase is required for NF-kappaB- dependent gene expression: the role of TATA-binding protein (TBP). J. Biol. Chem., 274, 30858–30863.

[9] Baldwin, A.S. Jr. (1996) The NF-kappa B and I kappa B proteins: new discoveries and insights. Annu. Rev. Immunol., 14, 649–683.

[10] Maniatis, T. (1997) Catalysis by a multiprotein IkappaB kinase complex. Science, 278, 818–819.

[11] Gupta, S., Hastak, K., Afaq, F., Ahmad, N. and Mukhtar, H. (2004) Essential role of caspases in epigallocatechin-3-gallate-mediated inhibition of nuclear factor kappa B and induction of apoptosis. Oncogene, 23, 2507–2522.

[12] Kaufman, C.K. and Fuchs, E. (2000) It's got you covered. NF-kappaB in the epidermis. J. Cell Biol., 149, 999–1004.

[13] Peto, R., Darby, S., Deo, H., Silcocks, P., Whitley, E. and Doll, R. (2000) Smoking, smoking cessation and lung cancer in the UK since 1950: combination of national statistics with two case-control studies. Br. Med.J., 321, 323–329.

[14] Cohen, V. and Khuri, F.R. (2002) Chemoprevention of lung cancer: current status and future prospects. Cancer Metastasis Rev., 21, 349–362.

14

The Serotonergic System and Neuroplasticity are Implicated in the Effect of Phytochemicals on Mood and Cognitive Disorders

Ying Xu[1*], Chong Zhang[1*] and William O. Ogle[2]
[1]*Department of Behavioral Medicine and Psychiatry, West Virginia University, WV,*
[2]*Crayton Pruitt Family Department of Biomedical Engineering and Evelyn F. & William L. Mcknight Brain Institute, University of Florida, Gainesville, FL, USA*

1. Introduction

Studies has been established in the 1930s that any environmental changes, whether internal or external, that disturbs the maintenance of homeostasis can cause stress response, including psychological, neuronal, endocrine and immune system reactivity (B E Leonard, 2005). During chronic stress or long-term exposure to external stress, glucocorticosteroids induce the hyperactivity of the Hypothalamic-Pituitary-Adrenal (HPA) axis, which produces an increase in plasma glucocorticoid level that then impairs the negative feedback mechanism, causing psychological disorders (Croes, Merz, & Netter, 1993; Henry, 1992). In stress-induced emotional and cognitive disorders, such as depression, anxiety and learning and memory impairment, the serotonergic system mainly exerts its regulatory functions through different subtypes of receptors. Research over the past decades have found that serotonin receptors, such as 5-HT_{1A}, 5-HT_{1B}, 5-HT_{2A}, 5-HT_{2C}, 5-HT_4, 5-HT_6, and 5-HT_7 subtypes, are closely related to depression and memory deficits. Moreover, clinical investigation suggests that some of the agonists or antagonists of the 5-HT receptor subtypes can be used for treatment of depression. However, the detailed roles of serotonin receptors in these disorders remain unclear.

Neuroplasticity has been described as the ability of the brain to reorganize itself and form new neuronal connections throughout life. Depression is associated with a neuronal loss in specific brain regions, which has been proven by functional brain imaging and other neurobiological techniques. The dendritic abnormalities seen in the hippocampus in animal models of depression and in patients with depression and Alzheimer's suggest changes in hippocampal circuitry are involved in disorders involving depression, anxiety and learning and memory impairment. The morphological and functional changes of neurons may be reversed after treatment with antidepressants, such as some natural compounds. In this review, a connection between neuroplasticity and the antidepressant-like effects of phytochemicals that are currently being studied is brought into attention. Some phytochemicals, such as curcumin, are found to reverse impaired hippocampal

---

* Equal contribution

neuroplasticity in chronically stressed rats by, for instance, increasing the dendritic length and the number of dendrites and axons. Compelling evidence now suggests a close relation between serotonin system and neuroplasticity in depression. For example, the reduced neuronal plasticity in chronically stressed rats is accompanied by down-regulation of 5-HT_{1A} receptor mRNA expression, which can be prevented by the administration of curcumin. Other intriguing findings suggest that 5-HT_7 receptor can even differentially regulate neuroplasticity in different brain regions after treatment with corticosterone and curcumin. With these findings, there has been a remarkable increase in interest regarding the use of phytochemicals in repairing the neuroplasticity related to central nervous system dysfunction.

Phytochemicals, particularly anti-oxidative natural compounds, are considered promising alternatives to conventional drugs, such as tricyclic antidepressants, monoamine oxidase inhibitors, serotonin reuptake inhibitors (SSRI), and norepinephrine and dopamine reuptake inhibitors. This is not only because they are extracted from fruits and vegetables and affect biological activities with high potency and low systemic toxicity, but also because they can bind to multiple targets. Studies in the early 90s had a general focus on long-term dietary supplementation. For example, foods supplemented with strawberry extracts and spinach had beneficial effects in retarding functional age-related mood and neurodegenerative diseases, due to their potent anti-oxidative properties. In the following years, phytochemicals have been isolated from the antioxidant-rich foods and their biological activities are gradually being elucidated. Typical phytochemicals that are being studied include curcumin, resveratrol, fisetin, and berberine.

This review summarizes the series of studies on the involvement of serotonin system and neuronal plasticity in treatment of mood and cognitive disorders using Chinese medicine.

2. The 5-HT system in mood and cognitive diseases

Serotonin (5-hydroxytryptamine, 5-HT) is an important neurotransmitter in the central nervous system (CNS). Through activation or inhibition of its receptor subtypes, studies have demonstrated that 5-HT has multiple physiological functions and dysregulation of serotonergic system can cause stress-related diseases such as Alzheimer's Diseases (AD), anxiety, depression and cognitive disorders (Goddard et al., 2010; Ramanathan & Glatt, 2009). The neurons of the raphe nuclei release the majority of 5-HT in the brain and project onto many other regions of the brain, exerting the regulatory function of 5-HT on physiology. 5-HT expression in developing raphe nuclei neurons and the preferential generation of the nerve fiber projecting terminals during the formation of neuronal synapses demonstrated that 5-HT affects not only morphology and neural activity of embryonic neurons, but also neurogenesis and neuroplasticity after neuronal maturation, including proliferation, translocation, differentiation and synapse formation (Veenstra-VanderWeele et al., 2000). 5-HT is also involved in the development of cerebral cortex in mammals; during the early stages of sensory cortex development, temporary serotonergic fiber projections were detected, indicating that 5-HT might be helpful in conjugation and integration of the developing cortex (Nayyar et al., 2009). Brain serotonin synthesis, packaging, transportation, targeting, release, reuptake and degradation all affect the concentration of 5-HT and its functions. Proteins and related genes that are involved in regulating these physiological functions include speed-limiting enzyme TPH-1 and TPH-2 (Illi et al., 2009), Vmat2 (Fukui et al., 2007; Zucker, Weizman, & Rehavi, 2005), serotonin transporter (SERT or 5-HTT), monoamine oxidase A (MAO-A) and 5-HT pre and post synaptic receptors (Paaver et al., 2007).

5-HT receptors are assigned to one of seven receptor families, 5-HT_{1-7}, comprising a total of fourteen structurally and pharmacologically distinct mammalian 5-HT receptor subtypes. With the exception of 5-HT_3 receptor, a ligand-gated ion channel, all receptors (5-HT_{1A-E}, 5-HT_{2A-C}, 5-HT_4, 5-HT_5, 5-HT_6, 5-HT_7) are G protein-coupled receptors (GPCR) that activate an intracellular second messenger cascade to produce an excitatory or inhibitory response. Activation of the specific G-protein can affect enzymes, such as adenylate cyclase, phospholipase A and C, mitogen-activated protein kinase, and cation channels, especially K^+ and Ca^{2+} (Kushwaha & Albert, 2005). Recent literature has shown, in intact brain, the unequivocal participation of 5-HT receptors in specific physiological responses, ranging from modulation of neuronal activity and transmitter release to behavioral change, especially in psychological disorders like depression, anxiety, obsessive-compulsive disorder, and panic disorder (Ayala, 2009). Among the receptor subtypes, 5-HT_{1A}, 5-HT_{1B}, 5-HT_{2A}, 5-HT_{2C}, 5-HT_4, 5-HT_6, 5-HT_7 are associated with chronic stress-induced neural diseases, inhibition of learning and memory, and cognitive disorders (King et al., 2008; Meneses, 2007; Pérez-García et al., 2006).

3. Role of neuroplasticity in mood and cognitive disabilities: Protective effects of herbal medicines

Neuroplasticity is referred to as the ability of the nervous system to respond and adapt to environmental challenges as a result of one's experiences. It encompasses a series of functional and structural adaptation mechanisms that may lead to neuronal remodeling, including adding, removing or changing the strength of connections between nerve cells and glial cells. Failure of such adaptations might enhance the susceptibility to environmental challenges and ultimately lead to psychopathology. The brain may become more vulnerable by losing the ability to maintain homeostasis. In the case of depression, it is now well accepted to be characterized by profound alterations in brain function and responsiveness, which might be closely linked with neuroplasticity and the ability to modulate a cascade of events from intracellular signaling mechanisms to gene expression.

3.1 Structure change in mood and cognitive disorders

Recent neuroimaging and post-mortem morphometric studies of several brain regions, including limbic and non-limbic circuits, in individuals with mood disorders have begun to demonstrate that depression is accompanied by morphological changes at both the macro-anatomical and histological levels (Miguel-hidalgo & Rajkowska, 2002). Some researchers applying the most sensitive structural neuroimaging techniques to the brains of patients with major depressive disorder (MDD) or bipolar disorder have shown that they are associated with an enlargement of the lateral ventricles, reduction in the volume of grey and white matter in the prefrontal cortex, shrinkage of the hippocampus and decreased volume of the amygdala. Due to the scant access to post-mortem studies on patients, whether treated or untreated, with mood disorders, information on possible morphological alterations of brain regions is limited. Instead, cytomorphological changes associated with mood disorders in animal models, such as the number of neurons, the size and shape of their cell bodies, as well as dendritic and axonal components, have been greatly studied.

Studies in rodents and nonhuman primates demonstrate that exposure to stress can cause alterations in cytomorphology of neurons. Layer II/III pyramidal neurons in the medial prefrontal cortex showed dendritic retraction and reduction in spine number after several weeks of glucocorticoid administration or restraint stress (S. C. Cook & Wellman, 2004). In the hippocampus, repeated stress is reported to cause atrophy of CA3 pyramidal neurons and dentate gyrus. This is supported by a decrease in the number and length of apical tree, but not base tree (R S Duman, 2002). Volume reduction and, more importantly, a shift from neuronal processes to glial processes to make up for the volume decrease have also been observed. Distinct from the CA3 hippocampal region, 24 hr after a single forced swim stress rather than a 3-week period, apical dendrites showed fewer branches in medial prefrontal cortex (mPFC) (Izquierdo, Wellman, & Holmes, 2006). Moreover, the hippocampus is one of the first brain regions to suffer damage from Alzheimer's disease. The comparison of multiple brain regions provides an even more convincing proof of the relationship between neuroplasticity and stress-induced mood disorders: while chronic stress induces significant regression of the apical dendrites in both hippocampus and prefrontal cortex (PFC), it enhances synaptic plasticity in amygdala (Pittenger & Ronald S Duman, 2008). The latter change could both result from and contribute to over-activation of neuronal circuits within amygdala that control fear, anxiety, and emotion. These findings in the animal models with regard to cytomorphological alterations are consistent with several structural imaging studies in human patients with major depression or anxiety.

In learning and memory, synaptic plasticity is even more thoroughly studied. The theory postulating that changes at synapses within the brain underlie learning and memory was formalized in the 1950s. Two crucial terms involved in this theory are long-term potentiation (LTP) and long-term depression (LTD) (Howland & Y. T. Wang, 2008). LTP is a long-lasting enhancement in signal transmission between two neurons that results from stimulating them synchronously. LTD, on the other hand, is an activity-dependent reduction in the efficacy of neuronal synapses lasting hours or longer and occurs in many areas of the CNS. Both of them describe the ability of chemical synapses to change their strength, which is considered one of the major cellular mechanisms that underlies learning and memory. Cytomorphology of individual neurons and macro-morphology of brain support the normal functioning of synaptic plasticity which plays a direct role in regulating cognitive functions.

The underlying mechanisms of morphological alterations during the onset and treatment of mood and cognitive disorders have not yet been clearly understood. However, a few studies show that in patients with MDD and bipolar disorder, there are changes in synaptic proteins that might be associated with morphological changes in related brain regions (Jørgensen & Riederer, 1985). It has also been revealed that antidepressant treatment have a reversing effect on the intracellular signaling, transcription factors and target genes. Neurotophic factors (NTFs), particularly the neurotrophin family such as BDNF, are one of the activity-regulated gene expressions responsive to neuronal activity. It is possible that these treatments could oppose the adverse cellular effects, which may be regarded as a loss of neural plasticity, by blocking or reversing the atrophy of neurons and by increasing cell survival and function.

3.2 Herbal medicines able to restore neuroplasticity in some CNS malfunction

Antidepressant medications may act by correcting the dysfunction of neuronal adaptive responses, namely neuroplasticity. The most likely immediate cause of depressive symptoms turns out to be changes in the synaptic availability of the monoamines such as noradrenaline (norepinephrine), serotonin and dopamine, or in the activity of their receptors. As a result, the best accepted pharmacological treatments for depression have been those that increase the availability of monoamines, particularly serotonin.These antidepressants also greatly correct dendritic abnormalities of patients with mood disorders. Dendrites and their spines undergo morphological changes after treatment with some antidepressants. For example, treatment with the selective serotonin reuptake inhibitors (SSRIs) produces a significant increase in dendritic spine density and total length of secondary dendrites in the CA1 region and dentate gyrus of the hippocampus (Norrholm & Ouimet, 2000).

Beyond the classical antidepressants, herbal medicines have been receiving mounting attention due to their ability to reverse or halt impaired neuroplasticity. A wide variety of herbal plants, including Panax ginseng, Zukomei-to (ZMT), Gongjin-dan (GJD), their extracts, compounds and so on have, to date, already presented beneficial results when tested against known pathological neuronal morphology in some mood and cognitive disorders.

Ginsenosides are extracts from Panax ginseng root that are widely used as a tonic medicine throughout the world and in the treatment of amnesia. In animal models, such as brain-damaged rats and aged rats, a significant improvement in learning and memory has been observed using ginseng powder, which contains the major ginseng saponins, ginsenoside Rb1 and Rg1 (Zhong et al., n d). Beyond all doubt, change of neuronal cells morphology underlies the above-mentioned beneficial effects of ginseng saponins. In the 1980s, Sugaya et al. was one of the earliest groups to show that ginseng saponins can improve neurite extension (A. Sugaya et al.,1988). In their study, rat cerebral cortex neurons were cultured. Cytochalasin-B induced disappearance of the growth cone and looping phenomenon were both blocked by administration of crude saponin extract. A proliferative effect of neurite extension, about 1.5 fold in ganglioside content, of cultured neurons was observed, indicating that ginsenosides can promote neurite extension and protect neurons against cytochalasin-B-induced cell lesion. However, this study did not clarify which component within the crude saponin extract of ginseng roots played the most significant role. Later studies screened out ginsenoside Rb1, Rb3, notoginsenosideR4 and Fa as the active compounds that caused the outgrowth and maturation of neurites and they could possibly recover the function of degenerated brains (Nishiyama, Cho, Kitagawa, & Saito, 1994; Tohda, N. Matsumoto, Zou, Meselhy, & Komatsu, 2002).

Zukomei-to (ZMT, or Xu Ming Tan in Chinese), composed of traditional Chinese and Japanese herbal drugs, has long been used in treating postapopletic sequelae, clinically indicating that it might reactivate neuronal function in degenerated neuronal circuits. Based on this speculation, the effects of ZMT on memory impairment and synaptic loss in an Alzheimer's mouse model were investigated (Tohda et al., 2003). In this study, synaptophysin, a vesicle protein located at the presynaptic membrane, was used as a marker for synaptic loss. Mice brain slices stained with anti-synaptophysin antibody showed that ZMT prevented synaptic loss induced by Aβ (25-35) in the CA1 region and dentate gyrus of the hippocampus and the parietal cortex. Neuron densities were also measured in CA1, CA3, and dentate gyrus of the hippocampus and the parietal cortex of mice brains treated with Aβ (25-35) only or both AMT and Aβ (25-35). However, no significant difference was observed, suggesting that synaptic reconstruction rather than neuronal death was involved here.

Gongjin-dan (GJD) is a multi-herbal formula containing different parts of up to six botanicals. It has been used clinically in Korea as an anti-fatigue and anti-aging agent for hundreds of years. GJD was proven to have beneficial effects not only on promoting neurite outgrowth but also on preventing neuronal cell death (Moon et al., 2009). GJD was used on PC12 cells and stressed mice models either as a mimetic or inducer of nerve growth factor (NGF), a small protein commonly reported to stimulate cholinergic neurons, improve memory loss, and increase long-term potentiation and learning tasks. PC12 cells exhibited extended neurite outgrowth after treatment with GJD, although not as obvious as after treatment with NGF. Moreover, NGF level in the cell culture media was elevated. The effect of GJD on survival of neurons was examined by immunostaining microtubule-associated protein-2 (MAP-2), which is a key player in neurogenesis. In the hippocampus of immobilization stressed rats, neuronal cell death was greatly triggered, and GJD was able to decrease this neuronal loss. Since NGF is also required for the survival of the neurons, it is highly possible that GJD exert its neuroprotective function, both in neuroplasticity and neuronal cell survival, by activating the secretion of NGF or simply acting as a mimetic of NGF.

Herbal medicines that have similar effects on the shape and structure of the CNS are not limited to the above-mentioned examples. In later sections of this chapter, more natural compounds, such as curcumin, resveratrol and others, will be discussed with respect to their tonic effects on CNS and operating mechanisms, especially when the 5-HT system is involved. Most of them appear to prevent morphological alterations induced by stress insults. Even though individual studies might have slightly different outcomes due to different cell types or animal models, herbal medicine generally proves to be a promising in treating CNS-related disorders.

4. The antioxidative effects of neuroprotective natural compounds

4.1 Oxidative stress and the 5-HT system

Oxidative stress is a result of a build-up of reactive oxygen species (ROS) due to reduced ability of a biological system to detoxify the reactive intermediates or to repair the resulting damage. ROS are a group of chemically-reactive molecules containing oxygen. They are generated by enzymatic and non-enzymatic reactions in the mitochondria and cytoplasm. In humans, oxidative stress is involved in many diseases including those in the CNS. Oxygen radicals initiate neurotoxicity such as build up of Abeta, leading to neurodegenerations. For example, neurodegenerative diseases, such as Alzheimer's disease (AD), Parkinson's disease (PD), and stroke, are commonly accompanied by oxidative stress markers. Environmental stress can lead the body into pathological conditions, in which ROS levels can increase dramatically, activating enzymes including proteases, phospholipases, and nucleases that result in significant damage to cell morphology. As a result, there is increasing attention to develop nutritional therapies to combat these age-related oxidative processes. Mounting focus has been placed on compounds extracted from botanicals in vegetables, fruits, grains, roots, flowers and so on. Polyphenolics, like resveratrol from grape and red wine and curcumin from turmeric, are becoming recognized for their antioxidative effects against neurodegenerative diseases, possibly by restoring the neuronal cell morphology, as mentioned earlier in this chapter.

The 5-HT system is involved with the oxidative process in several aspects. First, the process interferes with 5-HT system's precursor tryptophan. ROS and reactive nitrogen species (RNS), excluding NO, oxygen and superoxide anion, rapidly react with many tryptophan derivatives, thus gradually eliminating the important neurotransmitter serotonin (Peyrot & Ducrocq, 2008). Second, serotonin and oxidative stress have a counterbalance effect in synthesizing NO. NO, as an endothelium-derived relaxing factor, is synthesized by the endothelial isoform of nitric oxide synthase (eNOS). This process involves pertussis-toxin-sensitive G protein that responses to serotonin and can be inhibited by oxidative stress (Michel & Vanhoutte, 2010). Third, 5-HT receptor subtypes interact with components of the oxidative process. For example, NADPH oxidase is necessary for the activation of 5-HT_2 receptors (MacFarlane et al., 2011). NADPH oxidase is recognized for its dual-edge roles in health and disease. Altered NADPH oxidase function has been linked to neurological disorders such as AD, as it is present in Abeta-induced ROS production (Lambeth, 2007). Superoxide produced by NADPH oxidase may interact with NO to form the toxic peroxynitrite, which is normally associated with neuronal death (Brown, 2007). All in all, oxidative stressors impair neuronal plasticity while concurrently altering neurotransmission, contributing to CNS diseases.

4.2 Natural compounds as antioxidants

Plant-derived supplements for improving mental health are gradually gaining popularity because they are natural and thus considered to be safer and produce fewer side effects than chemically synthesized antioxidants. One of the most commonly studied type is the polyphenols, which have a wide array of phenol ring structures, as one of the first antioxidative natural compounds to catch attention. They are divided into different groups according to the number of phenol rings and the chemical groups attached to them, among which flavonoids are the largest and most well-known group. The capacity of flavonoids to act as an antioxidant, i.e. scavenging free radicals, depends on their molecular structure. In general, polyphenols are rapidly converted to their glucuronide derivatives upon ingestion and transported to the circulatory system, where they can cross the blood brain barrier.

4.2.1 Resveratrol

Dietary supplement of polyphenols extracted from grape skin and seeds had been reported to ameliorate oxidative damage in synaptic membrane of brain cells (G. Y. Sun et al., 1999). Later on, trans-resveratrol was found to be the most effective extract from grape skin and seed, as well as a variety of other plants such as peanuts and berries, that produces beneficial health effects. To assess its role as an antioxidant, resveratrol was compared with the classical antioxidative vitamins C and E in a 1977 study (Chanvitayapongs et al., 1997). In this study, oxidative stress was induced by addition of Fe2+ and t-butyl hydroperoxide to the cultured PC12 cell medium. Even though the combination of the three antioxidants exhibited the greatest effect, when used alone, resveratrol is more effective than vitamins C and E combined.

Several studies have demonstrated the ability of resveratrol to protect neurons against Abeta-induced oxidative toxicity in vitro. In a rat model of sporadic AD induced by intracerebroventricular streptozotocin, in which both oxidative stress and cognitive impairment were present, trans-resveratrol significantly prevented the cognitive deficits (Sharma & Gupta, 2002). Red wine, with a high content of resveratrol, was also reported to markedly attenuate AD-type deterioration of spatial memory function and Abeta neuropathology (Jun Wang et al., 2006). The mechanism by which resveratrol fights against Abeta-induced oxidative stress mainly lies in its ability to inhibit not only the secretion of

Abeta, but also formation and extension of Abeta fibrils and to destabilize the fibrilized Abeta (Marambaud et al., 2005; Ono et al., 2006).

The antidepressant-like activity of resveratrol, which involves the inhibition of monoamine oxidase (MAO) isoform activity, also attributes to its potent antioxidative effects (Ying Xu et al., 2010). MAOs are mitochondrial-bound isoenzymes that catalyze the oxidative deamination of dietary amines and monoamine neurotransmitters, such as 5-HT, noradrenaline, dopamine and other trace amines. In a PCPA-induced serotonin-depleted mice model, treatment with resveratrol significantly improved the performance of mice in forced swimming and tail suspension tests. In the meantime, serotonin levels were dramatically increased, accompanied by inhibition of MAO-B activity. The involvement of 5-HT system in neuroprotective effects of resveratrol was also confirmed by an electrophysiological study (Lee et al., 2011). It was reported that resveratrol is able to mediate current flow in the cell by regulating 5-HT_3 receptor activity, possibly through interactions with the N-terminal domain of the receptor.

There are different modes of administration of resveratrol, such as i.p. injection or supplemention with grape powder formulation. Studies to examine bioavailability indicate that resveratrol is rapidly conjugated to its glucuronide derivative and can be transported to the circulatory system. Once in the circulatory system, it can pass through the blood brain barrier. This renders a possibility that resveratrol can be developed into drugs for use in clinical trials.

4.2.2 Curcumin

The learning and memory deficits associated with chronic stress may be alleviated by novel therapeutic strategies involving dietary and medicinal phyto-antioxidants. One such nutraceutical is turmeric, which has been used throughout Asia as a food additive and a traditional herbal medicine. The active substance in turmeric is curcumin, the yellow pigment extracted from the rhizoma of Curcuma longa (Ying Xu et al., 2009). In this study, the effects of curcumin on restraint stress-induced spatial learning and memory dysfunction in a water maze task were investigated, and related neuroendocrine and plasticity changes were measured. The results showed that memory deficits were reversed with curcumin in a dose-dependent manner, as were stress-induced increases in serum corticosterone levels. These effects were similar to those seen with positive antidepressant imipramine. Additionally, curcumin prevented adverse changes in the dendritic morphology of CA3 pyramidal neurons in the hippocampus, as assessed by the changes in branch points and dendritic length. Moreover, curcumin protected primary hippocampal neurons against corticosterone-induced toxicity.

Curcumin supplementation has also been recently considered as an alternative approach to reduce oxidative damage associated with AD (Wu et al., 2006). High-fat diet has been shown to induce oxidative stress as an intrinsic component that can exacerbate the damage caused by traumatic brain injury (TBI). The group of rats feeding on curcumin supplemented high-fat diet performed better in the cognition tests than the group of rats feeding on high-fat diet only, when both groups were subjected to a mild fluid percussion injury. Synaptic plasticity also changed in accordance with the cognition results. Brain-derived neurotrophic factor (BDNF) was shown involved in this neuroprotective effect of curcumin. Detailed mechanisms by which curcumin regulate the expression of BDNF will be discussed in a later section of this chapter. Moreover, curcumin, but not ibuprofen, a conventional non-steroidal anti-inflammatory drug, was also able to prevent the synaptic loss related to Abeta-induced oxidative damage (Frautschy et al., 2001).

The impact of curcumin on the 5-HT system has been extensively studied. One study showed that curcumin protected against arsenic-induced neurobehavioral toxicity by modulating oxidative stress and dopaminergic functions in rats; the serotonin level was restored to normal if the rats were treated with both curcumin and arsenic, compared with the group of rats treated with arsenic only (Yadav et al., 2010). A similar phenomenon was found in a stressed mice model (Ying Xu et al., 2005): neurochemical assays showed that curcumin produced a marked increase in serotonin levels at 10 mg/kg in both the frontal cortex and hippocampus.

Alterations in 5-HT transmission are associated with changes in adult cell proliferation, since 5-HT depletion results in significant decreases in the number of newborn cells in the hippocampus. In order to further clarify the mechanism by which curcumin interacts with the 5-HT system and affects neuronal cells morphology, different 5-HT receptor subtypes were studied. A study aimed to investigate the effects of curcumin on hippocampal neurogenesis in chronically stressed rats used an unpredictable chronic stress paradigm (Ying Xu et al., 2007). It found that 5, 10 and 20 mg/kg, p.o. chromic treatment for 20 days could alleviate or reverse the effects of stress on adult hippocampal neurogenesis, denoted by BrdU labeling. This result was similar to 10 mg/kg, i.p. classic antidepressant imipramine treatment. In addition, curcumin significantly prevented the stress-induced decrease in 5-HT_{1A} mRNA and BDNF protein levels in the hippocampal subfields. These results suggest that curcumin treatment overcomes the stress-induced behavioral abnormalities and hippocampal neuronal damage by increasing cell proliferation and neuronal populations.

Moving on to neuroplasticity, the 5-HT system also plays a significant role in the neuroprotective effects of curcumin. In a 2011 study, exposure of cortical neurons to corticosterone resulted in decreased mRNA levels for the 5-HT receptor subtypes 5-HT_{1A}, 5-HT_{2A} and 5-HT_4, but no change for the 5-HT_{1B}, 5-HT_{2B}, 5-HT_{2C}, 5-HT_6 and 5-HT_7. Pretreatment with curcumin reversed this decreased mRNA level for the 5-HT_{1A} and 5-HT_4 receptors, but not the 5-HT_{2A} receptor. Moreover, curcumin exerted a neuroprotective effect against corticosterone-induced neuronal death. This observed effect was partially blocked with the separate application of 5-HT_{1A} receptor antagonist p-MPPI and 5-HT_4 receptor antagonist RS 39604, and completely blocked with the simultaneous application of the two antagonists. Curcumin was also found to regulate corticosterone-induced morphological changes, such as increases in soma size, dendritic branching and dendritic spine density, as well as elevate synaptophysin expression in cortical neurons. Again, p-MPPI and RS 39604 reversed these effects of curcumin to prevent the morphological changes of neurons (Ying Xu et al., 2011).

4.2.3 EGCG

Green tea polyphenols (GTPs) are the most active antioxidative constituents in green tea. Among the 5 isoforms of GTPs, EGCG has the greatest potential beneficial effects in the CNS. In male Wistar rats undergoing restraint stress for 3 weeks, EGCG-treated groups performed better in the open field test and step-through test than the stress group. Similar results were observed in the crude GTP-treated group. Moreover, plasma levels of serotonin in both EGCG- and GTP- treated groups were elevated closer to the normal groups, compared to the stress group (Chen et al., 2010). This supports the involvement of the 5-HT system in the mechanism of the antioxidative effects of many neuroprotective herbals.

4.2.4 Other herbal supplements

Ginkgo biloba, also known as the maiden tree, contains compounds with antioxidant properties that protect neuron membranes, regulate neurotransmitters and retard cell degeneration. Standardized Ginkgo biloba extract EGb 761 was shown to improve neurogenesis and cognitive function in both young and old transgenic mice model TgAPP/PS1 with AD (Tchantchou et al., 2007). Later studies however suggested that Ginkgo biloba aids cognition only when subjects have AD rather than preventing AD. The neuroprotective effects of EGb 761 pertaining to the serotonin system and depression were also examined (P. Rojas et al., 2011). Not surprisingly, EGb 761 exerted its antidepressant property, as assessed by the forced swimming test, via its antioxidative effects. Moreover, serotonin level in the midbrain was increased in the EGb 761-treated group of mice, compared to the stress group. This indicates that ginkgo biloba can modulate serotonergic neurotransmission. A recent study suggests that ginkgo biloba is able to block the 5-HT3 receptor channel, further attesting to its function on the serotonin system (Thompson et al., 2011).

Huperzine A (HupA) is an alkaloid compound extracted from the Chinese moss Huperzia serrata. Besides its role as a natural acetylcholinesterase inhibitor in treating AD, HupA also has potent antioxidative effects. It has been found to protect against Abeta-induced cell lesion and abnormal morphology in the primary cultured rat cortical neurons (Xiao et al., 2002) HupA treatment reduced ROS formation and caspase 3 (a protein regulating cell apoptosis) activity in a dose-dependent manner in cortical neurons. In PC12 cells, cell death triggered by oxygen-glucose deprivation (OGD) was alleviated by HupA treatment as well (Zhou et al., 2001). Moreover, it prevented the change in cell morphology caused by OGD. After 30 min OGD exposure, PC12 cells developed a mild cell body swelling and neurites retraction or even complete loss. Cells pre-treated with HupA, however, maintained their morphology almost at the same level as normal control. Regarding cognitive behavior, HupA also exhibited beneficial effects. For instance, daily administration of HupA produced significant reversals of the Abeta-induced deficit in learning and memory tasks (R. Wang et al., 2001).

There are other natural antioxidants outside of the above-mentioned ones that are being used to treat or prevent some CNS diseases, such as withania somnifera from a small evergreen shrub; apocynin from Picrorhiza kurroa, a creeping plant native to the mountains of India, Nepal, Tibet and Pakistan; and Coenzyme Q, enriched in a number of diets, all of which have neuroprotective effects via oxidative stress reduction in mammalian brains. Natural antioxidants are advantageous for use, because they can cross the blood brain barrier, have low toxicity to the overall health being, and can be easily administered. Many antioxidant studies have indicated their interactions with the 5-HT system, including serotonin and the 5-HT receptor subtypes. More attention to these interactions may bring promise to the development of drugs treating depression and neurodegenerative diseases caused by oxidative stress.

5. Beyond the antioxidants

Even though the biological actions of most neuroprotective natural compounds have been attributed to their antioxidant properties, namely their abilities to scavenge free radicals or through their impact on the intracellular redox status, studies have also argued that at least some of these compounds' bioactivity in vivo is not due to their classical H-donating antioxidant property. This is mainly because of their relatively low level in the brain. Instead, the neuroprotective actions might be exerted through the modulation of the expression of genes that control neuronal survival, death and differentiation; interactions with mitochondria; structural similarities to other hormones in the body and so on.

5.1 Natural compounds used as estrogen replacement

Natural estrogen, also known as the female sex hormone, is a group of compounds belonging to the steroid hormones that exist in humans and other animals. The actions of estrogen are mediated by the estrogen receptors (ER). One of the key functions of estrogen in women is the maintenance of mental health. Withdrawal and fluctuating or low levels of estrogen correlate with significant mood lowering. For example, animal behavioral studies have shown that ovariectomy may lead to the development of cognitive dysfunction, accompanied by changes in neuronal architecture. And estrogen replacement can prevent these changes (Birge, 1996). As a result, there has been increasing interest in the cognitive preserving effects of soybean isoflavones, mainly in post-menopausal women, due to their structural similarity to estrogen and ability to mimic the actions of estrogen in the brain (Henderson, 2006; Kritz-Silverstein et al., 2003). Resveratrol, like soy products and other polyphenols, has free hydroxyl groups and phenolic ring structures that are important for estrogen receptor binding. Indeed, resveratrol can ameliorate neuronal damage induced by acute and chronic stress in different neuronal cell types by interacting directly with both estrogen receptors alpha and beta, though stronger with ER-beta (Robb & Stuart, 2010). Ginsenoside Rb1 also proved to have comparable effects with estrogen on improving behavioral performance in ovariectomized mice (K. Hao et al., 2011). After treatment with ginsenoside Rb1, there were increased TPH (an enzyme in the synthesis of 5-HT) level, decreased MAO activities, and finally elevated 5-HT levels in the mice brains, all to a similar extent observed using estrogen treatment. Additionally, estrogen receptor clomiphene blocked the effects of both ginsenoside Rb1 and estrogen, confirming that ginsenoside Rb1 shares similar pathways with estrogen.

5.2 Increase in the expression of growth factors

Neurotrophic factors are a family of proteins responsible for the growth and survival of developing neurons, thus maintaining the normal function and integral plasticity of the brain. There are three families involved: neurotrophins, glial cell-line derived neurotrophic factor family ligands (GFLs), and neuropoietic cytokines, among which neurotrophins is the most commonly studied. In this family, nerve growth factor (NGF), brain-derived neurotrophic factor (BDNF), neurotrophin-3 (NT-3), and neurotrophin-4/5 (NT 4/5) are basic components. Regulated by the transcriptional factor CREB, BDNF plays a central role in brain development and plasticity by opposing neuronal damage and promoting neurogenesis and cell survival. Similar to classical antidepressant imipramine, chronic curcumin treatment prevented stress-induced decreases in BDNF levels and neurogenesis across all hippocampal subfields (Y. Xu et al., 2007). Malonylginsenoside Rb1 (GRb1-m) extracted from dried root of Panax ginseng C.A. Meyer and ginsenoside Rb1 had a synergizing effect on NGF (Nishiyama et al., 1994). They potentiated the effect of NGF on promoting the neurite outgrowth, eliminating the glial cells when they are co-cultured with neurons, and prolonging the duration of neuronal survival.

Vascular endothelial growth factor (VEGF) is an important signaling molecule that induces proliferation and migration and reduces apoptosis of endothelial cells. It has also gained attention for its beneficial effect on the physiological function of the brain, such as increasing angiogenesis in the ischemic area and enhancing neurogenesis in the hippocampus, which leads to improved cognitive performances (Q. Zhao et al., 2010). Kangen-karyu, a traditional Chinese medicine prescription consisting of six different herbs, upregulates not only BDNF, but also VEGF levels in SAMP8 mice brains. As a result, anxiety-like behaviors as observed in the elevated plus-maze test and impairment in learning and memory as measured in the object recognition/location tests were reduced.

5.3 Increase in blood flow

Learning and memory have long been connected with neurogenesis, i.e. new neuronal growth, increases in the spine density and morphology, especially in the hippocampal area. New hippocampal cells are not only observed to be stimulated by neurotrophic factors, but also cluster near blood vessels, where they proliferate in response to vascular growth factors (Palmer et al., 2000). A brain imaging study showed that cocoa flavanol are able to enhance the cortical blood flow, indicating its potential ability to increase angiogenesis and neurogenesis (Dinges, 2006). Indeed, though flavanol (-)epicatechin did not increase the number of new born cells in the dentate gyrus of the hippocampus in this case, it was reported to increase angiogenesis and neural spine density (H. van Praag et al., 2007). In this study, behavioral tests were also conducted to confirm the effects of neurogenesis. Retention of spatial memory in the water maze test increased in both sedentary and wheel-running performance. Cognition, too, was enhanced, though to a greater extent in the wheel-running group.

6. The signaling pathways

Synaptic plasticity is often involved in stress-induced brain injury, neuroinflammation, and neurocognitive performances. There are several signaling pathways linked with the neuroprotective effects of natural compounds that preserve normal synaptic plasticity. It is likely that the neuroprotection process is carried through selective activation or inhibition of different components, as well as change of gene expression, within a number of protein kinase and lipid kinase signaling pathways, including the mitogen-activated protein kinase (MAPK), protein kinae A (PKA), phosphatidylinositol-3 kinase (PI3K), protein kinase C (PKC) and CaMK pathways. The activation of these pathways commonly result in the activation of the cAMP response element-binding protein (CREB) and a variety of downstream responses, including neurotrophin expression, dendritic spine remodeling and synaptic plasticity such as LTP. Moreover, most flavonoids can bind to the ATP-binding sites of a large number of proteins (Conseil et al., 1998), such as mitochondrial ATPase and Ca2+ plasma membrane ATPase. This binding leads to a three-dimensional structural change, followed by series of kinase inactivation, thus preventing the formation of pro-apoptotic proteins in the neurons.

6.1 Mitogen-activated protein kinase (MAPK) signaling cascade

MAPK is mainly responsible for transducing various extracellular stimuli into intracellular responses. There are three levels of regulation: a MAP kinase kinase kinase (MAPKKK), a

MAP kinase kinase (MAPKK) and a MAPK, each regulating the following element. Each MAPKK can be activated by more than one MAPKKK, thus increasing the complexity and diversity of MAPK signaling. The three best characterized pathways involved in the neuroprotective effects of most natural compounds are: the mitogenic extracellular signal-regulated protein kinase (ERK) pathway, the stress activated, c-Jun N-terminal kinase (JNK) pathway, and the p38 pathway (Schroeter et al., 2002). The activation of these MAP kinases phosphorylates their downstream proteins and transcription factors, leading to change in gene expression, as well as neuronal activities.

6.1.1 ERK1/2

ERK1/2 are usually associated with pro-survival signaling such as upregulation of the anti-apoptotic protein Bcl-2. ERK1/2 are activated by upstream MAPKKs, such as MEK1/2, and MAPKKKs, such as c-Raf. Phosphorylation of ERK usually occurs at 2 sites, threonin 202 and tyrosin 204, within the tripeptide motif TEY, and activates a series of transcription factors that regulate neuronal cell differentiation, survival and plasticity. Flavonoids have not only been reported to modulate the phosphorylation state of ERK1/2, but also to have an effect on upstream kinases and membrane receptors. This might be due to their structural homology to specific inhibitors of the ERK signaling. For example, PD 098059 is a flavone that has the ability to bind to the inactive MEK, preventing its activation by upstream MAPKKK and thus inhibiting the pro-survival process (Alessi et al., 1995). Compared to the neurotoxic properties of flavones through the ERK1/2 pathway, the neuroprotective effects are even more intriguing. Curcumin, mentioned multiple times previously, also has an influence on the ERK1/2 pathway. Adminstration of curcumin alleviated corticosterone-induced cytotoxicity in PC12 cells, with an increase in the ERK1/2 phosphorylation (H. Zhou et al., 2009). Moreover, elevation of phosphorylated ERK1/2 was only visible at a certain time period, 15-90 min in this case, indicating that other mechanisms are also involved in the ERK-regulated cell morphology. There is also evidence of the involvement of 5-HT system in this pathway: serotonin was able to increase ERK1/2 phosphorylation, possibly involving 5-HT1A, 5-HT2B and 5-HT2C receptors (Debata et al., 2010; B. Li et al., 2010).

6.1.2 JNK

JNK is considered to oppose the effects of ERK, in that they generally promote neuronal apoptosis rather than neuronal survival. JNK cascade is strongly activated by stress signals such as oxidative stress, inflammatory cytokines and UV radiation. Regulated by GTPases such as Rac1, MAPKKKs such as MEKK1/4 and ASK1 activate MAPKKs, such as MKK4/7, which go on to regulate the JNK1/2/3. Activated JNK then enters the nucleus and activates or inhibit a series of downstream gene expression, including c-jun and AP-1 proteins that transduce the apoptotic signaling. Similar to ERK, JNK is dually phosphorylated at threonin138 and tyrosine185 within the motif pTPpY. Since changes in the cellular redox status may result in the activation of JNK, and oxidative stress can more or less be alleviated by many antioxidative plant extracts, massive studies are investigating whether JNK pathway is involved in the neuroprotective process of these plant extracts. Oxidized low-density lipoprotein (oxLDL) can be used to induce oxidative stress in cultured striatal neurons (H Schroeter et al., 2001). The neurotoxicity was characterized by the activation of JNK, which phosporylates c-jun, as measured by western blots. Flavonoid epicatechin strongly inhibited this activation. JNK is also necessary for the serotonin-induced cell proliferation, for this was blocked with exposure to a specific JNK inhibitor. Furthermore, 10min of serotonin addition maximally activated of JNK. Blockade of 5-HT1B and 2A receptors abolished the stimulatory effect of serotonin in JNK (Wei et al., 2010).

6.1.3 P38

p38 shares some of the upstream MAPKKKs with the JNK, i.e. MEK1/4 and ASK1, which regulates MKK3/4/6 (MAPKKs). Downstream transcription factors include ATF-2, Max and MEF2. p38 MAP kinase is activated by cellular stresses, including osmotic shock, inflammatory cytokines, UV radiation and growth factors. An isoflavonoid from soybean, genistein, was found to induce the activation of p38, followed by downregulation of Cdc25C, thus preventing the dividing MCF-10F, a nonmalignant human mammary epithelia cell line, from entering mitosis. In other words, genistein can inhibit cell proliferation by activating p38, indicating that it may be able to induce neural effects via this pathway (Frey & Singletary, 2003). However, the precise sites of action within the p38 pathway and the specific elements involved in regulating stress-induced neuronal death remain unknown.

6.2 PKA pathway

PKA is a family of enzymes that have several functions in the cell by phosphorylating other proteins and altering their function. It is also known as cAMP-dependent protein kinase, because its activity is only dependent on the level of cyclic AMP (cAMP). In the activation process, activated alpha subunit of G-protein binds to the enzyme adenylyl cyclase (AC), which catalyzes the conversion of ATP into cAMP, which further leads to the activation of PKA. Once PKA is activated, a series of proteins gets phosphorylated, including the transcription factor CREB. Since PKA exists in different types of cell, where they exert different biological functions, it is plausible that the same compound may have different regulatory effects on the activity of PKA. Curcumin was reported to inhibit the growth of several tumor cell types, in which hyperactivated PKA might play an important role in unlimited cell division, prompting a study on the mechanism by which curcumin may inhibit different types of phosphatases (Reddy & Aggarwal, 1994). Indeed, curcumin was able to inhibit the activity of PKA in tumor cells, even though not to a very high extent. However, in neurons, curcumin activated the PKA pathway rather than inhibited it,and this effect involved the 5-HT system (Y Xu et al., 2011). Treatment of the primary cortical cultured neurons with curcumin significantly increased the cAMP level, PKA activity and pCREB level, compared with the corticosterone-treated only group. Cell morphology parameters, including the soma size, total number of branching points, dendritic length and spine density, were also positively regulated by curcumin compare with the corticosterone-treated group. Addition of 5-HT4 receptor antagonist, RS 39604, blocked the elevation of cAMP level, while 5-HT1A antagonist, p-MPPI, inhibited the increase in PKA activity and pCREB. These findings suggest that the neuroprotection and modulation of neuroplasticity exhibited by curcumin might be mediated, at least in part, via the 5-HT receptor-cAMP-PKA-CREB signal pathway.

6.3 PI3K/Akt signaling cascade (PKB pathway)

PI3Ks are a family of enzymes involved in cellular functions, such as cell survival, growth, proliferation, differentiation and motility. Activation of PI3K by extracellular signals catalyzes the production of phosphatidylinositol-3,4,5-triphosphate (PIP3), phosphatidylinositol-4-phosphate (PIP) and phosphatidylinositol-4,5-bisphosphate (PIP2). PIP3 then activates phosphoinositide-dependent protein (PDK1/2), which plays a role in many signal transduction pathways by activating Akt (also known as protein kinase B, or PKB). Akt can promote cell survival mainly by inhibiting some important apoptosis-inducing proteins such as Bad (Cardone et al., 1998; Zha et al., 1996). Querctin has been reported to dose dependently regulate neuronal cell fate. At lower doses, quercetin may activate the MAPK pathway and exert its protective mechanism. However, high concentrations of quercetin inhibit the PI3K pathway and thus stimulate the pro-apoptotic pathway (Kong et al., 2000). The relationship between serotonin and PI3K/Akt signaling has also been studied. 5-HT-induced phosphorylation of Akt in different cell types was blocked either by PI3K inhibitors or 5-HT_{1A} antagonist, indicating the necessary presence of both elements in the proliferation and migration activities of cells (Dizeyi et al., 2011).

6.4 PKC pathway

PKC is a family of enzymes responsible for phosphorylating other proteins at the hydroxyl groups of serine and threonin residues, and plays an important role in several signal transduction cascades that regulate growth, differentiation and tumorigenesis. Signals such as an increase in the diacylglycerol or Ca^{2+} levels can initiate this signal cascade. The PKC pathway shares some components with the PI3K/Akt pathway, such as the intracellular signaling molecules PI3K and PDK1. Flavonoids have been reported only to have an inhibitory effect on the PKC activity, rather than activation or a dual effect. TPA is a potent tumor promoter often employed to activate PKC, and consequently PKC is considered as a cellular receptor for TPA. In a brain-purified mixture of PKC isoenzymes, flavonols, in particular fisetin, quercetin and myricetin, and flavones, in particular luteolin, were found to be the most potent inhibitors for PKC. They also inhibited PI3K activity (Agullo et al., 1997; Ferriola et al., 1989). Since PKC is expressed in different cell types, the same compound may have varying extent of inhibitory effects on its activity (Y. T. Huang et al., 1996).

6.5 CaMK pathway

Ca^{2+}/calmodulin-dependent protein kinases II or CaM kinases II are serine/threonine-specific protein kinases that are regulated by the Ca^{2+}/calmodulin complex. CaMKII is intricately involved in memory formation and synaptic plasticity in the hippocampus. The phosphorylation of CaMKII at Thr286 switches the kinase into an active biochemical state required for synaptic plasticity and learning, including spatial learning. However, CaMKII over phosphorylation may produce some degree of neurotoxicity to the cells and alter some biochemical pathways involved in memory processing. It should be noted that mice that expressed a constitutively active CaMKII lacked low frequency LTP and were not able to form stable place cells within the hippocampus (Ying Xu et al., 2009). In hippocampal neurons, pCaMKII levels were significantly increased in response to corticosterone exposure, though no changes were found in total CaMKII levels. These results are similar to the changes elicited by the immobilization stress, which was previously reported (Suenaga et al., 2004). This elevation of pCaMKII was reversed by curcumin administration at different dose ranges from 0.62 to 2.5 mM (Ying Xu et al., 2009).

6.6 Other cascades

Signaling cascades involved in the neuroprotection effect of natural compounds may not be limited to the above-mentioned pathways. Besides the common transcription factor CREB of these pathways, there is FoxO1, an important target for insulin and growth factor signaling in the regulation of metabolism and cell proliferation. FoxO1 can mediate an autofeedback loop regulating SIRT1 expression (Xiong et al., 2011), a protein previously discussed to be regulated by resveratrol as well. A lot of the flavonoids also modulate the functions of the mitochondria by binding to the ATP-binding sites (Conseil et al., 1998). More or less, these pathways involve the 5-HT system, as well as its different receptor subtypes, and together they regulate gene expressions that are responsible for neuronal cell survival or inhibition of abnormal cell proliferation under stress insults. Other than behavioral tests, the most effective way to observe their function is to assess the cell morphology. Indeed, most neuroprotective natural compounds are able to morphologically restore the neurons close to normal conditions.

7. References

Acker, S. A. van, Berg, D. J. van den, Tromp, M. N., Griffioen, D. H., Bennekom, W. P. van, Vijgh, W. J. van der, et al. (1996). Structural aspects of antioxidant activity of flavonoids. *Free radical biology & medicine*, *20*(3), 331-42.

Agullo, G., Gamet-Payrastre, L., Manenti, S., Viala, C., Rémésy, C., Chap, H., et al. (1997). Relationship between flavonoid structure and inhibition of phosphatidylinositol 3-kinase: a comparison with tyrosine kinase and protein kinase C inhibition. *Biochemical pharmacology*, *53*(11), 1649-57.

Alessi, D. R., Cuenda, A., Cohen, P., Dudley, D. T., & Saltiel, A. R. (1995). PD 098059 is a specific inhibitor of the activation of mitogen-activated protein kinase kinase in vitro and in vivo. *The Journal of biological chemistry*, *270*(46), 27489-94.

Ayala, M. E. (2009). Brain serotonin, psychoactive drugs, and effects on reproduction. *Central nervous system agents in medicinal chemistry*, *9*(4), 258-76.

Birge, S. J. (1996). Is there a role for estrogen replacement therapy in the prevention and treatment of dementia? *Journal of the American Geriatrics Society*, *44*(7), 865-70.

Brown, G. C. (2007). Mechanisms of inflammatory neurodegeneration: iNOS and NADPH oxidase. *Biochemical Society transactions*, *35*(Pt 5), 1119-21.

Cardone, M. H., Roy, N., Stennicke, H. R., Salvesen, G. S., Franke, T. F., Stanbridge, E., et al. (1998). Regulation of cell death protease caspase-9 by phosphorylation. *Science (New York, N.Y.)*, *282*(5392), 1318-21.

Chanvitayapongs, S., Draczynska-Lusiak, B., & Sun, A. Y. (1997). Amelioration of oxidative stress by antioxidants and resveratrol in PC12 cells. *Neuroreport*, *8*(6), 1499-502.

Chen, W.-Q., Zhao, X.-L., Wang, D.-L., Li, S.-T., Hou, Y., Hong, Y., et al. (2010). Effects of epigallocatechin-3-gallate on behavioral impairments induced by psychological stress in rats. *Experimental biology and medicine (Maywood, N.J.)*, *235*(5), 577-83.

Conseil, G., Baubichon-Cortay, H., Dayan, G., Jault, J. M., Barron, D., & Di Pietro, A. (1998). Flavonoids: a class of modulators with bifunctional interactions at vicinal ATP- and steroid-binding sites on mouse P-glycoprotein. *Proceedings of the National Academy of Sciences of the United States of America*, *95*(17), 9831-6.

Cook, S. C., & Wellman, C. L. (2004). Chronic stress alters dendritic morphology in rat medial prefrontal cortex. *Journal of neurobiology*, *60*(2), 236-48.

Croes, S., Merz, P., & Netter, P. (1993). Cortisol reaction in success and failure condition in endogenous depressed patients and controls. *Psychoneuroendocrinology, 18*(1), 23-35.

Debata, P. R., Ranasinghe, B., Berliner, A., Curcio, G. M., Tantry, S. J., Ponimaskin, E., et al. (2010). Erk1/2-dependent phosphorylation of PKCalpha at threonine 638 in hippocampal 5-HT(1A) receptor-mediated signaling. *Biochemical and biophysical research communications, 397*(3), 401-6.

Dinges, D. F. (2006). Cocoa flavanols, cerebral blood flow, cognition, and health: going forward. *Journal of cardiovascular pharmacology, 47 Suppl 2*, S221-3.

Dizeyi, N., Hedlund, P., Bjartell, A., Tinzl, M., Austild-Taskén, K., & Abrahamsson, P.-A. (n.d.). Serotonin activates MAP kinase and PI3K/Akt signaling pathways in prostate cancer cell lines. *Urologic oncology, 29*(4), 436-45.

Dröge, W., & Schipper, H. M. (2007). Oxidative stress and aberrant signaling in aging and cognitive decline. *Aging cell, 6*(3), 361-70.

Duman, R S. (2002). Pathophysiology of depression: the concept of synaptic plasticity. *European psychiatry : the journal of the Association of European Psychiatrists, 17 Suppl 3*(October), 306-10.

Ferriola, P. C., Cody, V., & Middleton, E. (1989). Protein kinase C inhibition by plant flavonoids. Kinetic mechanisms and structure-activity relationships. *Biochemical pharmacology, 38*(10), 1617-24.

Frautschy, S. A., Hu, W., Kim, P., Miller, S. A., Chu, T., Harris-White, M. E., et al. (n.d.). Phenolic anti-inflammatory antioxidant reversal of Abeta-induced cognitive deficits and neuropathology. *Neurobiology of aging, 22*(6), 993-1005.

Frey, R. S., & Singletary, K. W. (2003). Genistein activates p38 mitogen-activated protein kinase, inactivates ERK1/ERK2 and decreases Cdc25C expression in immortalized human mammary epithelial cells. *The Journal of nutrition, 133*(1), 226-31.

Fukui, M., Rodriguiz, R. M., Zhou, Jiechun, Jiang, S. X., Phillips, L. E., Caron, M. G., et al. (2007). Vmat2 heterozygous mutant mice display a depressive-like phenotype. *The Journal of neuroscience : the official journal of the Society for Neuroscience, 27*(39), 10520-9.

Goddard, A. W., Ball, S. G., Martinez, J., Robinson, M. J., Yang, C. R., Russell, J. M., et al. (2010). Current perspectives of the roles of the central norepinephrine system in anxiety and depression. *Depression and anxiety, 27*(4), 339-50.

Hao, K., Gong, P., Sun, S.-Q., Hao, H.-P., Wang, G.-J., Dai, Y., et al. (2011). Beneficial estrogen-like effects of ginsenoside Rb1, an active component of Panax ginseng, on neural 5-HT disposition and behavioral tasks in ovariectomized mice. *European journal of pharmacology*. [Epub ahead of print]

Henderson, V. W. (2006). Estrogen-containing hormone therapy and Alzheimer's disease risk: understanding discrepant inferences from observational and experimental research. *Neuroscience, 138*(3), 1031-9.

Henry, J. P. (n.d.). Biological basis of the stress response. *Integrative physiological and behavioral science : the official journal of the Pavlovian Society, 27*(1), 66-83.

Howland, J. G., & Wang, Y. T. (2008). *Synaptic plasticity in learning and memory : stress effects in the hippocampus. Progress in Brain Research* (Vol. 169, pp. 145-158). Elsevier.

Inhibitions of protein kinase C and proto-oncogene expressions in NIH 3T3 cells by apigenin. *European journal of cancer (Oxford, England : 1990), 32A*(1), 146-51.

Izquierdo, A., Wellman, C. L., & Holmes, A. (2006). Brief uncontrollable stress causes dendritic retraction in infralimbic cortex and resistance to fear extinction in mice. *The Journal of neuroscience : the official journal of the Society for Neuroscience, 26*(21), 5733-8.

Jørgensen, O. S., & Riederer, P. (1985). Increased synaptic markers in hippocampus of depressed patients. *Journal of neural transmission*, *64*(1), 55-66.

Kaneda, Y. (2009). Verbal working memory and functional outcome in patients with unipolar major depressive disorder. *The world journal of biological psychiatry : the official journal of the World Federation of Societies of Biological Psychiatry*, *10*(4 Pt 2), 591-4.

King, M. V., Marsden, C. A., & Fone, K. C. F. (2008). A role for the 5-HT(1A), 5-HT4 and 5-HT6 receptors in learning and memory. Trends in pharmacological sciences, 29(9), 482-92.

Kong, A. N., Yu, R., Chen, C., Mandlekar, S., & Primiano, T. (2000). Signal transduction events elicited by natural products: role of MAPK and caspase pathways in homeostatic response and induction of apoptosis. *Archives of pharmacal research*, *23*(1), 1-16.

Kritz-Silverstein, D., Von Mühlen, D., Barrett-Connor, E., & Bressel, M. A. B. (n.d.). Isoflavones and cognitive function in older women: the SOy and Postmenopausal Health In Aging (SOPHIA) Study. *Menopause (New York, N.Y.)*, *10*(3), 196-202.

Kushwaha, N., & Albert, P. R. (2005). Coupling of 5-HT1A autoreceptors to inhibition of mitogen-activated protein kinase activation via G beta gamma subunit signaling. *The European journal of neuroscience*, *21*(3), 721-32.

Lambeth, J. D. (2007). Nox enzymes, ROS, and chronic disease: an example of antagonistic pleiotropy. *Free radical biology & medicine*, *43*(3), 332-47.

Le Poul, E., Laaris, N., Hamon, M., & Lanfumey, L. (1997). Fluoxetine-induced desensitization of somatodendritic 5-HT1A autoreceptors is independent of glucocorticoid(s). *Synapse (New York, N.Y.)*, *27*(4), 303-12.

Lee, B.-H., Hwang, S.-H., Choi, S.-H., Shin, T.-J., Kang, J., Lee, S.-M., et al. (2011). Resveratrol enhances 5-hydroxytryptamine type 3A receptor-mediated ion currents: the role of arginine 222 residue in pre-transmembrane domain I. *Biological & pharmaceutical bulletin*, *34*(4), 523-7.

Lee, B.-H., Lee, Jun-Ho, Yoon, I.-S., Lee, Joon-Hee, Choi, S.-H., Shin, T.-J., et al. (2007). Mutations of arginine 222 in pre-transmembrane domain I of mouse 5-HT(3A) receptor abolish 20(R)- but not 20(S)-ginsenoside Rg(3) inhibition of 5-HT-mediated ion currents. *Biological & pharmaceutical bulletin*, *30*(9), 1721-6.

Leonard, B E. (2005). The HPA and immune axes in stress: the involvement of the serotonergic system. *European psychiatry : the journal of the Association of European Psychiatrists*, *20 Suppl 3*, S302-6.

Li, B., Zhang, S., Li, M., Hertz, L., & Peng, L. (2010). Serotonin increases ERK1/2 phosphorylation in astrocytes by stimulation of 5-HT2B and 5-HT2C receptors. *Neurochemistry international*, *57*(4), 432-9.

MacFarlane, P. M., Vinit, S., & Mitchell, G. S. (2011). Serotonin 2A and 2B receptor-induced phrenic motor facilitation: differential requirement for spinal NADPH oxidase activity. *Neuroscience*, *178*, 45-55.

Marambaud, P., Zhao, Haitian, & Davies, P. (2005). Resveratrol promotes clearance of Alzheimer's disease amyloid-beta peptides. *The Journal of biological chemistry*, *280*(45), 37377-82.

Meneses, A. (2007). Stimulation of 5-HT1A, 5-HT1B, 5-HT2A/2C, 5-HT3 and 5-HT4 receptors or 5-HT uptake inhibition: short- and long-term memory. *Behavioural brain research*, *184*(1), 81-90.

Michel, T., & Vanhoutte, P. M. (2010). Cellular signaling and NO production. *Pflügers Archiv : European journal of physiology*, *459*(6), 807-16.

Miguel-hidalgo, J. J., & Rajkowska, G. (2002). Morphological Brain Changes in Depression Can Antidepressants Reverse Them ? *CNS Drugs, 16*(6), 361-372.

Moon, E., Her, Y., Lee, J. B., Park, J.-H., Lee, E. H., Kim, S.-H., et al. (2009). The multi-herbal medicine Gongjin-dan enhances memory and learning tasks via NGF regulation. *Neuroscience letters, 466*(3), 114-9.

Morikawa, H., Manzoni, O. J., Crabbe, J. C., & Williams, J. T. (2000). Regulation of central synaptic transmission by 5-HT(1B) auto- and heteroreceptors. *Molecular pharmacology, 58*(6), 1271-8.

Nayyar, T., Bubser, M., Ferguson, M. C., Neely, M. D., Shawn Goodwin, J., Montine, T. J., et al. (2009). Cortical serotonin and norepinephrine denervation in parkinsonism: preferential loss of the beaded serotonin innervation. *The European journal of neuroscience, 30*(2), 207-16.

Nishiyama, N., Cho, S. I., Kitagawa, I., & Saito, H. (1994). Malonylginsenoside Rb1 potentiates nerve growth factor (NGF)-induced neurite outgrowth of cultured chick embryonic dorsal root ganglia. *Biological & pharmaceutical bulletin, 17*(4), 509-13.

Norrholm, S. D., & Ouimet, C. C. (2000). Chronic fluoxetine administration to juvenile rats prevents age-associated dendritic spine proliferation in hippocampus. *Brain research, 883*(2), 205-15.

Ono, K., Naiki, H., & Yamada, M. (2006). The development of preventives and therapeutics for Alzheimer's disease that inhibit the formation of beta-amyloid fibrils (fAbeta), as well as destabilize preformed fAbeta. Current pharmaceutical design, 12(33), 4357-75.

Paaver, M., Nordquist, N., Parik, J., Harro, M., Oreland, L., & Harro, J. (2007). Platelet MAO activity and the 5-HTT gene promoter polymorphism are associated with impulsivity and cognitive style in visual information processing. *Psychopharmacology, 194*(4), 545-54.

Palmer, T. D., Willhoite, A. R., & Gage, F H. (2000). Vascular niche for adult hippocampal neurogenesis. *The Journal of comparative neurology, 425*(4), 479-94.

Peyrot, F., & Ducrocq, C. (2008). Potential role of tryptophan derivatives in stress responses characterized by the generation of reactive oxygen and nitrogen species. *Journal of pineal research, 45*(3), 235-46.

Pittenger, C., & Duman, Ronald S. (2008). Stress, depression, and neuroplasticity: a convergence of mechanisms. *Neuropsychopharmacology : official publication of the American College of Neuropsychopharmacology, 33*(1), 88-109.

Praag, H. van, Lucero, M. J., Yeo, G. W., Stecker, K., Heivand, N., Zhao, C., et al. (2007). Plant-derived flavanol (-)epicatechin enhances angiogenesis and retention of spatial memory in mice. *The Journal of neuroscience : the official journal of the Society for Neuroscience, 27*(22), 5869-78.

Pérez-García, G., Gonzalez-Espinosa, C., & Meneses, A. (2006). An mRNA expression analysis of stimulation and blockade of 5-HT7 receptors during memory consolidation. *Behavioural brain research, 169*(1), 83-92.

Ramanathan, S., & Glatt, S. J. (2009). Serotonergic system genes in psychosis of Alzheimer dementia: meta-analysis. *The American journal of geriatric psychiatry : official journal of the American Association for Geriatric Psychiatry, 17*(10), 839-46.

Reddy, S., & Aggarwal, B. B. (1994). Curcumin is a non-competitive and selective inhibitor of phosphorylase kinase. *FEBS letters, 341*(1), 19-22.

Ribes, D., Colomina, M. T., Vicens, P., & Domingo, J. L. (2010). Impaired spatial learning and unaltered neurogenesis in a transgenic model of Alzheimer's disease after oral aluminum exposure. *Current Alzheimer research*, *7*(5), 401-8.

Robb, E. L., & Stuart, J. A. (2010). trans-Resveratrol as a neuroprotectant. *Molecules (Basel, Switzerland)*, *15*(3), 1196-212.

Rojas, P., Serrano-García, N., Medina-Campos, O. N., Pedraza-Chaverri, J., Ogren, Sven O, & Rojas, C. (2011). Antidepressant-like effect of a Ginkgo biloba extract (EGb761) in the mouse forced swimming test: Role of oxidative stress. *Neurochemistry international*.

Schroeter, H, Spencer, J. P., Rice-Evans, C, & Williams, R J. (2001). Flavonoids protect neurons from oxidized low-density-lipoprotein-induced apoptosis involving c-Jun N-terminal kinase (JNK), c-Jun and caspase-3. The Biochemical journal, 358(Pt 3), 547-57.

Schroeter, Hagen, Boyd, C., Spencer, J. P. E., Williams, Robert J, Cadenas, E., & Rice-Evans, Catherine. (n.d.). MAPK signaling in neurodegeneration: influences of flavonoids and of nitric oxide. *Neurobiology of aging*, *23*(5), 861-80.

Sharma, M., & Gupta, Y. K. (2002). Chronic treatment with trans resveratrol prevents intracerebroventricular streptozotocin induced cognitive impairment and oxidative stress in rats. *Life sciences*, *71*(21), 2489-98.

Suenaga, T., Morinobu, S., Kawano, K.-I., Sawada, T., & Yamawaki, S. (2004). Influence of immobilization stress on the levels of CaMKII and phospho-CaMKII in the rat hippocampus. *The international journal of neuropsychopharmacology / official scientific journal of the Collegium Internationale Neuropsychopharmacologicum (CINP)*, *7*(3), 299-309.

Sugaya, A., Yuzurihara, M., Tsuda, T., Yasuda, K., Kajiwara, K., & Sugaya, E. (n.d.). Proliferative effect of ginseng saponin on neurite extension of primary cultured neurons of the rat cerebral cortex. *Journal of ethnopharmacology*, *22*(2), 173-81.

Sun, G. Y., Xia, J., Xu, J., Allenbrand, B., Simonyi, A., Rudeen, P. K., et al. (1999). Dietary supplementation of grape polyphenols to rats ameliorates chronic ethanol-induced changes in hepatic morphology without altering changes in hepatic lipids. *The Journal of nutrition*, *129*(10), 1814-9.

Tchantchou, F., Xu, Yanan, Wu, Y., Christen, Y., & Luo, Y. (2007). EGb 761 enhances adult hippocampal neurogenesis and phosphorylation of CREB in transgenic mouse model of Alzheimer's disease. *The FASEB journal : official publication of the Federation of American Societies for Experimental Biology*, *21*(10), 2400-8.

Thompson, A. J., Jarvis, G. E., Duke, R. K., Johnston, G. A. R., & Lummis, S. C. R. (n.d.). Ginkgolide B and bilobalide block the pore of the 5-HT(3) receptor at a location that overlaps the picrotoxin binding site. *Neuropharmacology*, *60*(2-3), 488-95.

Tohda, C., Matsumoto, N., Zou, K., Meselhy, M. R., & Komatsu, K. (2002). Axonal and dendritic extension by protopanaxadiol-type saponins from ginseng drugs in SK-N-SH cells. *Japanese journal of pharmacology*, *90*(3), 254-62.

Tohda, C., Tamura, T., & Komatsu, K. (2003). Repair of amyloid beta(25-35)-induced memory impairment and synaptic loss by a Kampo formula, Zokumei-to. *Brain research*, *990*(1-2), 141-7.

Uc, E. Y., McDermott, M. P., Marder, K. S., Anderson, S. W., Litvan, I., Como, P. G., et al. (2009). Incidence of and risk factors for cognitive impairment in an early Parkinson disease clinical trial cohort. *Neurology*, *73*(18), 1469-77.

Veenstra-VanderWeele, J., Anderson, G. M., & Cook, E. H. (2000). Pharmacogenetics and the serotonin system: initial studies and future directions. *European journal of pharmacology*, *410*(2-3), 165-181.

Wang, Jun, Ho, L., Zhao, Z., Seror, I., Humala, N., Dickstein, D. L., et al. (2006). Moderate consumption of Cabernet Sauvignon attenuates Abeta neuropathology in a mouse model of Alzheimer's disease. *The FASEB journal : official publication of the Federation of American Societies for Experimental Biology*, *20*(13), 2313-20.

Wang, R., Zhang, H Y, & Tang, X C. (2001). Huperzine A attenuates cognitive dysfunction and neuronal degeneration caused by beta-amyloid protein-(1-40) in rat. *European journal of pharmacology*, *421*(3), 149-56.

Wei, L., Liu, Y., Kaneto, H., & Fanburg, B. L. (2010). JNK regulates serotonin-mediated proliferation and migration of pulmonary artery smooth muscle cells. *American journal of physiology. Lung cellular and molecular physiology*, *298*(6), L863-9.

Wu, A., Ying, Z., & Gomez-Pinilla, F. (2006). Dietary curcumin counteracts the outcome of traumatic brain injury on oxidative stress, synaptic plasticity, and cognition. *Experimental neurology*, *197*(2), 309-17.

Xiao, X. Q., Zhang, Hai Yan, & Tang, Xi Can. (2002). Huperzine A attenuates amyloid beta-peptide fragment 25-35-induced apoptosis in rat cortical neurons via inhibiting reactive oxygen species formation and caspase-3 activation. *Journal of neuroscience research*, *67*(1), 30-6.

Xiong, S., Salazar, G., Patrushev, N., & Alexander, R. W. (2011). FoxO1 mediates an autofeedback loop regulating SIRT1 expression. *The Journal of biological chemistry*, *286*(7), 5289-99.

Xu, Y, Zhang, C., Wang, R., Govindarajan, S S, Barish, P A, Vernon, M M, et al. (2011). Corticosterone induced morphological changes of hippocampal and amygdaloid cell lines are dependent on 5-HT7 receptor related signal pathway. *Neuroscience*, *182*, 71-81.

Xu, Ying, Ku, B.-S., Yao, H.-Y., Lin, Y.-H., Ma, X., Zhang, Y.-H., et al. (2005). The effects of curcumin on depressive-like behaviors in mice. *European journal of pharmacology*, *518*(1), 40-6.

Xu, Ying, Ku, B., Cui, L., Li, Xuejun, Barish, P. a, Foster, T. C., et al. (2007). Curcumin reverses impaired hippocampal neurogenesis and increases serotonin receptor 1A mRNA and brain-derived neurotrophic factor expression in chronically stressed rats. *Brain research*, *1162*, 9-18.

Xu, Ying, Li, S., Vernon, Matthew M, Pan, Jianchun, Chen, Ling, Barish, Philip A, et al. (2011). Curcumin prevents corticosterone-induced neurotoxicity and abnormalities of neuroplasticity via 5-HT receptor pathway. *Journal of neurochemistry*.

Xu, Ying, Lin, Dan, Li, S., Li, G., Shyamala, S. G., Barish, P. a, et al. (2009). Curcumin reverses impaired cognition and neuronal plasticity induced by chronic stress. *Neuropharmacology*, *57*(4), 463-71.

Xu, Ying, Wang, Z., You, W., Zhang, X., Li, S., Barish, P. a, et al. (2010). Antidepressant-like effect of trans-resveratrol: Involvement of serotonin and noradrenaline system. *European neuropsychopharmacology : the journal of the European College of Neuropsychopharmacology*, *20*(6), 405-13.

Yadav, R. S., Shukla, R. K., Sankhwar, M. L., Patel, D. K., Ansari, R. W., Pant, A. B., et al. (2010). Neuroprotective effect of curcumin in arsenic-induced neurotoxicity in rats. *Neurotoxicology*, *31*(5), 533-9.

Yamada, N., Araki, H., & Yoshimura, H. (2011). Identification of antidepressant-like ingredients in ginseng root (Panax ginseng C.A. Meyer) using a menopausal depressive-like state in female mice: participation of 5-HT(2A) receptors. *Psychopharmacology*, , 216(4): 589-99.

Zha, J., Harada, H., Yang, E., Jockel, J., & Korsmeyer, S. J. (1996). Serine phosphorylation of death agonist BAD in response to survival factor results in binding to 14-3-3 not BCL-X(L). *Cell*, *87*(4), 619-28.

Zhao, Haifeng, Li, Q., Zhang, Z., Pei, X., Wang, Junbo, & Li, Y. (2009). Long-term ginsenoside consumption prevents memory loss in aged SAMP8 mice by decreasing oxidative stress and up-regulating the plasticity-related proteins in hippocampus. *Brain research*, *1256*, 111-22.

Zhao, Q., Yokozawa, T., Yamabe, N., Tsuneyama, K., Li, Xiaohan, & Matsumoto, K. (2010). Kangen-karyu improves memory deficit caused by aging through normalization of neuro-plasticity-related signaling system and VEGF system in the brain. *Journal of ethnopharmacology*, *131*(2), 377-85.

Zhong, Y. M., Nishijo, H., Uwano, T., Tamura, R., Kawanishi, K., & Ono, T. (n.d.). Red ginseng ameliorated place navigation deficits in young rats with hippocampal lesions and aged rats. *Physiology & behavior*, *69*(4-5), 511-25.

Zhou, H., Li, Xuejun, & Gao, M. (2009). Curcumin protects PC12 cells from corticosterone-induced cytotoxicity: possible involvement of the ERK1/2 pathway. *Basic & clinical pharmacology & toxicology*, *104*(3), 236-40.

Zhou, J, Fu, Y., & Tang, X C. (2001). Huperzine A and donepezil protect rat pheochromocytoma cells against oxygen-glucose deprivation. *Neuroscience letters*, *306*(1-2), 53-6.

Zucker, M., Weizman, A., & Rehavi, M. (2005). Repeated swim stress leads to down-regulation of vesicular monoamine transporter 2 in rat brain nucleus accumbens and striatum. *European neuropsychopharmacology : the journal of the European College of Neuropsychopharmacology*, *15*(2), 199-201.

15

Targeting Effect of Traditional Chinese Medicine

Rui-Zhi Zhao
Second Affiliated Clinical College, Guangzhou University of Chinese Medicine, Nei Huan XiLu, Guangzhou Daxue Cheng, Guangzhou, China

1. Introduction

Most drugs have a widespread distribution in vivo, and effects beyond the disease site need to be avoided. As to herbs, it contains many components with different structure and varied effects, how to achieve the desired effect at the required site is a great challange. In ancient China, people usually get this goal by co-administration of other drugs, and in thousands of years, the experience was summarized as meridian guide theory. Since meridian guide theory is based on meridian distribution and compatibility, therefore, we should give a brief review about meridian, meridian distribution, and meridian guide drug.

In ancient China, diseases were treated by many methods, such as acupuncture, stone needle, drug, medicated bath, application, fumigate, and surgery. Concept of meridian was raised with acupuncture. In <Huangdi's Internal Classics>, the first monograph of China published at about 200 BC, diseases were divided according to their meridian, "meridian belongs to entrails inside and artus outside". There are 12 meridians, named as lung meridian, large intestine meridian, pericardium meridian, San Jiao meridian, heart meridian, small intestine meridian, spleen meridian, stomach meridian, liver meridian, gallbladder meridian, kidney meridian and urinary bladder meridian. Name of meridian is based on the main entrails the disease correlate and the route it will pass. And in <Huangdi's Internal Classics>, there are descriptions about the position, shape and weight of liver, heart, spleen, lung, kidney, intestine, stomach, gallbladder and urinary bladder, which are similar to that of modern anatomy. However, in ancient times, the anatomy was rough, and some version is different from modern views. For example, kidney is the main organ in kidney meridian, the function of "kidney" in traditional Chinese medicine includes kidney and genitical gland located near kidney. At that time, disease diagnosis and treatment especially in acupuncture was based on their meridian, such as taiyang diseases, yangming diseases, etc.

In Han dynasty, the famous physician Zhang Zhong-Jing described a method of diagnose - analyse and differentiate febrile diseases in accordance with the theory of six pairs of channels in his book < Treatise on Febrile Diseases> (Fu, 1990). Thereafter, drug use was summarized according to syndrome- differentiation of the six meridians. For example, nutgrass galingale rhizome is used to treat liver diseases, therefore, its meridian belongs to liver; fritillariae tuber is used to treat lung diseases such as cough, asthma, therefore, its meridian belongs to Lung; borneol is used to treat heart diseases, its meridian distribution is heart, etc. Some drugs have a wide use, its meridian distribution may be two or three entrails. For example, bupleuriradix is used to treat diseases of liver, Sanjiao, arcula cordis, and it belonges to these three meridians. And this is the basis for the formation of meridian distribution theory. In Tang and Song dynasty, there were some descriptions about drug orient and site-direct effect in books <Shi Liao Ben Cao>, <Supplement to the Herbal>, <Amplification on Canon of Materia Medica> and <Su Shen Liang Fang>. Thereafter, in Jin and Yuan dynasty, the famous physician Zhang Jie-Gu summarized these results and combined with his own experiment, raised the concept of meridian distribution. In his book <Zhen Zhu Lang>, and <Yi Xue Qi Yuan>, he summarized the experience of drug use according to meridian channels, such as "drug used to remove fire in ZANG FU-organ", "Meridian Guide drug of channels", and described meridian distribution as an important item of drug property. He thought that drug effect is related to its channal, and when used properly, the effect would be great. For example, Coptis chinensis, schtellaria, paeoniae radix, anemarrhenae, caulis hocquartiae, phellodendricortex, and gypsum all had the effect of purging pathogenic fire, however, Coptis chinensis is mainly used to purge the sthenic heart-fire, scutellaria is mainly used to purte the White, paeoniaeradix is mainly used to purge the sthenic liver-fire, caulis hocquartiae is used to rush down the fire in small intestine, phellodendricortex is mainly used to purge the fire in bladder. His disciple, famous physician Li Dong-Yuan and Wang Hao-Gu inherited his theory and developed it. In the book <Yong Yao Fa Xiang> of Li Dong-Yuan and <Materia Medica of Decoction> of Wang Hao-Gu, meridian distribution theory was used and improved. In <Materia Medica of Decoction>, there were 242 different kinds of drugs, among them, 80 were described as drugs with meridian distribution. In this book, drugs with meridian distribution were summarized in a table, named as "Guide profiles of various meridians". Due to its effectiveness in choosing drugs to formulate prescription, as it appeared, it was accepted by many physicians and more and more experience about drug meridian distribution was summarized. Then, in Ming dynasty, two famous physicians Liu Wen-Tai and Jia Ru-Li described meridian distribution as an indispensable content of drug property in their book <Ben Cao Pin Hui Jing Yao> and <Yao Pin Hua Yi> respectively. Li Shi-Zhen, a famous physician and pharmacist in Ming dynasty, inherited and developed the theory of meridian distribution of Zhang Jie-Gu in his world-famous book <Compendium of Materia Medica>, and indicated that "Chinese lovage is TaiYang meridian drug", "gypsum is cold Yangming meridian drug" etc. The meridian distribution of herbs was introduced when discussing drug property, such as "ephedra herb is the herb for lung meridian specially, when treating lung diseases, it is usually used." "frenugreek, herbs of right kidney, when kidney-YANG is deficient, it is used when cold-QI incubate in body and could not return to Yuan", "gastrodiarhizome is Qifen herbs belonging to liver meridian, in <Huangdi's Internal Classics>, it was indicated that all kinds of dazzling belongs to liver meridian, therefore, gastrodiarhizome could treat dizzy." Afterwards, meridian distribution was extensively described in books <Ben Cao Jing Shu> of Liao Xi-Yong, <Lei Gong Pao Zhi Yao Xing Jie> and <Ben Cao Tu Jie> by Li Zhong-Zi, , and more and more people accepted meridian distribution theory.

Meridian guide theory is the combination of meridian distribution and compatibility. It is first proposed in Qin and Han dynasty, and was developed in Tang and Song dynasty, formed at Jin and Yuan dynasty, completed in Ming and Qing dynasty. At 200 BC, in the first herb book <Shennong's herbal>, there was description that "Jun Gui is the message of other drugs". In Wei and Jin dynasty, famous physician Tao Hong-Jing described in his book <Ming Yi Bie Lu> that "cinnamomicortex guides other drugs". In Bei Song dynasty, Kou Zong-Shuang described in his book <Amplification on Canon of Materia Medica> that "Zhang Zhong-Jing used *Alismae rhizoma* in "Ba Wei Wan", just used it to guide cinnamomicortex and aconite root into kidney meridian, and no other means". In Jin and Yuan dynasty, Zhang Jie-Gu raised the concept of meridian guide drug. In his book <Zhen Zhu Lang>, he called drugs which could enforce other drugs effect at the meridian of its own as meridian guide drug, and listed meridian guide drug for twelve meridians. His disciple Li Dong-Yuan developed this idea and the theory. And then, in the book <Compendium of Materia Medica>, Li Shi-Zhen summarized the work of previous physicians, combined his and his father's experience in treating diseases, and revised the meridian guide drug of twelve channels. Also in this book, it is said that "ramuluscinnamomi guides other drugs to arm", "achyranthisradix guides other drugs to the lower part of the body" etc. Afterwards, many physicians exercised this method for diseases treatment, and got good results.

The twelve meridian guide drugs are: platycodonradix, angelica root, cimicifugae for lung meridian, gypsum and angelica root for large intestine meridian, cortex moutan and bupleuriradix for pericardium meridian, forsythia suspensa and bupleuriradix for San Jiao meridian, coptis chinensis, asariradix and borneol for heart meridian, Chinese lovage and phellodendri for small intestine meridian, atractylodes and cimicifugae for spleen meridian, angelica root, gypsum and pueraria for stomach meridian, vinger-baked bupleuriradix, evodiaefructus, and green tangerine peel for liver meridian, green tangerine peel and bupleuriradix for bladder meridian, cassia and anemarrhenae for kidney meridian, and incised notopterygium rhizome for urinary bladder meridian. There are some crossovers in meridian guide drug among different channels, for example, bupleuriradix and cimicifugae are meridian guide drugs for four channels, angelica root is the meridian guide drug for three channels. Besides twelve meridian guide drugs, there are some drugs for site targeting, such as chuanxiong for headache; ramulus cinnamomi and mulberry twig for Brachialgia; achyranthisradix for melosalgia; notopterygiirhizoma for cervical part disease etc. Many physicians practised meridian guide method in treating diseases and had a good effect, and they recorded their thoughts in their books. You Zai-Jing, a famous physician, said in his book <Yi Xue Du Shu Ji> that "soldiers could not reach enemies' place if there is not a guide, and drugs could not reach the disease site if there is not a meridian guide drug". Another physician in Qing dynasty, Shen Shi-Pao said that " meridian guide drug could induce other drugs to the disease site, and a great effect could be achieved with less drug used". Many famous prescriptions contained meridian guide drug, such as bupleuriradix in "Xiao Chai Hu Tang", gypsum in "Bai Hu Tang", kudzuvine root in "Ge Gen Qin Lian Tang", platycodiradix in "Sen Ling Bai Zhu San", and evodiaefructus in "Zuo Jin Wan", achyranthisradix in "San Miao San" and "Hu Qian Wan". Even in modern times, many famous physicians indicated that using meridian guide drug is an effective way for drug targeting (R.Z. Zhao et al, 2005).

Nowdays, more and more drugs are found to have side effects, and these effects affected clinical results especially for cancer treatment, about 30% patients give up treatment due to serious side effects of anticancer drugs. Many technologies are used to increase the therapeutic effect and reduce the side effect. However, site-directed pharmaco-delivery is a desirable but elusive goal. Although there are great achievements in target delivery, the clinical results were beyond people's expectation due to the difference between animals and human beings. The concept of meridian guide drug is similar to that of target delivery system, may be a new way for targeting delivery. Therefore, some studies had been carried out to demonstrate the meridian guide theory by experiment.

2. Modern study of meridian guide drug

At present, two methods are usually used to study meridian guide theory. One is pharmacokinetics method. This method demonstrated the effect of meridian guide drug by comparing drug distribution before and after co-administration with meridian guide drugs. This method is based on the hypothesis that drug effect is dependent on its concentration. The second method is pharmacological method. Meridian guide effect was investigated by comparing the target site effect between drug and their co-administration with meridian guide drugs. This method is based on the clinical definition of meridian guide drug. Vinegar-baked bupleuriradix, meridian guide drug of liver, platycodiradix, meridian guide drug of lung, borneol, meridian guide of heart meridian, and achyranthisradix, meridian guide drug of legs have been studied.

2.1 Study of liver meridian guide drug: vinegar-baked bupleuriradix

Bupleuriradix, is the dry radix of *Bupleurum Chinense DC*, and *B. Scozoneri folium wide.* It tastes acrid, and belongs to liver, cholecyst, Sanjiao and pericardium meridian. It is usually used in the treatment of influenza, fever, malaria, hepatitis, jaundice, nephritis, dizziness, bitter taste in the mouth, lung disease, cancer, and menstrual disorders in China, Japan, and other Asia. Pharmacological study showed that it had the effect of anti-inflammatory (S.M.Chen et al, 2008), antiviral activities (Chiang, 2003), antioxidant and hepatoprotective effect (B.J. Wang et al, 2004) etc. It is the meridian guide drug of liver, pericardium, gall bladder and Sanjiao meridian. In traditional Chinese medicine theory, it is regarded that drugs with sour taste enters liver first, and when baked with vinegar, it is the liver meridian guide only. It is described in the book <Ben Cao Zheng Yi> that "…besides, there is stagnation in collaterals and subcollaterals of liver, add few of bupleuriradix, the effect is quick".

Li Xiao-Dong and Nie Sa et al studied the effect of vinegar on pharmacological and chemical of bupleuriradix. The results showed that both pharmacological effect and components in the drug changed a little bit due to the vinegar-baked procedure (X.D. Li, 2000; S.Nie et al; 2008). It was demonstrated that vinegar-baked bupleuriradix had a much stronger effect on acesodyne and bile secretion than that of the bupleuriradix (J.Wu, 2008; S.Q Nie et al; 2002). Therefore, vinegar-baked bupleuriradix was extensively used in the liver diseases treatment medicines (Kou et al, 2006), such as DA Chai Hu Tang, Xiao Yao San, Xiao Chai Hu Tang etc. The study method was pharmacokinetics based.

2.1.1 Vinegar-baked bupleuriradix affected drug distribution

Four components were chosen in studying the liver targeting effect of vinegar-baked bupleuriradix, these are resveratrol (R.Z. Zhao et al., 2009), rhein (R.Z. Zhao et al., 2010), oxymatrine (unpublished data), and gentiopicroside (unpublished data). Their structure belongs to chrysophenine glycoside, anthraquinone, alkaloid and iridoid glycode respectively. In these studies, except resveratrol, animals were divided into two large groups according to dose of the components, and in each large group, animals were divided into four groups based on the dose of vinegar-baked bupleuriradix. For resveastrol, there was only one large group, and subgroup was similar to that of the other studies.

The detail of the experiment is listed in Table 1. For oral administration, components were suspended in solutions containing 1% sodium carboxymethylcellulose or in vinegar-baked bupleuriradix solutions containing 1% sodium carboxymethylcellulose. At predetermined time points, six animals were taken out from each group and blood was collected via heart puncture. Tissues of interest (heart, liver, spleen, lung, and kidney) were collected immediately after cervical dislocation and were blotted dry with tissue paper. Plasma and tissue samples were frozen at -80°C until analysis.

Component	Animal	Detection method	Detected components	subgroups	Drug dose (mg/kg)	Dose of vinegar-baked bupleuriradix (mg/kg)
resveratrol	mice	HPLC	resveratrol	4	200	300, 600,1200
rhein	rats	HPLC	Rhein and conjugated rhein	8	80, 40	300, 600, 1200
oxymatrine	mice	HPLC-MS	Oxymatrine and matrine	8	80, 10	400, 800, 1200
gentiopicroside	mice	HPLC-MS	gentiopicroside	8	100, 50	400, 800,1200

Table 1. Experiment design of liver targeting effect of vinegar-baked bupleuriradix

In all the studied animal groups, vinegar-baked bupleuriradix showed liver targeting effects for all the components with different degree. This effect is dependent on the dose of vinegar-baked bupleuriradix, components and its structure. Table 2 listed the most effective group within the study.

Vinegar- baked bupleuriradix enhanced other drugs liver distribution by three ways. First, it increased the Cmax of other drugs in liver, this indicated that vinegar-baked bupleuriradix enhanced liver uptake of other drug. This effect is component structure related. Among these four components, rhein is the most sensitive drug to the effect of vinegar-baked bupleuriradix, the maximal increased Cmax ratio in liver was 565%; second sensitive component is oxymatrine, the maximal increased Cmax ratio in liver was 89%, the third is gentiopicroside, the maximal increased Cmax ratio was 21%; and resveratrol is the least sensitive to the effect of vinegar baked bupleuriradix, its Cmax had marginal change. AUC is a parameter determined by Cmax and elimination rate. When using AUC as the evaluation criteria, rhein is still the most sensitive component to the effect of vinegar-baked bupleuriradix, second is oxymatrine. However the third is resveratrol, the increased AUC in liver was 79%, and gentiopicroside was the most insensitive component to the effect of vinegar-baked bupleuriradix. It should be indicated that although vinegar-baked bupleuriradix had marginal effect on the uptake of resveratrol, it decreased the elimination rate of resveratrol in liver significantly, also induced an increase in AUC.

Second, vinegar-baked bupleuriradix decreased AUC and Cmax of these components in other tissues. Rhein is the most sensitive components to the effect of vinegar-baked bupleuriradix. Low dose of vinegar-baked bupleuriradix decreased the distribution of rhein in other tissues except liver, and the decreased AUC ratio was 82%, 57%, 30%, 25% and 15% for spleen, heart, blood, lung and kidney respectively. The second sensitive component was resveratrol, high dose of vinegar-baked bupleuriradix decreased the distribution of resveratrol in kidney, spleen, heart and lung significantly, the decreased AUC ratio was 30%, 30%, 32% and 30% respectively. The third sensitive component was oxymatrine, medium dose of vinegar-baked bupleuriradix decreased the distribution of oxymatrine in blood, spleen, heart, and lung, the decreased AUC ratio was 33%, 27%, 17% and 19%, the least sensitive components was gentiopicroside, medium dose of vinegar-baked bupleuriradix only decreased the AUC of gentiopicroside in blood and lung, the decreased ratio was 17% and 18% respectively.

Drugs	AUC Changed extent in liver	Cmax Changed extent in liver	AUC Changed extent in other tissues	Cmax Changed extent in other tissues	Drug distribution original
resveratrol	79%	No significance	-44% in lung, 58% in heart, and 42% in kidney	-46% in kidney, -23% in lung, and -16% in heart	Kidney> liver> lung> blood> heart> spleen
rhein	264%	226%	-72%, -57%, -30%, -25%, -15% in spleen, heart, blood, lung and kidney respectively	- 31% in heart, and -65% in spleen	Kidney> lung> blood> liver> spleen> heart
Conjugated rhein	21%	No significance	-53%, -48%, -43%, -39% and -30% in lung, heart, spleen, kidney, and blood respectively	-36% in heart, and -23% in kidney	Spleen> lung> kidney> heart > liver≈blood
oxymatrine	152%	89%	-33%, -17%, -27%, -19% in blood, heart, spleen and lung respectively	56% in kidney, -36% in lung, -15% in blood	Blood> lung> spleen> kidney> liver≈ blood
matrine	32%	20%	-73%,-37%, -35%, -16% in lung, blood, heart, and kidney respectively	-63%,-46%,-41%, 35%,-28% in heart, kidney, blood, spleen, and lung respectively	Blood> liver> kidney> spleen≈ heart≈ lung
Gentio-picroside	No significance	20%	-39%, -27%, -27%, -18% in kidney, heart, spleen, lung respectively	-35% ,-36% -15% in heart, spleen and kidney respectively	Kidney> blood> liver> lung> heart> spleen

Table 2. The results of vinegar-baked bupleuriradix on the AUC, Cmax of other components, listed results were the most effective groups when using relative targeting ratio as evaluation index.

Third, vinegar-baked bupleuriradix decreased the elimination rate of all these four components in liver, but increased their elimination rate in other tissues. This may be another reason for AUC increase in liver and AUC decrease in other tissues.

The liver targeting effect of vinegar-baked bupleuriradix also depended on drug and vinegar-baked bupleuriradix dose. For resveratrol and gentiopicroside, medium dose of vinegar-baked bupleuriradix had the strongest effect. For rhein, in high rhein dose group, low dose of vinegar-baked bupleuriradix had the strongest effect, but in low rhein dose group, high dose of vinegar-baked bupleuriradix had the strongest effect. For oxymatrine, in high oxymatrine dose group, high and medium dose of vinegar-baked bupleuriradix had the strongest effect. For gentiopicroside, rhein and oxymatrine, all components were sensitive to the effect of vinegar-baked bupleuriradix at their high dose than that at low dose.

In the study of rhein and oxymatrine, effects of vinegar-baked bupleuriradix on the distribution of their metabolites were also studied. Interestingly, similar phenomenon was observed when the index is conjugated rhein and matrine. Vinegar-baked bupleuriradix increased not only their distribution in liver, but also decreased their distribution in other tissues, also showing a liver targeting effect. Compared the sensitivity of rhein, oxymatrine together with their metabolites to the effect of vinegar-baked bupleuriradix, rhein metabolite was less sensitive than its native form, and rhein dose had marginal effect. However, the sensitivity of oxymatrine to the effect of vinegar-baked bupleuriradix was dependent on its dose, in high dose group of oxymatrine, oxymatrine was more sensitive than its metabolite, anyhow, in low dose group of oxymatrine, matrine was more sensitive than its native form.

When comparing their own distribution and the effect of vinegar-baked bupleuriradix, it is found that for the components which are sensitive to the effect of vinegar-baked bupleuriradix, their main distribution is not in liver. For rhein and oxymatrine, liver distribution was only 5% and 3.8% of the total drug in vivo respectively. However, the two components were less sensitive to the effect of vinegar-baked bupleuriradix, their distribution in liver was relatively high, AUC in liver was 17% and 17.9% for gentiopicroside and resveratrol respectively.

2.1.2 Liver targeting effect mechanism of Vinegar-baked bupleuriradix

Effect of vinegar-baked bupleuriradix on drug distribution implied that vinegar-baked bupleuriradix may affect cell uptake of the drug and this is related with membrane constituents. Therefore, the effect of vinegar-baked bupleuriradix on membrane permeability, membrane constituents, pHi and morphology of BRL cell line were investigated (unpublished data). In these studies, samples were divided into four groups according to the concentration of vinegar-baked bupleuriradix, 10 mg/mL, 2 mg/mL, 0.4 mg/mL and drug free group, respectively. In each group, samples were further divided into 3 h, 6 h, 10 h, 18 h, 24 h, 48 h and 72 h subgroups according to the culture time for permeability study (n=5), and 3, 6, 12, 24, 48 h for membrane constituents study (n=5), and 12 h sample for morphology study. Each experiment was repeated five times. Membrane permeability was determined by flow cytometry, membrane morphology of BRL was observed by electronic microscope, and constituents were determined by automatic biochemistry analysator and thin layer chromatography scanning method.

Vinegar-baked bupleuriradix increased the BRL membrane permeability significantly, and this effect was vinegar-baked bupleuriradix concentration dependent, at all the time points, high concentration vinegar-baked bupleuriradix had a stronger effect than that of low concentration, and as the culture time prolonged, the effect of vinegar-baked bupleuriradix concentration on the permeability was more obvious. Further study showed that the membrane permeability increase was not due to membrane breakage, but prompting the growth of BRL cell. Morphology study showed that compared with the control group, the cell surface was much smoother after co-cultured with medium and high dose of vinegar-baked bupleuriradix, the effect was drug dose dependent. In order to study the reason, the content of cholesterol, protein and lipids were determined. Vinegar-baked bupleuriradix had marginal effect on the content of cholesterol, and the effect of vinegar-baked bupleuriradix on the lipids and protein content was dependent on the culture time and drug dose.

Cholesterol/phospholipids reflected cell integrity and permeability, when it decreased, the increase of permeability is toxic to cells, in this study, however, compared to the control group, high and medium dose of vinegar-baked bupleuriradix increased the ratio at 3, 12, 24 h, only decreased the ratio at 6 h, low dose of vinegar-baked bupleuriradix had marginal effect on the ratio.

Proportion among lipids is related with membrane fluidity, and it is related with membrane permeability, especially phosphatidylcholine/phosphatidyl ethanolamine ratio. Like cholesterol/phospholipids ratio, when it is decreased, cells are under danger. However, vinegar-baked bupleuriradix increased the ratio before 12 h, and thereafter, it had marginal effect on it. Membrane constituents were related with transporters, and the effect of vinegar-baked bupleuriradix on the activity of P- glycoprotein in BRL cell line was also studied, and the results showed that vinegar-baked bupleuriradix inhibited the activity of P-glycoprotein, this is in accordance with the results of morphological and membrane constituents results, and indicated that liver targeting effect of vinegar-baked bupleuriradix may be related with transporters.

2.2 Study of lung meridian guide drug: platycodiradix

Platycodiradix is the root of *Platycodon grandiflorum* A. DC, and it is widely used in treating diseases of lung and respiratory system, such as laryngopharyngitis, bronchitis, asthma, pulmonary tuberculosis, and pneumonia in clinics in China. Pharmacological research showed that it is responsible for diverse effects including anti-inflammation, anti-allergy, anti-tumor, augmentation of immune response, anti-obesity, anti-oxidation, hypoglycemic activity etc (Y.Tai et al, 2009). It is described in book <Ben Cao Qiu Zhen> that platycodiradix could promote the function of lung, and guide other drugs to lung. Therefore, it is the meridian guide drug of lung.

The lung target enhancing effect of platycodiradix was studied by pharmacokinetics method. Animals were divided into two groups, drug alone group and drugs co-administration with platycodiradix. Drug concentration and the target evaluation were listed in Table 3. The studied components included levofloxadin (Y.L, Li et al., 2006), florenicol (Y.L. Li et al., 2008), and roxithromycin (Y.L. Li et al., 2005).

component	animal	Detection method	Detected components	Drug dose	Target evaluation
levofloxacin	chicken	HPLC	levofloxacin	10mg/kg	Cmax, AUC
Florfenicol	rabbit	HPLC	florfenicol	30mg/kg	Cmax, AUC
roxithromycin	chicken	Biological effect method	roxithromycin	8,10,12mg/kg	Cmax, AUC

Table 3. Experiment design of lung targeting effect of platycodiradix

Platycodiradix increased the distribution of levofloxacin, florfenicol in lung significantly and this effect is platycodiradix dose dependent and components property related. The most sensitive component was levofloxacin. When co-administered with platycodiradix, Cmax of levofloxacin in lung increased 4.4 times; and its AUC increased 470%, although platycodiradix also increased the AUC of levofloxacin in heart and kidney, the increased extent was far less than that in lung. Florfenicol was less sensitive than levofloxacin. Platycodiradix increased Cmax and AUC of florfenicol in lung. However, it also increased the distribution of florfenicol in liver. Meanwhile it decreased Cmax of florfenicol in blood and kidney with the decreased extent of 28% and 44% respectively.

Drugs	AUC Changed extent in lung	Cmax Changed extent inlung	AUC Changed extent in other tissues	Cmax Changed extent in other tissues	Drug distribution original	Distribution ratio of drug in lung
levofloxacin	440%	470%	-15% in liver, 50% in kidney, 44% in heart	-14% in liver, 72.7% in heart, 103% in kidney	Kidney>=liver >heart=lung	8.5%
Florfenicol	50%	59.7%	-26% in blood, 76.8% in liver	-28% in blood, -44% in kidney 110% in liver,	Kidney> lung≈ liver> heart	10.4%
Roxithro-mycin	No significance	36%	_	_	_	_

Table 4. Results of lung targeting effect of Platycodiradix, _ represent no data

Effect of platycodiradix on the distribution of roxithromycin was a little different from that of others. Although at 10mg/kg dose, platycodiradix increased Cmax of roxithromycin, it had marginal effect on AUC, platycodiradix enhanced drug absorption, Tmax of roxithromycin was 3 or 4 h for medium and low dose respectively, when co-administered with platycodiradix, Tmax was 0.75 h and 1.5 h respectively. In control group, drug was absorbed slowly, and there were 3 peaks, but in experimental group, there was only 1 peak. Multi-peak usually indicated liver-intestine cycle, and platycodiradix may be able to inhibit this cycle and induce a rapid elimination. Since effect of platycodiradix on drug distribution in other tissues was not studied, effect of platycodiradix on roxithromycin is not complete. This limited our knowledge.

2.3 Effect of borneol on brain targeting

Borneol, a simple bicyclic monoterpene with acrid-bitter flavor, belongs to heart, spleen and lung meridian, it has the effect of communicating holes and scattering stagnant fire, detumescencing and relieving the pain. It is frequently used in the treatment of encephalopathy, such as stroke, epilepsy and headache. Pharmacological study showed that borneol had the effect of anti-excitation of central nerve induced by picrotoxin, prolong the delitescence of hyperspasmia, prolong the survival time of mice under oxygen deficiency, and prolong the awareness of tired rats (S.R.Wu & G.Cheng et al, 2001).

In the book "Amplification on Canon of Materia Medical", it is said that "borneol is weak when used alone, it strengthens the therapeutic action of other herbs when it is used as an adjuvant and message drug", it also had the effect of "commanding other drugs". In <Plain Questions of Huangdi's Internal Classic>, it is said that "Heart, King of organs, mind efferens", "heart controls mental and emotional activities", that is to say, brain function in ancient China was listed as "Heart". Therefore it is the meridian guide drug of brain.

2.3.1 Borneol increased drug concentration in brain

Brain targeting effect of borneol was studied by determining drug concentration in brain and pharmacological method. Drugs studied using the first method included sodium ferulate (Z.Z. Lin et al, 2008), carbamazepine (H.Y. Zhou et al, 2008), tetramethylpyra (Y.

Wang et al, 2006), methotrexat (Gao et al, 2009), rifampici (S.R. Wu et al, 2004), Panax pseudo-ginsing (S.X. Wang et al, 2009), puerarin (C.Y. Gao et al, 2010), gastrodin (Cai et al, 2008), cidomycin (Q.D. Liu et al, 1994), danshensu (J. Liu et al, 2008) et al. The study design was listed in Table 5.

Drugs	Animal	Detection method	Detected components	Drug dose g/kg	Meridian guide drug dose (g/kg)	Target evaluation
Sodium ferulate	mice	HPLC-MS	Sodium ferulate	0.2	0.05,0.002	Concentration in brain and blood
Carbamazepine	mice	HPLC	Carbamazepine, 10,11- epoxide carbamazepine		0.75	Cmax, AUC
Tetramethyl-pyrazine	rat	HPLC	Tetramethyl-pyrazine	0.0034	0.034	Concentration in blood and brain
methotrexat	Rabbit	HPLC	Methotrexat	0.1	0.75	Concentration in brain
Cidomycin	rat	Enzyme immu-nization	cidomycin	0.035	1.0	Concentration in brain
rifampici	Mice	HPLC	rifampici	0.182	0.6	AUC
notoginsenoside R1	rabbit	HPLC	notoginseng R1	15.0	0.085	Concentration in tissues
Ginsenoside Rg1	rabbit	HPLC	ginsenoside Rgl	15.0	0.085	Concentrationin tisues
Ginsenoside Re	rabbit	HPLC	ginsenoside Re	15.0	0.085	Concentration in tissues
Puerarin	Rats	HPLC	puerarin	0.0625	0.3	AUC in brain
gastrodin	mice	HPLC	gastrodin	0.2	0.4, 0.6	AUC in brain and blood
danshensu	rabbit	HPLC-MS	Danshnsu	10	0.18	Concentration in tissues

Table 5. Experiment design of brain targeting effect of borneol

Among these drugs, cidomycin is aminoglycoside antibiotic, puerarin is a kind of flavonoid, notoginsenoside R1, ginsenoside Rg1 and Re are saponin, rifampici is rifomycins antibiotics, methotrexat is antifolate drug. Borneol increased their distribution in brain, and this effect is borneol dose dependnt and chemical structure related. In the study of borneol to the distribution of gastrodin, 40 and 60 mg/kg borneol increased the distribution of gastrodin in brain significantly. However, 20 mg/kg had marginal effect on the distribution of gastrodin. Among the reported study, Ginsenoside Rg1 was the most sensitive compound to the effect of borneol, and drug concentration increase in brain was 2438%. Although it also increased drug concentration in other tissues, the increased ratio was far less than that in brain. The second sensitive component was notoginsenoside R1, the increased ratio of drug concentration in brain was 523%, and borneol also increased drug concentration in other tissues in the meantime. The originally distribution of these two components in brain was very low. Borneol also had the effect of decreasing drug concentration in non-target tissues. For example, borneol decreased the concentration of tetramethylpyrazine in blood, and decreased the concentration of rifampici in liver and kidney.

Drugs	% Change of AUC in Brain	% Change of Con-centration in brain	AUC Change in other tissues	Cmax Change in other tissues	Drug distribution original
Sodium ferulate	66%	47%	No significance	46% in blood	_
Carbamazepine	24.5%	129%	-9%~- 37% in lung, liver, heart and kidney	14%~29%, in liver, lung, blood, heart, muscle, 175% in spleen	Lung> brain> fat> liver> blood> kidney> spleen >heart > muscle
epoxide carbamazepine	174.5%	56%	-52~- 40% in lung, liver and heart	146% in spleen, -38%, -20.5%,-53% in lung, liver and heart respectively	Lung>heart> liver> kidney> blood> brain> fat> spleen> muscle
Tetramethylpyrazine	30%	26 %	-15% in blood	-10%	_
methotrexat	75%	56.5%	No significance	No significance	_
Cidomycin	-	142%	-	22.8	_
rifampici	99%	79%	-12%, -17%, 64%, 46% in liver, kidney lung and blood respectively	-40%,-24% 75% in liver , kidney and lung respectively	Liver> kidney> lung> blood> brain
notoginsenoside R1	--	523%	--	497% , 227% , 36% 20% in liver, lung, heart, kidney	Heart> kidney> lung> liver> brain
ginsenoside Rgl	_	2438%	_	927%, 567% and 491% in heart, kidney, liver	lung> liver >kidney >heart >brain
ginsenoside Re	_	71%	_	264%, 251%, 85% 73% in, liver, lung, heart, kidney	Kidney >heart > brain= liver > lung
Puerarin	191%	-	-	-	Lung>>kidney> pancreas> liver> heart> spleen> brain
gastrodin	109%	80%	No significance	No significance	
Danshensu	_	355%		-100%, 158%, 104%in heart, liver, kidney respectively	Kidney> heart> brain >liver

Table 6. Effect of borneol on drug distribution of other drugs

Among these studies, only in the study of carbamazepine, the effect of borneol on the metabolite of carbamazepine was studied. Borneol also increased the distribution of the metabolite of carbamazepine in brain, and decreased its distribuion in lung, liver and heart, also showed a brain targeting effect. However, since most of these studies only pay attention to the blood-brain barrier, effect of borneol on drug distribution in other tissues was neglected, and this limited our knowedge of borneol on the absorption, distribution, elimination and excretion of the studied drugs.

2.3.2 Brain action enhancing effect of borneol

Besides pharmacokinetics study, pharmacological method was also used to demonstrate the effect of borneol. Ischemic reperfusion usually induces brain injury. Although some drugs are effective for ischemic reperfusion, low drug concentration in brain limited their effect. Sodium ferulate is one of these drugs.

Chen Xiao-Hong et al studied the brain curative enhancing effect of borneol on sodium ferulate by ischaemia reperfused model (X. H. Chen et al, 2010). Mice were randomly divided into 6 groups (n = 6): sham-treated, which was administered 10% ethanol, treated group included sodium ferulate 100 mg/kg per day, sodium ferulate 400 mg/kg per day, borneol 10 mg/kg per day, sodium ferulate 100 mg/kg +10 mg/kg borneol per day, sodium ferulate 400 mg/kg +10 mg/kg borneol per day. Therapy was initiated 30 min before or after ischaemia reperfused. To evaluate the treatment effects, tissues of the mice were collected for brain oedema analysis after 24 h of ischaemia reperfusion, for BBB permeability detection after 48 h and for Morris water maze test after 4 days of ischaemia reperfusion. Ischemic reperfusion model was made by the bilateral common carotid artery occlusion method. The results showed that compared with sham-operated group, the ischaemia reperfused mice were associated with long-lasting spatial learning deficits in the absence of other behavioral impairments and with neurodegeneration in the hippocampal CA1 region. However, the histological injuries were significantly attenuated by oral co-administration of sodium ferulate with borneol. Furthermore, combined treatment with sodium ferulate and borneol resulted in a significant reduction in brain oedema, gliofibrillar acid protein-positive cells, and blood–brain barrier permeability, but an increase in superoxide dismutase activity, indicating a brain targeting enhancing effect.

Artherosclerosis is the patho-basis for coronary disease and stroke. Dioscin, a component from plants of dioscoreaceae, lilium and pulse family, is usually used to treat coronary disease but due to blood- brain barrier, it is seldomly used to treat stroke. Wang Guang-Jian et al investigated the cure effect of dioscin on stroke when co- administered with borneol (G.J. Wang, 2010).

Rats were divided into five groups randomly, that is control group (sham operation group), model group, dioscin group (0.2g / kg), dioscin (0.2g / kg) co-administered with borneol (0.01g/kg) and dioscin (0.2g / kg) co-administered with borneol (0.02g/kg). Animals were administered drugs or equal volume of isotonic Na chloride (for control and model group). After 7 days, besides control group, animals in other groups were made into cerebral ischemia model by block arteria cerebri media. After the animals were recovered, their neurology was given a mark. Thereafter, animals were sacrificed, brain were taken out, dyeing and calculated the ratio of cerebral infarction.

The results showed that no neurologic impairment was found in control group. Animals in model group appeared ptosis, enophothamos, the neurology mark increased significantly, and cerebral infarction ratio was 12.9%. Compared with model group, cerebral infraction ratio and neurology mark of animals in dioscin and dioscin co-administration with low dose of borneol group had a tendency of decreasing, however, dioscin co-administered with high dose of borneol decreased the cerebral infarction ratio and neurology mark significantly, indicating a very obvious synergy effect.

2.3.3 Mechanism study of borneol

The most accepted thought is that low drug concentration in brain is due to blood- brain barrier. And mechanism studies about borneol were focused on the blood- brain barrier and its tight junction. Zhao Bao-Sheng and Liu Qi-De studied the effect of borneol on blood-brain barrier, and compared its effect with the blood-brain opening under pathological condition (B.S.Zhao & Q.D. Liu, 2002). The activity of anti-induce nitric oxide synthetase antibody (iNOS) in capillary endotheliocyte of brain was determined by streptomycin-bioepiderm - oxidase linking method. Compared with normal control group, iNOS in normal animals administered with borneol did not increase, while in animals with brain injured iNOS increased significantly, indicating that the opening of blood-brain barrier induced by borneol was different from that under pathological conditions. Ultrastructure of the blood-brain barrier influenced by borneol were also studied (Ge et al, 2008). It was showed that compared with the control group, borneol loosened the tight junction and some of the tight junction was not continuous. After 24h, the ultrastructure turned to normal, also indicating a reversible effect.

Since many factors are not easily controlled in vivo, people studied the effect of borneol on tight junction of BBB using different cell models. Chen Yan-Ming & Wang Ning-Sheng et al studied effect of borneol on the BBB model constructed by MDCK cell line (Y.M. Chen and N.S. Wang, 2004). First, borneol was administrated to rabbits for 4 consective days, and blood were taken out, the concentration of borneol in serum determined by GC-MS was 133 μg/ mL. Study was carried out by comparing the BBB among MDCK cells co-cultured with serum at different time and concentration, containing or not containing borneol. After 4 h co-culture with serum containing 0.086 μmol/L borneol, the tight junction was open, after 24h co-culture with serum containing borneol at the same concentration, the number and volume of pinocytosis vesicles in the BBB cells increased significantly, thus accelerating the transport of substances by cell pinocytosis. However, 24h after removing serum contained borneol, effect of borneol disappeared and there was no difference in morphology when compared with normal cell. This is in accordance with the in vivo effect, also indicating a reversible effect.

P-glycoprotein is multidrug resistant protein. There are lots of P-glycoprotein in BBB, and some people think it is one of the reasons that BBB restrains other drugs from getting into the brain. Chen Yan-Ming & Wang Ning-Sheng studied the effect of borneol on the vinblastine toxicity in MDCK and Hela cell line, verapamil was the positive control. It was found that borneol increased the toxicity of vinblatine in both cell lines significantly, and the increased degree was similar to that of verapamil, indicating that borneol may be able to inhibit the activity of P-glycoprotein (Y.M Chen. & N.S.Wang, 2003).

Histamine and 5- hydroxytryptamine take part in the regulation of BBB, therefore, Li Wei-Rong et al studied the effect of borneol on the content of histamine and 5-hydroxytryptamine. The results showed that borneol increased the contents of histamine and 5-hydroxytryptamine in brain significantly, indicating that effect of borneol on BBB may be related with histamine and 5-hydroxytryptamine (W.R. Li et al, 2006).

2.4 Meridian guide effect of achyranthisradix

Achyranthisradix is the radix of *Achyranthes bidentata BI.* It tastes sweet, a little bitter and sour, belongs to kidney, liver meridian. It had the effect of enforcing the function of liver and kidney, strengthening bones and muscle, inducing float fire to descend and promoting diuresis for stranguria. In clinic, it is usually used to treat gonarthritis, swelling of throat caused by flaring up of stomach fire, and gingivitis etc. A famous physician Wang Ang in Qing dynasty said in his book <Essentials of Metea Medica> that "achyranthisradix induces fire to descend". Zhang Xi-Chun said in his book <Yi Xue Zhong Zhong Can Xi Lu> that "achyranthisradix induces fire and blood to descend". In book <Han Wen Tiao Bian>, it is described that "achyranthisradix, when used without baking, its property descends quickly, it could cure emia and amenia, induce other drugs to descend". In book <Ben Cao Feng Yuan>, it was reported that "achyranthisradix induces other drugs to the lower part, arthrolithiasis of bones and muscles at the lower part should use it". It is the meridian guide of lower limb.

Pharmacological study revealed that achyranthisradix enhanced lympholeukocyte to reproduce, and increased the secretion of IL-2, decreased the Sil-2 content in old rats. It also increased the SOD activity, LPO content in old and feeble rats. Besides, it had the effect of anti-tumor, anti- inflammatory, anti- bacteria, and analgesic (Meng & Li, 2001). Its meridian guide effect was studied by pharmacokinetics combined with pharmacological method.

Rats were divided into five groups randomly, that is normal control group, model control group, achyranthisradix group (5g/kg), diclofenac sodium (10mg/kg) group, achyranthisradix (5g/kg) co-administered with diclofenac sodium group (10mg/kg for diclofenac sodium). Besides normal group, Freud's compete adjuvant (0.1mL) were injected at right voix pedis of rats in other groups, and made the inflammatory model for 28 days by measuring weights and the volume of voix pedis each week. At the 22 day, drugs were administered to rats and the drug administration continued to the 28 day. On the last day, after measuring weight and volume of voix pedis, rats were anesthetized, and blood was collected from hepatic portal vein. Afterwards rats were sacrificed, right voix pedis was cut down and the skin was removed, the soft tissues were weighed and homogenized, the content of diclofenac sodium in blood, and voix pedis was determined by high performance liquid chromatography, the content of PGE2 was determined by kit., the content of IL-1β was determined by radio-immunity kit.

Compared with normal control group, right voix pedis in model group swelled significantly ($P<0.01$), both PGE and IL-1β increased significantly. In the study of diclofenac sodium, compared to the model group, both diclofenac sodium and its co-administration with achyranthisradix inhibited the swell significantly, achyranthisradix alone had marginal effect on the swell. Compared with diclofenac sodium, effect of inhibited swell was more effective in the group co-administered with achyranthisradix, showing a synergistic effect. Diclofenac sodium decreased both the PGE content in blood and inflammatory tissues significantly, and there was no difference between the decreased ratio in blood and inflammatory tissues. Achyranthisradix had marginal effect on PGE content, however when co-administered with diclofenac sodium, it decreased PGE content both in blood and inflammatory tissues significantly, and the decreased ratio in inflammtory tissues was more obvious, and this is different from the effect of diclofenac sodium. Same results was obtained when comparing the content of IL-1β. Both diclofenac sodium alone and co-administration with achyranthisradix decreased the content of IL-1β significantly, the latter had no significance when compared with normal control group, all these results showed that achyranthisradix could enhance the effect of diclofenac sodium. Besides, compared with model group, diclofenac sodium decreased the weight of rats significantly, when co-

administered with achyranthisradix, the weight of rats increased, indicating that achyranthisradix decreased the side effect of diclofenac sodium (Y.Q Lin, 2009).
Drug concentration in tissues gave a clue for the pharmacological results. When co-administered with achyranthisradix, concentration of diclofenac sodium in blood decreased, and drug concentration in inflammatory site increased significantly, the decreased and increased extent were 75% and 10% respectively.

3. Meridian guide drug and transporters

Above results showed that meridian guide drug enhanced the curative effect of the co-administered drugs and this effect was induced by the increased distribution of other drugs in target site or decreased distribution in non-target site. This is in accordance with modern theory, and demonstrated that meridian guide drug could be used as a target delivery method.
Drug concentration in tissues is a balance of uptake and elimination. Uptake could be reflected by Cmax. Almost all the results in pharmacokinetics studies showed that meridian guide drug increased a Cmax of other drugs in target site, this indicated that increasing the uptake is one of the ways for the effect of meridian guide drug. Elimination rate could be calculated by the concentration- time profile. Meridian guide drug usually increased the elimination in non- target site in above studies. Usually, drug uptake into cells and efflux to outside through two methods, one is passive diffusion, the other is active transport. Passive diffusion mainly depends on the property of the drugs, and fewer factors could affect it. Active transport is different, since it needs the help of carriers, factors which affected the activity directly or indirectly would affect its transport efficiency. Above results indicated that the effect of meridian guide drug may be related with influx and efflux transporters.
Mechanism study also gives some clues for meridian guide drug with transporters. In cell surface, there are lots of lipid raft related with the transport of xenobiotics and endogenous metabolites. Vinegar-baked bupleuriradix increased the permeability of BRL cell line, and in high dose the cell surface changed smoothly, indicating a change at transport capability. Further study indicated that this change was due to membrane constituents change.
Transporters is a kinds of protein resides in membrane and is responsible for the across of xenobiotics and endogenous metabolites into cells. Transporters could be divided into two families according to their transport directions, and they are influx transporters and efflux transporters. Influx transporters include organic anion transport protein (OAT), organic anion transport polypeptide (OATP), organic cation transport protein (OCT) and organic cation transport polypeptide (OCTP). Efflux transporters, also named as ATP- binding cassette (ABC) transporter super-family, include P- glycoprotein (P-gp), the multi-drug resistance protein family (MRP1-9), the breast cancer resistance protein (BCRP). There are many excellent reviews about them (H. Miyazaki et al, 2004; Kusuhara & Sugiyama, 2002; Shirata et al, 2006; M. L. Elaine et al, 2005; S. Gergely, 2008). The distribution of transporters is vary with different tissue, and the results are listed in Table 8. For example, OAT1 was expressed in kidney, brain, uterus, but OCT 1 was predominantly expressed in liver, and had trace amount in kidney; OAT3 was expressed in kidney, liver, brain, and eye; MRP1 was extensively expressed in most organs, and had a high expression in lung, testicle, kidney, musculi skeleti, peripheral blood mononuclear cell etc, but had a relatively low expression in liver (B. Hagenbuch & C. Gui, 2008; M. Huls et al, 2009; M. Elaine, 2005; C. J. Endres, 2006). More and more studies showed that transporters play a major role in drug absorption, distribution, toxicity, efficacy, elimination and excretion. And it is a main reason

for drug-drug interaction. Some drugs affected the activity of transporters and as a consequence affected the distribution of the substrate of transporters (S. Eberl et al, 2007; A.Y. Coban et al, 2004 ; A. Seithel, et al, 2007, Sikri et al, 2004). Most of the meridian guide drugs had the effect of inhibiting the activity of P-gp (Q. Wu, 2005), and many drugs studied above such as resveratrol (A.Lancon et al, 2004, Juan et al, 2010), rhein (Garbap, 2002), levofloxacin (T. Ito et al, 1997), danshensu (P.F.Yu et al, 2011) are the substrate of P-gp or Mrp, indicating that meridian guide drug may influence the activity of these transporters and affect drug distribution and its pharmacological action.

By analyzing the pharmacokinetics data, this hypothesis could be further elucidated. Cmax is a parameter reflecting drug absorption. The increase in Cmax suggested an uptake increase and efflux decrease in intestine. Levofloxacin is the substrate of OATP (T. Maeda et al, 2007), P-gp (T. Ito et al, 1997) and MRPs (H. Polache et al, 2010), which are located in intestine, platycodiradix inhibited the activity of P-gp and Mrps and may also increase the activity of OATP, the Cmax of levofloxacin increased 470%. Resveratrol is the substrate of MRP2 (M. E. Juan et al, 2010; Lancan A, 2004), which transported drug from the liver to blood and induced a significantly increased blood concentration. Drug distribution and elimination is the balance of drug affinity to different tissues. As shown in Table 8, different tissues had different transporters or different content of the same transporters, and the affinity with different transporters was determined by the influx and efflux rate of the drug and as a sequel, the balance in different tissues determined distribution, elimination, and excretion of the drug.

Transporters	Gene	Transporter distribution	Substrates	Inhibitors
P-gp	ABCB1	**brain**, intestine, liver, kidney, placenta, lung, stomach, colon, pancreatic gland, oesophagus	danshensu, roxithromycin, quinolone, levofloxacin, berberine, rifampicin, ofloxacin	Bupleuri Radix, cimicifugate, cortex moutan, coptis chinensis, cortex phellodendri, anemarrhenae, Tetramethylpyrazine, platycodiradix, borneol, berberine, matrine, saikosaponin, paeoniflorin, baicalin, Roxithromycin, puerarin
Mrp1	*ABCC1*	Testicle, skeletal muscle, heart, kidney, lung, Brain, intestine, liver (trace)	rhein, methotrexate	puerarin
Mrp2	*ABCC2*	liver, gut, kidney, brain, placenta	Methotrexate resveratrol diclofenac baicalein	Tetramethylpyrazine, puerarin
Mrp3	ABCC3	Adrenal gland, Intestine, Pancreas, Gallbladder	Methotrexate	Tetramethylpyrazine, puerarin,
Mrp4	*ABCC4*	Placenta, Liver,	Methotrexate	

Transporters	Gene	Transporter distribution	Substrates	Inhibitors
		Kidney, Prostate Ovary, Testis, **Kidney**, Lung, Prostate		
MRP5	ABCC5	Liver, Testis, Skeletal and Cardiac Muscle, Brain		Tetramethylpyrazine
MRP6	ABCC6	Kidney, **keratinocytes**, liver tracheal, bronchial, epithelium, intestinal mucosa, corneal epithelium, smooth muscle cell		
BCRP	ABCG2	**Placenta, colon, intestine,** liver, heart, brain, kidney, prostate, ovary	Methotrexate, resveratrol Ofloxacin	
OAT1	SLC22A6	**Kidney**, brain, eye, placenta		Cidomycin, diclofenac, Methotrexate
OAT2	SLC22A7	**Liver**, kidney		Methotrexate
OAT3	SLC22A8	Liver, intestine, liver, Blood cerebrospinal fluid barrier, placenta		Methotrexate
OAT4	SLC22A11	Liver, placenta, kidney, adrenals		Methotrexate
OAT5	SLC22A	Liver, kidney		Methotrexate
OAT10	SLC22A13	Kidney, brain, heart, colon		
OCT1	SLC22A1	**Liver**, intestine, lung, heart, placenta		
OCT2	SLC22A2	Liver, **kidney**, brain, intestine		
OCT3	SLC22A3	**Liver**, intestine, placenta, brain,heart		
OCTN1	SLC22A4	Kidney, liver, testis, muscle, heart		

Transporters	Gene	Transporter distribution	Substrates	Inhibitors
OCTN2	SlC22A5	Kidney, liver, brain, intestine, testis		
OATP1A2	SLCO1A2	**Brain**, liver, kidney, eye	Levofloxacin Methotraexate	rifampicin
OATP2B1	SLCO2B1	Brain, **liver**, kidney, placenta, **intestine**	levofloxacin	Roxithromycin, rifampicin
OATP1B1-3	SLCO1B	**Liver**	Rifampicin, methotrexate	Rifampicin cimicifugae
OATP3A1	SLCO	ubiquitous	Rifampicin, methotraexate	Rifampicin
OATP4A1	SLC	ubiquitous		Rifampicin
OATP1C1	SLC	Brain, testis, heart, lung, eye		Rifampicin
OATP1AB3	SLC	**Liver**		Rifampicin
PEPT1	SLC	Liver, kidney, **intestine**		
PEPT2	SLC	**Kidney**, brain, lung, spleen, lacteal gland		

Table 8. Distribution, substrate, and inhibitors of transporters.

The activity and expression of transporters could be affected by many factors, such as xenobiotics, diseases, stress, metabolism enzyme, microenvironment change. And as a sequence, meridian guide drug may affect drug distribution by affecting these factors directly or indirectly. Efflux transporters are usually ATP dependent, drugs affecting ATP enzyme would affect activity of transporters and then affect drug effectiveness and toxicity (MunićV. et al, 2010; Regev et al, 1999). Bupleuriradix inhibited the activity of Na-K ATP enzyme (Q.L. Zhou et al, 1996), and may indirectly affected the activity of transporters.

Different transporters may be affected by different factors, and a factor may have different effect on different transporters. MRP is affected by many factors, and even in this family, despite of a great homology in family members, factors had different effect on different MRPs. Drugs may affect transporters by affecting the factor and thereafter affected other drugs distribution. For example, MRP1 is a glutathione dependent transporter, but other transporters of MRP family are glutathione independent. Water extract of bupleuriradix increased the glutathione content (M.H. Yen et al, 2005), and enhanced the activity of MRP1. MRP1 is expressed widely in other tissues but less in liver, leading to a fast elimination rate in other tissues, while it had marginal effect on drug elimination in liver. This may be one of the reasons for its toxicity reducing effect.

In spite of above well known transporters there are some transporters such as Mate1-2, RLIP76, and aquaporin, may play a role in meridian guide effect (Tanihara 2007, Ohta et al, 2009; Singhal, 2009). For example, carbamazepine is an active drug for epilepsy, and it has drug-resistant phenomenon. P-gp was first considered as the reason, however, study showed it is not the substrate of P-gp (Maines, 2005). Further studies showed that it is also not the substrate of MRP (Luna-Tortós et al, 2010; F. Rivers, 2008), BCRP (L. Cerveny et al,

2006). Recently, Awasthi et al found that RLIP76, a multifunctional modular protein, was involved in its drug-resistance (S. Awasthi et al, 2005). Borneol increased the brain concentration of carbamazepine, probably by inhibiting the activity of RLIP76.

Besides transporters, drug metabolism enzyme had an important effect on drug absorption, distribution, elimination and excretion. Most of meridian guide drug affected the activity of metabolism enzyme, such as pueraria, cassia bark, incised notopterygium rhizome, coptis chinensis, cortex phellodendri, evodiaefructus, angelica root, forsythia suspensa, paeoniaeradix and bupleuriradix, angelica dahurica etc. And this also may be one of reasons for its meridian guide effect (Yang et al, 2002; Mao et al, 2007, X.L. Bi et al, 2010). However, there are many herbs which could affect drug transporters and metabolism enzyme and they are not the meridian guide drug. For example, ginseng is drug usually used to invigorate vital energy, the main components of it not only affected drug metabolism but inhibited P-gp as well (C.H. Choi et al, 2003; S.W. Kim et al, 2003; S. Kitagwa Et al, 2007; Y.R. Pokharel, 2010); many herbs contained flavone, such as sophoraeflos, Chinese hawthom, soybean which also could affect drug metabolism enzyme and transporters (R.X. Zhu et al, 2011; Y.H. Liu et al, 2011) and only few of them are meridian guide drug, therefore, there must be other factors co-operating this effect and further study is required.

4. Conclusion

In summary, meridian guide drug had the effect of synery and attenuation, and this effect is based on drug concentration at target-site. Meridian guide effect had a close relationship with drug transporters and metabolism enzymes. Different components had different affinity to transporters or enzymes, and meridian guide effect is a combination of all components in meridian guide drug. Therefore, it is necessary to investigate the exact effect of main components of meridian guide drug on transporters and metabolism enzymes, establish the relationship between its dose and its effect as well as effects on different kinds of diseases. As we know more about the relationship among components in meridian guide drug, kinds of transporters and metabolism enzymes, activity in nomal and disease state, we could design target delivery system freely as desired.

5. Acknowledgements

This research was financially supported by the found of National Science Foundation of China (Grant No. 30672668, 81073063)

6. References

Awasthi S., Hallene K. L, Fazio V., Singhal S. S , Cucullo L., Awasthi Y. C , Dini G. and Janigro D. (2005). RLIP76, a non-ABC Transporter, and Drug Resistance in Epilepsy, *BMC Neuroscience,* VOL. 6, *No.* 61, doi:10.1186/1471-2202-6-61

Bi X.L., Du Q, Di L.Q., (2010). Important Application of Intestinal Transporters and Metabolism Enzymes on Gastrointestinal Disposal of Active Ingredients of Chinese Materia Medica, *Zhongguo Zhongyao Zazhi,* Vol.35, No.3, (February, 2010), ISSN 1001-5302

Cerveny L., Pavek P., Malakova J., Staud F., and Fendrich Z., (2006). Lack of Interactions between Breast Cancer Resistance Protein (BCRP/ABCG2) and Selected Antiepileptic Agents, *Epilepsia,* Vol.47, No.3, pp.461–468, ISSN 0013-9580

Chen S.M., Sato N., Yoshida M., Satoh N., Ueda S. (2008). Effects of *Bupleurum scorzoneraefolium, Bupleurum falcatum,* and Saponins on Nephrotoxic Serum Nephritis in Mice. *Journal of Ethnopharmacology,* No 116 , (November, 2008) ,pp. 397–402, ISSN 0378-8741

Chen X. H., Lin Z.Z., Liu A.M, Ye J.T., Luo Y.Y, Mao X.X., Liu P.Q. and Pi R.B., (2010). The Orally Combined Neuroprotective Effects of Sodium Ferulate and Borneol Against Transient Global Ischaemia in C57 BL/6 Mice, *Journal of Pharmacy and Pharmacology,* No.62, (July, 2010), 915–923, ISSN 0022-3573

Chen Y.M., Wang N.S., (2004). Effect of Borneol on the Intercellular Tight Junction and Pinocytosis Vesicles in vitro Blood·Brain Barrier, *Zhongguo Zhongxiyi Jiehe Zazhi,* Vol.24, No. 7,(July, 2004), pp.632-634, ISSN 1003-5370

Chen Y.M., Wang N.S., (2003). Effect of Borneol on P-gp, *Zhongyao Xinyao Yu Linchuang Yaoli,* Vol.14, No.2, (April, 2003), pp.96-99, ISSN 1003-9783

Chiang L.C., Ng L.T., Liu L.T., Shieh D., Li C.C., (2003). Cyctoxicity and Anti-Hepatitis B Virus Activities of Saikusaponins from Bupleurum, *Planta Med,* No.69, pp. 705-709, ISSN 0032-0943

Coban A. Y., Ekinci B., Durupinar B., (2004). A Multidrug Efflux Pump Inhibitor Reduces Fluoroquinolone Resistance in *Pseudomonas aeruginosa* isolates, *Chemtherapy,* No.50, pp.22-26. ISSN 0009-3157

Eberl S., Renner B., Neubert A., Reisig M., Bachmakov I., König J., Dörje F., Thomas E. M, Ackermann A., Dormann H., Gassmann K.G., Hahn E. G., Zierhut S., Brune K. and Fromm M. F. (2007). Role of P-Glycoprotein Inhibition for Drug Interactions Evidence from In Vitro and Pharmacoepidemiological Studies, *Clin Pharmacokinet,* Vol.46, No,12, pp.1039-1049, ISSN 0312-5963

Elaine M. Leslie, Roger G. Deeley, Susan P.C. Cole, (2005). Multidrug Resistance Proteins: Role of P-glycoprotein, MRP1, MRP2, and BCRP (ABCG2) in Tissue Defense, *Toxicology and Applied Pharmacology,* No.204, pp.216– 237, ISSN 0041-008X

Endres C. J., Hsiao P., Chung F. S., Unadkat J.D., (2006). The Role of Transporters in Drug Interactions, *European journal of pharmaceutical sciences,* No. 27, pp. 501–517, ISSN 0928-0987

Fu W. K., (1990). *History of Chinese medicine* (1st), ShangHai Zhongyi Xueyuan Publishing Company, Shanghai, China. ISBN 7-81010-093-9

Gao C., Gao M., Shi W.Z., Zhao Z.G, Sun H., Zhao X.L., (2009). Experimental Study on the Effect of Borneol for Methotrexate Penetrating Across Blood Brain Barrier, *Zhongguo Linchang Yaolixue Zazhi* Vol.25, No.2, (April, 2009), pp. 134-137, ISSN 1001-6821

Gao C.Y, Li X.R., Li Y.H., Wang L.J. and Xue M., (2010). Pharmacokinetic Interaction Between Puerarin and Edaravone, and Effect of Borneol on the Brain Distribution Kinetics of Puerarin in Rats. *Journal of pharmacy and pharmacology,*No.62, (March, 2010), pp.360-367, ISSN 0022-3573

Ge C.L, Han M.F, Bai R.T., Yu C.,(2008). Effect of Borneol Oil the Ultrastructure of Promoting Blood Brain Barriar Open, *Zhongxiyi Jiehe XinNao Xueguanbing Zazhi,* Vol.6, No. 10, (October, 2008), pp. 1183-1185, ISSN 1672-1349

Gergely S., Andras V., Csilla O.L.，and Balazs S. (2008). The Role of ABC Transporters in Drug Absorption, Distribution, Metabolism, Excretion and Toxicity (ADME-Tox)，*Drug Discovery Today,* Vol.13, No. 9/10, pp.379-393, ISSN 1359-6446

Gorkom BAP van, Timmer-Bosscha H., Jong S de, Kolk DM van der, Kleibeuker JH and Vries EGE de (2002). Cytotoxicity of Rhein, the Active Metabolite of Sennoside

Laxatives, is Reduced by Multidrug Resistance-associated Protein 1, *British Journal of Cancer*, No. 86, pp.1494 – 1500, ISSN 0007-0920

Hagenbuch B. & Gui C., (2008). Xenobiotic Transporters of the Human Organic Anion Transporting Polypeptides (OATP) Family, *Xenobiotica*, Vol.38, No.7–8, (July–August, 2008), pp.778–801, ISSN 0049-8254

Huls M., Russel F. G. M., and Masereeuw R., (2009). The Role of ATP Binding Cassette Transporters in Tissue Defense and Organ Regeneration, *The Journal of Pharmacology and Experimental Therapeutics*, Vol. 328, No.1, (January, 2009), pp. 3-9, ISSN 0022-3565

Ito T, Yano I, Tanaka K., and Inui, (1997), Transport of Quinolone Antibacterial Drugs by Human P-glycoprotein Expressed in Kidney Epithelial Cell Line, LLC-PK, *The journal of Pharmacology and Expermental Therapeutics*, No. 282 pp. 955-960, ISSN 0022-3565

Juan M. E., Gonzalezález-Pons E., and Planas J. M., (2010). Multidrug Resistance Proteins Restrain the Intestinal Absorption of trans-Resveratrol in Rats, *The Journal of Nutrition;* Vol.140, No.3, (March, 2010), pp.489-495, ISSN 0022-3166

Kim S.W., Kwon H.Y., Chi D.W., et al, (2003). Reversal of P-glycoprotein- Mediated Multidrug Resistance by Ginsenoside Rg3, *Biochem Pharmacol*, No.65, pp.75-82, ISSN, 0006-2952

Kitagwa S., Takahshi T., Nabekura T., Tagchikawe, and Hasegawa H, (2007). Inhibitory Effects of Ginsenosides and Their Hydrolyzed Metabolites on Daunorubicin Transport in KB-C2 Cells, *Biol. Pharm. Bull.*, Vol.30. No. 10, pp.1979—1981, ISSN 1347-5215

Kou W-M., 2006. Effect of Radix Bupleuri Processing Method on the Drug Action and its Rule in Clinical Use, *Shizhen Guoyi Guoyao*, Vol.17, No. 10 (October, 2006), pp. 1998-1999, ISSN 1008-0805

Kusuhara H., Sugiyama Y., (2002). Role of Transporters in the Tissue-Selective Distribution and Elimination of Drugs: Transporters in the Liver, Small Intestine, Brain and Kidney, *Journal of Controlled Release* No.78, pp.43–54, ISSN 0168-3659

Lancon A., Delmas D., Osman H., J.-P. , Thenot, and Jannin B., Latruffe N., (2004). Human Hepatic Cell Uptake of Resveratrol: Involvement of Both Passive Diffusion and Carrier-mediated Process, *Biochemical and Biophysical Research Communications* No.316, (February, 2004), pp. 1132–1137, ISSN 0006-291X

Lin Y.Q.,Sun B., Yang S.Y., Lv L., Liu Y., (2009). Therapeutic Effect of Radix Achyranthis Bidentatae Guiding Function on Diclofenac Sodium Induced Adjuvant Rats Arthritis, *Zhongyao Xinyao Yu Linchuang Yaoli*, Vol.20, No.5, (October, 2009), pp. 408-411, ISSN 1003-9783

Lin Z.Z, Yao M.C., Lan M. X., Liu P.Q., Zhong G.P., Pi R. B., (2008). Effects of Borneol on Distribution of Sodium Ferulate in Plasma and in Brain Regions of Mice, *Zhong Cao Yao*, Vol.39, No.4, (April, 2008), pp.551-556, ISSN 0253-2670

Liu J., Li X., Hu S.S., Yu Q.L, Sun W.J., Zheng X.H., (2008). Studies on the Effects of Baras Camphor on the Tissue Distribution of *Salvia miltiorrhiza Bge.* in Complex Danshen Prescription in Rabbits, *Yaowu Fenxi Zazhi*, Vol.28, No.10, (October, 2008), pp.1612-1615, ISSN 0254-1793

Liu Q.D., Liang M.R, Chen Z.X., (1994). The Influence of Borneol on the Passing of Gentamycin through Blood-Brain Barrier, *Guangzhou Zhongyiyao Daxue Xuebao* Vol.11, No.1, (January, 1994), pp.87-90, ISSN 1007-3213

Liu Y.H., Mo S.L., Bi H.C., Hu B.F., Li C.G., Wang Y.T., Huang L., Huang M., Duan W., Liu J.P., Wei M.Q., Zhou S.F., (2011). Regulation of Human Pregnane X Receptor and its Target Gene Cytochrome P450 3A4 by Chinese Herbal Compounds and a Molecular Docking Study, *Xenobiotica*. Vol.41, No.4, (April, 2011), pp.259-80, ISSN 0049-8254

Li W.R., Yao L.M., Mi S.Q., Wang N.S., (2006). Relation of Openness of Blood-Brain Barrier by Borneol with Histamine and 5-Hydroxytryptamine, *Zhongguo Linchuang Kangfu*, Vol.10, No.3, pp.167-169, ISSN 1671-5926

Li X.D., (2000). Comparative Analysis of Active Composition of Radix Bupleuri Before and After Being Processed, *Zhong YI Yao Xue Bao, Vol.* 22, No.7 (July, 2000), pp.483-484, ISSN 1002-2392

Li Y. L., Cui H.M., Chen H. W., (2008). Effect of Platycodon Grandiflorum on Pharmacokinetics of Florfenico, *Zhongguo ShouYi Xuebao*, Vol. 28, No.10 (October, 2008), pp. 1203-1207, ISSN 1005-4545

Li Y. L, Jiang Z. G., He X. L. (2006). Effect of Chinese Herb Platycodon Grandiflorum Leading Action on Distribution of Levofloxacin in Chickens After Oral Administration, *Zhongguo ShouYi Xuebao* Vol.26, No.5, (May, 2006), pp.541-543, ISSN 1005-4545

Li Y. L., Lu S. M., Jian M., (2005). Effect of Chinese Herb Platycodon Grandiflorum on Roxithromycin Concentration of Lung Tissue, *Zhongguo ShouYi Xuebao*, No. 3, (March, 2005), pp.3-6 ISSN 1005-4545

Luna-Tortós C., Fedrowitz M. , Löscher W., (2010). Evaluation of Transport of Common Antiepileptic Drugs by Human Multidrug Resistance-Associated Proteins (MRP1, 2 and 5) that Are Overexpressed in Pharmacoresistant Epilepsy, *Neuropharmacology*, No. 58, (January, 2010), pp 1019-1032, ISSN 0028-3908

Maeda T., Takahashi K., Ohtsu N., Oguma T., Ohnishi T. Atsumi R., and Tamai I., (2006). Identification of Influx Transporter for the Quinolone Antibacterial Agent Levofloxacin, *Molecular Pharmaceutics*, Vol. 4, No. 1, (October, 2007), pp.85-94, ISSN 1543-8384

Maines L. W., Antonetti D. A., Wolpert E. B., Smith C.D., (2005). Evaluation of the Role of P-Glycoprotein in the Uptake of Paroxetine,Clozapine, Phenytoin and Carbamazapine by Bovine Retinal Endothelial Cells, *Neuropharmacology* No.49, pp. 610-617, ISSN 0028-3908

Mao X.Q, Xie H.T., Zhou H.H, (2007). MDR- and CYP3A4- Mediated Drug-herb Interactions, *Zhongguo Linchuang Yaolixue Yu Zhiliaoxue*, Vol 12, No 7 (July, 2007), pp 728-734, ISSN 1009-2501

Meng D.L. & Li X., (2001). The Research Development of Achyranthesbidentata B1, *Zhongguo Yaowu Huaxue Zazhi*, Vol. 40, No.2, (February, 2001): 120-124, ISSN 1005-0108

Miyazaki H., Sekine T. and Endou H., (2004). The Multispecific Organic Anion Transporter Family: Properties and Pharmacological Significance, *TRENDS in Pharmacological Sciences*, Vol.25, No. 12, pp. 654-662, ISSN 0165-6147

Nie S., Liu X.P., Chen Sh.W, Li K., (2008). Study on Fingerprint of Bupleurum Chinese and Vinegar-baked Bupleurum Chinese in Hubei Province, *Zhong Yao Cai, Vol* .31, No.5, (May, 2008), pp. 657-659，ISSN 1001-4454

Nie S.Q, Yang Q., Li L.F, Huang L.Q, (2002). Pharmacokinetics Comparisons of Bupleurum Root and Red Peony Root, Vinegar-baked Bulpeurum Root and White Reony Root between Compatibility and Single Application, *Zhongguo Shiyan Fangji Xue Zazh, Vol.*8, No.3, (March, 2002), pp. 11-14, ISSN 1005-9903

Ohta K.Y., Imamura Y., Okudaira N., Atsumi R., Inoue K., and Yuasa H., (2009). Functional Characterization of Multidrug and Toxin Extrusion Protein 1 as a Facilitative Transporter for Fluoroquinolones, *The Journal of Pharmacology and Experimental Therapeutics*, Vol. 328, pp.628–634, ISSN 0022-3565

Pokharel Y.R., Kim ND, Han HK, Oh WK, Kang KW, (2010). Increased Ubiquitination of Multidrug Resistance 1 by Ginsenoside Rd. *Nutr Cancer.* Vol.62, No.2, pp.252-9, ISSN 1531-7914

Choi C.H., Kang G., Min Y.D, (2003). Reversal of P-glycoprotein-mediated Multidrug Resistance by Protopanaxatriol Ginsenosides from Korean Red Ginseng.*Planta Med.*, Vol.69, No. 3 (Mar,2003), pp.235-40, ISSN 0032-0943

Regev R., Assaraf Y. G. and Eytan G. D., (1999). Membrane Fluidization by Ether, Other Anesthetics, and Certain Agents Abolishes P-glycoprotein ATPase Activity and Modulates Efflux from Multidrug-resistant cells, *Eur. J. Biochem.* 259, 18-24, ISSN 0014-2956

Rivers F., ÓBrien T. J., Callaghan R., (2008). Exploring the Possible Interaction between anti-Epilepsy Drugs and Multidrug Efflux Pumps; in vitro Observations, *European Journal of Pharmacology* No.598, (September, 2008),pp 1–8, ISSN 0014-2999

Seithel A., Eberl S., Singer K., Auge D., Heinkele G., Wolf N. B., Dorje F., Fromm M.F., and Konig J., (2007). The Influence of Macrolide Antibiotics on the Uptake of Organic Anions and Drugs Mediated by OATP1B1 and OATP1B3, *Drug Metabolism and Disposition*, No.35, (May, 2007) pp.779–786, ISSN 0090-9556

Shitara Y., Horie T., Sugiyama Y., (2006). Transporters as a Determinant of Drug Clearance and Tissue Distribution, *European Journal of Pharmaceutical Sciences*, No.27, pp. 425–446, ISSN 0928-0987

Sikri V., Pal D., Jain R., Kalyani D., and Mitra A. K., (2004). Cotransport of Macrolide and Fluoroquinolones, a Beneficial Interaction Reversing P-glycoprotein Efflux, *American Journal of Therapeutics* No. 11, pp.433–442, ISSN 1075-2765

Singhal S.S., Yadav S., Roth C., Singhal J., (2009). RLIP76: A Novel Glutathione-conjugate and Multi-drug Transporter Biochemical Pharmacology, No. 77, pp. 761– 769, ISSN 0006-2952

Tai Y., Hou J. P., Meng J.G., Xu W.W., Wang Q., (2009). Pharmacological Development of Platycodiradix, *Xiandai Zhongyiyao,* No.6, (June, 2009), pp. 74-75, ISSN 1672-0571

Tanihara Y., Masuda S., Sato T., Katsura T., Ogawa O., Inui Ken-ichi, (2007). Substrate Specificity of MATE1 and MATE2-K, Human Multidrug and Toxin Extrusions/H+-Organic Cation Antiporters, *Biochemical Pharmacology,* No.74, pp.359– 371, ISSN 0006-2952

Wang B.J., Liu C.T., Tseng C.Y, Wu C.P., Yu Z.R., (2004). Hepatoprotective and Antioxidant Effects of Bupleurum Kaoi Liu (Chao et Chuang) Extract and Its Fractions Fractionated Using Supercritical CO2 on CCl4-induced Liver Damage, *Food and Chemical Toxicology*, No. 42, (November, 2004) , pp. 609–617, ISSN 0278-2915

Wang G. J., Zhang B., Zhang X. S., Zhang E. H., (2010). Effect of Dioscin Co-administration with Borneol on Cerebral Ischemia Induced by MCAO, *Zhongyao Yaoli Yu Linchuang* Vol. 26, No. 5, (October, 2010), pp. 54-55, ISSN 1001-859X

Wang S. X., Miao W. L., Fang M. F., Nan Y. F., Meng X., Yu J., Zheng X. H., (2009). Effect of Borneol on the Tissue Distribution of Notoginseng R1, Ginsenoside Rgl and Re in

Rabbits, *DiSi Junyi Daxue Xuebao, Vol.* 30, No.23, (December, 2009), pp. 2750-2752, ISSN 1000-2790

Wang Y., Zhang Z.Y., Xu F., Wang B.J., Zhang S.Y., (2006). Effects of Borneol on Concentration of Tetramethylpyrazine in Blood and Distribution in Brain of Rat, *Zhongguo Yaoye*, Vol.15, No.1, (January, 2006), pp.30-31, ISSN 1006-4693

Wu J., (2008). Effect of Process on Components and Pharmacological of Radix Bupleurum, *Hubei Zhongyi Zazhi* Vol. 30, No. 9, (September, 2008), pp.60-61, ISSN 1000-0704

Wu S. R., Cheng G., He Y.X., Hao X. H., Wang L., Sun J., (2004). Studies on the Effects of Borneol on the Distribution of Rifampicin in Mice, *Zhongguo Yaoxue Zazhi* , Vol. 39, No.4 (April, 2004), pp. 289-291, ISSN 1001-2494.

Wu Q., (2005). Effect of Meridian Guide Drug on P-gp, *Xiandai Yufang Yixue*, Vol.32, No.7, (July, 2005), pp.855-856, ISSN 1003-8507

Wu S.R., Cheng G.,(2001). Pharmacological Development of Borneol, *Zhong Cao Yao*, Vol.32, No.12, (December, 2001), pp.1143-1145, ISSN 0253-2670

Yang X. F., Wang N. P., Zeng F. D., (2002) Effect of the Active Components of Some Chinese Herbs on Drug Metabolizing- Enzymes, *Zhongguo Zhongyao Zazhi*, Vol. 27, No. 5 (May, 2002), pp. 325-328, ISSN 1001-5302

Yu P.F., WangW. Y., Eerdun G., WangT., Zhang L.M., Li C., and Fu F.H,2011. The Role of P-Glycoprotein in Transport of Danshensu across the Blood-Brain Barrier, *Evidence-Based Complementary and Alternative Medicine* Vol. 2011, Article ID 713523, 5 pages doi:10.1155/2011/713523

Zhao B.S., Liu Q. D, (2002). Difference Between Borneol and Pathological on Blood-Brain Barrier, *Zhongyao Xinyao Yu Linchuang Yaoli*, Vol.13, No. 5, (October, 2002), pp. 287-288, ISSN 1003-9783

Zhao R.Z., Liu S.J, (2005). TCM Tradicinal Guide Theory and Target-tropism Administration, *Zhong Yi Za Zhi*, volume 46, No. 9, (September, 2005), pp. 643-645, ISSN 1001-1668

Zhao R.Z., Liu S.J., Mao S. R., Wang Y.J., (2009). Study on Liver Targeting Effect of Vinegar-baked Radix Bupleuri on Resveratrol in Mice, *Journal of Ethnopharmacology*, No.126, (September, 2009), pp.415-420, ISSN 0378-8741

Zhao R.Z., Yuan D, Liu S.J., Chen YJ., Liu L.J. Zhao Y. (2010). Liver Targeting Effect of Vinegar-baked Radix Bupleuri on Rhein in Rats, *Journal of Ethnopharmacology*, No. 132, (October, 2010), pp. 421-428, ISSN 0378-8741

Zheng C., Xiang H. S., Li Y. B., Zhao B. B., Yang Z. X., Xu S.G., Pu J.X., (2008). Effect of Borneol on the Distribution of Gastrodin to the Brain in Mice via Oral Administration, *Journal of Drug Targeting*, Vol.16, No.2, (February, 2008), pp178–184, ISSN 1061-186X

Zhou H. Y., Chen X. Y., Huang C. K., Jiang W. G., Hu G. X.. (2008), Effect of Borneol on Distribution of Carbamazepine in Mice, *Wenzhou Yixueyuan Xuebao*, Vol.38, No.4, (July, 2008), pp.300-305, ISSN 1000-2138

Zhou Q.L., Zhang Z.Q., Nagasawa T., and Hiai S., (1996). The Structure Activity Relationship of Saikosaponins and Glycyrrhizin Derivatives for Na+, K+ ATPase Inhibiting Action, *Yaoxue Xuebao*, Vol.31, No.7, (July, 1996), pp 496-501, ISSN 0253-3707

Zhu R.X., Hu L.W., Li H.Y., Su J.,Cao Z.W., and Zhang W.D.,(2011) Novel Natural Inhibitors of CYP1A2 Identified by *in Silico* and *in Vitro* Screening, *Int J Mol. Sci.* Vol. 12, No.5, (May, 2011), pp.3250–3262, doi: 10.3390/ijms12053250, ISSN 2306-2321

16

Knowledge-Based Discovery of Anti-Fibrotic and Pro-Fibrotic Activities from Chinese Materia Medica

Qihe Xu et al.*
King's College London, Department of Renal Medicine, The Rayne Institute, London, United Kingdom

1. Introduction

Fibrosis, also known as scarring, sclerosis or cirrhosis, is characterised by excessive accumulation of extracellular matrix (ECM) proteins leading to tissue contraction, disruption of tissue architecture and eventually chronic organ failure (Wynn, 2007; Xu et al., 2007). Research and development of anti-fibrotic drugs are generally based on two distinct but interactive strategies, with one based on mechanism studies and another based on exploring efficacy. In principle, the mechanism-based strategy begins with identification of molecular targets through mechanistic studies, and then development of inhibitors or enhancers targeting the molecules. On the other hand, efficacy-based strategy starts with screening drug candidates in disease models to identify activities and efficacy, with less reliance on analysis of mechanisms of action. There are certain limitations in both the mechanism-based strategy and the efficacy-based strategy, which largely account for the lack of success in development of anti-fibrotic drugs. The former is often associated with identification of multiple molecular targets impeding development of a single drug that tackles multiple targets, while the latter is often hampered by establishment of apt models ideal for efficacy-driven drug screens.

Efficacy-based strategy has been employed in development of both traditional and modern medicines. In the context of traditional medicine, the knowledge about efficacy of a given drug is largely derived from a trial-and-error process, namely by assessing patients' response upon treatment with natural drug candidates. However, in modern medicine, it is impossible to directly test any new drugs in patients. Solid scientific evidence on efficacy and safety of a given drug in experimental models is required prior to clinical trials. Understandably, quality of these models would determine the specificity and efficiency of the tested drug.

---

* Yuen Fei Wong[1], Shanshan Qu[1], Qingyang Kong[1], Xiu-Li Zhang[2], Xin-Miao Liang[2], Qin Hu[1], Mazhar Noor[1] and Bruce M. Hendry[1],
[1]*King's College London, Department of Renal Medicine, The Rayne Institute, London, United Kingdom*
[2] *Multi-Component TCM Group, Dalian Institute of Chemical Physics, Chinese Academy of Sciences, Dalian PR China*

In vivo models are invaluable research tools but not without its limitation, especially in the development of drugs targeting fibrosis given the complex aetiologies and inflammatory processes involved in this pathological condition. In particular, drug leads displaying effectiveness in *in vivo* models of fibrosis may stem from (i) inhibition of the primary aetiological factors, (ii) inhibition of inflammation, a common inciting factor of fibrosis, (iii) inhibition of fibrosis *per se*, or (iv) a net effect of any combinations of the aforementioned.

For the initial development of drugs with specific anti-fibrotic effects independent of anti-inflammatory actions and any specific aetiological factors, *in vitro* models of fibrosis appear to be more appropriate. Our laboratory recently reported transforming growth factor-β1 (TGF-β1)-induced inflammation-free *in vitro* models of fibrosis in mesenchymal cells, featuring 2-dimentional (2D) ECM protein accumulation reflecting net collagen accumulation, and 3-dimentional (3D) nodular formation following ECM protein-induced disruption of cell monolayer, which can both be objectively quantified. By coating specific matrix on 96-well plates, which determines the 2D or 3D nature of the models, we are able to quantify readouts more reliably, permitting high-throughput screening of compounds with anti-fibrotic activities (Xu et al., 2007).

In contrast to the lack of "anti-fibrotics" in Western medicine clinics, there is accumulating evidence suggesting anti-fibrotic effects of Chinese materia medicas (CMMs), i.e., medicinal materials used in traditional Chinese medicine (TCM) (Hu et al., 2007). However, most of these conclusions were drawn from animal models or patients and hence it was not clear whether the reported efficacy of those CMMs was secondary to inhibition of aetiological factors or inflammation, or whether they exerted genuine anti-fibrotic activities (Hu et al., 2009). We hypothesised that at least some of the "anti-fibrotic" herbal derivatives reported in the literature are indeed anti-fibrotic by antagonising TGF-β1-specific pro-fibrotic pathways or common pathways of fibrosis. By employing the 2D *in vitro* model (Xu et al., 2007), we tested the anti-fibrotic activity of 21 CMM-derived compounds, 11 methanolic extracts of single CMMs and 27 formulae that contained two or more CMMs as mixtures, and found that five compounds, three single CMM extracts and 16 formulae had *in vitro* anti-fibrotic activities (Hu et al., 2009). Among the five CMM-derived compounds, three flavonoids (quercetin, baicalin and baicalein) showed similar dose-dependent *in vitro* anti-fibrotic activities while two non-flavonoids (salvianolic acid B and emodin) showed varied *in vitro* anti-fibrotic activities with poor dose dependency. Among the three CMM extracts showing significant *in vitro* anti-fibrotic activities, Huangqin (root of *Scutellaria baicalensis* Georgi) is rich in baicalin and baicalein, Danshen (root of *Salvia miltiorrhiza* Bunge) is rich in salvianolic acid B and Dahuang (root of *Rheum palmatum* L.) is rich in emodin. Among the 16 herbal formulae with *in vitro* anti-fibrotic effects, eight contained neither Huangqin, Danshen nor Dahuang, while the remaining eight contained at least one of the three CMMs (Hu et al., 2009).

Following successful identification of *in vitro* anti-fibrotic activities in herbal entities, we have extended our work to focus on TCM knowledge-based discovery of novel anti-fibrotic drug leads from natural sources, especially CMMs. In TCM, fibrosis is diagnosed as a kind of "Jie Zheng" which means "lump or clot". Based on this concept, two senior TCM practitioners were invited to choose a collection of 27 CMMs, including 26 medicinal plant parts and one medicinal fungus, which they would consider using in patients with fibrotic diseases. Based on the traditional categories of CMMs, the 27 CMMs fall into three functional subgroups, namely "Huo Xue Hua Yu" ("promoting the circulation and resolving the clot"), "Hua Tan" ("resolving the sputum") and "Bu Xu" ("tonifying the deficiency"), where "clot" and "sputum" in TCM do not mean the same as the terms in Western medicine. In addition to the 27 CMMs, Chuanwutou, an unprocessed herb with well-known toxic effects, was also tested to serve as a control for cytotoxic effects, if any. In fact, owing to its strong "Qu Feng Shi" ("dispelling the wind and damp" or anti-rheumatic function) property, Chuanwutou is rather commonly prescribed to patients with diseases complicated by fibrosis, although only processed Chuanwutou is allowed for clinical use.

The aim of this project was to examine the *in vitro* anti-fibrotic and pro-fibrotic activities of these 28 CMMs (Table 1) and herein we report that eight CMMs (Baibeiyegen, Liedang, Gusuibu, Jixueteng, Lingzhi, Meiguiqie, Moyao and Shiliuhua) have *in vitro* anti-fibrotic activities while three (Chuanwutou, Dangshen and Yimucao) have pro-fibrotic activities.

2. Materials and methods

2.1 CMMs and extraction methods

Liedang was authenticated according to the criteria described in *Jilin Zhongcaoyao* (Changchun TCM College Revolutionary Committee (Ed.), (June 1970), *Jilin Chinese Herbal Medicine,* Jilin People's Press, Changchun, China) and all other CMMs were authenticated according to Chinese Pharmacopeia (2005 Edition). Voucher specimens were deposited at Dalian Institute of Chemical Physics, Chinese Academy of Sciences, Dalian, China. Individual CMM was grounded into fine powder, from which 85 g was precisely weighed out and added to 600 ml of 80% ethanol. The mixtures were boiled for 2 h and filtrated, after which the residual ethanol was evaporated. Ethanolic extracts were then concentrated and dried in an oven, and were stored at room temperature before use. For experimental purpose, ethanolic extracts were reconstituted in dimethyl sulfoxide (DMSO, Sigma-Aldrich Company Ltd., Dorset, UK) and were stored in freezer at -20 °C until use.

2.2 TGF-β1, Alk5 inhibitor and PPAR antagonists

Human TGF-β1 in lyophilised powder form (R&D Systems Europe Ltd., Abingdon, UK) was reconstituted in filter-sterilised buffer consisting of 1 mg/ml bovine serum albumin in 4 mM HCl, to a final concentration of 10 μg/ml and kept frozen at -80 °C before experiments. IN-1130, a selective inhibitor of TGF-β type I receptor (Alk5), was a kind gift from Dr Dae Kee Kim, Ewha Women's University, Korea, and was used as a positive control for *in vitro* anti-fibrotic activity (Moon et al., 2006). Peroxisome proliferator-activated receptor (PPAR) antagonists, including PPARα antagonist GW6471 (Xu et al., 2002), PPARβ/δ antagonist GSK0660 (Shearer et al., 2008) and PPARγ antagonist T0070907 (Lee et al., 2002) were purchased from Sigma-Aldrich.

2.3 Cell culture, TGF-β1-induced *in vitro* models of fibrosis and related assays

A normal rat kidney fibroblast cell line (NRK-49F) was purchased from European Collection of Cell Cultures (ECACC, Health Protection Agency, Salisbury, UK). The cells were maintained in Dulbecco's Modified Eagle Medium (DMEM, PAA Laboratories Ltd., Somerset, UK) supplemented with 100 U/ml of penicillin G (PAA), 100 μg/ml of streptomycin (PAA), 0.25 μg/ml of amphotericin B (Invitrogen Ltd., Paisley, UK) and 5% foetal calf serum (FCS, Sigma-Aldrich), in Falcon tissue culture flasks (Marathon Laboratory supplies, London, UK), and incubated at 37 °C and 5% CO2. During routine maintenance,

Functional group	Pinyin name	Part, Latin name and authority	Authenticator	Extraction yield (%)	Voucher number
"Bu Xu"	Baibeiyegen	Dried roots of *Mallotus apelta* (Lour.) Muell.-Arg.	SJS*	21	B012081
	Liedang	Dried whole plants of *Orobanche coerulescens* Steph.	SJS	28.5	C013081
	Dangshen	Dried roots of *Codonopsis pilosula* (Franch.) Nannf.	SJS	58.7	D001081
	Gancao	Dried roots and rhizomes of *Glycyrrhiza uralensis* Fisch.	SJS	81.7	G010081
	Roucongrong	Dried fleshy stem with scales of *Cistanche deserticola* Y. C. Ma	SJS	82.2	R002081
	Yinyanghuo	Dried rootless plants of *Epimedium brevicornum* Maxim.	SJS	42.1	Y006081
"Bu Xu" & "Hua Tan"	Lingzhi	Dried mushroom of *Ganoderma lucidum* (Leyss. Ex Fr.) Karst.	SJS	8.33	L003081
"Hua Tan"	Baiguo	Dried ripe seeds of *Ginkgo biloba* L.	HXR**	7.9	B013041
	Jiegeng	Dried roots of *Platycodon grandiflorum (Jacq.)* A. DC.	SJS	12.3	J009081
	Meiguiqie	Dried flowers of *Hibiseus sabdariffa* L.	SJS	37.6	M004081
	Tiannanxing	Dried tuberous roots of *Arisaema erubescens* (Wall.) Schott.	SJS	2.34	T001081
"Hua Tan" and "Huo Xue Hua Yu"	Yinxingye	Dried leaves of *Ginkgo bilobla* L.	SJS	65	Y009081
"Huo Xue Hua Yu" & "Qing Re Jie Du"***	Baihuasheshecao	Dried plants of *Oldenlandia diffusa* (Willd.) Roxb.	HXR	18	B010041
"Huo Xue Hua Yu"	Ezhu	Dried rhizomes of *Curcuma kwangsiensis* S. G. Lee et C. F. Liang	HXR	60.1	E001041
	Gusuibu	Dried rhizomes of *Drynaria fortunei* (Kunze) J. Sm.	SJS	27	G007081
	Jixueteng	Dried stem of *Spatholobus suberectus* Dunn	SJS	33.9	J001081
	Maqianzi	Dried ripe seeds of *Strychnos nux-vomica* L.	SJS	7.7	M003081
	Moyao	Dried resin of *Commiphora myrrha* Engl.	SJS	33.7	M002081
	Niuxi	Dried roots of *Achyranthes bidentata* Bl.	SJS	9.9	N002081

Functional group	Pinyin name	Part, Latin name and authority	Authenticator	Extraction yield (%)	Voucher number
	Ruxiang	Dried oleogum resin of *Boswellia carterii* Birdw.	SJS	60.6	R001081
	Sanleng	Dried tuberous roots of *Sparganium stoloniferum* Buch.-Ham.	SJS	25.1	S003081
	Sheputaogen	Dried roots of *Ampelopsis (Miq.)* W. T. Wang	SJS	14	S011081
	Shiliuhua	Dried flowers of *Punica granatum* L.	SJS	88	S012081
	Taoren	Dried ripe seeds of *Prunus persica (L.)* Batsch.	SJS	35.6	T004081
	Yanhusuo	Dried tuberous roots of *Corydalis yanhusuo* W. T. Wang	HXR	69.5	Y010041
	Yimucao	Dried rootless plants of *Leonurus japonicus* Houtt.	SJS	12.8	Y005081
	Zhenzhumei	Dried bark of the stems of *Sorbaria sorbifolia (L.)* A. Brown.	SJS	33.1	Z004081
"Qu Feng Shi"	Chuanwutou	Dried main roots of *Aconitum carmichaeli* Debx.	SJS	18.2	C005081

Table 1. Functional groups, species names and parts, authenticators, extraction yield and voucher numbers of the 28 test materials. * SJS: Shi Jian Sa, Tong De Chinese Materia Medica Co. Ltd., Anguo, Hebei, China; ** HXR: He Xi Rong, Institute of Chinese Materia Medica, China Academy of Chinese Medical Sciences, Beijing, China; *** "Qing Re Jie Du" means "clearing heat and detoxifying".

NRK-49F cells were sub-cultured before they became confluent to prevent transformation. The 2D model was employed for experiments in this project. Cells were seeded in collagen type I-coated 96-well plates (BD Biosciences, Oxford, UK) at a density of 1×10^4 cells per well in 200 μl DMEM supplemented with 2.5% FCS and 2.5% Nu-Serum™ V serum replacements (NU, BD Biosciences). After three days, the medium was changed to serum-free DMEM supplemented with 1% insulin-transferrin-selenium liquid media supplement (ITS, Sigma-Aldrich) for four days, and then changed to fresh ITS-supplemented serum-free medium containing 5 ng/ml TGF-β1 in the presence of different concentrations of herbal extracts or a vehicle control (an equal volume of DMSO) for 48 h. In all the experiments, 1 μM IN-1130 was used as a positive control for anti-fibrotic activities. For initial screening, the concentrations of CMM extracts tested were 10, 20, 40, 80, 160 and 200 μg/ml, 3-6 wells per group, and the screening was repeated at least twice. For follow-up confirmation studies, four herbal extracts were selected based on the results from initial screening studies, and their effects were further confirmed using three different concentrations, 3-6 wells per group. Each follow-up experiment was performed four times.

2.4 Cell detachment index (CDI) and lactate dehydrogenase (LDH) release assay

For the screening studies, *in vitro* cytotoxicity at the end of 48 h treatment was assessed by phase-contrast microscopy using the same CDI criteria that we reported before (Hu et al.,

2009). In brief, CDI reflects cell monolayer disruption, including cell detachment from the adherent surface and disorganisation of cell monolayer. Scores of 0, 0.5, 1, 1.5, 2, 2.5, 3, 3.5 and 4 represented an area of 0, 5%, 10%, 20%, 30%, 40%, 60%, 80% and 100%, respectively, of the total adherent surface not covered by cells. This method was used to approximate cytotoxicity, as well as to ensure the reliability of subsequent picro-Sirius red (PSR) staining results, which required minimum cell (and matrix) detachment and disruption of cell monolayer. For follow-up studies, LDH release assay was used to assess *in vitro* cytotoxicity at the end of 48 h treatment. Fifty microlitre of supernatant from each well was collected and tested for LDH release according to the manufacturer's instructions (Promega, Southampton, UK). LDH release was measured using a Dynex Technologies MRX spectrophotometer (Prior Laboratory Supplies Ltd., East Sussex, UK), at optical density (OD) value of 490 nm.

2.5 Microscopic examination

Microscopic examination was performed on a Nikon Eclipse TE2000-S microscope (Nikon Instruments Europe B.V., The Netherlands). Bright-field and phase-contrast images were captured with a DXM1200F Nikon digital camera (Nikon UK Limited, Surrey, UK) and processed with Adobe Photoshop (Adobe System Europe Ltd., London, UK).

2.6 PSR staining and spectrophotometric analysis

Total collagen accumulation was assessed qualitatively by microscopic examination of PSR-stained cells and quantitatively by spectrophotometric analysis of PSR staining. After CDI determination and conditioned medium collected for LDH release assay, cell monolayer in 96-well plates were fixed in ice-cold methanol (200 μl per well) overnight at –20 °C. Cells were carefully washed twice (5 min each) with 1x phosphate buffered saline (PBS, 200 μl per well) and then stained with 0.1% w/v PSR solution (200 μl per well, Sigma-Aldrich) at room temperature for 4–6 h. The staining solution was then removed and excessive PSR stain was carefully washed off with 0.1% v/v acetic acid (200 μl per well, VWR International Ltd, Lutterworth, UK) three times (5 min each). The stained wells were left to air dried for 24–48 h. PSR stain was then observed under bright-field microscopy and microscopic pictures were taken. Finally, PSR stain was eluted in 0.1 N NaOH (200 μl per well) on a rocking platform at room temperature for 1 h. The plate was then subjected to spectrophotometric analysis of OD at 540 nm on a Dynex Technologies MRX spectrophotometer (Hu et al., 2009).

2.7 PPARα, PPARβ/δ and PPARγ agonistic activities of Shiliuhua extract and effect of Shiliuhua extract in the presence of PPAR antagonists

We commissioned Tebu-bio Laboratories, Le Perray en Yvelines, France, to perform a pilot test on Shiliuhua extract for its isotype-specific PPAR activation. In brief, the assay was carried out *in vitro* in three HeLa cell lines stably expressing a chimeric protein containing the yeast transactivator GAL4 DNA binding domain fused to ligand binding domain regions of human PPARα, PPARβ/δ or PPARγ, and a luciferase reporter gene driven by a pentamer of the GAL4 recognition sequence in front of the β-globin promoter (Seimandi et al., 2005). The PPAR reporter cell lines were seeded in a 96-well plate in triplicates, and treated with 40 μg/ml Shiliuhua extract, or an equal volume of DMSO as negative control, for 24 h. Luciferase activity was determined with a luminometer and relative light units (RLU) were recorded. Three independent experiments were performed and the fold changes of RLU were normalised to the mean of negative control.

The effect of PPAR antagonism on Shiliuhua extract treatment was assessed following the protocol as described in sections 2.3-2.6. Cells were treated with 40 μg/ml Shiliuhua extract with and without PPARα antagonist, GW6471 (0.01-10 μM), PPARβ/δ antagonist, GSK0660 (0.001-1 μM), or PPARγ antagonist, T0070907 (0.1-25 μM). Three independent biological experiments were performed, 3-6 wells per group.

2.8 Statistical analysis

Results of PSR and LDH OD values were expressed as mean ± SEM unless stated otherwise. Statistical differences were computed with Prism 4.0 (GraphPad Software, San Diego, CA, USA), by one-way analysis of variance and Dunnett post test for comparison between a control group and all other groups; for PPAR reporter activity, one-tail paired *t* test was performed on log-transformed fold changes. $p<0.05$ was regarded as statistically significant.

3. Results

3.1 Initial screening

The screening results of CMM extracts were summarised in Table 2. Anti-fibrotic and pro-fibrotic effects were defined as PSR OD values significantly lower and higher than that of TGF-β1-treated group, respectively; cytotoxicity was defined as CDI significantly higher than that of TGF-β1-treated group. Doses at which extracts exhibited reproducible effects were indicated in the table. The CMMs were categorised into four groups, i.e., eight in Group A showed *in vitro* anti-fibrotic activities; three in Group B showed pro-fibrotic activities; six in Group C showed prominent cytotoxicity; 11 in Group D did not have profound effects on total collagen accumulation nor integrity of cell monolayer. In Group A, Liedang, Meiguiqie and Gusuibu extracts were well-tolerated agents with anti-fibrotic activities noted within the range of 80-200 μg/ml; extracts of Shiliuhua, Baibeiyegen, Jixueteng, Moyao and Lingzhi showed anti-fibrotic effects at concentrations ranging from 10–80 μg/ml, beyond which cytotoxicity was noted. In Group B, Chuanwutou showed a pro-fibrotic effect at concentrations as low as 20 μg/ml whereas pro-fibrotic effect of Dangshen and Yimucao were observed only at higher concentrations (160–200 μg/ml).

3.2 Follow-up studies

Based on the initial screening results, Shiliuhua (SLH), Liedang (LD), Meiguiqie (MGQ) and Chuanwutou (CWT) extracts were selected for follow-up studies in view of their minimum CDI changes indicating low cytotoxicity, and the results are shown in Fig. 1. In contrast to SLH, LD and MGQ extracts, which showed varying degrees of *in vitro* anti-fibrotic effects, CWT extract exhibited a marked pro-fibrotic effect. Representative effects of SLH, LD, MGQ and CWT extracts on PSR staining, relative PSR OD values and LDH release are shown in Fig. 2 and Fig. 3.

3.3 Activation of PPARs by SLH extract

As SLH extract is one of the CMM extracts with the most potent *in vitro* anti-fibrotic activity and it was previously reported to interfere with the PPAR signalling pathway (Li et al., 2008), we hypothesised that the anti-fibrotic effect of SLH extract was at least in part mediated by activation of one or more PPAR receptors. Indeed, SLH extract induced PPARα- and PPARγ-mediated reporter activity; it also marginally activates PPARβ/δ but the induction of reporter activity was just above the threshold of significance (p=0.066) (Fig. 4a). In order to determine if the agonistic effect of SLH extract has an impact on TGF-β1-induced fibrogenesis, cells were treated with SLH extract and individual PPAR antagonists. PPARβ/δ antagonist, GSK0660 (IC_{50} 160 nM) (Shearer et al., 2008), did not affect the anti-fibrotic activity of SLH extract at all concentrations tested (up to 6.25-fold higher than its IC_{50}); PPARα antagonist, GW6471 (IC_{50} 240 nM) (Xu et al., 2002), also did not show any significant effect at concentrations up to 4.2-fold of its IC_{50}, but at 10 μM (42-fold higher than its IC_{50}), it did moderately suppress the anti-fibrotic activity of SLH extract; PPARγ antagonist, T0070907 (IC_{50} 1 nM in inhibiting rosiglitazone binding to PPARγ and 3.2-24.3 μM in inhibiting proliferation of different cancer cell lines) (Lee et al., 2002; Burton et al., 2007), did not show any significant effect at concentrations of 0.1, 1 and 10 μM, but further increased the anti-fibrotic effect of SLH extract at 25 μM (Fig. 4b).

Group	Pinyin name	Anti-fibrotic or pro-fibrotic doses (μg/ml)	Changes at optimum doses compared to TGF-β1 treated group	Cytotoxic doses (μg/ml)
A. Anti-fibrotic	Baibeiyegen	20-40	-81.4% (40 μg/ml) -63.3% (20 μg/ml)	≥80
	Liedang	80-160	-61.2% (160 μg/ml) -59.3% (80 μg/ml)	200
	Gusuibu	160-200	-36.8% (200 μg/ml) -30.0% (160 μg/ml)	–
	Jixueteng	10-40	-75.0% (20 μg/ml) -63.0% (10 μg/ml)	≥80
	Lingzhi	10-80	-34.9% (80 μg/ml) -47.4% (40 μg/ml)	≥160
	Meiguiqie	160-200	-28.0% (200 μg/ml) -21.0% (160 μg/ml)	–
	Moyao	10-40	-57.2% (40 μg/ml) -67.9% (20 μg/ml)	≥80
	Shiliuhua	10-40	-78.0% (40 μg/ml) -61.2% (20 μg/ml)	≥80
B. Pro-fibrotic	Chuanwutou	≥20	+90.2% (40 μg/ml) +68.5% (20 μg/ml)	–
	Dangshen	200	+32.4% (200 μg/ml)	–
	Yimucao	160-200	+65.7% (200 μg/ml) +53.9% (160 μg/ml)	–
C. Cytotoxic	Baihuasheshecao (≥80 μg/ml), Ruxiang (≥10 μg/ml), Sheputaogen (≥80 μg/ml), Tiannanxing (≥80 μg/ml), Yinxingye (≥20 μg/ml), Zhenzhumei (≥40 μg/ml).			
D. Inert	Baiguo, Ezhu, Gancao, Jiegeng, Maqianzi, Niuxi, Roucongrong, Sanleng, Taoren, Yanhusuo, Yinyanghuo.			

Table 2. Initial screening results of CMMs in TGF-β1-induced *in vitro* fibrogenesis. Minus (-) and plus (+) percentages represent relative reduction and increase in TGF-β1-induced PSR OD values, respectively. " – ": Cytotoxicity, assessed from CDI, was not significantly different from TGF-β1-treated group at all concentrations tested (10-200 μg/ml).

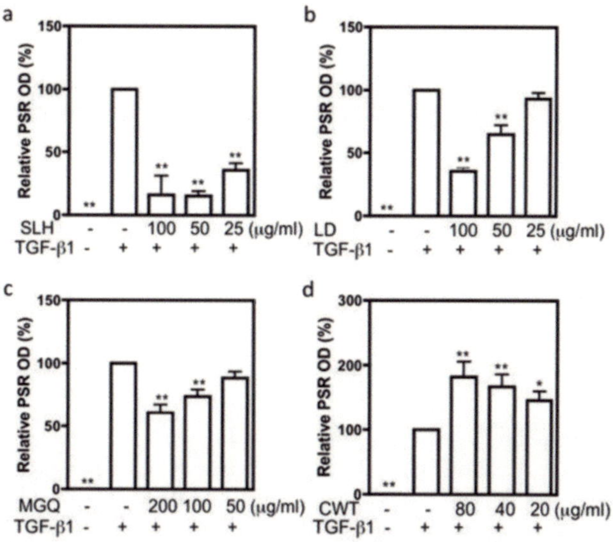

Fig. 1. *In vitro* anti-fibrotic and pro-fibrotic effects of four selected extracts, Shiliuhua (SLH) (a), Liedang (LD) (b), Meiguiqie (MGQ) (c) and Chuanwutou (CWT) (d) at three selected concentrations. Shown here are relative PSR OD changes of four independent experiments. The CDI changes were minimum and not shown. The average PSR OD values of negative control group and TGF-β1-treated group were normalised to 0 and 100%, respectively, and changes in percentage of herbal extract-treated groups were relative to the TGF-β1 only group. *, **: $p<0.05$ and $p<0.01$ vs TGF-β1 only group.

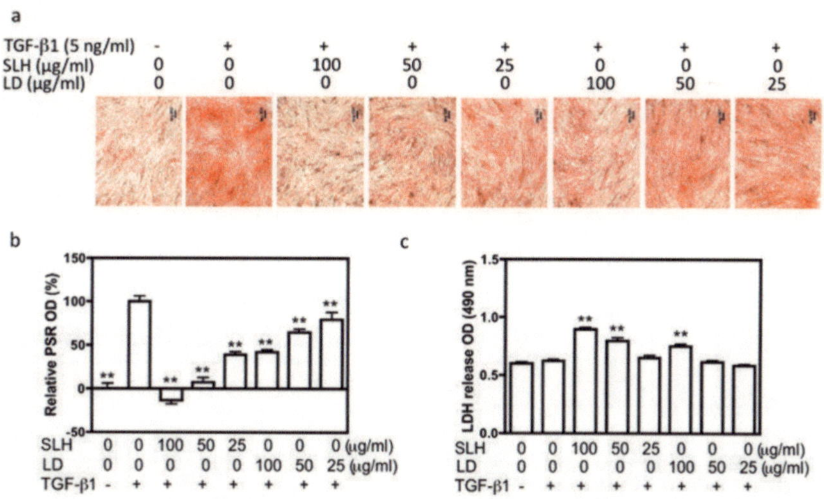

Fig. 2. Effects of Shiliuhua (SLH) and Liedang (LD) extracts on PSR staining (a), relative PSR OD values (b) and LDH release (c). Results in (b) and (c) shown here are in Mean ± SEM from one representative experiment, ** $p<0.01$ vs TGF-β1 only group, n=6 wells. The average PSR OD values of negative control group and TGF-β1 only group were normalised to 0 and 100%, respectively, and changes in percentage of herbal extract-treated groups were relative to the TGF-β1 only group.

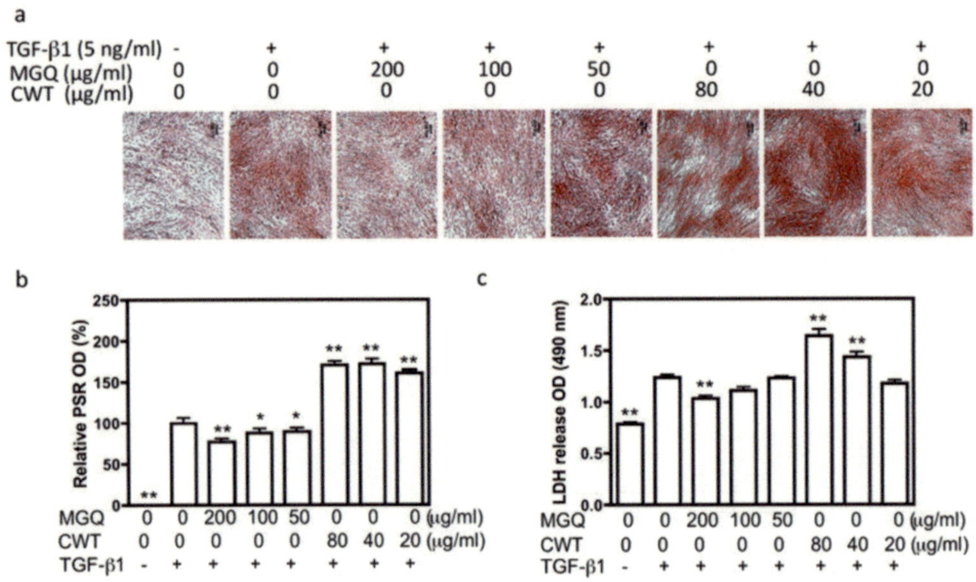

Fig. 3. Effects of Meiguiqie (MGQ) and Chuanwutou (CWT) extracts on PSR staining (a), relative PSR OD values (b) and LDH release (c). Results in (b) and (c) shown here are in Mean ± SEM from one representative experiment, *, ** $p<0.05$, $p<0.01$ vs TGF-β1 only group, n=6 wells. The average PSR OD values of negative control group and TGF-β1 only group were normalised to 0 and 100%, respectively, and changes in percentage of herbal extract-treated groups were relative to the TGF-β1 only group.

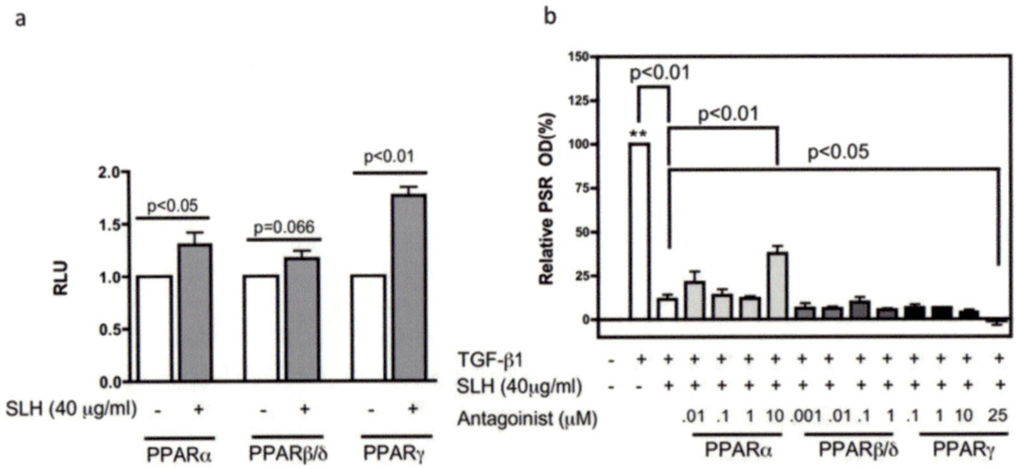

Fig. 4. Regulation of PPARα, PPARβ/δ and PPARγ activation by Shiliuhua (SLH) extract and effects of PPARα, PPARβ/δ and PPARγ antagonists on the anti-fibrotic effect of SLH extract. a. Effects of SLH extract on PPARα, PPARβ/δ and PPARγ activation, n=3 independent biological experiments; b. effects of increasing doses of PPARα, PPARβ/δ and PPARγ antagonists on the anti-fibrotic effect of SLH extract. ** $p<0.01$ vs control group, n=3 independent biological experiments. Other statistical results are as indicated in the figures.

4. Discussion

4.1 Knowledge-based discovery of anti-fibrotic activities from CMMs

Further to the evidence-based approach that we used in our earlier screens (Hu et al., 2009), in which we selected CMMs that had been reported to reduce fibrotic lesions *in vivo*, we used a knowledge-based approach in this study, namely, to screen candidate CMMs that were believed to be beneficial in treating fibrotic diseases based on the theory and practice of TCM. Of the 28 CMM extracts examined, eight (28.5%) showed reproducible *in vitro* anti-fibrotic activities, *i.e.*, Baibeiyegen, Liedang, Gusuibu, Jixueteng, Lingzhi, Meiguiqie, Moyao and Shiliuhua. Identification of these CMMs with anti-fibrotic activities *in vitro* underscores their inflammation-independent activities to inhibit TGF-β1-induced total collagen accumulation, perhaps through inhibiting TGF-β1-specific signalling or common pathways of fibrogenesis.

Among the eight CMM extracts with anti-fibrotic activities, Baibeiyegen (Zhao et al., 2002), Lingzhi (Lin et al., 2006; Wang et al., 2009; Wu et al., 2010), Meiguiqie (Liu et al., 2006), Moyao (Massoud et al., 2004) and Shiliuhua (Huang et al., 2005) have been reported anti-fibrotic in animal models of liver fibrosis or in hepatic stellate cells; Gusuibu was one of the weakest and its effect on fibrosis has never been previously reported either *in vivo* or *in vitro*; Liedang has not been reported on its effect on fibrosis either, but the ethanolic extract of its closely related family member *Boschniakia rossica* (Cham. & Schltdl.) B. Fedtsch. has been reported to mitigate liver fibrosis in a rat model of dimethylnitrosamine-induced liver fibrosis (Piao et al., 2005); Jixueteng is used in some herbal formulae, such as Huangqijixuetengtang (Li et al., 2006; Li et al., 2007) and Herbal Compound 861 (also known as Fufangdanshenheji) (Wang 2000; Wang et al., 2008), which were reported to be anti-fibrotic in patients and *in vitro*, but has never been reported as an individual anti-fibrotic herb.

Although only a quarter of the selected CMMs showed anti-fibrotic activities in our model, we do not exclude the possibilities that some of these CMMs might have a favourable effect in treating fibrotic diseases by interfering with other factors *e.g.* inflammation, TGF-β1 production and activation, molecules upstream of TGF-β1 signalling and TGF-β1-independent pro-fibrotic signalling pathways. Of note, CMMs which were identified as cytotoxic in the NRK-49F renal fibroblast model might be of therapeutic value in fibrotic diseases since loss of fibroblasts, the main producers of pathological matrices, may result in reduced ECM accumulation hence promoting regression of fibrosis. It is also worth reiterating that the results presented here were derived from extracts of CMMs in boiling 80% ethanol. Different extraction methods, including extraction solutions and efficiency, might have different impact on *in vitro* activities of the materials. Nevertheless, it would be of particular interest to isolate compounds contained in the eight ethanolic CMM extracts with *in vitro* anti-fibrotic activities, and to further test individual compounds for their *in vitro* anti-fibrotic activities.

4.2 *In vitro* anti-fibrotic activities and TCM categorisation of the CMMs

CMMs are traditionally characterised based on their function, nature, taste and channel tropism. By focusing on functional groups of the selected CMMs, we found that four out of 15 (27%) CMMs of "Huo Xue Hua Yu" group, two out of six (33%) CMMs of "Hua Tan" group and three out of seven (43%) CMMs of "Bu Xu" group, had *in vitro* anti-fibrotic activities. In view that "Hua Tan" and "Bu Xu"groups had rarely been the focus of previous evidence-based studies of anti-fibrotic CMMs, we consider our findings significant in guiding future studies of anti-fibrotic herbal medicines and in selecting therapeutic options in the clinic. However, due to the small sample numbers involved in this study, we do not intend to conclude that CMMs of certain functional groups have a higher chance of being anti-fibrotic than another. For example, results of Danshen, a drug in the "Huo Xue Hua Yu" group, was excluded from this project as it has been tested and reported elsewhere (Hu et al., 2009). In fact, Danshen is the most used herb in the 16 herbal formulae that showed *in vitro* anti-fibrotic activities (Hu et al., 2009). On the other hand, our results do not negate the fact that other functional groups of CMMs may possess anti-fibrotic activities. For example, Dahuang (root of *Rheum palmatum* L.) and Huangqin (root of *Scutellaria baicalensis* Georgi), both not in these three functional groups, had been previously reported to be anti-fibrotic and their activities had been confirmed in our earlier studies (Hu et al., 2009).

4.3 Shiliuhua and PPAR

In this study, Shiliuhua extract was one of the most potent CMMs in reducing TGF-β1-induced matrix accumulation. Extracts of Shiliuhua had been previously reported to activate PPARα and induce PPARγ expression. We found that ethanolic extract of Shiliuhua significantly activated both PPARα and PPARγ, which might account for its anti-fibrotic activity since agonists of PPARα (Toyama et al., 2004; Iglarz et al., 2003) and PPARγ (Milam et al., 2008; Kawai et al., 2008; Iglarz et al., 2003) were previously reported to suppress fibrosis of liver, lung, heart and kidney. Contrary to our hypothesis, we found that the anti-fibrotic activities of Shiliuhua extract can only be partially blocked by GW6471, a PPARα antagonist, at a dose 42-fold of its reported IC_{50}. Since the dose of PPAR antagonists were selected based on their IC_{50} reported in other cell types, it is possible that the doses we employed were sub-optimal in blocking PPARs in NRK-49F renal fibroblast cells. More interestingly, T0070907, a PPARγ antagonist, further increased the anti-fibrotic effect of shiliuhua extract when used at high dose (25 μM). Thus, it appears that Shiliuhua extract can activate both PPARα and PPARγ, but this property could not explain the anti-fibrotic activity of Shiliuhua in full. Further studies are required to elucidate the involvement of PPAR signalling pathway in anti-fibrotic activities of shiliuhua, for example to establish if these two PPAR isotypes have opposing functions in regulating fibrogenesis in renal fibroblasts in view that they did have opposing effects on monocyte chemotaxis in endometriosis (Hornung et al., 2001).

4.4 *In vitro* pro-fibrotic activities observed in this project

The *in vitro* pro-fibrotic activities of Chuanwutou, Dangshen and Yimucao deserve special attention. It rationalises pharmacovigilant studies to establish clinical relevance of these effects. Before clinical conclusions are drawn, it might be wise to avoid un-necessary, large-dose and long-term use of these herbs, especially in patients prone to fibrotic diseases. This issue is important because Dangshen and Yimucao are commonly used in formulae for fibrotic diseases (Yao et al., 2003) and Chuanwutou is indicated for conditions such as osteoarthritis, muscular diseases and stroke that often are complicated by fibrosis as well. As CMMs are rarely used individually, it is important to explore if their pro-fibrotic activities could be antagonised or eliminated when used in formulae. Of note, Yimucao had been reported in animal models to induce nephrotoxicity, including renal fibrosis, but its toxicity was reduced when used in formulae (Sun et al., 2005a, 2005b).

Among the three pro-fibrotic herbs, Chuanwutou appeared to be the most potent. Chuanwutou has well-known toxic effects that are believed to be reduced through a special processing procedure known as "Paozhi" (Chan et al., 1994; Singhuber et al., 2009), but as far as we know, this is the first report linking Chuanwutou to potent pro-fibrotic activities. The Chuanwutou we examined in this project was a raw material that had not undergone any "Paozhi" before ethanolic extraction. It is important to establish if the potent pro-fibrotic effect of this toxic herb could be reduced or even eliminated through traditional "Paozhi" and if this newly identified adverse effect contributes to any known clinical toxicity and adverse effects, in view that only processed Chuanwutou is allowed to be used in TCM practice according to the Chinese Pharmacopeia.

Interestingly, while extract of Dangshen, the root of *Codonopsis pilosula* (Franch.) Nannf. was found pro-fibrotic in this study, pollen of the same plant had been previously reported to be effective in preventing carbon tetrachloride-induced liver damage including fibrosis (Xiao et al., 1989). Furthermore, Fuzi, the daughter roots of the same plant as Chuanwutou, is a CMM categorised into a different functional group. We examined Fuzi in our *in vitro* model but it did not show any pro-fibrotic, anti-fibrotic or apparent cytotoxicity (data not shown). Thus, different parts of the same plant might have different and even opposite effects in regulating fibrogenesis.

5. Conclusion

Among the 28 herbal and fungal materials tested, eight showed *in vitro* anti-fibrotic activities while another three, especially Chuanwutou, showed pro-fibrotic activities. These results warrant further prudent investigations of their potential translation into clinical efficacy and their adverse effects.

6. Acknowledgements

We thank Ms. Dan Jiang (Acu-herb Clinic Sheffield, Sheffield, UK) and Professor Dunxu Wu (Shanghai University of Traditional Chinese Medicine) for recommending CMMs screened in this project. We are grateful to Dr Dae Kee Kim (Ewha Women's University Korea) for his kind gift of IN-1130, a selective inhibitor of TGF-β type I receptor (Alk5). The project was funded by Innovation China UK, Kidney Research UK, as well as European Union's Framework Programme 7 Coordination Action grant, Good Practice in Traditional Chinese Medicine Research in the Post-genomic Era.

7. References

Burton, J.D.; Castillo, M.E.; Goldenberg, D.M. & Blumenthal, R.D. (2007). Peroxisome proliferator-activated receptor-γ antagonists exhibit potent antiproliferative effects versus many hematopoietic and epithelial cancer cell lines. *Anticancer Drugs*, Vol. 18, No. 5, (June 2007), pp. 525-34, ISSN 0959-4973

Chan, T.Y.; Tomlinson, B.; Tse, L.K.; Chan, J.C.; Chan, W.W. & Critchley, J.A. (1994). Aconitine poisoning due to Chinese herbal medicines: a review. *Veterinary and Human Toxicology*, Vol. 36, No. 5, (October 1994), pp. 452-455, ISSN 0145-6296

Hornung, D.; Waite, L.L.; Ricke, E.A.; Bentzien, F.; Wallwiener, D. & Taylor, R.N. (2001). Nuclear peroxisome proliferator-activated receptors a and g have opposing effects on monocyte chemotaxis in endometriosis. *The Journal of Clinical Endocrinology & Metabolism*, Vol. 86, No. 7, (July 2001), pp. 3108-3114, ISSN 0021-972X

Hu, Q.; Jiang, D. & Xu, Q. (2007). In vitro models of fibrosis: Anti-fibrotic herbal medicines revisited. In: *Elements of fibrosis and the prevention and treatment of fibrosis in traditional Chinese medicine*, J. Niu, (Ed.), pp678-pp682, People's Health Press, ISBN 978-7-117-09337-8, Beijing, China

Hu, Q.; Noor, M.; Wong, Y.F.; Hylands, P.; Simmonds, M.S.J.; Xu, Q.; Jiang, D.; Hendry, B.M. & Xu, Q. (2009). *In vitro* anti-fibrotic activities of herbal compounds and herbs. *Nephrology Dialysis & Transplantation,* Vol. 24, No. 10, (October 2009), pp. 3033-3041, ISSN 0931-0509

Huang, T.H.; Yang, Q.; Harada, M.; Li, G.Q.; Yamahara, J.; Roufogalis, B.D. & Li Y. (2005). Pomegranate flower extract diminishes cardiac fibrosis in Zucker diabetic fatty rats: modulation of cardiac endothelin-1 and nuclear factor-κB pathways. *Journal of Cardiovascular Pharmacology,* Vol. 46, No. 6, (December 2005), pp. 856-862, ISSN 0160-2446

Huang, W. & Sun, R. (2010). Pathological damage mechanism of rats' nephrotoxicity caused by alcohol extracted components of Herba Leonuri. *Chinese Journal of Experimental Traditional Medical Formulae,* Vol. 16, No. 9, pp. 111-114, ISSN 1005-9903

Iglarz, M.; Touyz, R.M.; Viel, E.C.; Paradis, P.; Amiri, F.; Diep, Q.N. & Schiffrin, E.L. (2003). Peroxisome proliferator-activated receptor-alpha and receptor-gamma activators prevent cardiac fibrosis in mineralocorticoid-dependent hypertension. *Hypertension*. Vol. 42, No. 4, (October 2003), pp. 737-43, ISSN 0914-91IX

Kawai, T.; Masaki, T.; Doi, S.; Arakawa, T.; Yokoyama, Y.; Doi, T.; Kohno, N. & Yorioka, N. (2009). PPAR-γ agonist attenuates renal interstitial fibrosis and inflammation through reduction of TGF-beta. *Laboratory Investigation*, Vol. 89, No. 1, (January 2009), pp. 47-58, ISSN 0023-6837

Lee, G.; Elwood, F.; McNally, J.; Weiszmann, J.; Lindstrom, M.; Amaral, K.; Nakamura, M.; Miao, S.; Cao, P.; Learned, R.M.; Chen, J.L. & Li, Y. (2002). T0070907, a selective ligand for peroxisome proliferator-activated receptor γ, functions as an antagonist of biochemical and cellular activities. *Journal of Biological Chemistry*, Vol. 277, No. 22, (May 2002), pp. 19649-19657, ISSN 0021-9258

Li, R. & Zhao, M.Y. (2006). Effects of Huangqijixueteng decoction on TGF-β1, CTGF and PDGF-BB expression in experimental rat liver fibrosis. *Proceeding of Clinical Medicine,* Vol. 15, No. 9, (2006), pp. 659-661, ISSN 1671- 8631

Li, R.; Lu W. & Zhao, M.Y. (2007). Preventive effect and mechanism of Huangqijixueteng decoction on hepatic fibrosis in rats. *Chinese Journal of Integrated Traditional and Western Medicine on Digestion*, Vol. 15, No. 2, (2007), pp. 99-103, ISSN 1671-038X

Li, Y.; Qi, Y.; Huang, T.H.; Yamahara, J. & Roufogalis, B.D. (2008). Pomegranate flower: a unique traditional antidiabetic medicine with dual PPAR-α/-γ activator properties. *Diabetes, Obesity and Metabolism* Vol. 10, No. 1, (January 2008), pp. 10-17, ISSN 1463-1326

Lin, W.C. & Lin, W.L. (2006). Ameliorative effect of Ganoderma lucidum on carbon tetrachloride-induced liver fibrosis in rats. *World Journal of Gastroenterology*, Vol. 12, No. 2, (January 2006), pp. 265-270, ISSN 1007-9327

Liu, J.Y.; Chen, C.C.; Wang, W.H.; Hsu, J.D.; Yang, M.Y. & Wang, C.J. (2006). The protective effects of Hibiscus sabdariffa extract on CCl4-induced liver fibrosis in rats. *Food and Chemical Toxicology*, Vol. 44, No. 3, (March 2006), pp. 336-343, ISSN 0278-6915

Massoud, A.M.; El Ebiary, F.H. & Abd El Salam, N.F. (2004). Effect of myrrh extract on the liver of normal and bilharzially infected mice. An ultrastructural study. *Journal of the Egyptian Society of Parasitology*, Vol. 34, No. 1, (April 2004), pp. 1-21, ISSN 1110-0583

Milam, J.E., Keshamouni, V.G.; Phan, S.H.; Hu, B.; Gangireddy, S.R.; Hogaboam, C.M.; Standiford, T.J.; Thannickal, V.J. & Reddy, R.C. (2008). PPAR-γ agonists inhibit profibrotic phenotypes in human lung fibroblasts and bleomycin-induced pulmonary fibrosis. *American Journal of Physiology - Lung Cellullar and Molecular Physiology*, Vol. 294, No. 5, (May 2008), pp. L891-901, ISSN 1040-0605

Moon, J.A.; Kim, H.T., Cho, I.S.; Sheen, Y.Y. & Kim, D.K. (2006). IN-1130, a novel transforming growth factor-β type I receptor kinase (ALK5) inhibitor, suppresses renal fibrosis in obstructive nephropathy. *Kidney International*, Vol. 70, No. 7, (October 2006), pp. 1234-1243, ISSN 0085-2538

Piao, X.-X.; Huang, H.-G. & Piao, D.M. (2005). Therapeutic role of ethanolic extract of Boschniakia Rossica in dimethylnitrosamine-induced liver fibrosis in rats. *World Chinese Journal of Digestology*, Vol. 13, No. 18, (September 2005), pp. 2205-2209, ISSN 1009-3079

Seimandi, M.; Lemaire, G.; Pillon, A.; Perrin, A.; Carlavan, I.; Voegel, J.J.; Vignon, F.; Nicolas, J.C. & Balaguer, P. (2005). Differential responses of PPARα, PPARδ, and PPARγ reporter cell lines to selective PPAR synthetic ligands. *Analytical Biochemistry*, Vol. 344, No. 1, (September 2005), pp. 8-15, ISSN 0003-2697

Shearer, B.G.; Steger, D.J.; Way, J.M.; Stanley, T.B.; Lobe, D.C.; Grillot, D.A.; Iannone, M.A.; Lazar, M.A.; Willson, T.M. & Billin, A.N. (2008). Identification and characterization of a selective peroxisome proliferator-activated receptor β/δ (NR1C2) antagonist. *Molecular Endocrinology*, Vol. 22, No. 2, (February 2008), pp. 523-529, ISSN 0888-8809

Singhuber, J.; Zhu, M.; Prinz, S. & Kopp B. Aconitum in traditional Chinese medicine: a valuable drug or an unpredictable risk? *Journal of Ethnopharmacology*, Vol. 126, No. 1, (October 2009), pp. 18-30, ISSN 0378-8741

Sun, R.; Wu, X.; Liu, J.; Sun, L. & Lv, L. (2005a). Experimental study of the rat renal toxicity of Tripterygium wilfordii, Caulis aristolochiae and Leonurus. *Pharmacology and Clinics of Chinese Materia Medica*, No. 2, 2005, pp. 26-28, ISSN 1001-859X

Sun, R.; Sun, L.; Wu, X. & Lv, L. (2005b). Formulation reduces the renal toxicity of Yimucao. *Chinese Journal of Pharmacovigilance*, No. 3, (June 2005), pp. 144-147, ISSN 1672—8629

Toyama, T.; Nakamura, H.; Harano, Y.; Yamauchi, N.; Morita, A.; Kirishima, T.; Minami, M.; Itoh, Y. & Okanoue, T. (2004). PPARα ligands activate antioxidant enzymes and suppress hepatic fibrosis in rats. *Biochemical and Biophysical Research Communications. Vol. 324, No. 2,* (November 2004), pp. 697-704, ISSN 0006-291X

Wang, B.E. (2000). Treatment of chronic liver diseases with traditional Chinese medicine. *Journal of Gastroenterology & Hepatology*, No. 15 Suppl, (May 2000), pp. E67-70, ISSN 0815-9319

Wang, L.; Wang, B.E.; Wang, J.; Xiao, P.G. & Tan, X.H. (2008). Herbal compound 861 regulates mRNA expression of collagen synthesis- and degradation-related genes in human hepatic stellate cells. *World Journal of Gastroenterology*, Vol. 14, No. 11, (March 2008), pp. 1790-1794, ISSN 1007-9327

Wang, G.J.; Huang, Y.J.; Chen, D.H.; Lin, Y.L. (2009). Ganoderma lucidum extract attenuates the proliferation of hepatic stellate cells by blocking the PDGF receptor. *Phytotherapy Research*, Vol. 23, No. 6, (June 2009), pp. 833-939, ISSN 0951-418X

Wu, Y.W.; Fang, H.L. & Lin, W.C. (2010). Post-treatment of Ganoderma lucidum reduced liver fibrosis induced by thioacetamide in mice. *Phytotherapy Research*, Vol. 24, No. 4, (April 2010), pp. 494-499, ISSN 0951-418X

Wynn, T.A. (2007). Common and unique mechanisms regulate fibrosis in various fibroproliferative diseases. *Journal of Clinical Investigation,* Vol. 117, No. 3, (March 2007), pp. 524-529, ISSN 0021-9738

Xiao, J.C.; Liu, H.J.; Han, D.; Li, Z.; Jiang, J.X. & Qing, C. (1989). Protective effects of the pollen of Codonopsis pilosula (Franch.) Nannf. on liver lesions at the ultrastructural level. *Zhongguo Zhong Yao Za Zhi*. Vol. 14, No. 3, (March 1989), pp. 42-44, ISSN 1001-5302

Xu, H.E.; Stanley, T.B.; Montana, V.G.; Lambert, M.H.; Shearer, B.G.; Cobb, J.E.; McKee, D.D.; Galardi, C.M.; Plunket, K.D.; Nolte, R.T.; Parks, D.J.; Moore, J.T.; Kliewer, S.A.; Willson, T.M. & Stimmel, J.B. (2002). Structural basis for antagonist-mediated recruitment of nuclear co-repressors by PPARα. *Nature* Vol. 415, No. 6873, (February 2002), pp. 813-817, ISSN 0028-0836

Xu, Q.; Norman, J.T.; Shrivastav, S.; Lucio-Cazana, J. & Kopp, J.B. (2007). *In vitro* models of TGF-β-induced fibrosis suitable for high-throughput screening of antifibrotic agents. *Am J Physiol Renal Physiol* Vol. 293, No. 2, (August 2007), pp. F631-40, ISSN 0363-6127

Yao, C.F. & Jiang, S.L. (2003). Prevention and treatment of pulmonary-fibrosis by traditional Chinese medicine. *Zhong Xi Yi Jie He Xue Bao*. Vol. 1, No. 3, (September 2003), pp. 234-238, ISSN 1672-1977

Zhao, J.; Lü, Z.; Wang, X. & Zhang, X. (2002). The study on the anti-oxidation effect of root of Mallotus apelta in the rat model of liver fibrosis. *Zhong Yao Cai*. Vol. 25, No. 3, (March 2002), pp. 185-187, ISSN 1001-4454

17

Chinese Medicine and Integrative Approaches in the Prevention of Breast Cancer – Acupuncture Meridian, Pulsed Eletromagnetic Field Test and Chinese Food Therapy

Lulu Fu and Hong Xu
Victoria University,
Endeavour College of Natural Health,
Australia

1. Introduction

A series of studies conducted demonstrate the integrative abilities of hormone regulation and subsequent preventative strategies with the use of Chinese Medicine (CM) in the prevention of breast cancer and balancing hormones.

These investigations studied the patterns of disharmony for groups of middle aged women and explored the relationship between the CM patterns of disharmony and specific bio-markers (Xu, 2004; Fu & Xu, 2011).

Chinese medicine assessment in Fu and Xu's study (2011) indicated that the participants felt correspondingly weaker and their health conditions also had adverse trends in their middle age. They commonly had mood swings which relates to *Liver Qi stagnation*. Peri-menopausal symptoms also affected their daily life. Data collected from these participants indicated that the adverse symptoms and relative signs changed after the treatment resulting in the levels of disharmony being reduced. The changes of patterns of disharmony indicated in the Chinese medicine assessment are relevant to the change of biomedical markers, which may be useful in western-medical assessment of hormones fluctuation and pre-clinical breast diseases. If Chinese medicine diagnostic methods indicate that *Liver Qi stagnation* and *Liver-Kidney Yin deficiency* are the main patterns of middle aged women hormone fluctuation or pre-clinical breast diseases, it is reasonable to argue that the treatment principle should be based on regulating *Qi* and nourishing *Yin*. This study has provided a repeatable evidence of using the Chinese kiwi fruit extract for the regulation of hormonal disorder and Chinese medicine patterns of disharmony.

The bio-markers used in these studies are the 2-hydroxyestrone and 16α-hydroxyestrone (2-OHE: 16α-OHE), they are both reliable and sensitive in order to investigate the hormone imbalance. These can be easily applied as early preventative strategies that integrate both CM and Western diagnostic methods. The selected Chinese kiwi fruit *(Actinidia chinensis var. deliciosa)* extract could benefit women with hormone imbalance or hormone related diseases (Xu & Xu, 2006). In another clinical trial, 16 participants, who were diagnosed with breast cancer and had just completed chemotherapy, were given this Chinese kiwi fruit drink (equal to 20g) daily over a seven day period. The results indicated that the rate of binucleate lymphocyte cells with micronuclei in these participants had significantly decreased. This may indicate the recovery of chromosome change in the breast tissue (Xu, 1999). Appropriate choice of nutritional products on the scientific basis is an important aspect in cancer patients' recovery (Xu & Xu, 2006).

This study focused on the relationships between the acupuncture meridian, Chinese food therapy and pulsed electromagnetic field test in the same population group, using a double-blind, placebo-controlled clinical trial.

1.1 Acupuncture meridian

In Chinese Medicine, all the primary 12 meridians passed the trunk area and over spread to peripheral extremities. The *Yang* meridians traverse the outer surface of the arm or leg and travel to the head and the back, in spite of the *Stomach Meridian* that are running the lateral side of the *Kidney Meridian*, at the anterior of the trunk. All *Yin* meridians traverse or bypass the breast area and the special superior lateral side of the breast. These meridians each correspond to different organ (*Zang Fu*) systems. Meridians harmonise the whole body's function if *Qi* and *Blood* could circulate well, they can also reflect the direct trauma and the *Zang Fu* function. Pathogens and diseases can make visible changes on the related meridians (Tang et al., 1999). The acupuncture meridians are important transportation channels, any blockage of the meridians will cause disease and disharmony in the body.

During the fourteenth century, Dr Dan-Xi Zhu summarized the etiology of breast cancer that a woman, who was worried and depressed, could suffer from an accumulation of stagnation. The stagnation could be the cause of *Liver Qi* rebels horizontally and the stagnation finally turns into nodules (Niu, 1996). Female hormonal related diseases and breast diseases are related to the *Liver* and *Kidney Meridians* (Fu & Xu, 2011).

1.2 Pulsed Electromagnetic Field (PEMF) test

Electromagnetic fields are present everywhere in our environment but are invisible to the human eye. One of the main characteristics which define an electromagnetic field is its frequency or its corresponding wavelength. Fields of different frequencies interact with the body in different ways (WHO, 2011). The equipment selected for the PEMF test is safe according to the WHO guideline. The magnetic field changes were measured by a noninvasive medical device, which has been supplied on the market for over 10 years. This magnetic test, using a polarized light can detect a defect at the cellular level (Gianni & Liberti, 2006).

Humans have an electromagnetic energy field, the human body is an aerial that can transmit and receive energy (William, 2002). When there is a disorder, the magnetic field could be alternated by the *Qi and Blood* stagnation in CM theory. Magnetic therapy has been used in CM practices from 200 BC according to CM history.

In the early stage study of electromagnetic models, the magnetic network was recognized similar to the acupuncture meridian (Omura, 1986). Later study indicated that the acupuncture meridians were related to the electromagnetic model of transmission lines (Yung, 2005). In this study, the polarized light was used to detect the magnetic field change near and along the acupuncture meridian.

1.3 Chinese Kiwi Fruit Extract

Chinese herbal formulae, food therapy and acupuncture have long been used to effectively regulate endocrinal disorders in Chinese clinical practice. One Chinese food therapy of interest is the Chinese food formula - Kiwi Fruit Extract (KFE), which has been used in practice for many years and related safety tests have also been conducted. Kiwi fruit extract is rich in vitamin C, vitamin E, vitamin K, folate, antithetic acid, niacin, lutein, zeaxanthin, arytenoids, falconoid, calcium, iron, manganese, selenium, zinc, copper, potassium, magnesium, fibre and amino acids (Collins et al., 2001).

Xu (2004) in his book *The Progress of Resource, Environment and Health* indicated that: Some varieties of kiwi fruit found in China have a strong anti-mutagenesis effect. When somatic cells change into cancer cells they will go through mutation, apoptosis of cells and loss of control of proliferation. Mutagenesis can be examined by gene mutation, chromosome aberration and DNA damage in laboratory experiments. High mutagenic rates can indicate the risk of cancer. There are many mutagens in the environment, e.g., coal, petroleum, tobacco, uncompleted burning of products benzo(a)pyrene etc. Polycyclic Aromatic Hydrocarbons (PAHs); over stir fried meat PhIP; peanuts, corn etc. produce aflatoxin in the damp heat environment polluted by mould; farm chemicals that pollute food like nitrous amine compound (nitrosamine), organic chlorine, toxic algae's toxins, organic pollutions in water e.g., methyl mercury; benzene, formaldehyde which are chemical pollutants in workshops and living room air; as well as overdoses of irradiation of ultraviolet ray and electromagnetic waves. The greater concern for cancer patients is some chemotherapy drugs e.g., cyclophosphamide, radiotherapy's radiation is also a mutagen.

To reduce the effects of the mutagen and the side effects of chemotherapy and radiotherapy it is beneficial to use therapeutic fruits, i.e., kiwi fruit and hawthorn fruit, which have broad anti-mutagenesis effects. Moreover, these fruits have the effect of increasing immune function. Of course, use of expansion agents to increase the size of the kiwi fruit can damage the quality of the kiwi fruit. To enhance kiwi fruit's health care effects, withdrawing the effective components, e.g., anti-cancer isoflavones, organic acids, polysaccharide and trace element, by formulation and scientific experiments to produce functional health care products, can enhance the whole anti-cancer defensive system, e.g., Hong En Health Drink (Xu & Xu, 2006).

KFE is used to improve the quality of life of women suffering from endocrine disorders (Xu, 2004; Fu & Xu, 2011). In this study, the effects of KFE on regulating the function of acupuncture meridians and unblocking the stagnation in these meridians were evaluated.

2. Research methodologies

Thirty-six middle aged peri-menopausal women living in Melbourne Australia were recruited and randomly assigned (using numbered order as they became available) into two groups, treatment group taking KFE and control group taking placebo. The group assignments were kept blind from the participants and data collectors. All the participants were in the age range from 40 to 55 year-old. They were not taking either contraceptive pills or hormone replacement therapy. None of them suffered from either breast cancer or liver and or kidney disease according to western medicine and they did not have any food allergies.

Participants took 10g of powder, either KFE or placebo each time, twice a day, mixed with 100ml of warm water. The powder was administered one hour before each breakfast and dinner meal, over an eight week period. The selected Chinese therapeutic food is a wild resourced Chinese kiwi fruit extract, Hong En No. 1 (also known as Hong En Health Drink) in powder form, provided by Professor Houen Xu of Peking University.

Pulsed electromagnetic field changes at pre and post trial were tested, at the trunk area, where the pass way of acupuncture meridians distributed. Each test lasted about 10 minutes to go through all the meridians on both the left and right side of the body, this short time exposure to the PEMF is not expected to cause any change to the body. No adverse events were reported by any of the participants in this study.

The Ultra-long Electromagnetic Wave technique, a pulsed electromagnetic field (TW-1) was selected, supplied by Health Link Food & Equipment Pty. A polarized light was used for detecting changes in the magnetic flux, the light turns off when the magnetic flux is blocked. The results were recorded on a map where there is an anatomical drawing of the human trunk. These include the depiction of any defective areas found in the two dimensions (length and width). A 0-10 scale is used to measure the portion of the blockage, "0" represents unblocked and "10" represents fully blocked. The tested area on the body was restricted between the mid-clavicular line and mid-axillary line, from the iliac crease to the clavicula and the axillary line at the trunk area, which matches the CM *Liver Meridian* area (See Figure 1).

The detailed steps of magnetic test were to:

- Obtain consents from participants to record the dots on their bodies and to take photographs as records for the first measurement and the last measurement.
- Explain the test purposes and procedure to the participant individually. Place the patient in supine position with the arm at 90 degree abduction.
- Measure the area of the magnetic test.
- Record the magnetic flux changes on the surface of the skin with a marker. The marks will show any defective areas found along the *Liver Meridian*.
- Use a tape measure to measure the magnetic flux changes area (width and length).
- Record the dots formed on a body map, which include the trunk area of the anatomy.
- Remove the marks on the skin, cleaning with ethanol swabs or wet cotton ball.

The study was approved by the related committees and the ethics approval was gained from the Human Research Ethics Committee of Victoria University, Australia. All participants received an explanation document and a consent form for completion.

3. Results and discussion

All the 36 participants (aged 48.38 ± 3.97 in the treatment group and 48.50 ± 5.15 in the control, $p > 0.05$) completed the tests (See Table 1), the magnetic test results were positive which indicated that blockage existed in the tested areas. The *Liver* and *Kidney* meridians in breast and flank areas are mostly affected. The average of the test results of both the left and right sides of the *Liver* and *Kidney* meridians, in both the treatment and the control group were analyzed using *t-test* by SPSS 19.

The pre-trial PEMF test results indicated that both the meridians of KFE and control groups were blocked at similar levels, there were no significant differences between the pre-trial comparisons in the two groups ($p > 0.05$) (Table 1).

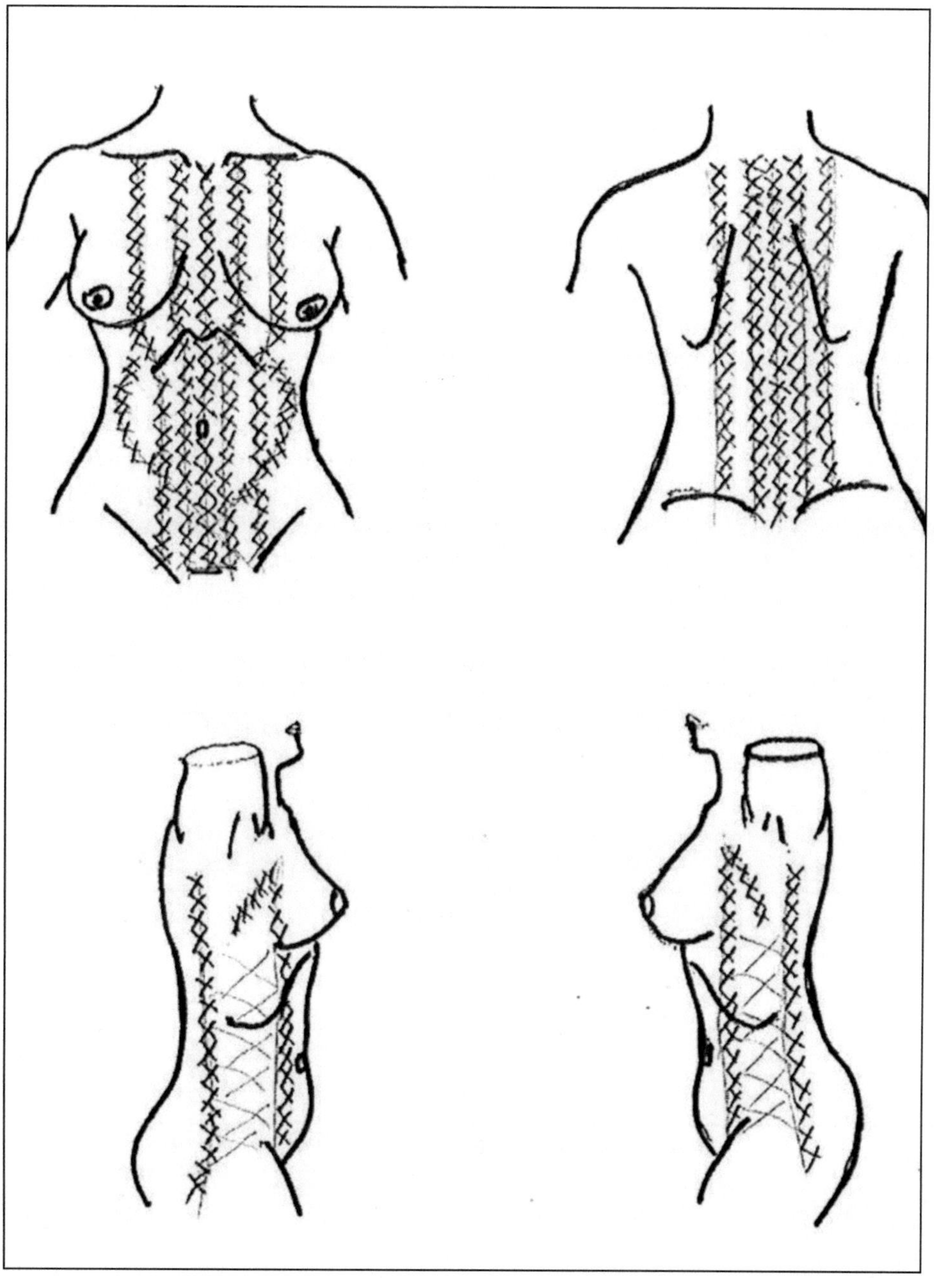

Fig. 1. PEMF test transmission lines

Groups	n	Age (years)	*Liver Meridian* PEMF test	*Kidney Meridian* PEMF test
Treatment	18	48.38 ± 3.97	7.64 ± 4.18	5.61 ± 4.99
Control	18	48.50 ± 5.15	6.11 ± 4.94	4.89 ± 4.86

Notes: *Participants in treatment group take Chinese kiwi fruit extract (Hong En No. 1) 10g X 2/days X 8 weeks; **Participants in control group take placebo
$p > 0.05$ between groups.

Table 1. Pre - trial base-line comparison of the age and PEMF test results (mean ± SD) between the treatment* and control** group of peri-menopausal women

After eight week's treatment, the results of the PEMF tests were significantly different between the two groups and between the pre and post treatment on the *Liver Meridian* (See Table 2). This indicates that KFE can improve *Liver Meridian*'s function. The results of the pre and post treatment comparison on the *Kidney Meridian* indicated a reduction of the meridian blockage while there was no change observed in the control group. However, this comparison did not achieve statistical significance (Table 3). According to common CM theory and practise, it could take much longer time to recover *Kidney* disorders, especially if the disorder is related to the pattern of deficiency. In the previous study (Fu & Xu, 2011), *Kidney* function can be improved by KFE indicated by the biomarker 2-OHE:16α-OHE change. It is therefore suggested that an integrative approach that incorporates different diagnostic methods may be a more effective way to identify and prevent breast diseases.

Groups	n	Pre-trial *Liver Meridian* PEMF test	Post-trial *Liver Meridian* PEMF test
Treatment*	18	7.64 ± 4.18	1.33 ± 2.68**
Control	18	6.11 ± 4.94	4.67 ± 4.95***

Notes: *Participants take Chinese kiwi fruit extract (Hong En No. 1) 10g X 2/days X 8 weeks. **Pre and post comparison in treatment group, $p = 0.000, t = 8.864$;
***Post-trial comparison between treatment and control groups, $p = 0.003, t = 3.252$¶

Table 2. Comparison of *Liver Meridian* PEMF test results (mean ± SD) of peri-menopausal women

Groups	n	Pre-trial *Kidney Meridian* PEMF test	Post-trial *Kidney Meridian* PEMF test
Treatment*	18	5.61 ± 4.99	4.58 ± 4.88
Control	18	4.89 ± 4.86	4.89 ± 5.00

Note: $p > 0.05$.

Table 3. Comparison of *Kidney Meridian* PEMF test results (mean ± SD) of peri-menopausal women

Most participants in the KFE group reported the improvement of general well-being after taking KFE, the details included: the decrease of hot flushes, mood swing, tiredness, abdominal distension and anger. However, these changes were not reported by the control group. There were no adverse events reported.

4. Conclusion

In this study, the pulsed electromagnetic field test is an effective diagnostic tool for the detection of acupuncture meridian disorder. The stagnation of the meridian is related to the magnetic field change. Chinese kiwi fruit extract could regulate the function of the acupuncture meridians which have been proved by the pulsed electromagnetic tests. These approaches can be easily applied as early preventative and diagnostic strategies that integrate both Chinese Medicine and contemporary therapies.

5. References

Xu, H.E. (2004). Chinese Kiwi Fruit and Health, In: *The Progress of Resource, Environment and Health in China - SCOPE China Publication Series III*, H.E. Xu, (Ed.), 113-133, Peking University Medical Press, ISBN 7-81071-559-3, Beijing, China

Fu, L.L. & Xu, H. (2011). A Preliminary Study of the Effectiveness of Chinese Therapeutic Food on Regulating Female Reproductive Hormones. *Integrative Medicine Insight,* Vol 6, (March 2011), pp. 7-12, ISSN 1177-3936

Xu, H. & Xu, H.E. (2006). Chinese Food and Cancer Healing. *Integrative Medicine Insights,* Vol 1, (Febuary 2007), pp. 1-5, ISSN 1177-3936

Xu, H.E. (1999). *Hong-En Health Drink – Development and Research*, Beijing Medical University Publishing House, pp. 11-21, ISBN 7-81034-975-9, Beijing, China

Tang, Y.X; Dang, Y. & Geng, E.G. (1999). *Acupuncture and Moxibustion*, Academy Press, pp. 462–480, ISBN 7-5077-1269-9, Beijing, China

Niu, J.Z. (1996). *Modern Gynecology of Traditional Chinese & Western Medicine,* China Science and Technology Publishing House, pp. 39-46. ISBN 9787504619402, Beijing, China

WHO, (2011). Electromagnetic Fields, Available from http://www.who.int/peh-emf/about/WhatisEMF/en

Gianni, M. & Liberti, M. (2006). Modeling Electromagnetic Fields Detectability in a HH-like Neuronal System: Stochastic Resonance and Window Behavior. *Biological Cybernetics,* Vol.94, No.2, pp. 118-127, ISSN 0340-1200

William, S. (2002). The Human Electromagnetic Energy Field: Its Relationship to Interpersonal Communication. *Journal of Theoretics,* Vol.4, No.2, ISSN 1529-3548

Omura, Y. (1986). Re-evaluation of the Classical Acupuncture Concept of Meridians in Oriental Medicine by the New Method of Detecting Meridian-like Network Connected to Internal Organs Using "Bi-Digital O-Ring Test". *Acupuncture & Electro-Therapeutic Research,* Vol.11, No.3-4, pp. 219-31, ISSN 0360-1293

Yung, K.T. (2005). A Birdcage Model for the Chinese Meridian System: Part III. Possible Mechanism of Magnetic Therapy. *The American Journal of Chinese Medicine,* Vol.33, No.4, pp. 589-597, ISSN 1793-6853

Collins, B.H.; Horská, A.; Hotten, P.; Riddoch, C. & Collins, AR. (2001). A Kiwifruit Protects Against Oxidative DNA Damage in Human Cells and in Vitro. *Nutrition and Cancer.* Vol.39, pp. 148-153, ISSN 1532-7914

18

Traditional Chinese Medical Criteria About the Use of Yongquan as a Life Support Maneuver

Adrián Angel Inchauspe
La Plata National University,
Argentina

1. Introduction

Although I consider the beginning of my formal Dim Mak education since 1993 -when Master Erle Montaigue spread out this theory in the western world *("Dim Mak -Death Point Striking")*, my first contact with K-1 Yongquan was in 1976, when I had the opportunity to explore some "almost secret" scripts about this subject.

I waited until 1987, during my surgical residence, to apply this knowledge in my first case - a cardiac arrest derived from a pulseless activity with no response of the life support therapy, but with great success using the K-1 maneuver.

Since then, my researches are continuous about the acupuncture-point Yongquan manipulation results after both basic and advanced Cardio-Pulmonar Resuscitation (CPR) protocol failure. It surprising results guide me to call this phenomenon the "Lazarus Effect".

It's necessary to describe briefly the principles that give sense to the K-1 Yongquan maneuver, in order to integrate them to western medical concepts.

2. *Jing:* Our energetic inheritance

The ancestral u original energy represents the value of our energetic inheritance, or *Jing*.

The *Innate Jing*, received from our parents is hidden in the Kidneys (Yin) and in the Mingmen (Yang) to generate the initial Qi for our vital processes (*Jing Yue Quan Shu – Zhang Jie Bin).*

The *Adquired Jing* gives the substrate of the anterior one. It is contained into the five *zhang* and the six *fu*, nurturing our vital substance.

The *Yin or Nurture Qi* enters in our energy system from the Earth through K-1 Yongquan; and it will be selected in its "pure form" by the Spleen before reaching the Lungs and Heart. In that way, the last organs will be able to elaborate *Zheng Qi* or Central (thoracic) energy for its vital priority of his active cardio-respiratory function.

3. Kidney and traditional Chinese medicine

In acupuncture, the Kidneys (Shen) represents Water, so that is the Yin organ "par excellence". Their main function, similar to the allopathic medical knowledge, is" *to control the body Water distribution*" (*Su Wen, chap. 34*). In the same way, it will be responsible of filtering wastes, eliminate toxins, the water intake excess and the mineral salts incorporated by diet, in order to regulate the blood Ph.

For the Chinese Medicine, the Kidney develops the following functions:

1. *"to store the Jing and dominate reproduction, growth and development"*

This includes the mastering of derived functions as birth, growing, development and reproduction, for Kidneys are our natural ancestral energy depot - the purified and condensed modality of Qi *(Jing)* - that will aid us to get each of the human development stages (*Su Wen ,chap.1).*

2. *"to produce the bone marrow" (Su Wen , chap.5).*

This statement involves the following properties:

- The control of the bones and their marrow *(Su Wen, chap.23).*
- To elaborate the blood –Xue-(were the Chinese intuitive about erythropoietin's existence?).
- To nurture the brain (for Chinese people, the brain represents the "Sea of Marrow").

We can see that the "Medullae concept" in TCM results very much transcendental than their western significance. Not only involves the bone marrow, but the matrix of the fundamental components of the Central Nervous System.

3. *"to dominate Water" (Su Wen, chap.34)*

This function has been analyzed before in this chapter. Is obvious to understand this meaning in the regulation of the methabolism of water and corporal fluids (*"Jin ye"*).

4. *"to control the reception of Qi"*

In the sense that Shen is the depot of the Ancestral energy or *Yuan Qi (Ling Shu.chap.5),* Kidneys are capable to captivate the Qi for recycle it energetically, taking influence over the following *zhang*:

- Over the Spleen and its "couple in Earth" Stomach, allowing the correct digestives procedures
- Over the Heart, getting the equilibrium in the Water. Fire harmony *(Kan Li)*
- Over the Lungs, helping to gather and descend the Qi during inspiration
- Over the Liver, ensuring a soft and harmonious Qi flux all around the body
- Over the Triple Heater, promoting the "Water transformation" through its energetic methabolism

5. *"It manifests in the hair".*

As indicated in *Su Wen (chap.5),* hair's characteristics show the internal sufficiency of the Qi of Shen.

6. *"to open the ears" (Ling Shu, chap.17).*

It was written in this chapter " *The Qi of the Kidneys go to the ears; when the Kidneys are in harmony, the ears can hear the Five Sounds"... _* thus referring not only to the five notes from the pentathonic Chinese music, but the effect of the Kidneys (Shen) over the other organs or *zhang.*

We must remember the hearing disorders as a consequence of treating patients with nephrotoxic drug (ej. antibiotics) to understand how advanced was the Chinese medical wisdom.

Among this, and searching for motives of the spectacular reaction through Yongquan in resuscitation, again in *Ling Shu* (chap. 10) appears the link between Kidney and Heart(by its internal vessel) and with the Lungs (by a secondary vessel),that justifying this powerful influence.

4. Specific analysis about the K-1 Yongquan acupuncture point

Its name means "Gushing spring" or "Bubbling well".The ancient book I-Ching instructs us about the Water ("Kan") trigram:"*...its correspondence is to Water; is the Water in movement, the spring that falls into deepness...*"

4.1 K1-Resuscitation maneuver: Chinese fundamentals

Located in the sole of the foot, in a depression where the sole makes its plantar flexion. Tracing a line from the base of the second toe up to the heel, and dividing it in three equal parts, the point is found at the junction between the anterior and the middle third.

Anatomically speaking, Yongquan´s precise ubication is between the second and third metatarsal bones, at the level of the plantar fascia. Medial to it are the longus and brevis flexor digitorum pedis tendons and the second lumbricalis pedis muscles.

In its deepest position, the point lay in the interossei plantaris muscles. It is innervated by the second common plantar digital nerve, and irrigated by the lateral plantar and the anterior tibial arteries anastomose in the plantar arch.

In the major acupuncture classical texts, K-1 Yongquan is considered the first and Jing (Tsing)-well point of the Kidney meridian. But through the *Ling Shu* analysis (chap.5),

K-1 is also hierarched as the "root" point of the *Shao Yin* .This energetical level, formed by the Kidneys and the Heart, is the most profound among all others, giving us a special reason why K-1 Yongquan can act as an effective cardiac pacemaker.

Moreover, Yongquan is the main place for the ascending Yin Qi from the Earth into our body. Therefore, this kind of energy will nurture the *zhang*, especially those placed in the most Yang part of the torso, in order to interact and compensate the Heavenly energy, essential for organs with a non-interruptable function to maintain our life, like the heart and the lungs. It can be read in *Ling Shu, chap 9:"Yin rules the organs, while Yang rules the viscus. Yin absorbs the Heavenly energy, while Yang absorbs the energy from the Five Organs"*. Thus, the Celestial Yang Qi provides them with continous motility in the Upper Jiao of our body, for a perfect vital equilibrium.

4.2 Main applications for K-1 Yongquan in TCM

Traditional Chinese Medicine "officially" recognizes the following as the main applications of K-1 Yongquan:

- Respiratory diseases	- Nasal obstruction - Epistaxis (nosebleed).
- O.R.L diseases	- Dry tongue – Amigdalitis – Swollen throat – Odinophagia –Vertigo
- Digestive diseases	- Abdominal colics -Vomits – Diarrhea – Difficult defecation
- Urinary conditions	- Difficult urination – Dysuria
- Genital conditions	- Functional sterility
- Psychiatric conditions	- Insomnia – Psychosis
- Cardiovascular diseases	- Arterial hypertension – Syncope
- Neurological conditions	- Blurred vision – Vertex headaches – Peripheral neuropathy – Infantile convulsions – Epilepsy – Lower limbs paralysis (Zheng Li)-Stroke – Loss of consciousness (Coma)

Among this indications, in relative recent times (2006), Chinese doctors added a case of subdural hematoma.
Since 1987, my specific and new use is as a rescue point against both basic and advanced CPR failure. Currently, a new paper has been sent to the World Journal of Critical Care Medicine in order to present a complete protocolization about K-1 uses during life- support maneuvers.

5. Bioenergetic survival axis

5.1 Valorative comparison between Oriental and Occidental axioms

In "Impending Death situation" patients, both Oriental and Western Medicines explain some biological reactions that make organs and viscus to take a peculiar concatenation that could be followed by a logical sequence. In this manner, we can understand this mutual cooperation as a result of K-1 stimulation in a dynamic way.

5.2 A common embryological origin

It is well known in Occident that both the skin and the Central nervous System recognize a common embryological origin.
In the beginning of the 3th week, a trilaminar embrion enhance its cranial extreme, and an axial depression appears in its ectoderm. This fissure is the Neural fold ;a structure that few days later will make the Neural tube ,and the first draught of raquis.
Over this, alternative medicines found arguments that support their action vehicled by the skin.This represents, in current neurological physiology ,the visceral-cutaneous reflex.

5.3 Survival axis components

Among the Kidneys, there are another organs to be integrated under the structure of what is presented as the "Survival Axis".
Integrated diagrams will configure this notions in a dynamic way.

SURVIVAL AXIS - Dr. Inchauspe

6. Suprarenal glands

Not only an anatomical relationship - for there are positioned over- entail them with the Kidneys, but also represent the Yang function of the mentioned channels (remember that Kidneys themselves maintain the Yin part of this balance).
In the mid 20th century, german investigator Hans Seyle described the "Stress reaction", while in North America, Cannon menctioned it as the "Fright, fight or flight" behaviour. Both were clearly coincident about the suprarenal response to an emergency state, producing glucocorticoids (the main one in primates is cortisol), mineralocorticoids (aldosteron) and androgens. The final release of catecholamines (L-dopa, ephynefrine, norephynefrine) will prepare our body to stress. All the last derive from phenylalanine´s molecule; so that it injection can enhance our alarm reaction.
This hypothesis is another evidence of the "Mother and son" rule from the Five Element´s theory in TCM.
K1-Yongquan hypothalamus-adrenal bio-feedbak

7. Brain

Above all emotions, **FEAR** is the natural response against any situation that put life into risk (is the emblematic emotion of the Water element). The sensorial perceptions are interpreted as a menace in the limbic system. From this site of the temporal lobe, signals will run down from the hypothalamus to hypofisis to stimulate suprarenal glands, preparing us to face **DANGER.**

Among all the cutaneous reflexes, the Babinski one is the best known and of utmost importance, because this plantar stimulation ,after the age of 2 ,can diagnose a pyramidal lesion with a patognomonic hallux extension –casualty scratching near the K-1 Yongquan!.

This evidence even more the axiom "*Kidney masters the Sea of Marrow*".

Interaction of the Water Element (Tai Yang Level)

8. Heart

Chinese related it with the Kidney by internal passways. Moreover, TCM considered this two organs conform the most profound energetic level in a human being: *The Shao Yin.*

Heart could be conceived in a Yin and a Yang phase: the "right heart" includes the right auricule and ventricle; same consideration can be made with the left side.

The right side acts as an "admission pump" the blood ***(Xue)*** follows a centripetal route towards the heart, so it can be understanded with a Yin nature.

The left auricle and ventricle transport oxygenated blood to the body, reaching them in a centrifugal travel impulsed by the systolic ejection. So this "propulsive part" of the Heart behaves as the Yang side.

In the right auricle, Keith & Flack´s sinoauricular node normally functions as our cardiac pacemaker. Because its same Yin polarity line of Kidney –and connected by profound collaterals -, it could be very influenced by it.

9. Kidneys and the Ancestral Energy

For the Chinese, they are the "Ancestral Energy Depot", and they also considered it as the "Prenatal Emperor" for their activity during pregnancy (perhaps they already knew that Kidneys are directly involved in the amniotic fluid production).

During the 3th week –in the vitelin sack, very near from the alantoid process -,a group of haploid cells travel through the inguinal stretch to testicles (or to ovaries) where will rest the cromosomic potential for our species perpetuation.

This essential energy, or *Yuan* is a kind to be convoked into emergency states, so that stimulating the route of our "Survival Axis".

In Traditional Chinese Medicine (TCM), it is generally accepted that, if the principal property from the Curious Vessels is to conduct the *Yuan* or ancestral energy into themselves, the reason is that all of this Particular Meridians have their origin in the Kidneys (Shen).

In chapter 9, *Ling Shu* tells us: "*Curious Vessels as Chong Mai and Ren Mai are connected to the Chao (Shao) Yin level*". So through the Chong Mai –the "*Mother of the Twelve Meridians*" - it can be understood in what way Kidney influences over the other body channels.

More specifically talking, those Curious Vessels of Yin nature (Yin Wei - Yin Qiao –Chong Mai) recognize their initial point in K-1 Yongquan, while the rest of them endowed with

Yang polarity (Yang Qiao - Yang Wei - Dai Mai) are born in the final point of the Yang descendent (centrifugal) channels in the inferior limbs. If you pay attention to the names of this points - ex.Gb 44: Zu Qiao Yin ("Passage to the Yin"); or B 67: Zhi Yin ("That who meets the Yin"), make us evident how close are they to contact the major Yin source ever known _ the terrestrial energy_ and their main entrance: the K-1 acupuncture point.
Yuan Considerations.

10. The *Shao Yin* level

The *Shao Yin* commands the vital functions, although the brain´s energy had been impaired. Up to the 60´s, cardiac activity´s suspension was evident by a fail in both breathing and pulse perception. Only this allowed the doctor to declare a clinical death.
With the development of the organ -transplantation therapy,death was not more the absence of vital signs,but a non - reactive EEG.So with the brain activity in suspension ,we are able to define a legally death patient, turning it into a "living donor".
In the *Shao Yin level* resides the last quantum of energy before life abandon us. For its connection with Earth -the most powerful Yin source available, K-1 Yongquan - the "root" point of the *Shao Yin* that enables the Terrestrial energy to rush up towards the cranial Yang pole - deserves the possibility of rescuing us with a simple maneuver, pressing the most dark and retired place of the body: in the sole of the foot!

11. Results

Since 1987, of a current statistic of 44 cases, 39 patients were admitted in hospital, while 5 external cases in "impending death situation" received life-support attention with failure of both basic and advanced CPR protocol.
The next table summarizes the demography and outcome of this people assisted with the "Lazarus Effect".

-	Stroke	7 cases	1 death
-	Severe hypertension	8 cases	no death
-	Electrocution	1 case	1 death
-	Chest crush	3 cases	1 death
-	Chest trauma with skull and bilateral femur fractures	1 case	1 death
-	Post-operative shock	4 cases	1 death
-	Intraoperative heart stoppage	6 cases	1 death
-	Pulseless activity	3 cases	1 death
-	Ventricular fibrillation	5 cases	1 death
-	Gas embolism	1 case	no death
-	Renal failure post-sepsis	2 cases	1 death
-	Anaphylactic shock (post oncology drugs)	3 cases	no death

12. Conclusions

Comparison between my first 30 patients against the best results of Emergency Services and Rescue Teams (around 19 % survival in CPR), justified its publication in the Resuscitation Journal (j.resus. 4183. JAN-2010; DOI information: 10.1016).

In October, 2010 I was invited to participate as speaker in the 8th International Congress of Drug Development, Science and Technology in the Convention Center of Beijing. There I exposed about the theoretical effect of phenylalanine inyection over K-1 Yongquan, based in its convertion into catecholamines and its action over the glomic micro-structure of the acupuncture point (Dr. Sergio Gutierrez Morales, Canarias). Hipothetically speaking, this allows the cardiac arrest victims to "respond" more effectively to the Yongquan maneuver, thus improving to higher survival rates.

Actuarial statistics show a mortality percentage in heart stoppage in aprox. 1,5/1000 healthy individuals. Translating this proportion to the current world population, nearly 8.000.000 deaths occur per year for this cause, a very much lethal situation that any epidemic or pandemic danger actually known. From them, only a limited 19% -it means, 1.520.000 persons - can be rescued.

The K-1 Yongquan resuscitation maneuver could raise up this rate to, at least, 38%.This signifies that more than 3.500.000 people could be potentially saved each year –as was informed in FILASMA Congress in Sevilla, in November 2010, where Dr.Enrique Ruffa summed another new 3 cases to the Yongquan resuscitation statistics. This number is comparable with the actual population of our neighbough country, Uruguay –aprox. 4.000.000 people.

Once the World Resuscitation Committee accepts this therapeutic maneuver, this whole theory will open the possibility of converting cardiac arrests victims into responders, allowing the K-1 Yongquan maneuver inclusion in the life-support protocols, upgrading the survival rates even much more.

13. References

Borison, R.L. et al: "Metabolism of amino acid with antidepressant properties". Res Commun Chem Pathol & Pharmacol, 1978; 21 (2):363-6.

Chamorro, C. et al: "Can heart donation exclusion factors be overcome?" Rev.Esp. Cardiol., 2006; 59:232-7.

Chamorro, C.: "Mantenimiento especifico del posible donante cardíaco". Conferencia como Coordinador de Transplantes - Servicio de Medicina Intensiva". Clinica "Puerta de Hierro", Madrid.

Gutierrez Morales, A.R.; Smith Agreda, V.: "Mecanismos de acción de la analgesia acupuntural: Biomedicina, practica clinica e investigación". Edit. Mandala, Madrid, 2001

Gray, B.: "The Advanced Iron Palm. Unique Publications, Burbank, California, 1995; (2), 11.

Huang Di: "Ling Shu, Yellow Emperor´s Canon of Acupuncture" 1° Edition, Madrid, 2002.

Huang Di: "Su Wen, Nan Jing"7° Edition, Ed. Plaza, Madrid, 2002.

Hsieh, D.: "Advanced Dim Mak". Meadea Enterprise Co., Inc. Republic of China, 1995; (7).87.

Inchauspe, A.: "Phenylalanine injection over K-1 Yongquan: a theoretical way of upgrading survival rates in CPR".speaker of the 8th IDDST Congress. Beijing, China. October 23-26th, 2010

Inchauspe, A.: "Traditional Chinese Medicine K-1 Yongquan and resuscitation: another Kind of "Lazarus phenomenon". Resuscitation (2010), doi: 10.1016/j. resuscitation. 2009.12.009.

Kitade, T.; Odahara, Y.; Shinohara, S. et al:"Studies on the enhanced effect of acupunture analgesia and acupuncture anesthesia by D-phenylalanine (2nd report)—schedule and administration and clinical effects in low back pain and tooth extraction". Acupunct. Electrother rev., 1990; 15 (2):121-35.

Len Kevin, MD.: ".DL-fenilalanina(DLPA):el agente analgesico y terapeutico natural". Conferencia como miembro de la Chemical Royal Society.

Long, H: "Advanced Dragon´s Touch - Anatomical targets and techniques. Paladin Press, Boulder, Colorado, 1995

Montaigue, E.: "Dim Mak -Death Point Striking", chap.4."The points and what they do". Paladin Press, Boulder, Colorado, 1993; 85.

Montaigue, E: "Advanced Dim Mak - The finer points of Death-Point Striking" chap. 8:"Point Power". Paladin Press, Boulder, Colorado, 1994, 198, fig.263 -264.

Poewe, W.: "Treatment for Parkinson disease---past achievements and current clinical Needs. Neurology, 2009.Feb.17; 72 (7 Suppl):s65-73.

Russell, A.L.; Mc Carthy, M.F.: "DL-phenylalanine markedly potentiates opiate analgesia - an example of nutrient/pharmaceutical up-regulation of the endogenous analgesic system.Med. Hypothesses.2000; 55 (4):283-8.

Sabelli, H.C.; Fawcett, J.; Gusovsky, F. et al.: "Clinical Studies on the phenylalanine hipótesis of affective disorders: urine and blood phenylacetic acid and phenylalanine dietary supplements".J. Clin Psychiatry, 1986; 47 :66-70.

Steven, D.; Ehrlich, NMD: "Solution Acupuncture, a private practice specializing in Complementary and Alternative Medicine". Verified Health Network.

Solorzano del Rio, H.."Funciones de la Fenilalanina".Conferencia como coordinador del Departamento de Medicinas Complementarias. Univ. Guadalajara, Mexico.

Szabo, G.: "Physiologic changes alter brain death".J. Heart Lung Transplant 2004; S223-6.

Walsh, N.E.; Ramamurthy, S.; Schoenfeld, L.; Hoffman, J."Analgesic effectiveness of D-phenylalanine in cronic pain patients".Arch. Phys. Med. Redhabil., 1986; 67(7):436-9.

Part 4

Pharmacodynamic Material Base Research

19

The MALDI-TOF Analysis of Aconitum Alkaloids in Proprietary Chinese Medicine and in the Concoction of Fuzi

Yong Wang and Chunhui Luo
College of Bioscience, Shenzhen University, Shenzhen
China

1. Introduction

In theory, the kinds and relative amounts of aconitum alkaloids in proprietary Chinese medicines should be consistent with those in Fuzi. However, this feature has not been noted enough and no direct experimental evidence to prove it. In this work MALDI-TOF-MS was used to analysis 19 kinds of proprietary Chinese medicines, benzoylmesaconine and hypaconitine have been proved to be the predominant monoester and diester alkaloids respectively. In addition, the MALDI-TOF analysis of the concoction of seven kinds of Chinese medicine has confirmed that the acidity of concoction will improve the aconitines contents and the toxicity of concoction, but this rule was not suited for Lonicera nitida, Rhizoma Chuanxiong or Chaenomeles sinensis.

The Aconitum plants are widely used in China as an analgesic, a cardiotonic, and an anti rheumatism treatment. Among all the species Aconitum, the lateral roots of Aconite (Aconitum Camicheali Debx, Fuzi), main roots of Aconite (Chuanwu) and roots of Aconitum kusnezoffii Reichb (Caowu) are the three kinds of plant medicines that are collected in Chinese Pharmacopoeia, and some of other Aconitum plants have been used as folk medicine. It is well known that diester diterpenoid aconitine (DDA) and its analogues isolated from Aconitum plants contribute to the bioactivity and the high toxicity for the heart and the central nervous system. Fortunately, aconitines are heat-unstable and will be conversed into less toxic monoester diterpenoid alkaloids (MDA) or lipo-alkaloids after processing [1], therefore, the amounts of highly toxic aconitine are lower than those of monoester diterpenoid alkaloids in processed aconite and proprietary Chinese medicines (PCMs).

For monitoring the possible toxicity of Chinese medicines, high-performance liquid chromatography (HPLC) has been frequently used for quantification analysis of aconitines. Generally, only aconitine, mesaconitine and hypaconitine three standards could be purchased and most of research was limited in these 3 alkaloids [2]. Therefore, qualitative analysis is also essential for PCM besides quantitative analysis. In contrast to chromatographic methods, matrix-assisted laser desorption time-of-flight mass spectrometry (MALDI-TOF-MS) determines the molecular mass of alkaloids, which represents an inherent physical property and is feasible for high-throughput analysis of different samples containing aconitines.

In this work, we have analyzed aconitum alkaloids in 19 kinds PCMs and found that hypaconitine is the dominant DDA in the 12 oral PCMs, which is somewhat different from previous quantitative results of aconitines in PCM reported by using HPLC method [3]. These PCMs include Guifudihuangwan (GFDHW), Fuzilizhongwan (FZLZW), Jinkuishenqiwan(JKSQW), Xiaohuoluowan (XHLW), Sanhanhuoluowan (SHHLW), Zuifengtouguwan (ZFTGW), Narusanwewan (NRSWW), Muguawan (MGW), Xiaojinwan (XJW), Haimabushenwan (HMBSW, Dahuoluowan (DHLW), Panlongqipian (PLQP), Fufangxuelianjiaonang (FFXLJN), Diedazhentonggao (DDZTG), Tiebangcuizhitonggao (TBCZTG), Guzengshengzhentonggao (GZSZTG), Shexiangzuifenggao (SXZFG), Zhentonglingding (ZTLD) and Shangtongding (STD).
On the other hand, the detoxification mechanism of aconite in concoction is far away from clear. For example, acidity is one of the factors to influence the hydrolysis of aconitines [4]. Here we have concocted Fuzi with 7 others herbal Medicines and analyzed the alkaloids in the concoction by MALDI-TOF-MS. We have found that acidity is not the only factor that affects the hydrolysis reaction of DDAs as well as the amounts of aconitines because of the complexity of Chinese medicine.

1.1 Experimental

Prepared root of aconite and all proprietary Chinese medicine (PCM) were purchased from drug store; 5g dried and powered aconite root or PCM were soaked with 60 mL ethanol for 48 h at room temperature, and the resulting solution of alkaloids was diluted with 50% ethanol for further analysis of MALDI-TOF.

1.2 Mass spectrometry

All experiments were performed using a Voyager DE-STR MALDI-TOF mass spectrometer (Applied Biosystems) The Voyager DE STR was operated in a positive reflector mode with the following parameters: acquisition mass range, 400-1000 Da; accelerating voltage, 20,000 V; grid voltage, 73%; mirror voltage ratio, 1.14; guide wire, 0.01%; low mass gate set at 300; extraction delay time, 150 ns; and the laser power attenuator set at 2700, total 100 shots/spectrum. Matrix solution was prepared by dissolving 8mg of α-cyano-4-hydroxycinnamic acid (CHCA) in 1 ml of 1:1 mixture of acetonitrile and 0.1% trifluoroacetic acid.

2. Results and discussions

2.1 The MALDI-TOF analysis of nineteen kinds of PCM

For aconitum alkaloids, protonated molecules $(M+H)^+$ were observed by MALDI-MS in positive ion mode. The structures of aconitum alkaloids are very similar and it is reasonable to assume that they have similar ionization efficiencies [5]. The alkaloids of 13 oral administration pills or tablets that using prepared aconite roots have been analyzed firstly. As shown in Fig.1-Fig.13, benzoylhypaconine (BHA, m/z 574), benzoylmesaconine (BMA, m/z 590) and benzoylaconine (BAC, m/z 604) were the major components, hypaconitine (HA, m/z 616) is the most main diester alkaloids, additionally, deoxyaconitine (DA, m/z 630), mesaconitine (MA, mz/ 632) and aconitine (AC, m/z 646) can also be observed. In all 13 PCMs, HMBSW exhibit the most high relative abundance of the highly toxic diester aconitines (Fig.12), however, different with some previous report that obtained by high performance liquid chromatography [3], it is HA other than MA is the dominant aconitine, in addition, 10-OH-MA (m/z 648) and 10-OH-AC (m/z 662) have been detected also. We believe our result is reasonable because MA is more prone to be hydrolyzed to BMA after boiling [1] and HA is the main aconitine in prepared aconite roots [5]. An exception is Daguoluowan, only BMA was detected with a weak signal. According to the ancient Chinese concept of Yin-Yang, Aconite is one of the most important herbal medicines that related Yang deficiency and relieving pain, so a certain amount of monoester aconitum alkaloids and diester alkaloids is essential for the treatment. Generally, in the mass region of m/z 400-500, talatizidine, talatisamine, neoline, fuziline and 14-acetyl- talatisamine can be detected at m/z 408, m/z422, m/z 438, m/z 545 and m/z 464 respectively owing to they also exist in prepared Fuzi [6]. Secondly, for the vitro dosage form such as plaster or tincture, some obvious changes have been observed. Aconitine at m/z 646 has been detected as the main alkaloids in DDZTG (Fig.14), TBCZTG (Fig.15), GZSZTG (Fig.16), and STD (Fig.17); thirdly, mesaconitine is the most high content alkaloids in SXZFG (Fig.18); fourthly, high abundance of HA, DA, MA and AC have been detected in ZTLD.

In sum, because of the high ionization efficiency of alkaloids, aconitines and their hydrolysis products can be easily analyzed by MALDI-TOF after extracted by chloroform, thus, MALDI-TOF mass spectrometry provides a rapid, sensitive, simple and specific method for the qualitative analysis of alkaloids mixtures in complex systems such as proprietary Chinese. By comparing the relative abundance of DDA and MDA, we can further acquire relatively quantitative information of aconitum alkaloids. Actually, as an analysis method that based on mass isolation, mass spectrometry method is especially suit for the well-known research system such as aconitum alkaloids.

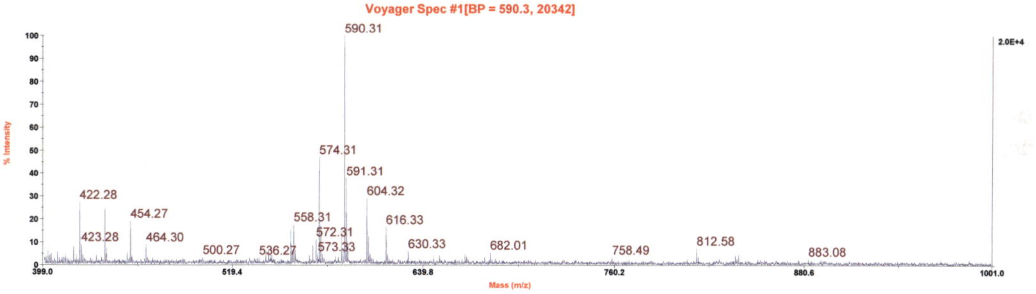

Fig. 1. MALDI-TOF spectrum of GFDHW

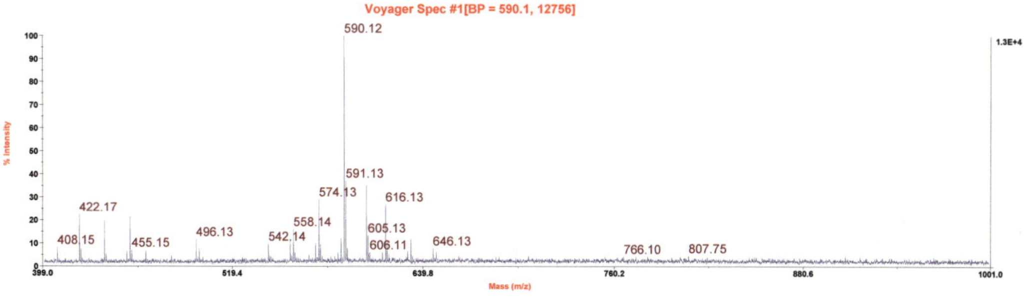

Fig. 2. MALDI-TOF spectrum of FZLZW

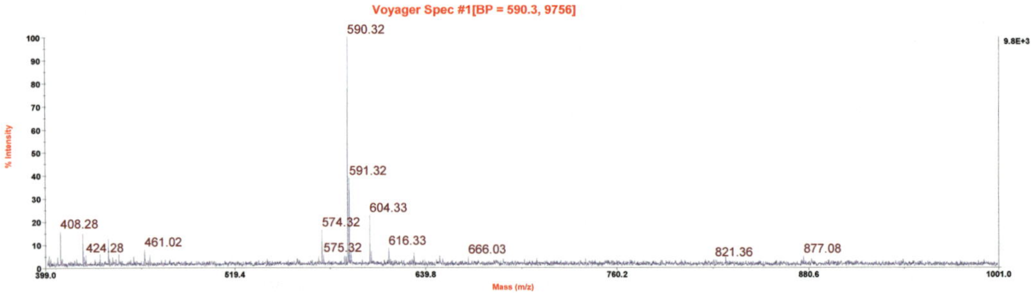

Fig. 3. MALDI-TOF spectrum of JKSQW

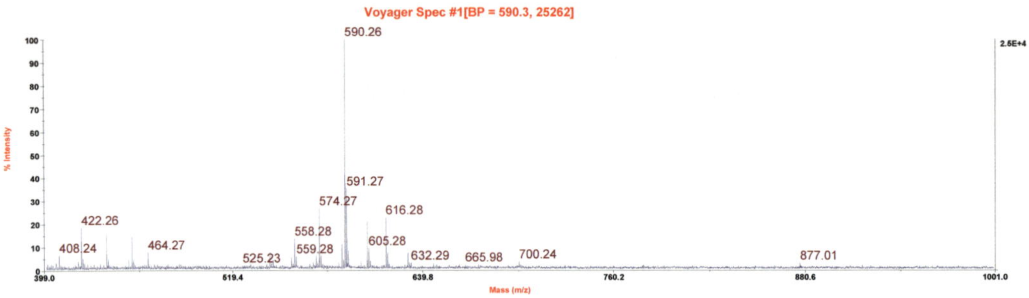

Fig. 4. MALDI-TOF spectrum of XHLW

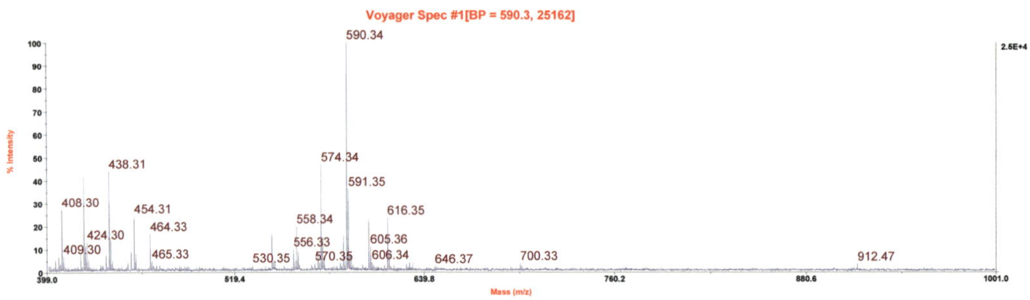

Fig. 5. MALDI-TOF spectrum of SHLLW

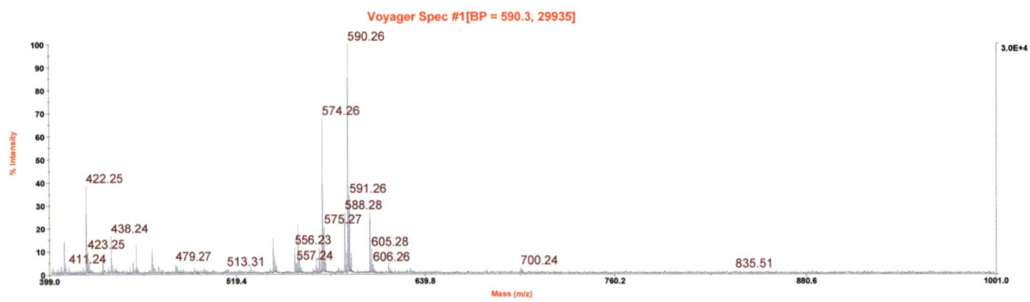

Fig. 6. MALDI-TOF spectrum of ZFTGW

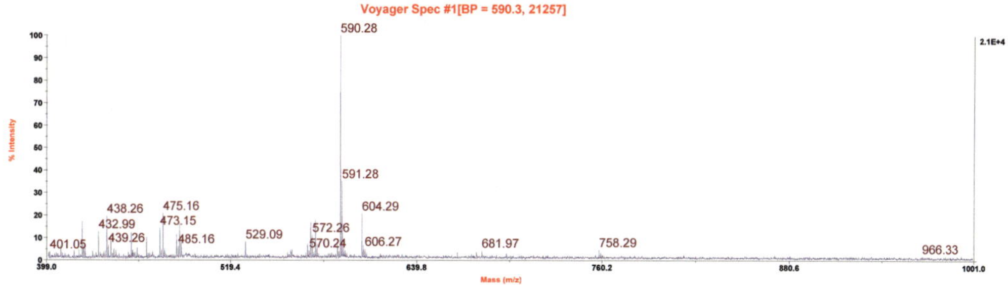

Fig. 7. MALDI-TOF spectrum of NRSWW

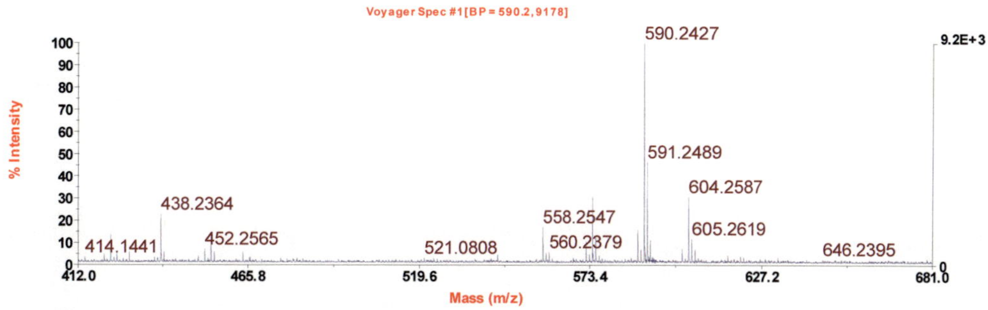

Fig. 8. MALDI-TOF spectrum of MGW

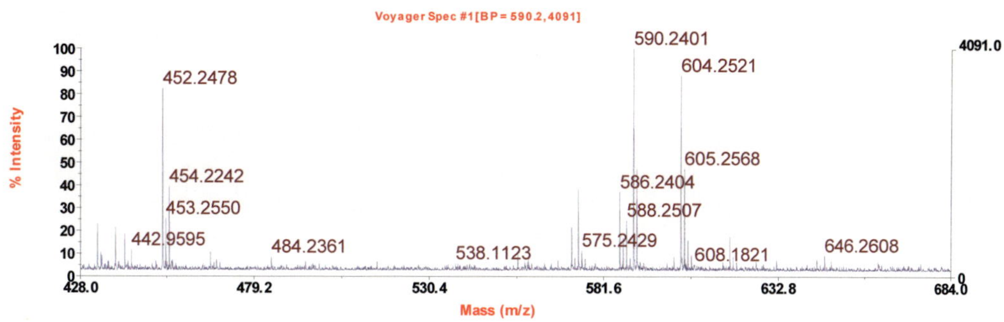

Fig. 9. MALDI-TOF spectrum of PLQP

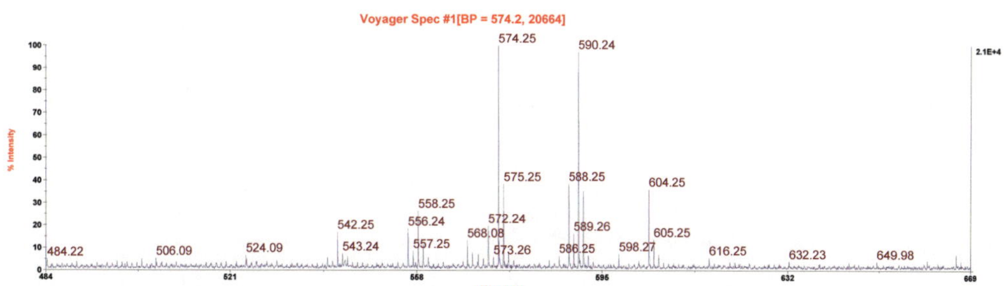

Fig. 10. MALDI-TOF spectrum of XJW

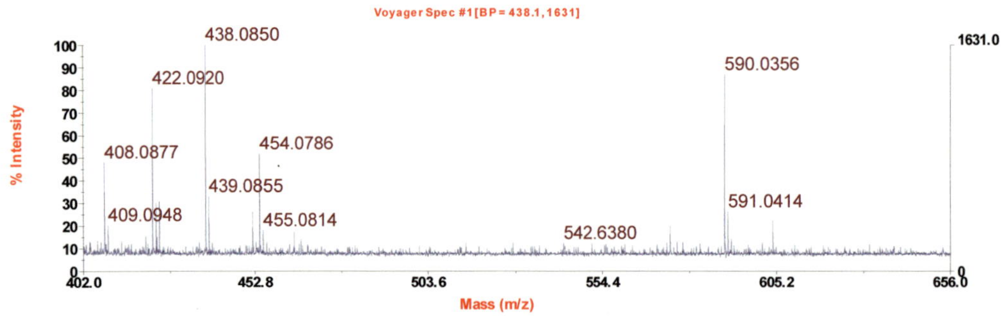

Fig. 11. MALDI-TOF spectrum of FFXLJN

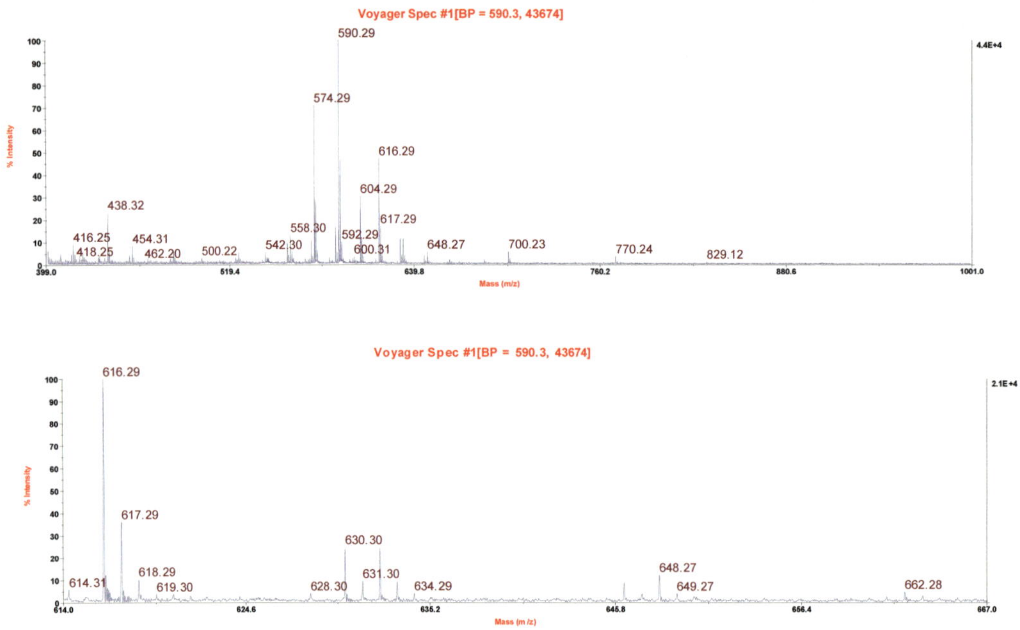

Fig. 12. MALDI-TOF spectrum of HMBSW

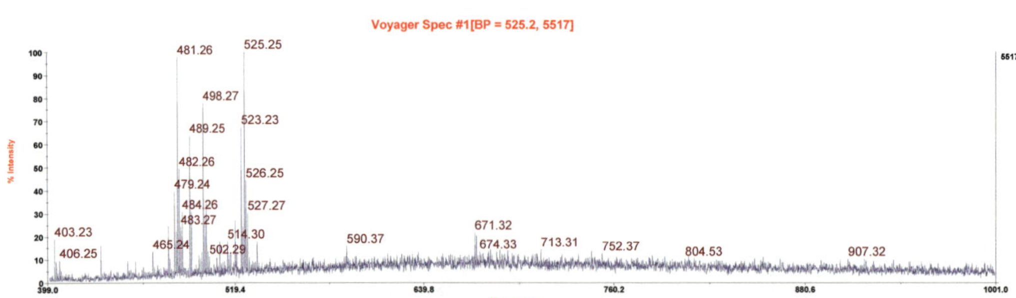

Fig. 13. MALDI-TOF spectrum of DHLW

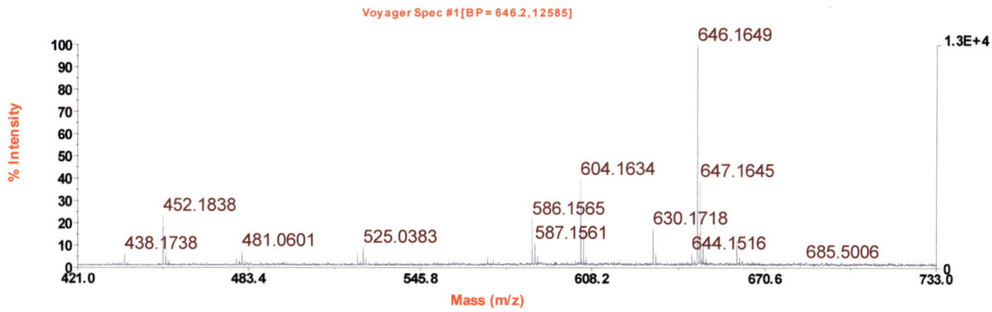

Fig. 14. MALDI-TOF spectrum of DDZTG

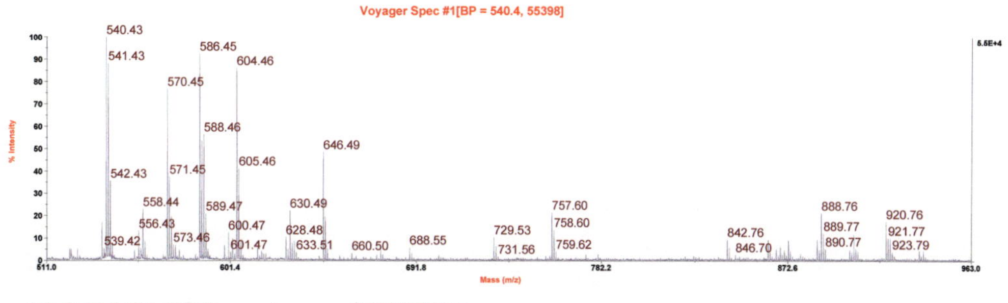

Fig. 15. MALDI-TOF spectrum of TBCZTG

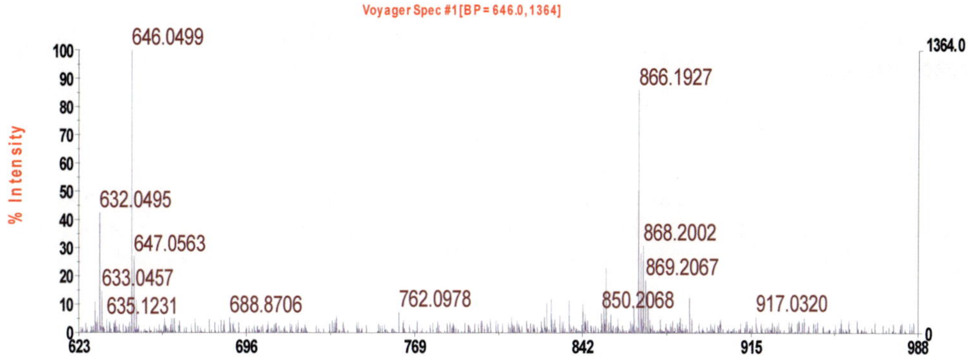

Fig. 16. MALDI-TOF spectrum of GZSZTG

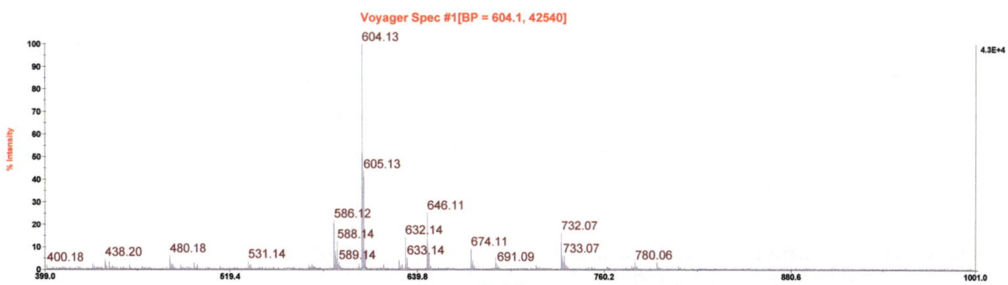

Fig. 17. MALDI-TOF spectrum of STD

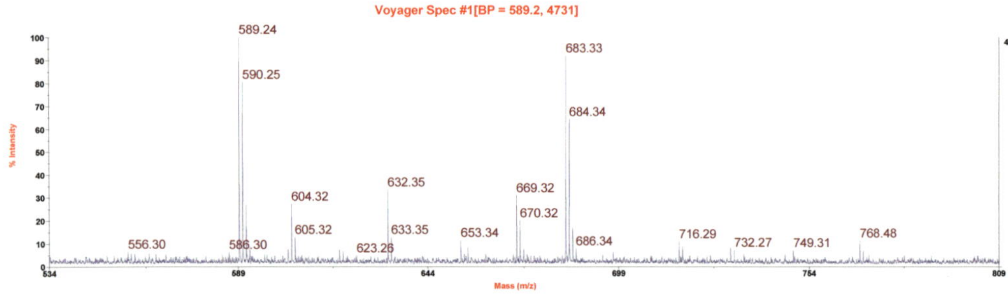

Fig. 18. MALDI-TOF spectrum of SXZFG

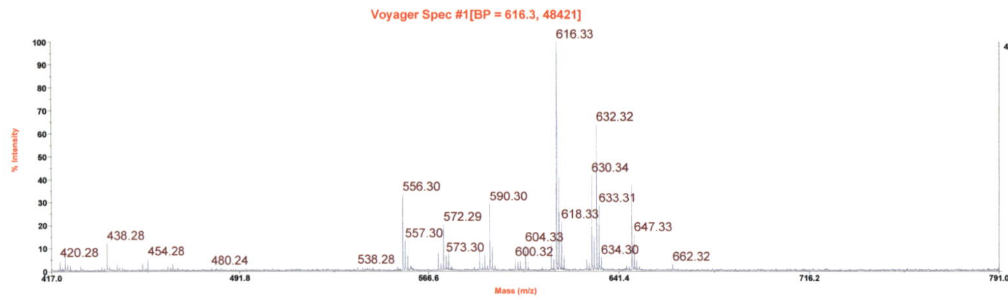

Fig. 19. MALDI-TOF spectrum of ZTLD

2.2 The MALDI-TOF analysis of alkaloids in the concoction of aconite roots with other Chinese medicine

To some extent, the combinational principles of Fuzi can be explained by the chemical reactions in the concoction, namely, DDA will be changed to MDA and lipo-alkaloids in boiling water [1]. In addition, the acidity of solution has played an important role for these chemical reactions and high acidity will inhibit the hydrolysis of aconitines [4]. However, it is still not clear that whether the acidity is the only factor for the amounts of aconitines in concoction. In this study, we have selected 7 kinds of Chinese medicines of which decoction are acidic to answer this question.

As shown in Table 1, the pH value of the Fuzi decoction is 4.73; the pH value of the decoction of Radix Glycyrrhizae is 5.54, the pH value of other 6 kinds of herbal medicine ranged from 3 to 4. The pH value of the concoction of aconite with others is similar with those of decoction.

2.3 The MALDI-TOF analysis of alkaloids in prepared Fuzi and the decoction of Fuzi

The MALDI-TOF spectrum of the ethanolic extract of prepared Fuzi provides a profile of the alkaloids. BHA, BMA and BAC are the main alkaloids in Prepared Fuzi, HA, DA, MA and 10-OH-AC has been observed as the main aconitines (Fig.20). After decocting, the relative amounts of highly toxic aconitines have been reduced because they are heat-unstable [5,6].

2.4 The MALDI-TOF analysis of alksloids in the concoction of Fuzi with Radix Glycyrrhizae, Lonicera nitida and Rhizoma Chuanxiong

It is well known that Radix Glycyrrhiza has the detoxify effect, so it is reasonable that almost no aconitines has been detected in the concoction of Fuzi with it except for low abundant

HA at m/z 616 (Fig.22). However, to our surprise, in the concoction of Fuzi with Lonicera nitida or Rhizoma Chuanxiong (Fig.23 and Fig.24), the relative intensity of aconitines is also low and other aconitines have been detected at noice lowel. Since the pH value of the concoction of Fuzi with Lonicera nitida and Rhizoma Chuanxiong is respective 3.54 and 3,75, these results have suggest that the acidity of concoction is not the only factor that effect the hydrolysis reactions of aconitines.

Aconite roots	4.73
Radix Glycyrrhizae (甘草)	5.54
Lonicera nitida (金银花)	3.54
Crateagus pinnatifida (山楂)	3.32
Chaenomeles sinensis (木瓜)	3.95
Rhizoma Chuanxiong (川穹)	3.75
Herba Potulacae Oleraceae (马齿苋)	3.84
Galla Chinensis (五倍子)	3.63
Aconite roots+ Radix Glycyrrhizae (A+RG)	5.12
Aconite roots+ Lonicera nitida (A+LN)	3.22
Aconite roots+ Crateagus pinnatifida (A+CP)	3.26
Aconite roots+ Chaenomeles sinensis (A+CS)	3.69
Aconite roots+ Rhizoma Chuanxiong (A+RC)	4.10
Aconite roots+ Herba Potulacae Oleraceae (A+HPO)	3.87
Aconite roots+ Galla Chinensis (A+GC)	3.65

Table 1. The pH value of the decoction of eight kinds of Chinese Medicine

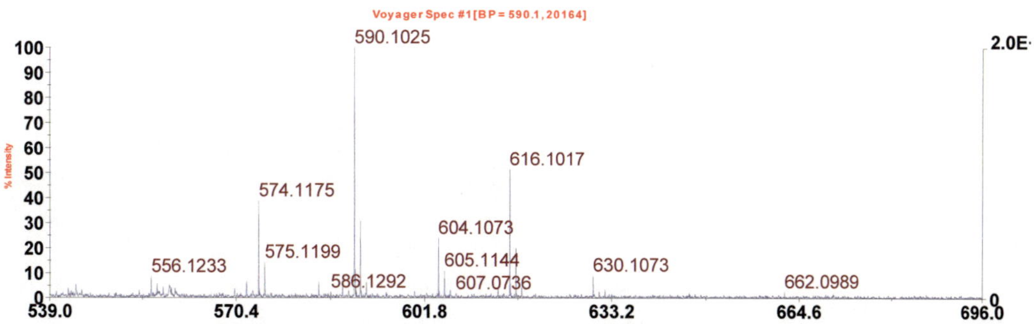

Fig. 20. MALDI-TOF spectrum of the ethanol extract of prepared Fuzi

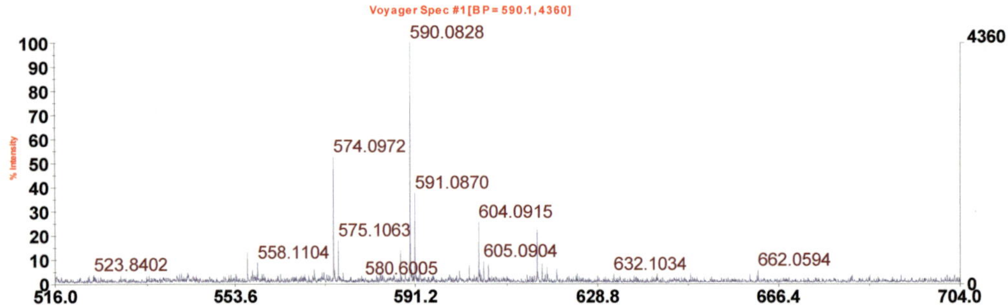

Fig. 21. MALDI-TOF spectrum of the decoction of prepared Fuzi

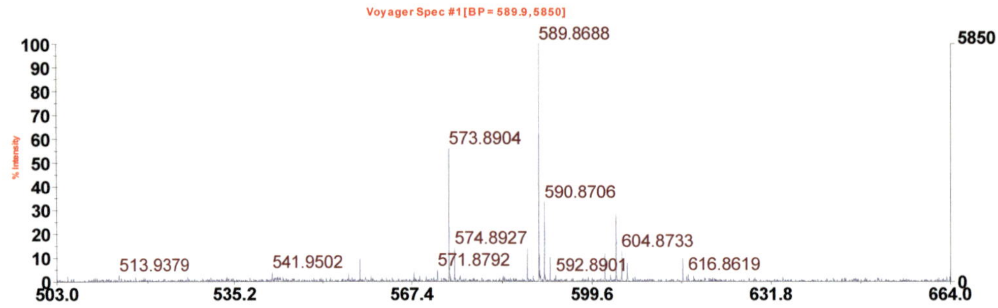

Fig. 22. MALDI-TOF spectrum of the concoction of prepared Fuzi with Radix Glycyrrhizae

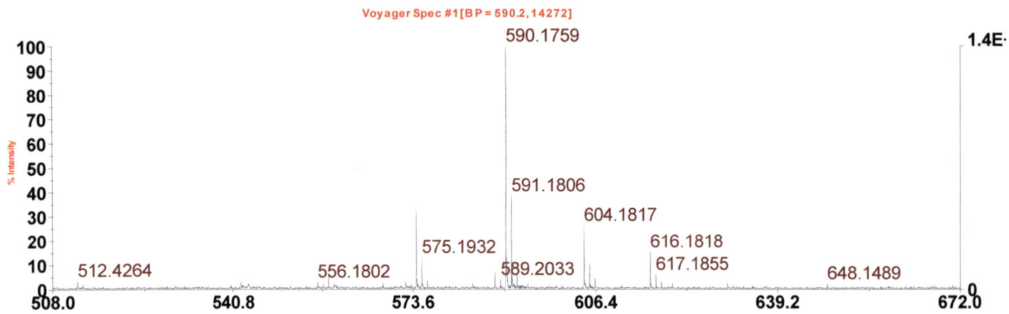

Fig. 23. MALDI-TOF spectrum of the concoction of prepared Fuzi with Lonicera nitida

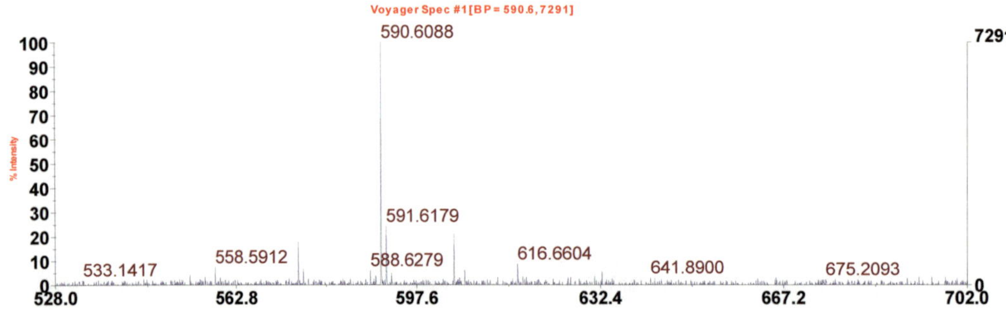

Fig. 24. MALDI-TOF spectrum of the concoction of prepared Fuzi with Rhizoma Chuanxiong

2.5 The MALDI-TOF analysis of alkaloids in the concoction of Fuzi with other 4 kinds of acidic herbal medicines

As shown in Fig.25-Fig.28, when Fuzi was concocted with Crateagus pinnatifida, Galla Chinensis, Chaenomeles sinensis or Herba Potulacae Oleraceae respectively, the relative amounts of DDA were higher that those in decoction, which suggested that these four herbal medicines should not be concocted with Fuzi. However, owing to the point-to-point difference of MALDI source, a statistical analysis is necessary. All the results have been shown in Table 3-Table 11 and summarized in Table 12.

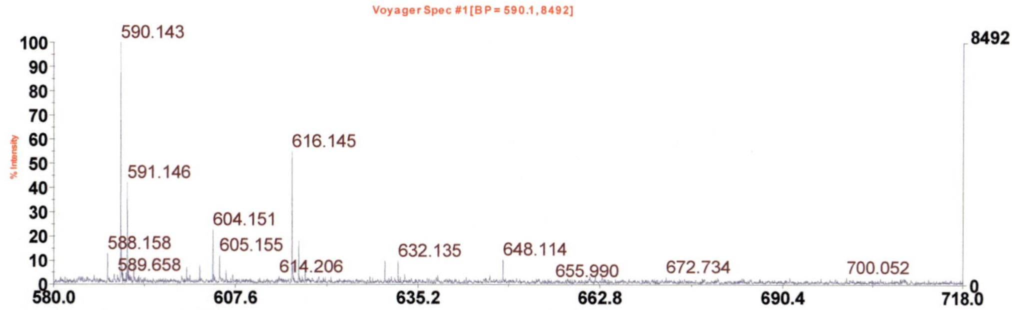

Fig. 25. MALDI-TOF spectrum of the concoction of prepared Fuzi with Crateagus pinnatifida

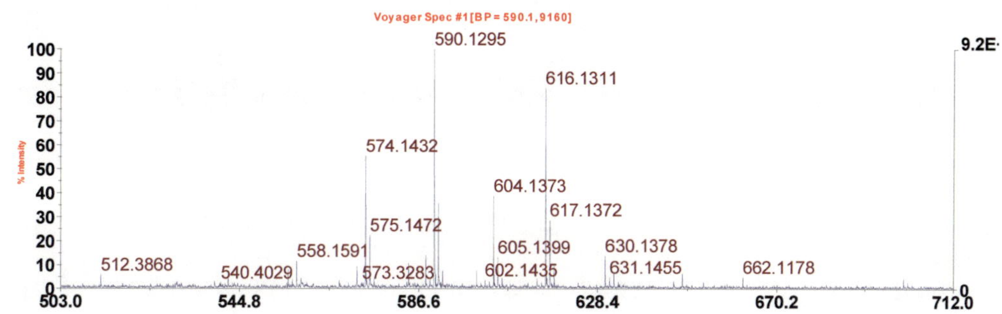

Fig. 26. MALDI-TOF spectrum of the concoction of prepared Fuzi with Galla Chinensis

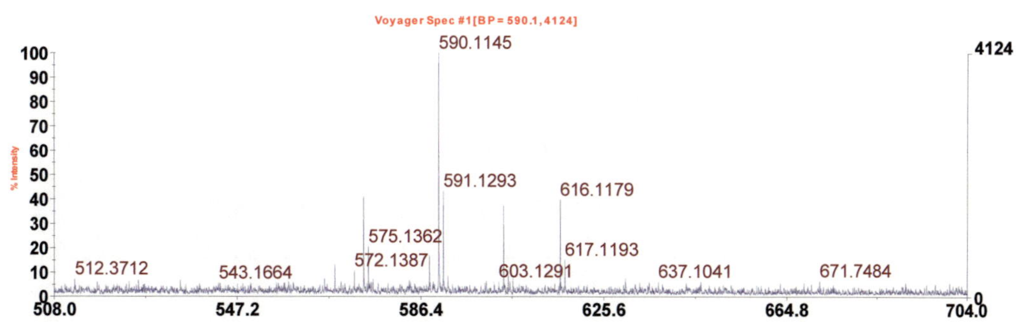

Fig. 27. MALDI-TOF spectrum of the concoction of prepared Fuzi with Chaenomeles sinensis

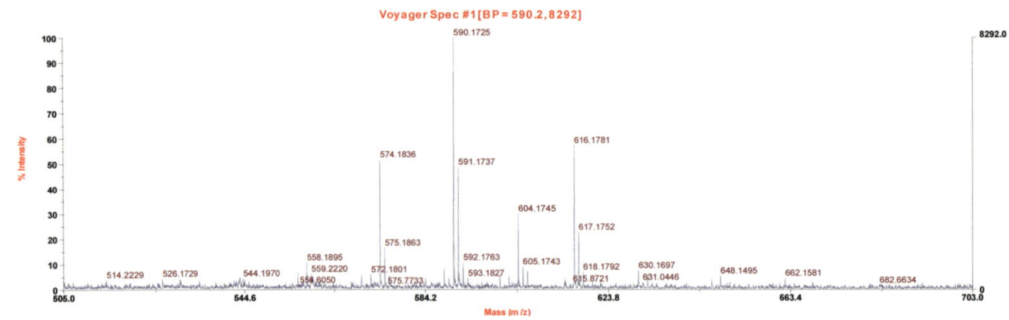

Fig. 28. MALDI-TOF spectrum of the concoction of prepared Fuzi with Herba Potulacae Oleraceae

Aconitum alkaloids	Relative intensities							Average value	RSD
	1	2	3	4	5	6	7		
Benzoylhypaconine (m/z574)	25.19	36.56	38.83	37.19	30.25	28.09	36.77	33.27	5.33
Benzoylmesaconine (m/z590)	100	100	100	100	100	100	100	100	0.00
Benzoylaconine (m/z604)	23.65	39.82	24.04	32.98	39.86	15.10	17.85	27.61	10.07
Hypaconitine (m/z616)	22.16	21.88	51.37	30.43	41.87	50.18	45.13	37.57	12.65
Deoxyaconitine (m/z630)	3.16	5.69	9.14	8.97	10.82	9.43	5.91	7.59	2.71
Mesaconitine (m/z632)	2.63	3.78	3.58	3.24	4.94	8.27	6.22	4.67	1.98
Aconitine (m/z646)	0.00	4.78	2.27	2.98	11.76	6.99	2.74	4.50	3.86
10-OH-mesaconitine (m/z648)	1.43	4.77	1.08	2.48	11.40	7.15	2.93	4.46	3.71
10-OH-aconitine (m/z662)	0.00	3.98	2.67	4.57	4.37	10.39	4.18	4.31	3.12

Table 3. The average value of relative intestines of the detected peaks from prepared Fuzi for seven times

Aconitum alkaloids	Relative intestines							Average value	RSD
	1	2	3	4	5	6	7		
Benzoylhypaconine (m/z574)	65.08	54.99	52.73	56.36	61.57	60.03	74.30	60.72	7.31
Benzoylmesaconine (m/z590)	100	100	100	100	100	100	100	100	0.00
Benzoylaconine (m/z604)	28.22	29.91	25.67	21.63	25.71	28.18	23.78	26.16	2.86
Hypaconitine (m/z616)	38.76	31.93	22.43	22.25	30.74	38.88	22.85	29.69	7.39
Deoxyaconitine (m/z630)	4.12	5.00	3.00	11.71	4.14	3.98	6.82	5.54	2.97
Mesaconitine (m/z632)	2.44	3.20	4.06	6.51	2.26	2.80	6.68	3.99	1.87
Aconitine (m/z646)	0.00	3.45	2.87	4.57	2.66	0.00	6.21	2.82	2.27
10-OH-mesaconitine (m/z648)	0.00	3.65	4.52	7.91	2.11	1.71	7.20	3.87	2.90
10-OH-aconitine (m/z662)	0.00	0.00	5.87	3.41	0.00	2.85	7.43	2.79	3.02

Table 4. The average value of relative intetie of the detected peaks from the detection of Fuzi for seven times

Aconitum alkaloids	Relative intestines							Average value	RSD
	1	2	3	4	5	6	7		
Benzoylhypaconine (m/z574)	57.73	40.16	40.63	51.59	55.97	53.19	52.16	50.20	7.04
Benzoylmesaconine (m/z590)	100	100	100	100	100	100	100	100	0
Benzoylaconine (m/z604)	23.91	24.03	21.44	38.33	28.22	28.27	36.77	28.71	6.53
Hypaconitine (m/z616)	31.67	5.56	11.75	28.82	9.85	17.67	23.82	18.45	9.97
Deoxyaconitine (m/z630)	9.91	0	0	8.33	0	0	2.62	2.98	4.33
Mesaconitine (m/z632)	8.08	0	0	3.7	0	0	6.08	2.55	3.42
Aconitine (m/z646)	5.51	1.91	2.13	2.21	0	0	4.13	2.27	2.02
10-OH-mesaconitine (m/z648)	6.71	0	1.63	2.21	0	0	5.65	2.31	2.80
10-OH-aconitine (m/z662)	4.4	0	2.2	2.5	0	0	10.13	2.75	3.66

Table 5. The average value of relative intestines of the detected peaks from the concoction of Fuzi with Radix Glycyrrhiza for seven times

Aconitum alkaloids	Relative intestines						Average value	RSD
	1	2	3	4	5	6		
Benzoylhypaconine (m/z574)	32.81	44.01	24.66	32.52	30.84	38.10	33.82	6.60
Benzoylmesaconine (m/z590)	100	100	100	100	100	100	100	0.00
Benzoylaconine (m/z604)	26.40	23.12	25.97	21.72	26.86	26.06	25.02	2.09
Hypaconitine (m/z616)	15.43	11.11	12.24	23.16	12.01	13.42	14.56	4.47
Deoxyaconitine (m/z630)	2.59	1.74	0.00	3.67	0.00	2.40	1.73	1.48
Mesaconitine (m/z632)	0.00	4.72	2.68	3.75	0.00	2.90	2.34	1.95
Aconitine (m/z646)	0.00	3.97	0.00	2.95	0.00	0.00	1.15	1.82
10-OH-mesaconitine (m/z648)	2.33	9.11	0.00	3.49	0.00	2.71	2.94	3.35
10-OH-aconitine (m/z662)	0.00	5.40	0.00	2.66	0.00	0.00	1.34	2.25

Table 6. The average value of relative intestines of the detected peaks from the concocction of Fuzi with Lonicera nitida for six times

Aconitum alkaloids	Relative intestines			Average value	RSD
	1	2	3		
Benzoylhypaconine (m/z574)	37.02	17.91	21.42	25.45	10.17
Benzoylmesaconine (m/z590)	100.00	100.00	100.00	100.00	0.00
Benzoylaconine (m/z604)	22.79	21.14	15.60	19.84	3.77
Hypaconitine (m/z616)	19.69	8.84	15.17	14.57	5.45
Deoxyaconitine (m/z630)	0.00	0.00	0.00	0.00	0.00
Mesaconitine (m/z632)	2.98	5.20	3.90	4.03	1.12
Aconitine (m/z646)	0.00	0.00	0.00	0.00	0.00
10-OH-mesaconitine (m/z648)	3.61	1.76	0.00	1.79	1.81
10-OH-aconitine (m/z662)	0.00	0.00	1.76	0.59	1.02

Table 7. The average value of relative intestines of the detected peaks from the concocction of Fuzi with Rhizoma Chuanxiong for three times

Aconitum alkaloids	Relative intestines						Average value	RSD
	1	2	3	4	5	6		
Benzoylhypaconine (m/z574)	35.39	38.94	21.33	40.68	40.24	28.24	34.14	7.79
Benzoylmesaconine (m/z590)	100.00	100.0 0	100.0 0	100.0 0	100.0 0	100.00	100.00	0.00
Benzoylaconine (m/z604)	22.79	18.42	21.20	22.46	21.01	24.09	21.66	1.95
Hypaconitine (m/z616)	54.98	56.09	38.57	80.39	51.51	53.42	55.83	13.61
Deoxyaconitine (m/z630)	9.86	5.56	8.57	7.49	13.16	12.54	9.53	2.94
Mesaconitine (m/z632)	9.92	8.74	11.58	10.90	6.60	9.80	9.59	1.76
Aconitine (m/z646)	3.86	3.56	2.42	4.54	3.85	4.56	3.80	0.79
10-OH-mesaconitine (m/z648)	10.46	6.37	5.08	6.64	6.01	7.20	6.96	1.85
10-OH-aconitine (m/z662)	3.71	4.33	0.00	3.62	4.71	3.06	3.24	1.69

Table 8. The average value of relative intestines of the detected peaks from the concocction of Fuzi with Crateagus pinnatifida for six times

Aconitum alkaloids	Relative intestines							Average value	RSD
	1	2	3	4	5	6	7		
Benzoylhypaconine (m/z574)	54.45	77.33	50.76	64.26	55.34	51.57	75.68	61.34	11.26
Benzoylmesaconine (m/z590)	89.18	98.06	84.35	84.77	100	100	81.59	91.14	8.03
Benzoylaconine (m/z604)	41.47	36.27	25.70	59.23	38.73	44.37	39.13	40.70	10.07
Hypaconitine (m/z616)	100	100	100	100	83.70	71.44	100	93.59	11.50
Deoxyaconitine (m/z630)	11.65	13.77	12.18	27.91	13.89	7.47	11.48	14.05	6.47
Mesaconitine (m/z632)	13.28	8.18	8.29	5.87	6.38	3.81	8.90	7.82	2.98
Aconitine (m/z646)	3.11	4.25	9.76	10.47	3.46	0.00	8.90	5.71	4.00
10-OH-mesaconitine (m/z648)	3.96	4.78	10.82	13.53	6.57	6.87	10.06	8.08	3.48
10-OH-aconitine (m/z662)	6.98	7.57	11.76	11.32	4.93	4.54	8.15	7.89	2.82

Table 9. The average value of relative intestines of the detected peaks from the concocction of Fuzi with Galla Chinensis for seven times

Aconitum alkaloids	Relative intestines							Average value	RSD
	1	2	3	4	5	6	7		
Benzoylhypaconine (m/z574)	41.22	33.60	25.68	29.67	48.78	44.39	33.30	36.66	8.34
Benzoylmesaconine (m/z590)	1000	100	100	100	1000	100	100	100	0.00
Benzoylaconine (m/z604)	37.32	23.85	39.65	27.92	27.20	18.33	33.73	29.71	7.60
Hypaconitine (m/z616)	39.79	15.07	24.40	26.92	24.88	15.75	19.98	23.83	8.39
Deoxyaconitine (m/z630)	7.76	2.94	9.67	6.85	4.92	6.86	8.78	6.83	2.29
Mesaconitine (m/z632)	5.29	2.26	5.82	6.61	4.02	3.64	2.73	4.34	1.62
Aconitine (m/z646)	6.28	2.90	7.55	9.68	4.84	3.85	2.00	5.30	2.71
10-OH-mesaconitine (m/z648)	4.97	2.61	6.57	7.25	6.26	5.04	3.95	5.24	1.61
10-OH-aconitine (m/z662)	3.59	2.84	5.97	8.17	5.83	2.78	4.09	4.75	1.99

Table 10. The average value of relative intestines of the detected peaks from the concocction of Fuzi with Chaenomeles sinensis for seven times

Aconitum alkaloids	Relative intestines					Average value	RSD
	1	2	3	4	5		
Benzoylhypaconine (m/z574)	30.49	51.63	20.61	43.12	30.06	35.18	12.19
Benzoylmesaconine (m/z590)	100	100	100	100	100	100	0.00
Benzoylaconine (m/z604)	15.28	30.10	18.81	19.65	18.81	20.53	5.61
Hypaconitine (m/z616)	33.70	57.20	34.36	92.86	46.45	52.91	24.34
Deoxyaconitine (m/z630)	5.85	7.59	9.45	8.27	14.36	9.10	3.21
Mesaconitine (m/z632)	5.56	5.71	4.61	7.46	10.20	6.71	2.21
Aconitine (m/z646)	0.00	4.29	5.57	4.02	4.30	3.64	2.12
10-OH-mesaconitine (m/z648)	3.21	5.45	5.76	4.79	3.32	4.51	1.19
10-OH-aconitine (m/z662)	2.95	4.55	6.10	5.93	4.16	4.74	1.31

Table 11. The average value of relative intestines of the detected peaks from the concoction of Fuzi with Herbal Potulacae Oleraceae for five times

	Relative Intensities								
Concoction	BHA	BMA	BAC	HA	DA	MA	AC	10-OH-MA	10-OH-AC
Fuzi	33.27±5.33	100	27.6±10.07	37.57±12.65	7.59±12.65	4.76±1.98	4.50±3.86	4.46±3.71	4.31±3.12
Fuzi decoction	60.72±7.31	100	26.16±2.86	29.69±2.86	5.54±2.97	3.99±1.87	2.82±2.90	3.87±2.90	2.79±3.02
Concoction of A+RG	50.20±7.04	100	28.71±6.53	18.45±9.97	2.98±4.33	2.55±3.42	2.27±2.02	2.31±2.80	2.75±3.66
Concoction of A+LN	33.82±6.60	100	25.02±2.09	14.56±4.47	1.73±1.48	2.34±1.95	1.15±1.82	2.94±3.35	1.34±2.25
Concoction of A+RC	25.4±10.17	100	19.84±3.77	14.57±5.45	0	4.03±1.12	0	1.79±1.81	0.59±1.02
Concoction of A+CS	36.66±8.34	100	29.71±7.60	23.83±8.39	6.83±2.29	4.34±1.62	5.30±2.71	5.24±1.61	4.75±1.99
Concoction of A+GC	61.3±11.26	91.1±8.03	40.7±10.07	93.56±11.50	14.05±6.47	7.82±2.98	5.71±4.00	8.08±3.48	7.89±2.82
Concoction of A+CP	34.14±7.79	100	21.66±1.95	55.83±13.61	9.53±2.94	9.59±1.76	3.80±0.79	3.69±1.85	3.24±1.69
Concoction of A+HPO	35.1±12.19	100	20.53±5.61	52.91±24.34	9.10±3.21	6.71±2.21	3.64±2.12	4.51±1.19	4.74±1.31

Table 12. The average value of relative intestines of the detected peaks from the concocction and decoction of Fuzi

Taken the ethanol extract of Fuzi as a standard, we will find that the DDAs have been reduced after decocting or concocting with Radix Glycyrrhizae, Lonicera nitida, Rhizoma Chuanxiong or Chaenomeles sinensis, respectively. Coincidentally, both Radix Glycyrrhizae and Lonicera nitida is the most popular medicine for detoxification. However, when Fuzi has been concocted with Crateagus pinnatifida, Galla Chinensis or Herba Potulacae Oleraceae, the relative amounts of all DDAs, especially of hypaconitine, have been increased significantly despite that the pH value of Lonicera nitida is smaller than that of Galla Chinensis and Herba Potulacae Oleraceae. The results have indicated that the detoxification mechanism of traditional Chinese medicine such as Fuzi is very complex and can not be explained by a simple reason such as pH value. In addition, our studies have suggested that although Crateagus pinnatifida, Galla Chinensis and Herba Potulacae Oleraceae is beyond the list that should not be combined with aconite according to traditional Chinese theory or experience, but they do increase the toxicity of Fuzi.

3. References

[1] Yong Wang, Lei Shi, Fengrui Song, Zhiqiang Liu and Shuying Li. Exploring the reaction of ester exchange for diester-diterpenoid alkaloids in the process of decocting aconite by electrospray ionization tandem mass spectrometry. Rapid Commun. Mass Spectrom, 2003, 17(4), 279-284

[2] Judith Singhuber, Ming Zhua, Sonja Prinz and Brigitte Kopp. Aconitum in Traditional Chinese Medicine—A valuable drug or an unpredictable risk? Journal of Ethnopharmacology, 2009, 126 , 18–30

[3] Ying Xie, Zhi Hong Jiang , Hua Zhoua, Hong Xi Xu, Liang Liu. Simultaneous determination of six Aconitum alkaloids in proprietary Chinese medicines by high-performance liquid chromatography. Journal of Chromatography A, 2005, 1093, 195–203

[4] Yong Wang, Fengrui Song, Zhiqiang Liu and Shuying Li. Study on the combination principles about aconite roots by electrospray ionization mass spectrometry. Acta Pharmaceutica Sinica (in Chinese).2003, 38(6): 451 - 454

[5] Yong Wang, Lei Shi, Dongming Jin, Fengrui Song, Zhiqiang Liu and Shuying Li. Stripping and hydrolyzing balance of aconitic alkaloids in processing of Sini Decoction. Chinese Traditional and Herbal Drugs. (in Chinese), 2003, 34(4): 311-314

[6] JiangshanWang, Rob van der Heijden, Gerwin Spijksma, Theo Reijmers, MeiWang, Guowang Xua, Thomas Hankemeier and Jan van der Greef. Alkaloid profiling of the Chinese herbal medicine Fuzi by combination of matrix-assisted laser desorption ionization mass spectrometry with liquid chromatography-mass spectrometry. Journal of Chromatography A, 2009, 1216 2169–2178

20

Therapeutic Effects of Lignans and Blend Isolated from *Schisandra chinesis* on Hepatic Carcinoma

Dae Youn Hwang
Pusan National University,
Republic of Korea

1. Introduction

Schisandra chinesis (*S. chinesis*) is widely used as one of the 50 fundamental herbs in traditional Oriental medicine; the species is a member of the *Schisandra* genus of shrub, which grows commonly in the native forests of Northern China, Korea, Japan and Russia. The *Schisandra* are deciduous climbers that thrive in any type of soil, so long as it is moist, shaded, and well-drained (Panossian and Wikman, 2008). The female *S. chinesis* plant can produce the fruit via fertilization with pollen from a male plant (Shilova, 1963). It is harvested in most countries, including Korea, by the cutting of half-matured berries between August and September. The berries of *S. chinesis* are called omija (translated as "five-flavor fruit") in Korea, because this fruit has all five of the basic flavors-salty, sweet, sour, pungent, and bitter (Gutnikova, 1951; Panossian and Wikman, 2008). Generally, its dried fruits have been used for a variety of purposes, including as a therapeutic drug, teas and wines. In many countries, it has been used as a therapeutic drug, and is purported to have liver-protective and immune-modulatory abilities. A variety of key constituents including schizandrin, deoxyschizandrin, gomisin, and pregomisin have been isolated from the seeds of the fruit. Additionally, *S. chinesis* berries have been used in the manufacture of several foods. A wine was using the berries of *S. chinesis* has been produced in China, whereas in Korea, the berries are made into a tea. Meanwhile, in Japan, these berries are referred to as "gomishin", and have been used for medicinal purposes, to treat colds and sea-sickness. In Russia, dozens of tons of berries are used annually in the commercial production of juices, wine, extracts and sweets (Gutnikova, 1951; Agejenko and Komisssarenko, 1960).

A variety of previous pharmacological studies have suggested that *S. chinesis* may exert beneficial biological effects on liver tissue, the central nervous system, the respiratory system, the cardiovascular system and the endocrine system (Table 1) (Panossian and Wikman, 2008). The major and characteristic components of *Schisandraceae* berries have been previously isolated, and are referred to as lignans. The lignans are categorized into the five following classes: dibenzocyclooctadiene lignans (type A), spirobenzofuranoid dibenzocyclooctadiene lignans (type B), 4-aryltetralin lignans (type C), 2,3-dimethyl-1,4-diarylbutane lignans (type D), and 2,5-diaryltetrahydrofuran lignans (type E)(Table 2)(Lu and Chen, 2009). Thus far, a total of 43 lignans have been isolated from *S. chinesis* in various studies; a list is provided in Table 2. Among these lignans, most of the lignans isolated from *S. chinesis* exhibit a dibenzocyclooctadiene lignan (type A) structure, with the exception of three lignans: pregomisin, meso-dihydroguaiaretic acid and nordihydroguaiaretic acid. The three lignans described in this chapter are of the type A structural group. Additionally, the dibenzocyclooctadiene lignans are further divided into two types based on their stereostructures-S- and R-biphenyl configuration. Structural elucidation studies have shown that the cyclooctene rings of dibenzocyclooctadiene lignans evidence a twist-boat-chair (TBC) or twist-boat (TB) conformation (Lu and Chen, 2009). Approximately half of the lignans from *S. chinesis* evidence an S-biphenyl configuration and the other half exhibit an R-biphenyl configuration. According to the conformation with cyclooctene rings, only four lignans exhibited a TB conformation, but the rest of the lignans had the TBC conformation. Among the three lignins described in this chapter, only gomisin N exhibits an S-biphenyl configuration, whereas tigloylgomisin H and schisandrin A has an R-biphenyl configuration.

Body system	**Regulatory system: stress-system**	**Pharmacological effect: adaptogenic effect**
Cardiovascular system	Central and vegetative nervous system	Stimulating effect
Gastrointestinal system	Endocrine system	Stress-mimetic and stress-protective effect
Respiratory system	Immune system	Stress-protective effect

Table 1. Summary of the pharmacological activities of *S. chinensis* (Panossian and Wikman, 2008).

Compounds	**Structure type**	**Configuration/ conformation**	**References**
Gomisin N	A	S/TBC	Ikeya et al., 1978a
Schizandrin C(wuweizisu C, schisandrin C)	A	S/TBC	Chen and Shu, 1976
(-)-Gomisin K1	A	S/TBC	Ikeya et al., 1980
Gomisin J	A	S/TBC	Ikeya et al., 1978b
(-)-Gomisin L2	A	S/TBC	Ikeya et al., 1982
(-)-Gomisin L1	A	S/TBC	Ikeya et al., 1982
Gomisin S	A	S/TBC	Ikeya et al., 1988
Epigomisin O	A	S/TBC	Ikeya et al., 1991; Ikeya et al., 1979
Tigloylgomisin P	A	S/TBC	Ikeya et al., 1990; Ikeya et al., 1980
Angeloylgomisin P	A	S/TBC	Ikeya et al., 1990; Ikeya et al., 1980
Gomisin D	A	S/TBC	Ikeya et al., 1976
Gomisin E	A	S/TBC	Ikeya et al., 1979
Gomisin O	A	S/TBC	Ikeya et al., 1979
6-o-benzoylgomisin O	A	S/TB	Chen et al., 1994
Angeloylgomisin O	A	S/TB	Ikeya et al., 1982

Angeloyl isogomisin O	A	S/TB	Ikeya et al., 1982
Benzoyl isogomisian O	A	S/TB	Ikeya et al., 1982
Schisandrene	A	S/TBC	Choi et al., 2006
Angeloylgomisin Q	A	S/TBC	Ikeya et al., 1979
Gomisin F	A	S/TBC	Taguchi and Ikeya, 1977
Gomisin G	A	S/TBC	Taguchi and Ikeya, 1977
Schisantherin A(gomisin C, wuweizi ester A)	A	S/TBC	Ikeya et al., 1990; Taguchi and Ikeya, 1977
Schisantherin B(gomisin B, wuweizi ester B)	A	S/TBC	Ikeya et al., 1990; Taguchi and Ikeya, 1977
Schisantherin D	A	S/TBC	Liu et al., 1978; Ikeya et al., 1982
Gomisin R	A	S/TB	Ikeya et al., 1982
Deoxyschizandrin (wuweizisu A, schisandrin A, deoxyschisandrin)	A	R/TBC	Chen and Shu, 1976; Yue et al., 1994
(+)-Gomisin K2	A	R/TBC	Ikeya et al., 1980
Schisanhenol [(+)-gomisin K3]	A	R/TBC	Ikeya et al., 1980; Ikeya et al., 1990
γ-Schizandrin(γ-schisandrin)	A	R/TBC	Liu et al., 1978
Schizandrin B(wuweizisu B, schisandrin B, (±)- γ-schizandrin)	A	R/TBC	Chen and Shu, 1976
(±)-Gomisin M1	A	R/TBC	Ikeya et al., 1982
(+)-Gomisin M2	A	R/TBC	Ikeya et al., 1982
Schizandrin(schisandrol A, schisandrin, wuweizi alcohol A)	A	R/TBC	Chen and Shu, 1976
Gomisin A(schisandrol B, wuweizi alcohol B)	A	R/TBC	Taguchi and Ikeya, 1977
Gomisin H	A	R/TBC	Ikeya et al., 1979
Angeloylgomisin H	A	R/TBC	Ikeya et al., 1979
Tigloylgomisin H	A	R/TBC	Ikeya et al., 1979
Benzoylgomisin H	A	R/TBC	Ikeya et al., 1979
Gomisin T	A	R/TBC	Ikeya et al., 1988
Isoschizandrin	A	R/TBC	Ikeya et al., 1991; Ikeya et al., 1988
Pregomisin	D	/	Ikeya et al., 1978
Meso-dihydroguaiaretic acid	D	/	Ikeya et al., 1979
Nordihydroguaiaretic acid	D	/	Sakurai et al., 1992

Table 2. Lignans isolated from the fruits of *S. chinensis*. A: Dibenzocyclooctadiene lignan; D: 2,3-dimethyl-1,4-diarylbutane lignan; S or R: the configuration of the biphenyl unit; TBC or TB: the conformation of the cyclooctane ring (Lu and Chen, 2009).

Meanwhile, hepatocellular carcinoma is a primary malignancy of the hepatocytes, and generally leads to death within 6-20 months. The disease is the fifth most common cancer in men and the eighth most common cancer in women worldwide (Bosch et al., 2004). Cirrhosis of any etiology is known to be the major risk factor for hepatocellular carcinoma (Adami et al., 2008). Thus far, approximately 80% of patients with newly diagnosed hepatocellular carcinoma have preexisting cirrhosis in the liver organ, caused mainly by excessive alcohol use, hepatitis C infection and hepatitis B infection (El-Serang and Mason, 2000). Additionally, many therapeutic strategies have been attempted to medically treat hepatocellular carcinoma, including surgical resection and liver transplantation, although the available treatment options depend on the specific characteristics of the tumor (Thomas and Zhu, 2005; Bruix and Sherman, 2005).

There has been some very interesting research conducted to determine whether the lignans isolated from *S. chinensis* may improve and prevent a variety of human diseases, including cardiac disease, respiratory disease, immune disease, endocrine disease and neuronal disease. However, only a few investigations have been conducted to determine the therapeutic effects of lignans isolated from *S. chinensis* on hepatic carcinoma. Therefore, this chapter describes the important results of an experiment using three lignans (gomisin N, tigloylgomisin H (TGH) and schisandrin A) and one blend (KY88 Liver-Livo) which may prove valuable in the development of a therapeutic drug for the treatment of hepatic carcinoma.

2. Therapeutic effects of lignans and blend isolated from *S. chinensis* on hepatic carcinoma

This main section described experimental data regarding the biological effects of three lignans and a blend on hepatic carcinoma, and the potential for the use of those lignins as therapeutic drugs.

2.1 Effects of gomisin N

Gomisin N (Fig. 1) is already well known as a member of the schisandrin B family, and the most abundant lignin in the fruit lignins of *S. chinensis*. Among the various functions of gomisin N, its ability to increase antioxidant capacity and protect against mitochondria decay was initially identified by a biochemical mechanism study (Ko and Lam, 2002). Additionally, gomisin N could induce an increase in heat shock protein, which performed an important function when cells and tissues were affected by a variety of stressful stimuli from the external environment. Recently, a stereoisomer of gomisin N, (-) schisandrin B, was identified and its function in cell protection was investigated. These results demonstrated that schisandrin B and (-) schisandrin B were the most potent in enhancing antioxidant protection. Therefore, these two lignans may be employed for the protection against and reversal of tissue damage induced by environmental hazards, physical exercise, and aging (Chiu et al., 2006). However, we found a new function of gomisin N, particularly its effects against hepatic carcinoma.

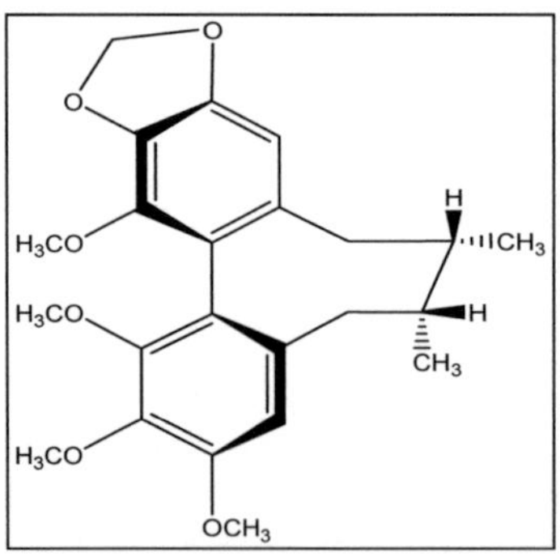

Fig. 1. Chemical structure of gomisin N isolated from *S. chinensis*.

2.1.1 Preparation of gomisin N

The dried fruits of *S. chinensis* (2.5 kg) were ground to a fine powder and were successively extracted at room temperature with *n*-hexane, EtOAc, and MeOH. The hexane extract (308 g) was evaporated under vacuum and chromatographed on a silica gel (40 μm, J.T. Baker, NJ, USA) column (70 x 8.0 cm) with a step gradient of 0%, 5%, 10%, 20%, and 30% EtOAc in hexane (each 1 L). Of these extracts, Fraction 11IA, one of 5 subfraction originated from fraction 11 was further purified by column chromatography on silical gel eluting with $CHCl_3$-acetone (19:1) to give a gomisin N (774 mg)(Yim et al., 2009).

2.1.2 Effects of gomisin N on cell proliferation

The therapeutic effects of gomisin N on hepatic carcinomas was initially suggested by Yim et al. (2009). First, they extracted lignans including gomisin N (Seo et al., 2004), schisandrin (Ikeya et al., 1979a), schisandrin C (Seo et al., 2004) and gomisin A (Ikeya et al., 1979b; Park et al., 2007) from *S. chinensis* via *n*-hexane, EtOAc and MeOH extraction techniques. Their structures were analyzed via LC-MS and NMR analysis for identification. Proliferation activity was screened for all groups that had received one of the four lignans of varying concentrations via an MTT assay to select the lignan with the highest apoptotic effect on hepatic carcinoma. For schisandrin C, the MTT assay demonstrated that this lignan induced cell proliferation rather than cell death in hepatic carcinoma cells in a concentration range of 40 μM to 160 μM, whereas the gomisin A-treated group maintained a stable cell population (Fig. 2). However, the MTT screening also demonstrated that two lignans, gomisin N and schisandrin, significantly induced cell death in relation to other lignans. In the gomisin N-treated group, cell proliferation in the 40 μM-treated groups was slightly increased compared to the vehicle. However, cell proliferation decreased rapidly in a gomisin N concentration range from 80 μM to 320 μM (Fig. 2). Schisandrin also induced cell death at the higher concentrations, but the cell death ratio was lower than that observed with gomisin N (Fig. 2). These results indicated that gomisin N treatment was highly effective in inducing the death of hepatic carcinoma cells at higher concentrations, but not at low concentrations. Yim et al. selected gomisin N as the candidate lignan for further analysis, owing to its anti-proliferation and pro-apoptosis functions.

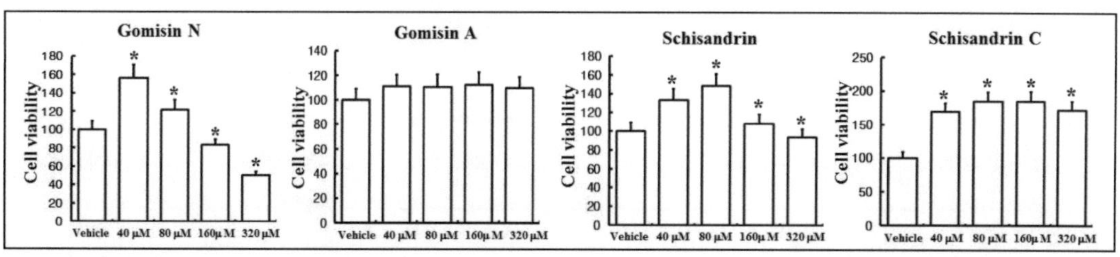

Fig. 2. Anti-proliferative effect of gomisin N, schisandrin, schisandrin C and gomisin A isolated from *S. chinensis* (Yim et al., 2009).

Additionally, phase-contrast microscope analysis was conducted to determine whether the cell death effects observed in the MTT assay were concurrent with the observed cell morphological changes. In the 40 μM-treated group, the number and morphology of hepatic carcinoma evidenced greater crowding than was observed in the vehicle-treated group. The hepatic carcinoma cell line in the 80 μM-treated groups evidenced a pattern similar to that observed with the vehicle-treated group. In the 160 μM-treated group, few dead cells were observed in the microscopic images of the hepatic carcinoma cell line. The numbers of these cells were increased markedly in the 320 μM-treated groups (Fig. 3). These results demonstrated that the results observed on cell morphology analysis under gomisin N-treated conditions were consistent with the results of an MTT assay under the same conditions (Yim et al., 2009).

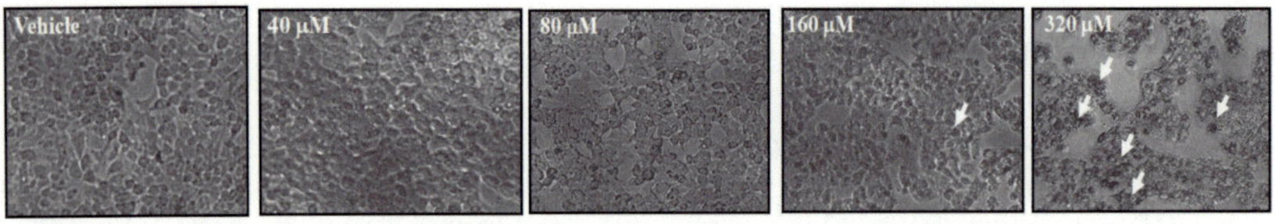

Fig. 3. Microscope images of hepatic carcinoma cell lines after 24 hrs of treatment with gomisin N at various concentrations (Yim et al., 2009).

2.1.3 Effects of gomisin N on apoptosis

Apoptosis, or programmed cell death, performs a critical role in a variety of physiological processes during fetal development and in adult life. Defects in the apoptotic process lead to the progress of many diseases involving progressive cell accumulation and cancer in most cases. Yim et al. (2009) further investigated the correlation between gomisin N and apoptosis. To achieve this, a hepatic carcinoma cell line treated with various concentrations of gomisin N were stained with FITC Annexin V, and fluorescence activity was determined via flow cytometry. Gomisin N significantly induced the increase in the number of cells undergoing apoptosis, from 15% to 98%, in 24 hrs. However, this reaction was induced even at low gomisin N concentrations, and this level of induction remained at a constant level up to and throughout higher concentrations (Fig. 4). Therefore, these results indicated that gomisin N could induce the apoptosis of hepatic carcinoma cell lines in a dose-independent manner. Specifically, gomisin N may induce the loss of plasma membrane asymmetry, one of the early events in the apoptosis process, for most cells treated at a concentration of 40 μM.

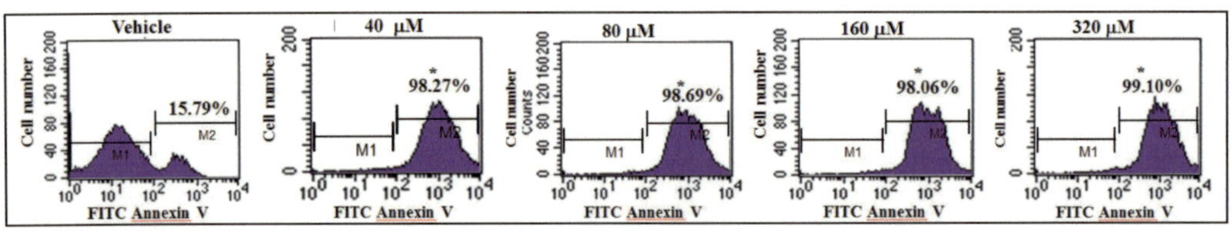

Fig. 4. Identifying apoptotic cells affected with gomisin N treatment. Hepatic carcinoma cells were incubated with gomisin N at various concentrations for 24 hrs, and stained with FITC Annexin V to detect the apoptotic cells (Yim et al., 2009).

Additionally, the apoptosis process involves many families of proteins. Among these proteins, the Bcl-2 proteins are one of the key molecules in inducing the anti-apoptotic process (Apakama et al., 1996). The results of previous studies have shown that this protein was overexpressed in many solid tumors, and that it contributes to chemotherapy resistance and radiation-induced apoptosis (Apakama et al., 1996; Joensuu et al., 1994). Unlike many other known human oncogenes, Bcl-2 exerts its influence by enhancing cell survival rather than by stimulating cell division (Joensuu et al., 1994). Yim et al. (2009) attempted to determine whether the expression level of Bcl-2 protein would be affected by gomisin N treatment in a hepatic carcinoma cell line. Additionally, Yim et al. (2009) assessed the effects of gomisin N treatment on proteins associated with the apoptosis signaling pathway. To achieve this, the expression levels of Bcl-2 and Bax proteins were determined in the vehicle-treated and gomisin N-treated groups via Western blot analysis. The expression level of Bcl-2 protein did not change in the low concentration range as compared to the vehicle. However, the high concentration range-namely the 160 μM and 320 μM-treated groups-evidenced higher levels of Bcl-2 protein expression than was observed in the low concentration range. In the case of Bax, the expression level of this protein was markedly increased only in the 320 μM treated group compared to the vehicle and the other concentration groups. Furthermore, in order to determine whether the tumor suppressor gene would be affected by gomisin N in the hepatic carcinoma cell line, the expression level of p53 protein was detected in the vehicle and gomisin N-treated groups. The expression level of p53 protein remained unchanged in the four treatment groups and the vehicle (Fig. 5). These results indicate that gomisin N may simultaneously induce an increase in the levels of the proteins associated with the anti-apoptotic and pro-apoptotic processes, but does not alter the level of expression of the tumor suppressor protein, p53.

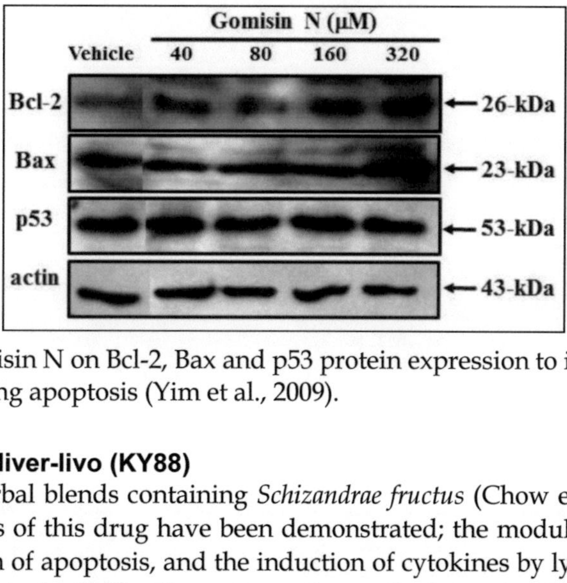

Fig. 5. Effects of gomisin N on Bcl-2, Bax and p53 protein expression to investigate the mechanism underlying apoptosis (Yim et al., 2009).

2.2 Effects of KY88 liver-livo (KY88)

KY88 was one of herbal blends containing *Schizandrae fructus* (Chow et al., 2001). Thus far, three major functions of this drug have been demonstrated; the modulation of the immune system, the induction of apoptosis, and the induction of cytokines by lymphocytes and liver cancer cells (Chow et al., 2004). However, a thorough determination of the therapeutic effects of KY88 against hepatic carcinoma will require further research into its action mechanism.

2.2.1 Preparation of KY88

KY88 is a blend containing the herbal extract of *Schizandrae fructus, Bupleuri radix, Artemisiae capillaris, Desmodii herba, Poria sclerotium, Lithospermi radix, Paeoniae radix, Phellodendri cortex, Scutellariae radix* and *Trichosanthis radix*. Ten grams of each of all ingredients of above herbs were primarily washed and concentrated and purified with the process of extraction. Then, the essence of the herbal extracts -KY88- was assembled. Also, this capsule had been verified by SGS Hong Kong Ltd (Socie´te´ Ge´ne´rale de Surveillance) to be free of heavy metals and microorganisms. Before the study for inhibition ability, KY88 (50 g) was extracted with three times using MeOH. The solid residue obtained from the crude extract was then dissolved in dimethyl sulphoxide to a concentration of 92 mg/ml and stored at 4°C until use (Loo et al. 2007).

2.2.2 Effects of KY88 on cell proliferation and HBeAg/HBsAg secretion

Loo et al. (2007) was the first to investigate whether KY88 has an ability to inhibit hepatocellular carcinoma cell proliferation and the secretion ability of HBsAg (hepatitis B virus surface antigen) and HBeAg (hepatitis B virus core antigen). For this assessment, KY88 was applied to the HB-8064 hepatocellular carcinoma cell line, and the cell proliferation rate and HBsAg/HBeAg secretion were measured on days 1, 3, 5 and 7. The MTT assay showed that the treatment of 0.1, 0.5 and 1 mg/ml KY88 for 7 days induced the significant suppression of hepatic carcinoma. Additionally, the cell proliferation rate of all KY88-treated cells was significantly lower than that of the control-treated group (Fig. 6). In particular, a remarkable suppression of cell proliferation was detected at three concentrations from day 5. Therefore, these data demonstrated that KY88 may potentially exert an effect in inhibiting the cellular proliferation of hepatocellular carcinoma.

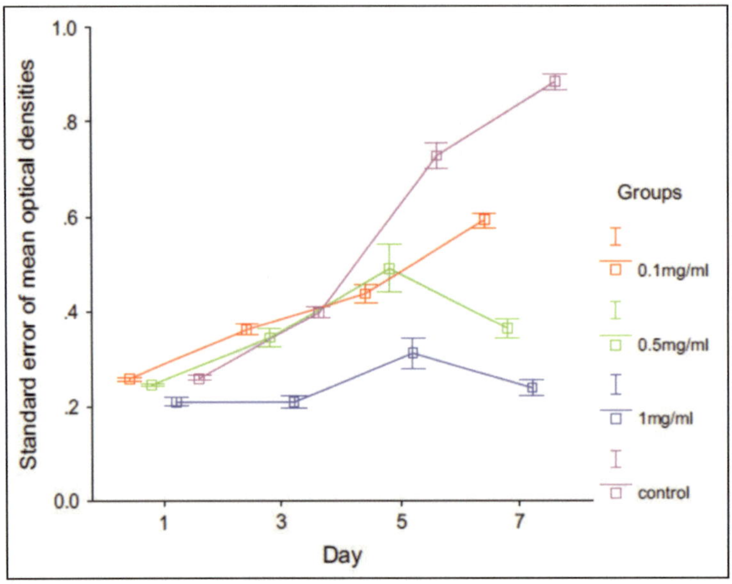

Fig. 6. Dose-dependent inhibition of cell proliferation at three concentrations of KY88 (Loo et al., 2007).

Furthermore, the secretions of HBsAg and HBeAg from the hepatocellular carcinoma cell line were dramatically inhibited by KY88 treatment (Fig. 7). The observation of HBsAg and HBeAg reflected the cell's infection with hepatitis B virus and their replication activity (Loo et al., 2007). This data indicated that KY88 may potentially have the ability to inhibit the proliferation of hepatocellular carcinoma cells, as well as the reduced secretions of HBsAg and HBeAg to restrict tumor growth.

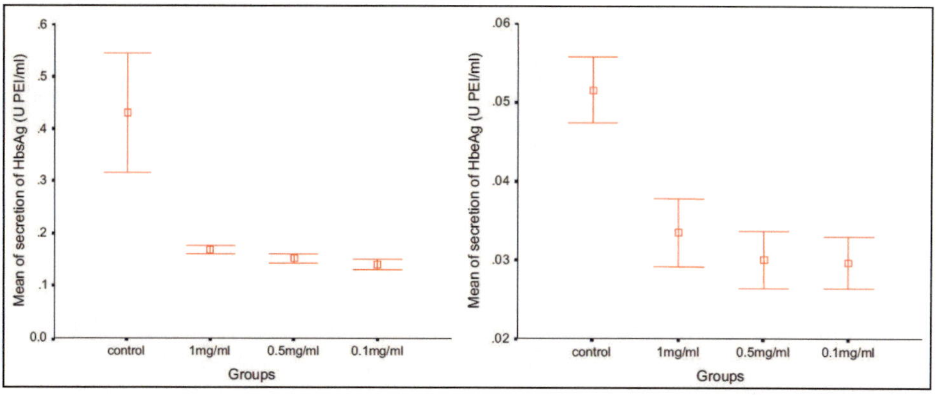

Fig. 7. Secretion level of HBsAg and HBeAg from hepatocellular carcinoma cell line after KY88 treatment (Loo et al., 2007).

2.2.3 Effects of KY88 on apoptosis and cytokine secretion

Chow et al. (2004) previously evaluated the effects and action mechanism of KY88 on liver cancer cells using methanol extracts of KY88 to develop a novel therapeutic drug for the treatment of hepatoma. After methanol extracts of KY88 were applied to a hepatocellular carcinoma cell line, the cell proliferation, DNA laddering and cytokine secretion were detected in these cells. KY88 induced a significant inhibition of cell proliferation and an increase in the DNA ladder pattern, which is a marker that indicates apoptosis in hepatocellular carcinoma cells (Fig. 8).

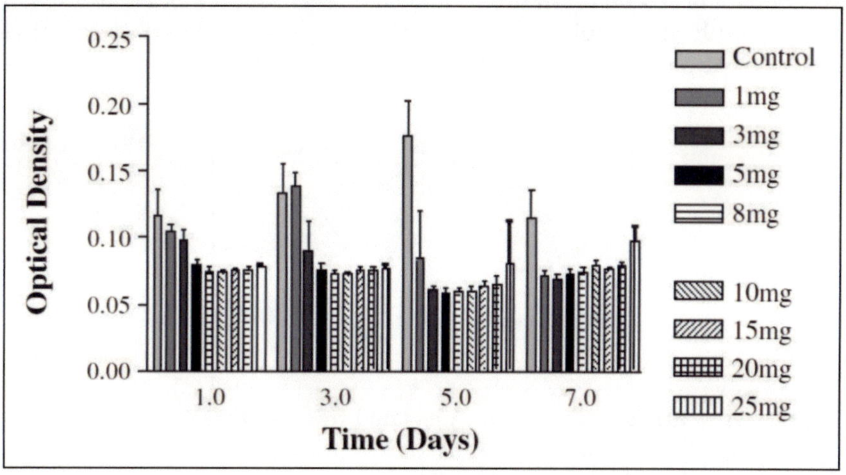

Fig. 8. Inhibition effect of KY88 methanol extracts on hepatocellular carcinoma cell (Chow et al., 2004).

Additionally, cytokine ELISA assay results demonstrated that IL-4 and TNF-α concentrations were increased significantly by KY88 treatment when compared against the control group at 24 hrs. However, IL-2, IL-6 and INF-γ concentrations were maintained at constant levels (Fig. 9). Therefore, this data indicates that the methanol extracts of KY88 may induce apoptosis via the regulation of IL-4 and TNF-α secretion.

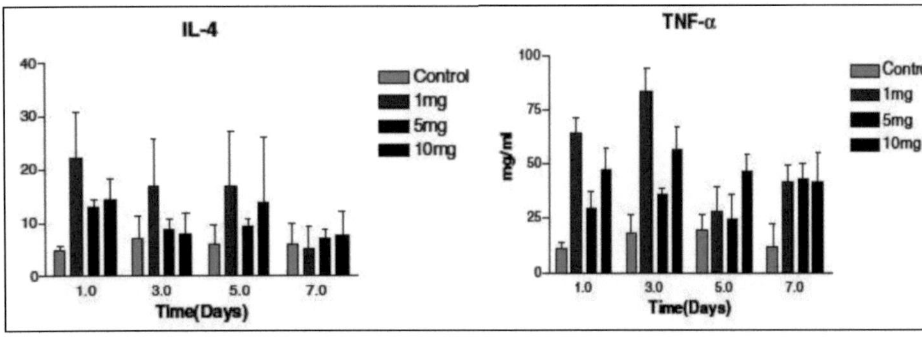

Fig. 9. Significant change of IL-4 and TNF-α level in hepatocellular carcinoma cell after KY88 treatment (Chow et al., 2004).

2.3 Effects of schizandrin A

Schizandrin A is referred to by several other names, including deoxyschizandrin, wuweizisu A, and deoxyschisandrin (Lu and Chen, 2009), and is one of the most effective lignins isolated from *S. chinensis* (Fig. 10). Previous studies have also demonstrated that schizandrin A may have the hepatoprotective, antioxidative, neurobiological performance-improving and anti-tumor activities (Deng et al., 2008; Huang et al., 2008). For the first time, the function of schizandrin A was found to protect against liver injuries, activate liver regeneration and supress liver carcinogenesis (Zheng et al., 1997). Additionally, this lignan was partially used as a Ca^{2+} modulator which induced the synchronization of Ca^{2+} oscillation via the influx inhibition of extracellular Ca^{2+} and the initiation of action potential (Fu et al., 2008). However, only a small amount of research has been conducted regarding the possible inhibitory effects of schizandrin A on hepatocellular carcinoma. This chapter also describes recent key results regarding the possible anti-liver cancer effects of schizandrin A.

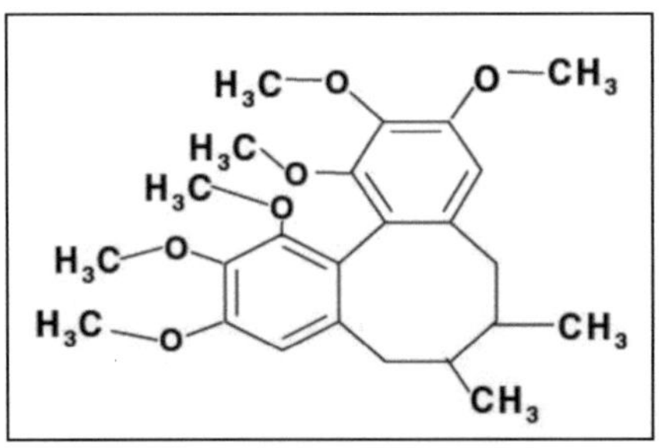

Fig. 10. Chemical structure of schizandrin A isolated from *S. chinensis.*

2.3.1 Preparation of schizandrin A

Generally, schizandrin A was prepared with a methods suggested by Chen et al. (1976) and Yue et al. (1994). Firstly, *S. chinensis* Baill (10 kg) was extracted with 50 L of hexane for 1.5 hr and the obtained extract was dried under a reduced pressure. The 978.8 g of hexane extract were dissolved in 9.8 L of hexane and sequentially extracted two times with 9.8 L of 60% (v/v) MeOH. The mixture obtained from above extraction was dried under a reduced pressure and finally 112.2 g of a fraction having a high lignan content were obtained. These fraction having a high lignan content was subjected to the fractionation high-speed liquid chromatography [column: Kiesel Gel 60 (230 to 400 mesh) supplied by Merk, diameter=10 cm, length=100 cm, moving phase: n-hexane/ethyl acetate (7/3), flow rate: 200 ml/min, apparatus: Waters Prep LC/System 500A]. Fractions eluted at 63 to 70 minutes in the fractionation high-speed liquid chromatography were combined and dried under a reduced pressure. The obtained residue (schizandrin A) was recrystallized from methanol to obtain 1.05 g of a colorless prism crystal.

2.3.2 Effects of schizandrin A and LCC (five schizandrins and crud extract from *Fructus shizandrae*) on human hepatocellular carcinoma

Huang et al. (2008) evaluated the reversal effects of five schizandrins (schizandrin A, schizandrin B, schizandrin C, schizandrol A and schizandrol B) and LCC on multidrug resistance (MDR) in several cancer cells, including hepatocellular carcinoma and epidermal carcinoma *in vitro* and *in vivo*. After treatment with various concentrations of five schizandrins and LCC into cancer cell lines, drug sensitivity, apoptosis, doxorubicin (Dox) accumulation and protein kinas C (PKC) expression were measured in cancer cell lines. Various levels of MDR reversal activity were noted at a 25 μM concentration of the five tested compounds. The most potent compound found was schizandrin A. The reversal activity of MDR was also induced by 25 μg/ml of LCC in KBV200, MCF-7/Dox cells, and human hepatic cellular carcinoma Bel7402 cells. The flow cytometry analysis results demonstrated that both schizandrin A and LCC treatment induced an increase in apoptosis in human hepatocellular carcinoma cells. As shown in Fig. 11, the sub-G1 peak, which is one of the characteristics of apoptosis, was increased significantly from 1.8% in the Bel7402 cells treated with Dox only to 10-14% in the schizandrin A + Dox-treated cells or the LCC + Dox-treated cells. Additionally, chromatin condensation, another marker of apoptosis, was enhanced in cells treated with schizandrin A + Dox or with LCC + Dox. Furthermore, downregulations of PKC and P-glycoprotein expression were noted in cells treated with schizandrin A + Dox or LCC + Dox (Fig. 11). These data showed that schizandrin A and LCC may induce a reversal of MDR in cancer cells via the inhibition of P-glycoprotein and PKC expression.

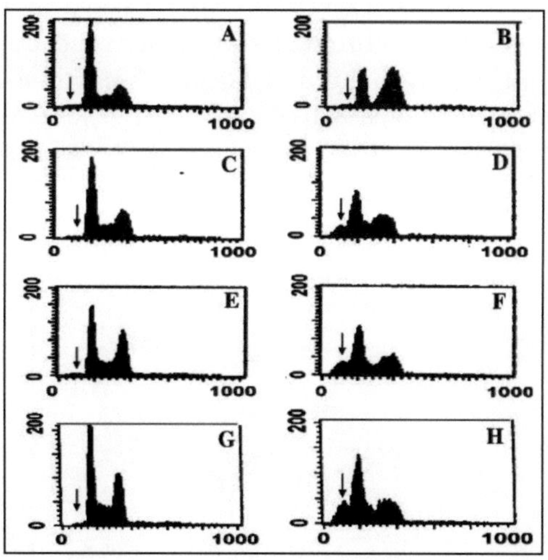

Fig. 11. Enhancing effects of schizandrin A and LCC on apoptosis in human hepatocellular carcinoma cells. **A** Control, **B** Dox 1,250 ng/ml, **C** Verapamil (VPL) 20 μM, **D** Dox 1,250 ng/ml + VPL 20 μM, **E** Schizandrin A 25 μM, **F** Dox 1,250 ng/ml + Schizandrin A 25 μM, **G** LCC 25 μg/ml, **H** Dox 1,250 ng/ml + LCC 25 μg/ml (Huang et al., 2008).

2.3.3 Effects of LCC on the tumor growth of mice

In order to confirm the MDR-reversing effects of LCC and schizandrin A detected *in vitro*, tumor growth was measured in nude mice bearing KBv200 xenografts. Following 10 days of vincristine injection, tumor growth was inhibited significantly-by approximately 12%-when tumor size was compared to that of the control group (Huang et al., 2008). Furthermore, co-treatment with LCC and vincristine at 100, 200 and 300 mg/kg BW increased the anti-tumor activity induced by vincristine in a dose-dependent manner (Fig. 12). In particular, LCC 300 mg/kg BW co-treatment for 15 days resulted in dramatic differences-most notably, a 41.9% inhibition of tumor size (Huang et al., 2008). These results indicate that LCC has potential for use in the development of a therapeutic drug for hepatoma *in vivo*.

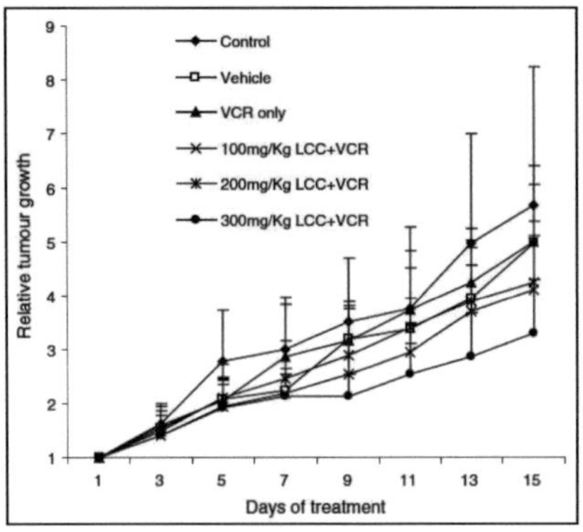

Fig. 12. Inhibition effects of LCC on vincristine-induced anti-tumor activity in nude mice bearing the KBv200 xenograft (Huang et al., 2008).

2.4 Effects of TGH

The structure of TGH (Fig. 13) was firstly assessed by Ikeya et al. (1978a). In Korea, this lignin was initially identified via gas chromatography/mass spectrometry (GC/MS) from *S. chinensis* harvested in Muju, Korea (Sohn and Bock, 1989). However, many things remain unknown regarding the functions of this lignan. Recently, several important study results suggesting a possible function of TGH in cancer therapy have caused an increase in interest in the compound.

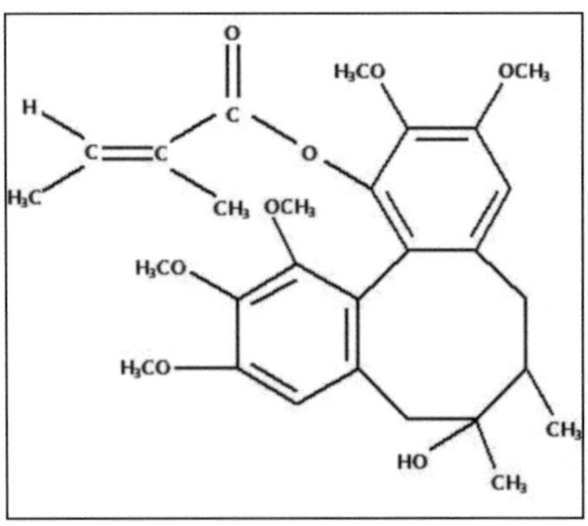

Fig. 13. Chemical structure of TGH isolated from *S. chinensis*.

2.4.1 Preparation of TGH

In order to prepare TGH, the fruit of *S. chinensis* (250 g) was firstly extracted three times using 500 mL of MeOH with sonication for 1 hr. The dried MeOH extract was collected from filtered solution with dryness under reduced pressure. Then, MeOH extract (50 g) was suspended in water and sequentially fractionated with *n*-hexane and CH_2Cl_2. The purified *n*-hexane fraction (10 g) was subjected to chromatography on an RP-18 column (4.5 x 20 cm, 5:5 - 9:1 MeOH:water, v/v) to yield fractions 1-8. Furthermore, fraction 4 (650 mg) was dissolved in MeOH and subjected to isocratic semi-preparative HPLC using an YMC J-sphere ODS column (20 x 250 mm, 4 μm; YMC). TGH was separated with MeCN-0.1% TFA in H2O (50:50 in 50 min, 10 mL/min, 254 nm) to yield 62.0 mg of compound 4 (93.65%). The identity of TGH was confirmed by 1H- and 13C-NMR spectroscopy (Lee et al., 2009).

2.4.2 Effects of TGH on cell survival

Lee et al. (2009) initially investigated the anti-cancer functions and action mechanisms of nine lignans isolated from the fruit of *S. chinensis*. Firstly, nine lignans including schisandrol A, schisandrol A, TGH, angeloylgomisin H (AGH), schisandrin A, schisandrin B, gomisin J, gomisin N and schisandrin C were isolated from *S. chinensis* and the effects of each lignin on the cell survival rate were determined. Among the nine lignans, TGH induced a reduction in cell survival at concentrations ranging from 31.3 μM to 250.0 μM, whereas the AGH samples maintained a steady level in terms of cell survival (Fig. 14). During this period, the quinone reductase activity was dramatically increased in hepatocarcinoma cells and evidenced a high chemoprevention index. Additionally, the mechanism study results demonstrated that the expression of genes mediated by the antioxidant response element (ARE), an important regulatory region in the promoter of the detoxification enzyme gene which is regulated by the nuclear accumulation of Nrf2, was enhanced significantly by TGH. Therefore, all study results appear to indicate that TGH may be considered as a potential liver cancer-preventive compound that specifically induces increases in antioxidant enzyme expression via the formation of the Nrf2-ARE binding complex.

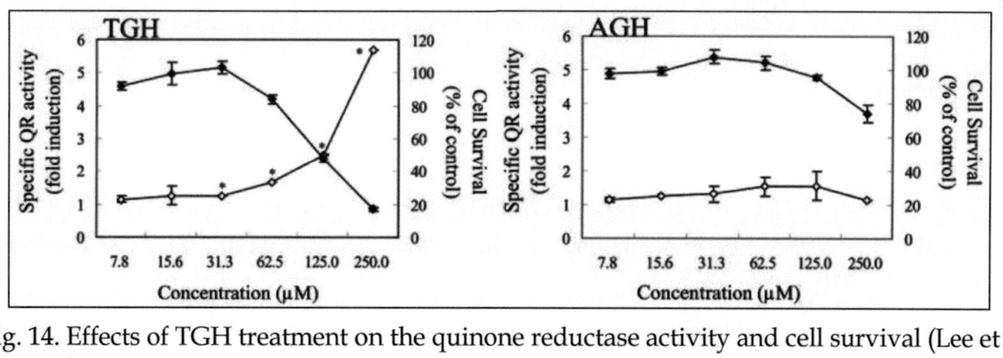

Fig. 14. Effects of TGH treatment on the quinone reductase activity and cell survival (Lee et al., 2009).

3. Conclusion

The development of novel therapeutic drugs for hepatic carcinoma is a very important objective in the field of pharmacological research. Among the variety of approaches thus far pursued to develop novel drugs, identification and screening of natural compounds from medical herbs has proven a very effective one-not least, because this method saves a great deal of time and cost. Recently, many institutes and companies in advanced countries have focused on an approach to novel drugs for hepatic carcinoma via the use of various lignins isolated from *S. chinensis.* This chapter introduces three lignans and one blend which may prove valuable in efforts to combat hepatic carcinoma. Gomisin A at high concentration was found to significantly induce anti-proliferative and pro-apoptotic effects in hepatic carcinoma. Schizandrin A markedly increased vincristine-induced hepatic carcinoma apoptosis and anti-tumor activity. Additionally, TGH induced the death of hepatic carcinoma cells and inhibited quinone reductase activity. Furthermore, KY88 was a blend composed of 10 herbal extracts and effects a dose-dependent inhibition of hepatocellular carcinoma cellular proliferation (Table 3).

Collectively, the results of these studies demonstrated that these lignins and the blend from *S. chinensis* were regarded as an anti-cancer drug candidate capable of inducing apoptosis and inhibiting the cell proliferation of hepatocellular carcinoma via a variety of mechanisms.

Compounds	**Function on hepatocellular carcinoma**	**References**
Gomisin N	· Induction of hepatic carcinoma apoptosis · Increase of Bcl-2 protein expression	Yim et al., 2009
KY88	·Dose-dependent inhibition of hepatocellular carcinoma proliferation and secretion of HBsAg and HBeAg ·Induction of hepatic carcinoma apoptosis and IL-4/TNF-α secretion	Loo et al., 2007 Chow et al., 2004
Schizandrin A	·Induction of hepatic carcinoma apoptosis and PKC down regulation ·Increase of anti-tumor activity induced by vincristine	Huang et al., 2008
TGH	·Induction of hepatic carcinoma death and inhibition of quinone reductase activity	Lee et al., 2009

Table 3. Summary therapeutic function of three lignins and one blend from *S. chinensis* on hepatocellular carcinoma.

4. Acknowledgments

I would like to express my gratitude to students, including JE Kim, SH Nam, SI Choi, IS Hwang, HR Lee and YJ Lee in our laboratory, for helping to compile this paper and with the graphics and charts herein.

5. References

Print Books

Adami, HO.; Hunter, D. & Trichopoulos, D. (2008): *Cancer of the Liver and Biliary Tract. In: Textbook of Cancer Epidemiology* (Second edition), Oxford University Press, ISBN 978-0-19-531117-4, Oxford England, pp. 308-332

Agejenko, AS. & Komissarenko, BT. (1960). *Schizandra and its Therapeutic Administration.* Sakhalinsk Book Press, Yuzhno-Sakhalinsk, p. 38

Gutnikova, ZI. (1951). Schizandra chinensis in the Far East. In: Lazarev,N.V. (Ed.), Materials for the Study of Ginseng and Schizandra Roots. Far East Branch of USSR Academy of Science, Vladivostok, pp. 23–43

Shilova, LM. (1963). *On the problem of sexual dimorphism and pollination in Schizandra chinensis. In: Brekhman, I.I., Belikov, I.F., Kuznetsova, G.E. (Eds.), Materials for the Study of Ginseng and Schizandra.* Far East Branch of the USSR Academy of Science, Primorsk Book Publisher, Vladivostok, pp. 267–270

Papers in Journals

Apakama, I.; Robinson, MC.; Walter, NM.; Charlton, RG.; Royds, JA.; Fuller, CE.; Neal, DE. & Hamdy, FC. (1996) Bcl-2 overexpression combined with p53 accumulation correlates with hormone refractory prostate cancer. *British Journal of cancer,* Vol. 74, No. 8, (October 1996), pp. 1258-1262, ISSN 0007-0920

Bosch, FX.; Ribes, J.; Díaz, M. & Clèries, R. (2004) Primary liver cancer: worldwide incidence and trends. *Gastroenterology,* Vol. 127, No. 5, (November 2004), pp. S5-S16, ISSN 0016-5085

Bruix, J. & Sherman, M. (2005) Management of hepatocellular carcinoma. *Hepatology,* Vol. 42, No. 5, (November 2005), pp. 1208-1236, ISSN 1527-3350

Chen, CC.; Shen, CC.; Shih, YZ. & Pan, TM. (1994) 6-O-Benzoylgomisin O, a New Lignan from the Fruits of Schizandra chinensis. *Journal of Natural Products,* Vol. 57, No. 8, (August 1994), pp. 1164-1165, ISSN 0163-3864

Chen, YY.; Shu, ZB. & Li, LN. (1976) Studies of Fructus schizandrae. IV. Isolation and determination of the active compounds (in lowering high SGPT levels) of Schizandra chinensis Baill. *Scientia Sinica,* Vol. 19, No. 2, (April 1976), pp. 276-290, ISSN 0250-7870

Chiu, PY.; Leung, HY.; Poon, MK.; Mak, DH. & Ko, KM. (2006) Effects of schisandrin B enantiomers on cellular glutathione and menadione toxicity in AML12 hepatocytes. *Pharmacology,* Vol. 77, No. 2, (April 2006), pp. 63-70, ISSN 0031-7012

Choi, YW.; Takamatsu, S.; Khan, SI.; Srinivas, PV.; Ferreira, D.; Zhao, J.P. & Khan I.A. (2006) Schisandrene, a Dibenzocyclooctadiene Lignan from *Schisandra chinensis*: Structure–Antioxidant Activity Relationships of Dibenzocyclooctadiene Lignans. *Journal of Natural Products,* Vol. 69, No. 3, (December 2005), pp. 356-359, ISSN 0163-3864

Chow, CW.; Loo, TY.; Sham, ST. & Cheung, NB. (2004) *Radix bupleuri* containing compound (KY88 liver-livo) induces apoptosis and production of interleukin-4 and tumor necrosis factor-alpha in liver cancer cells in vitro. *The American Journal of Chinese Medicine,* Vol. 32, No. 2, (February 2004), pp. 185-93, ISSN 0192-415X

Chow, LW.; Loo, WY. & Sham, JS. (2001) Effects of a herbal compound containing bupleurum on human lymphocytes. *Hong Kong Medical Journal,* Vol. 7, No. 4, (December 2001), pp. 408–413, ISSN 1024-2708

Deng, X.; Chen, X.; Yin, R.; Shen, Z.; Qiao, L. & Bi, K. (2008) Determination of deoxyschizandrin in rat plasma by LC-MS. *Journal of Pharmaceutical Biomedical Analysis,* Vol. 46, No. 1, (January 2008), pp. 121-126, ISSN 0731-7085

El-Serang, HB. & Mason, AC. (2000) Risk factors for the rising rates of primary liver cancer in the United States. *Archives of Internal Medicine,* Vol. 160, No. 21, (November 2000), pp. 3227-3230, ISSN 0003-9926

Fu, M.; Sun, ZH.; Zong, M.; He, XP.; Zuo, HC. & Xie, ZP. (2008) Deoxyschisandrin modulates synchronized Ca2+ oscillations and spontaneous synaptic transmission of cultured hippocampal neurons. *Acta Pharmacologica Sinica,* Vol. 29, No. 8, (August 2008), pp. 891-898, ISSN 1671-4083

Huang, M.; Jin, J.; Sun, H. & Liu, GT. (2008) Reversal of P-glycoprotein-mediated multidrug resistance of cancer cells by five schizandrins isolated from the Chinese herb Fructus Schizandrae. *Cancer Chemotherapy and Pharmacology,* Vol. 62, No. 6, (November 2008), pp. 1015-1026, ISSN 0344-5704

Ikeya, Y.; Kanatani, H.; Hakozaki, M.; Taguchi, H. & Mitsuhashi, H. (1988) The constituents of Schizandra chinensis Baill. XV. Isolation and structure determination of two new lignans, gomisin S and gomisin T. *Chemical & Pharmaceutical Bulletin,* Vol. 36, No. 10, (October 1988), pp. 3974-3979, ISSN 0009-2363

Ikeya, Y.; Miki, E.; Okada, M.; Mitsuhashi, H. & Chai, JG. (1990) Benzoylgomisin Q and benzoylgomisin P, two new lignans from Schisandra sphenanthera Rehd. et Wils. *Chemical & Pharmaceutical Bulletin,* Vol. 38, No. 5, (May 1990), pp. 1408-1411, ISSN 0009-2363

Ikeya, Y.; Ookawa, N.; Taguchi, H. & Yosioka, I. (1982b) The constituents of Schizandra chinensis Baill. XI. The structures of three new lignans, angeloylgomisin O, and angeloyl- and benzoylisogomisin O. *Chemical & Pharmaceutical Bulletin,* Vol. 30, No. 9, (September 1982b), pp. 3202-3206, ISSN 0009-2363

Ikeya, Y.; Sugama, K.; Okada, M. & Mitsuhashi, H. (1991) Two lignans from Schisandra sphenanthera. *Phytochemistry,* Vol. 30, No. 3, (March 1991), pp. 975-980, ISSN 0031-9942

Ikeya, Y.; Taguchi, H. & Litaka, Y. (1976) The constituents of Schizandra chinensis Baill. The structure of a new lignin, gomisin D. *Tetrahedron Letters,* Vol. 17, No. 17, (April 1976), pp. 1359-1362, ISSN 0040-4039

Ikeya, Y.; Taguchi, H. & Yosioka, I. (1979d) The constituents of Schizandra chinensis Baill. The cleavage of the methylenedioxy moiety with lead tetraacetate in benzene, and the structure of angeloylgomisin Q. *Chemical & Pharmaceutical Bulletin,* Vol. 27, No. 10, (October 1979d) pp. 2536-2538, ISSN 0009-2363

IKeya, Y.; Taguchi, H. & Yosioka, I. (1980a) The constituents of Schizandra chinensis Baill. VII. The structures of three new lignans, (-)-gomisin K1 and (+)-gomisins K2 and K3. *Chemical & pharmaceutical bulletin,* Vol. 28, No. 8, (August 1980a), pp. 2422-2427, ISSN 0009-2363

IKeya, Y.; Taguchi, H. & Yosioka, I. (1982a) The constituents of Schizandra chinensis BAILL. X. The structures of γ-schizandrin and four new lignans, (-)-gomisins L1 and L2, (±)-gomisin M1 and (+)-gomisin M2. *Chemical & pharmaceutical bulletin,* Vol. 30, No. 1, (January 1982a), pp. 132-139, ISSN 0009-2363

Ikeya, Y.; Taguchi, H. & Yosioka, I. (1982c) The Constituents of Schizandra chinensis BAILL. XII. Isolation and Structure of a New Lignan, Gomisin R, the Absolute Structure of Wuweizisu C and Isolation of Schisantherin D. *Chemical & Pharmaceutical Bulletin,* Vol. 30, No. 9, (September 1982c) pp. 3207-3211, ISSN 0009-2363

Ikeya, Y.; Taguchi, H.; Yosioka, I. & Kobayashi, H. (1978a) The constituents of *Schizandra chinensis* BAILL. The structures of two new lignans, pre-gomisin and gomisin J. *Chemical & Pharmaceutical Bulletin,* Vol. 26, No. 2, (February 1978a), pp. 682-684, ISSN 0009-2363

Ikeya, Y.; Taguchi, H.; Yosioka, I. & Kobayashi, H. (1978b) The Constituents of Schizandra chinensis BAILL. The Structures of Two New Lignans, Gomisin N and Tigloylgomisin P. *Chemical & pharmaceutical bulletin,* Vol. 26, No. 10, (October 1978b), pp. 3257-3260, ISSN 0009-2363

Ikeya, Y.; Taguchi, H.; Yosioka, I. & Kobayashi, H. (1979a) The constituents of *Schizandra chinensis* Baill. I. Isolation and structure determination of five new lignans, gomisin A, B, C, F and G, and the absolute structure of schizandrin. *Chemical & pharmaceutical bulletin,* Vol. 27, No.6, (November 1979a), pp. 1383-1394, ISSN 0009-2363

Ikeya, Y.; Taguchi, H.; Yosioka, I. & Kobayashi, H. (1979b) The constituents of Schizandra chinensis Baill. III. The structures of four new lignans, gomisin H and its derivatives, angeloyl-, tigloyl- and benzoyl-gomisin H. *Chemical & pharmaceutical bulletin,* Vol. 27, No. 7, (July 1979b), pp. 1576-1582, ISSN 0009-2363

Ikeya, Y.; Taguchi, H.; Yosioka, I. & Kobayashi, H. (1979c) The constituents of Schizandra chinensis Baill. IV. The structures of two new lignans, pre-gomisin and gomisin J. *Chemical & Pharmaceutical Bulletin,* Vol. 27, No. 7, (July 1979c) pp. 1583-1588, ISSN 0009-2363

Ikeya, Y.; Taguchi, H.; Yosioka, I. & Kobayashi, H. (1979e) The constituents of Schizandra chinensis Baill. V. The structures of four new lignans, gomisin N, gomisin O, epigomisin O and gomisin E, and transformation of gomisin N to deangeloylgomisin B. *Chemical & Pharmaceutical Bulletin,* Vol. 27, No. 11, (December 1979e), pp. 2695-2709, ISSN 0009-2363

Ikeya, Y.; Taguchi, H.; Yosioka, I.; Yosioka, I. & Kobayashi, H. (1980b) The constituents of Schizandra chinensis Baill. VIII. The structures of two new lignans,tigloylgomisin P and angeloylgomisin P. *Chemical & Pharmaceutical Bulletin,* Vol. 28, No. 11, (November 1980b), pp. 3357-3361, ISSN 0009-2363

Joensuu, H.; Pylkkänen, L. & Toikkanen, S. (1994) Bcl-2 protein expression and long-term survival in breast cancer. *The American Journal of pathology,* Vol. 145, No. 5, (May 1994), pp. 1191-1198, ISSN 0002-9440

Ko, KM. & Lam, BY. (2002) Schisandrin B protects against tert-butylhydroperoxide induced cerebral toxicity by enhancing glutathione antioxidant status in mouse brain. *Molecular & Cellular Biochemistry,* Vol. 238, No. 1-2, (September 2002), pp. 181-186, ISSN 0300-8177

Lee, SB.; Kim, CY.; Lee, HJ.; Yun, JH. & Nho, CW. (2009) Induction of the phase II detoxification enzyme NQO1 in hepatocarcinoma cells by lignans from the fruit of Schisandra chinensis through nuclear accumulation of Nrf2. *Planta Medica,* Vol. 75, No. 12, (October 2009), pp. 1314-1318

Liu, CS.; Fang, SD.; Huang, MF.; Kao, YL. & Hsu JS. (1978) Studies on the active principles of Schisandra sphenanthera Rehd. et Wils. The structures of schisantherin A, B, C, D, E, and the related compounds. *Scientia Sinica,* Vol. 21, No. 4, (July-August 1978), pp. 483-502, ISSN 0250-7870

Loo, WT.; Cheung, MN. & Chow, LW. (2007) Fructus schisandrae (Wuweizi)-containing compound inhibits secretion of HBsAg and HBeAg in hepatocellular carcinoma cell line. *Biomedicine & Pharmacotherapy,* Vol. 61, No. 9, (October 2007), pp. 606-610, ISSN 0753-3322

Lu, Y. & Chen, DF. (2009) Analysis of Schisandra chinensis and Schisandra sphenanthera. *Journal of Chromatography A,* Vo. 1216, No. 11, (March 2009), pp. 1980-1990, ISSN 0021-9673

Panossian, A. & Wikman, G. (2008) Pharmacology of Schisandra chinensis Bail.: an overview of Russian research and uses in medicine. *Journal of Ethnopharmacology,* Vol. 118, No. 2, (July 2008), pp. 183-212, ISSN 0378-8741

Park, JY.; Lee, SJ.; Yun, MR.; Seo, KW.; Bae, SS.; Park, JW.; Lee, YJ.; Shin, WJ.; Choi, YW. & Kim, CD. (2007) Gomisin A from *Schisandra chinensis* induces endothelium-dependent and direct relaxation in rat thoracic aorta. *Planta Medica,* Vol. 73, No. 15, (December 2007), pp. 1537-1542, ISSN 0032-0943

Sakurai, H.; Nikaido, T.; Ohmoto, T.; Ikeya, Y. & Mitsuhashi, H. (1992) Inhibitors of adenosine 3',5'-cyclic monophosphate phosphodiesterase from Schisandra chinensis and the structure activity relationship of lignans. *Chemical & Pharmaceutical Bulletin,* Vol. 40, No. 5, (May 1992), pp. 1191-1195, ISSN 0009-2363

Seo, SM.; Lee, HJ.; Park, YK.; Lee, MK.; Park, JI.; Paik, KH. & Park, JI. (2004). Lignans from the fruits of *Schizandra chinensis* and their inhibitory effects on dopamine content in PC12 cells. *Natural Product Sciences,* Vol.10, No.3, (June 2004), pp. 104-108, ISSN 1226-3907

Sohn, HJ. & Bock, JY. (1989) Identification of lignan compounds in fruits of *Schizandra chinensis* BAILLON by gas chromatography/mass spectrometry. *Journal of the Korean Agricultural Chemical Society,* Vol. 32, No. 4, (December 1989), pp. 344-349, ISSN 0368-2897

Taguchi, H. & Ikeya, Y. (1977) The Constituents of Schizandra chinensis BAILL. The Structures of Two New Lignans, Gomisin F and G, and the Absolute Structures of Gomisin A, B, and C. *Chemical & Pharmaceutical Bulletin,* Vol. 25, No. 2, (February 1977), pp. 364-366, ISSN 0009-2363

Thomas, MB. & Zhu, AX. (2005) Hepatocellular carcinoma: the need for progress. *Journal of Clinical Oncology,* Vol. 23, No. 13, (May 2005), pp. 2892-2829, ISSN 0732-183X

Yim, SY.; Lee, YJ.; Lee, YK.; Jung, SE.; Kim, JH.; Kim, HJ.; Son, BG.; Park, YH.; Lee, YG.; Choi, YW. & Hwang, DY. (2009) Gomisin N isolated from Schisandra chinensis significantly induces anti-proliferative and pro-apoptotic effects in hepatic carcinoma. *Molecular medicine reports,* Vol. 2, No. 5, (October 2009), pp. 725-732, ISSN 1791-2997

Yue, JM.; Jun, X. & Chen, YZ. (1994) Triterpenoids of Schisandra sphenanthera. *Phytochemistry,* Vol. 35, No. 4, (April 1994), pp. 1068-1069, ISSN 0031-9422

Zheng, RL.; Kang, JH.; Chen, FY.; Wang, PF.; Ren, JG. & Liu, QL. (1997) Difference in antioxidation for schisandrins and schisantherin between bio- and chemo-systems. *Phytotherapy Research,* Vol. 11, No. 8, (December 1997), pp. 600-602, ISSN 1099-1573

21

Study on Metabolism of Natural Medical Components *In Vivo*: Metabolism Study in Rat After Oral Administration of Rhubarb Decoction and Characterization, Identification of the Rat Metabolite of *Scutellaria baicalensis*

Chenggang Huang et al.*
Shanghai Institute of Materia Medica, Chinese Academy of Sciences, Shanghai, China

1. Introduction

Rheum palmatum L., one of the commonly used Traditional Chinese Medicines (TCMs), which is called Dahuang in Chinese, has been successfully used in China for thousands of years. The crude material of *R. palmatum* called rhubarb was widely used as laxative to treat constipation. Furthermore, it has various other pharmacological actions, such as antibacterial [1, 2], anti-inflammatory [3, 4], antiviral [5], anti-angiogenic [6], antioxidative [7], immunomodulatory [8], protecting effects in rat with chronic renal failure [9] and anti-diabetic effects on diabetic mice [10]. Although many investigations have been conducted in the fields of pharmacology, clinical trials, and phytochemistry about rhubarb, researchers still do not know what its effective constituents are, how many compounds are absorbed into blood after intragastric administration of the decoction, and what the fate of the decoction in the body is. The limited knowledge about the metabolism of rhubarb decoction restricts the deeper pharmacological mechanism study and wider clinical use of rhubarb.

It was well accepted that TCMs expressed its effects through multi-components and multi-targets. Rapid, sensitive and selective analytical method is needed to simultaneous determine of multiple components of TCMs in biological matrix with low concentrations. In recent years, HPLC/ESI/MS^n has been proved to be a modern and powerful method for the identification of compounds in biosamples or TCM extracts [11, 12]. Metabolism of rhubarb has been reported [13], but data on pharmacokinetics are scanty. So, our interest was to utilize a solid phase extraction (SPE) and HPLC/ESI/MS^n techniques for the detection of potentially active compounds in urine, plasma and tissue samples and for the

* Bin Wu[1], Shuyun Liu[1,2], Shuang Liu[3], Zhixiong Li[1], Longhai Jian[4], Yihong Tang[1], Zhaolin Sun[1] and Ke Wang[4]
[1]*Shanghai Institute of Materia Medica, Chinese Academy of Sciences, Shanghai, China*
[2]*Shuguang Hospital, Shanghai University of Traditional Chinese Medicine, Shanghai, China*
[3]*Haerbin University of Commerce, Haerbin, China*
[4]*Shanghai Institute for Food and Drug Control, Shanghai, China*

pharmacokinetic study of rhubarb. Total of 39 compounds were identified as absorbed bioactive constituents. The excretion of M22 and M39 reached more than 1000 μg in urine samples after intragastric administration of the decoction.

2. Experiments

2.1 Chemicals and materials

Standards of the rhapontin, aloe-emodin, chrysophanol, emodin, rheochrysidin and rhein were obtained from the National Institute for the Control of Pharmaceutical and Biological Products (NICPBP) (Beijing, China). The plasma, urine and tissue samples were extracted using Supelco™ LC-18 solid-phase extraction (SPE) tubes (1ml/100mg, USA). Acetonitrile (HPLC grade) was purchased from the Dikma Company (Dikma, USA). Water was deionized and double distilled. All other chemicals were of analytical grade. Blank rat plasma (drug free) was prepared in our laboratory.

2.2 Equipment

An HPLC-MS system (Agilent 1100, Agilent Technologies, Wilmington, DE, USA) with an electrospray ionization (ESI) ion source was used. The LC/MSD Trap software (version 5.3) was used for data acquisition and processing. An API 4000 triple quadrapole instrument (Applied Biosystems, Toronto, Canada) was used for the mass spectrometric detection using an electrospray ionization (ESI) source in the negative mode. A high-speed bench-top centrifuge (Sorvall ST16, Thermo Fisher Scientific, Germany) was used for centrifuge biological samples.

2.3 Preparation of rhubarb decoction

200 g rhubarb was immerged in 2000 mL distilled water and then refluxed for 1 h at 100°C. The aqueous extract was filtered and the residue was refluxed for 30 min with another 2000 mL of distilled water under the same conditions. The two water extracts were combined and condensed to 200 mL and stored at 4°C until use.

2.4 Standard preparation

The standard of rhapontin, aloe-emodin, chrysophanol, emodin, rheochrysidin and rhein were dissolved in methanol at a concentration of 100 μg/ml to obtain the standard stock solutions.

2.5 Animals

30 male Sprague-Dawley rats (200±20 g) were obtained from the Animal Center of Shanghai Institute of Materia Medica, Shanghai, China. They were kept under standard laboratory conditions (12/12 h light/darkness, 22±2°C room temperature, 50-60% humidity) for one week prior to the experiments. All animal experiments were carried out according to the Guidelines for the Care and Use of Laboratory Animals, and were approved by the Animal Ethics Committee of Shanghai Institute of Materia Medica.

Six male rats were orally administered a single dose of rhubarb decoction at 10 g/kg. After dosing, the rats were housed in separate glass metabolic cages with free access to water. Urine was collected at -8 to 0 h predose and during 0-2, 2-4, 4-6, 6-8, 8-24, 24-36, 36-48 h postdose.

Other 24 male rats were divided into four groups at random. They were used in determining the concentration of rhubarb in blood and tissues. One group of rats was killed predose to provide control blood and tissues for analysis. Other three groups of rats were orally administrated of rhubarb decoction at a dosage of 17.6 g/kg. Six rats each were anesthetized with ether and blood samples were collected from abdominal aorta of the rats at 1.0, 2.0, and 3.0 h after dosing, respectively. The following tissues and organs were collected and weighed at the time of killing for determination of rhubarb concentration: heart (HE), liver (LV), spleen (SP), lung (LU), kidney (KI), brain (BR), small intestine (SI), large intestine (LI), stomach (ST), and testis (TE). The whole tissues were homogenized with PBS to yield final concentration of 20% w/v. All the homogenates were stored at -80°C.

2.6 Extraction of rat biological samples

All samples were centrifuged at 3000×g for 10 min. The supernatants were loaded onto a C18 SPE cartridge. Before use, an SPE column was conditioned and washed with 2 ml of methanol and then 2 ml of deionized water. Then 600 µl of the selected supernatant sample was applied to the SPE well. The SPE well was washed with 1 ml of water, and then the analytes were eluted with 1 ml of methanol. The eluent was evaporated at 37°C under a gentle stream of nitrogen. The dry residue was then reconstituted with 200 µl methanol and vortex-mixed for 20 s. The solution was then centrifuged at 14000×g for 10 min, and an aliquot of 10 µl supernatant was injected into the HPLC/ESI/MS system for analysis.

2.7 HPLC condition

The metabolites of rhubarb decoction were separated on a Grace Apollo C18 reversed-phase column (250 mm×4.6 mm, 5 µm) equipped with an EasyGuard Kit C18 (4×2 mm) guard column. The column was maintained at 25°C. The mobile phase consisted of 0.5% formic acid-water (A) and acetonitrile (B) and was delivered at a flow rate of 1.0 ml/min. The detection wavelengths were set at 190-400 nm. Gradient elution was used as follows: a linear gradient from 35% to 100% B in the first 30 min, followed by 100% B for 10 min, and finally a linear gradient to 35% B at 45 min that was held for 5 min. The total run time was 50 min.

2.8 Mass spectrometry analysis for qualitation

The HPLC system used was an Agilent 1100 series LC/MSD Trap mass spectrometer (Agilent Technologies, Wilmington, DE, USA), connected to an Agilent 1100 HPLC instrument via an electrospray ionization (ESI) source. The LC/MSD Trap software (version 5.3) was used for system operation and data collection. The operating parameters in the negative ion mode were as follows: collision gas, ultra-high purity helium (He); nebulizing gas, high purity nitrogen (N_2); capillary voltage, 3.5 kV; end plate offset, 500 V; nebulizer, 30 psi; drying gas flow rate, 10 l/min; drying gas temp., 350°C. Trap: ICC, target, 30000, max accu. time, 300.00ms, averages, 5. Auto Ms. 4; MS/MS frag. ampl., 1.00V; auto MS (n>2): frag. ampl., 0.77V. Smart frag: start ampl., 30.0%; end ampl., 200%. For full-scan MS analysis, the spectra were recorded in the range of *m/z* 50-1500.

2.9 Mass spectrometry analysis for quantitation

An API 4000 Qtrap mass spectrometer (Applied Biosystems, Toronto, Canada) equipped with a pneumatically assisted ESI interface was linked with the HPLC system. Initially optimization of the parameters for the ESI/MS and ESI/MS/MS analyses of the standards and the samples was performed by direct infusion into the ES ionization source. The operating parameters were as follows: negative ion scan mode, curtain gas (CUR) 30 psi, collision gas (CAD) medium, ion source gas 1 (GC1) 45 psi, ion source gas 2 (GC2) 45 psi, ion spray voltage (IS) 5000 V, entrance potential (EP) 10 V, declustering potential (DP) 160 V, collision energy 60 V, collision cell exit potential (CXP) 3 V and temperature (TEM) 350°C.

3. Results

3.1 Optimization of HPLC and MS conditions

To obtain HPLC chromatograms with good separation and peak shape, different mobile phase compositions were screened. Given the acidity of phenolic compounds, it was found that acetonitrile and 0.5% aqueous formic acid were the most suitable eluting solvent system. The proposed method was acceptable as well as adequate for further MS/MS analysis. To acquire maximum sensitivity for most compounds, MS parameters such as spray voltage, capillary temperature, sheath gas and auxiliary gas pressure, source CID, collision gas pressure and collision energy were optimized using methanol extraction of rhubarb decoction by flow injection analysis (FIA). It was found that the negative ion mode was more sensitive than positive ion mode for most of the compounds.

3.2 System suitability

The system suitability test is performed to assure that the analytical method can be executed with the existing HPLC system. A system suitability test of the chromatographic system was performed before each validation run. Five replicate injections of a system suitability/calibration standard (at concentration of 10 μg/ml) were made. Area and retention time relative standard deviation, asymmetry factor t_a and efficiency (as plate number N) for the five injections was determined. For all samples analyses, the asymmetry factor t_a was≤1.4, efficiency≥3000 and area % R.S.D.≤1.0%.

3.3 Optimization of sample preparation

Solid-phase extraction was used as an important step of the sample preparation. Quantitative elution of standard samples from SPE cartridge are apparent after 1.0 ml of methanol. The reproducibility and recovery of solid-phase extraction was determined from five repetitions. The reproducibility expressed as R.S.D. was 0.6-0.9% and recovery was 84.8-97.2% for concentration of 10 μg/ml of standard samples.

3.4 Limits of detection (LOD)/ linearity/accuracy/precision for related substances

The limit of detection of the six standard components (based on a detector signal-to-noise ratio 3:1) was 0.1 μg/ml. The method was found to be linear with correlation coefficients (R^2) of 0.986-0.997 for the six standard components, with slops near unity and y-intercepts near zero for these low-level determinations. Accuracy and precision for the standard components were satisfactory at three concentrations studied. Accuracy and intra-day and inter-day precision of the six standard components were less than 10%.

3.5 Stability of standard and sample solutions

Prepared samples and standards have been shown to be stable for at least 2 weeks when stored refrigerated. Additionally, the standard solutions have been shown to be stable while in use for assays for at least 72 h. The stability of the six standard sample solutions was evaluated after 1 and 2 weeks under refrigerated condition. The results obtained for refrigerated standard solution were 100.1 to 101.2% of the initial concentration for 1 and 2 week time points, respectively. The result for the refrigerated sample solution were 102.1 to 96.8% of its initial concentration after 1 and 2 week's storage, respectively. No degradation products were observed for any of the solutions tested. The standard solutions that had been held at room temperature for 72 h were stable with responses of 98.7-100.9%.

3.6 Fragmentation behavior of the parent compounds

To interpret the mass spectra of the metabolites using the LC/MS^n technique, it is necessary to fully understand the fragmentation behavior of the parent compound. Rhapontin, aloe-emodin, chrysophanol, emodin, rheochrysidin and rhein were selected as representative parent compounds in this study. It was found that the negative ion mode was more sensitive than positive ion mode for most of the compounds with triple quadrupole mass spectrometer, so negative ion mode was chosen. The HPLC/ESI/MS^n spectra of $[M-H]^-$ ion of the six parent compounds were shown in Fig.1. As most of these metabolites remained the structural features of the parent compounds, the analysis of the fragmentation pathways greatly facilitated the identification of metabolites from rhubarb decoction.

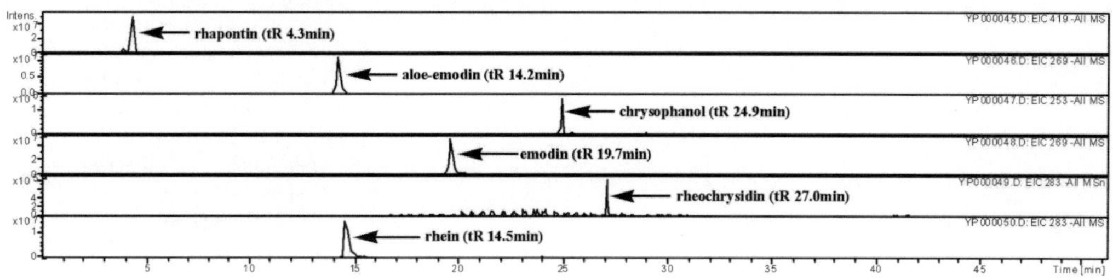

Fig. 1. The HPLC/ESI/MS spectra of the parent compounds

3.7 Identification of metabolites

Possible metabolite structures were considered based on the parent structure and the known metabolic pathways. As for MS detection, the potential metabolites were detected by comparison of the chromatograms of the drug-containing samples with those of blank samples. The retention time of each potential metabolite was ascertained by employing its mass to generate its extracted ion chromatogram (EIC) of the drug-containing sample. Compared with blank samples, a total of 39 compounds were detected in extracted ion chromatograms from the drug-containing urine, plasma and tissue samples (Table 1).

The identification of the metabolites and elucidation of their structures were performed mainly based on their MS^n fragmentations. Possible metabolite structures were considered based on the parent structure and the known metabolic pathways. Then, rat urine, plasma and tissue samples after i.g. administration of rhubarb decoction were analyzed and compared with blank samples by HPLC/ESI/MS^n in negative mode. Typical chromatograms resulting from the analysis of various biological samples are shown in Fig.2. Ultimately, the 39 metabolites could be generally divided into three groups: glucoside, glucuronidation and sulfation metabolites. The MS^2 spectra of the 39 compounds were shown in Fig. 3. Metabolite M4, M10 and M20 were selected as examples and the structural elucidations of the other metabolites were carried out similarly. The postulated fragmentation pathways of M4, M10 and M20 were shown in Fig.4.

Metabolites	t_R (min)	[M-H]$^-$	UR	PL	Tissues										ESI-MS data (% base peak) (*m/z*)
					HE	LV	SP	LU	KI	BR	SB	LB	ST	TE	
M1	3.3	591	+	-	-	-	-	-	-	-	-	-	-	-	MS^2[591]:253(100),175(14.4) MS^3[253]:253(100)
M2	3.3	383	+	-	-	-	-	-	-	-	-	-	-	-	MS^2[383]:303(34.7).207(100),113(52.1) MS^3[207]:207(52.8),163(100),122(10.8)
M3	3.3	445	-	-	-	-	-	-	-	-	-	-	+	-	MS^2[445]:427(8.0),283(100),175(4.5) MS^3[283]:283(100),239(17.4)
M4	3.4	479	+	-	-	-	-	-	-	-	-	-	-	-	MS^2[479]:303(100),174(20.9) MS^3[303]:303(100),259(9.8)
M5	3.4	417	+	-	-	+	-	-	-	-	-	-	-	-	MS^2[417]:373(100),330(12.5),241(41.0), 175(3.7) MS^3[373]:373(9.1),330(100)
M6	3.5	313	+	-	-	-	-	-	-	-	-	-	-	-	MS^2[313]:313(12.8),233(100),175(3.6) MS^3[233]:233(100),189(11.2)
M7	3.5	459	+	+	-	-	-	-	+	-	-	-	-	-	MS^2[459]:283(100),175(3.6) MS^3[283]:283(100),239(9.1)
M8	3.7	475	-	-	-	-	-	-	-	-	-	-	+	-	MS^2[475]:431(7.2),311(57.0),269(100) MS^3[269]:269(100)
M9	3.8	287	+	-	-	-	-	-	-	-	-	-	-	-	MS^2[287]:287(8.3),207(100) MS^3[207]:207(85.5),163(100)
M10	4.1	621	-	+	-	-	-	-	-	-	-	-	-	-	MS^2[621]:575(3.5),445(100),269(21.3) MS^3[445]:311(7.8),269(100)
M11	4.1	375	-	-	+	-	-	-	-	-	-	-	-	-	MS^2[375]:332(18.8),243(100) MS^3[243]:243(100)
M12	4.2	445	+	-	-	-	-	-	-	-	-	-	-	-	MS^2[445]:269(100),175(2.1) MS^3[269]:269(100)
M13	4.2	268	+	-	+	-	-	-	+	-	-	-	-	-	MS^2[269]:189(100)
M14	4.3	417	+	+	-	-	-	-	-	-	-	-	-	-	MS^2[417]:399(8.1),241(5.1),175 (100) MS^3[175]:113(100)
M15	4.5	435	-	-	-	-	-	-	-	-	-	-	+	-	MS^2[435]:273(100),167(4.3) MS^3[273]:273(100),167(53.0)
M16	4.6	431	-	-	-	-	-	-	-	-	-	-	+	-	MS^2[431]:269(100) MS^3[269]:269(100)
M17	4.6	459	+	-	-	-	-	-	-	-	-	-	+	-	MS^2[459]:283(100) MS^3[283]:283(100),257(1.9)
M18	4.7	297	+	+	+	-	-	+	+	-	-	-	-	-	MS^2[297]:175(83.7),113(100) MS^3[113]:95(80.0),85(100)
M19	4.9	401	-	+	-	+	-	+	+	-	+	-	-	-	MS^2[401]:358(100),296(4.2),225(32.4), 174(60.5) MS^3[358]:313(13.5),174(100)
M20	5.2	525	-	+	-	-	-	-	-	-	-	-	-	-	MS^2[525]:445(100),349(20.3),269(73.5) MS^3[445]:269(100)
M21	5.3	349	+	-	-	-	-	-	-	-	-	-	-	-	MS^2[349]:269(100) MS^3[269]:269(100),240(5.8)
M22	5.3	363	+	-	-	-	-	-	-	-	-	-	-	-	MS^2[363]:283(100) MS^3[283]:283(100),239(7.0)
M23	5.4	433	-	+	-	-	-	-	-	-	-	-	-	-	MS^2[433]:415(7.4),257(100),175(60.5) MS^3[257]:257(100)
M24	5.6	321	-	+	+	+	-	-	-	-	-	+	-	-	MS^2[321]:241(100),121(87.7) MS^3[241]:241(12.3),121(100)
M25	6.0	473	-	+	-	-	-	-	-	-	-	-	-	-	MS^2[473]:426(6.2),335(9.5),297(87.7), 253(100) MS^3[253]:253(100)

M26	6.0	363	+	+	+	-	-	-	+	-	-	-	-	-	MS²[363]:283(100) MS³[283]:283(100),239(4.7)
M27	6.3	407	-	-	-	-	-	-	-	-	-	-	+	-	MS²[407]:369(18.7),245(100) MS³[245]:245(100),230(50.4)
M28	6.6	431	-	-	-	-	-	-	-	-	-	-	+	-	MS²[431]:340(3.3),269(100) MS³[269]:269(100)
M29	6.6	429	+	+	-	-	-	-	+	-	-	-	-	-	MS²[429]:253(100),175(6.8) MS³[253]:253(100)
M30	6.8	415	-	-	-	-	-	-	-	-	-	-	+	-	MS²[415]:253(100) MS³[253]:253(100)
M31	7.0	429	+	+	+	+	-	+	+	-	-	-	-	-	MS²[429]:253(100),175(6.8) MS³[253]:253(100)
M32	8.2	313	-	-	-	-	-	-	-	-	-	-	+	-	MS²[313]:269(100),201(5.4) MS³[269]:269(100)
M33	8.4	445	+	+	+	+	-	-	+	-	-	-	-	-	MS²[445]:269(100) MS³[269]:269(100)
M34	8.4	459	+	-	-	-	-	-	-	-	-	-	-	-	MS²[459]:283(100),175(7.0) MS³[283]:283(100)
M35	10.2	443	-	-	-	-	-	-	-	-	-	-	-	-	MS²[443]:411(100),267(87.5),253(91.5), 157(10.9) MS³[411]:335(30.2),267(100),253(88.9)
M36	11.5	297	+	+	+	+	-	-	+	-	+	-	+	-	MS²[297]:253(100) MS³[253]:253(100)
M37	12.9	349	+	-	-	-	-	-	-	-	-	-	+	-	MS²[349]:269(100) MS³[269]:269(100)
M38	14.3	561	+	-	-	-	-	-	-	-	-	-	-	-	MS²[561]:269(100),240(9.5) MS³[269]:269(100)
M39	14.6	283	+	+	+	+	-	+	+	-	+	-	+	+	MS²[283]:257(100),239(66.9) MS³[257]:257(100),239(41.0)

tR: retention time; +:found; -:not found; [M-H]: negatively charged molecular ion

Table 1. The metabolites detected in rat urine, plasma and tissues after intragastric administration of rhubarb decoction

M4, which was only detected in plasma samples produced a $[M-H]^-$ at *m/z* 479 with a retention time of 3.4 min. It was found that the $[M-H-176]^-$ ion plus the ion at *m/z* 303 were observed in its MS² spectrum. So, M4 was identified as the metabolite that conjugated with one molecule of glucuronic acid (GlcA). The ion at *m/z* 303 could produce fragment ion at *m/z* 259. The spectroscope (MS^n) data of M4 was different from those reported in the published literature before [14]. According to the data above, M4 was conjectured to be glucuronide conjugate of methyl catechin.

M10 gave a $[M-H]^-$ signal at *m/z* 621 in the mass spectrum and fragmentation of the ion with the peak at *m/z* 621 gave the ion peak at *m/z* 445 (-176 Da), involving the loss of glucuronic acid. Then, the MS³ fragmentation yielded the ion peak at *m/z* 269 (-176 Da), involving another loss of glucuronic acid. The quasi-molecular ion of *m/z* 621 lost a 46 Da and a 30 Da fragmentation sequentially forming the product ions at *m/z* 575 and 591, suggesting that the mother nucleus was aloe-emodin, and the hydroxymethyl was not conjugated. Therefore, the compound M10 was identified as bisdesmoside conjugate of aloe-emodin.

The mass spectrum of the compound M20 displayed a signal at *m/z* 525 ($[M-H]^-$). A product ion spectrum of M20 displayed fragment ion at *m/z* 445, 400, 349 and 269. Fragmentation of the ion at *m/z* 525 gave the ion peak at *m/z* 349 (-176 Da), suggesting the loss of glucuronic acid. Meanwhile, fragmentation of the quasi-molecular ion yielded an ion peak at *m/z* 445 (-80 Da), involving the presence of sulfate. Glucuronic acid group and sulfate were not conjuncted with hydroxymethyl of the parent compound, which was judged by sequential loss of 44 Da and 46 Da. Therefore, the structure of M20 was conjectured to be glucuronide and sulfate conjugate of aloe-emodin, glucuronic acid group and sulfate occurred at the 1 and 8-hydroxy, respectively.

Based on the discussions above, the proposed metabolic pathways of rhubarb in rats are shown in Fig.5. The parent compound rhein was found in urine, plasma and most of the tissue samples.

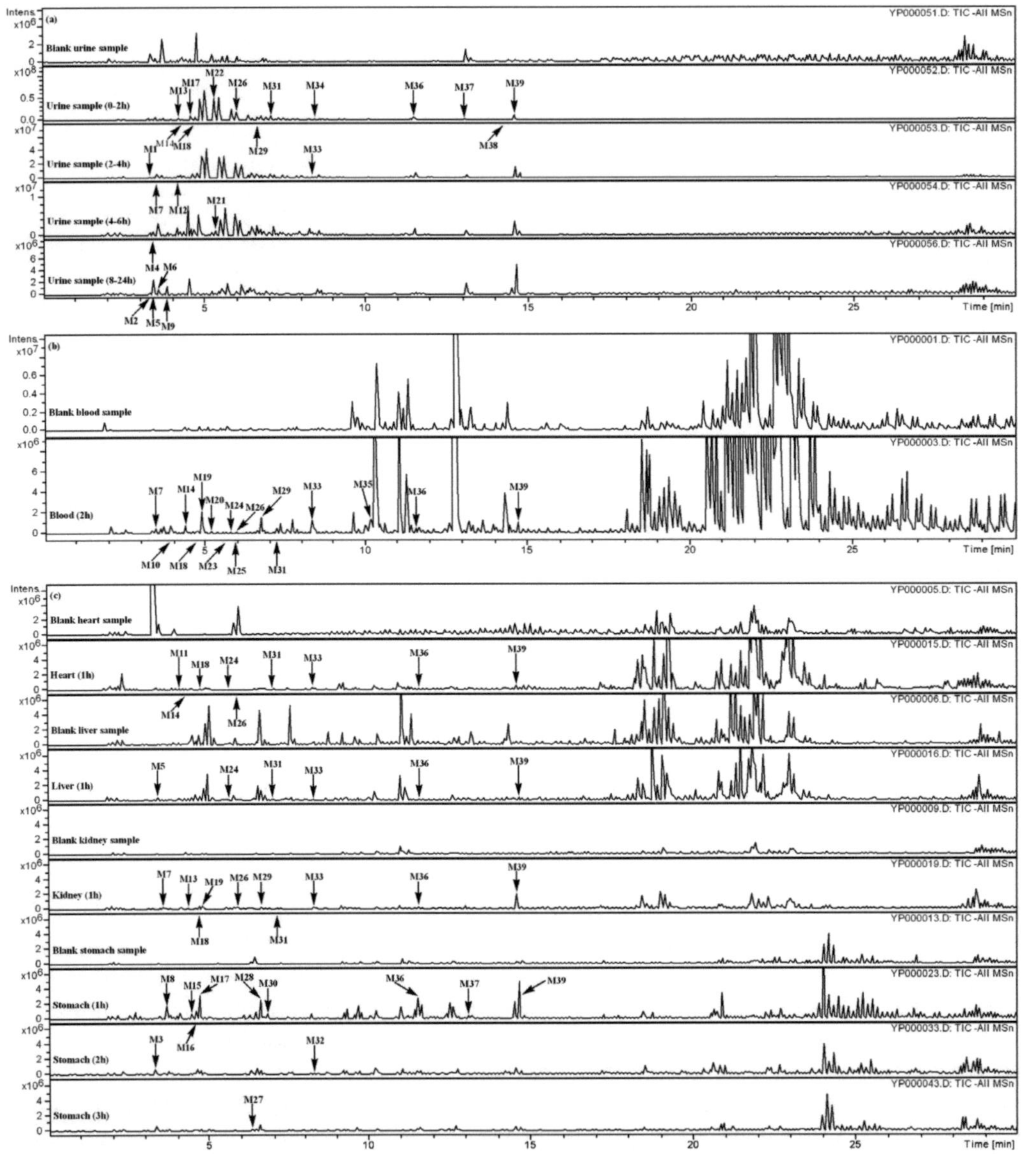

Fig. 2. Typical chromatograms of biological samples (a) chromatograms of urine samples after i.g. administration of 10 g/kg rhubarb decoction; (b) chromatograms of plasma samples after i.g. administration of 17.6 g/kg rhubarb decoction; (c) chromatograms of some tissue samples after i.g. administration of 17.6 g/kg rhubarb decoction

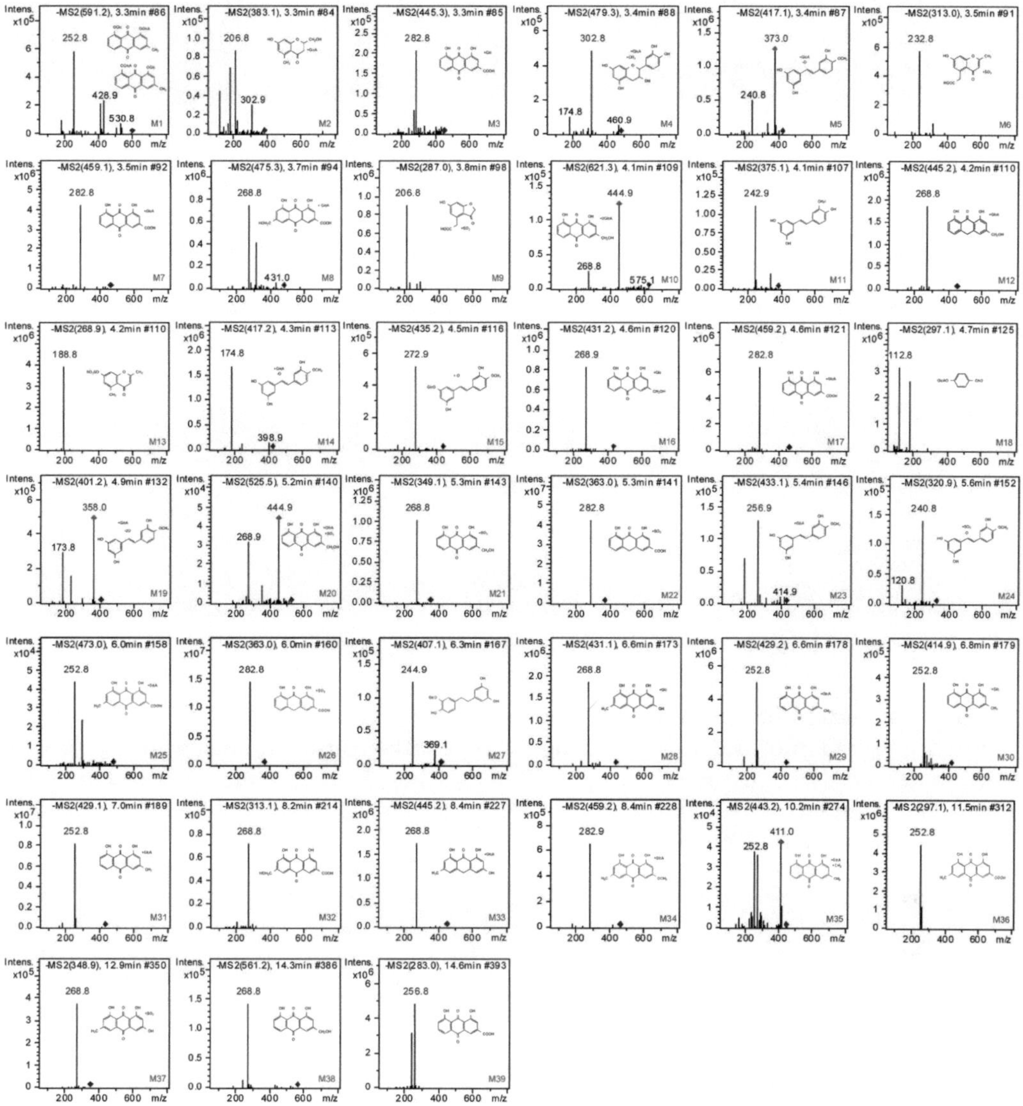

Fig. 3. The MS2 spectra of the 39 compounds

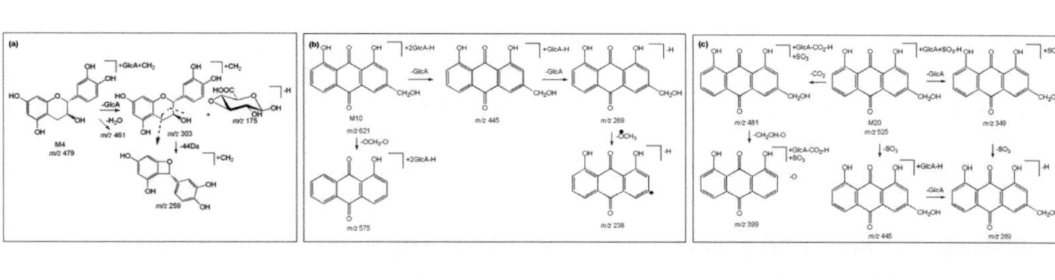

Fig. 4. Postulated fragmentation pathways of the selected metabolites (a) M4; (b) M10; (c) M20

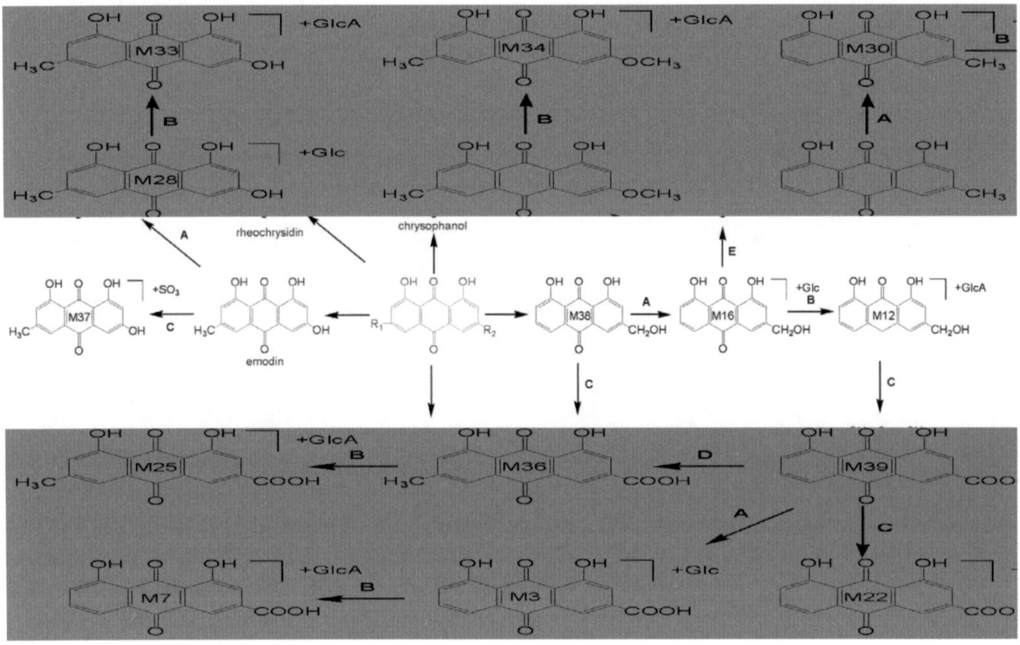

Fig. 5. The proposed transformation pathway of rhubarb in rats

3.8 Urinary excretion of rhubarb

The urinary excretion of rhubarb following a single intragastric administration of rhubarb decoction to rats is summarized in Fig.6. Among the 21 compounds detected in urine samples, the excretion of M22 and M39 were the largest, reaching more than 1000 µg in 48 h, the excretion of M5 and M26 has reached more than 500 µg.

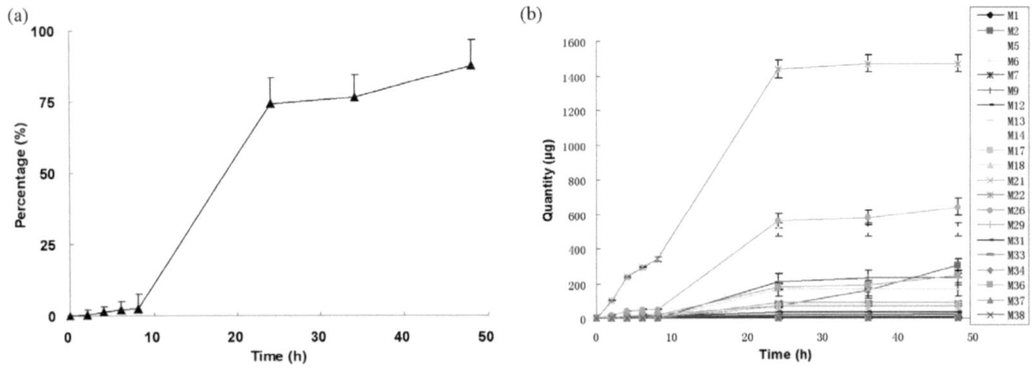

Fig. 6. Cumulative excretion curves of rhein (M39) and the metabolites of rhubarb following the intragastric administration of 10 g/kg rhubarb decoction to SD rats (a) the prototype component M39; (b) metabolites detected in urine samples

3.9 Plasma concentration of rhubarb and the metabolites

Among the 16 constituents detected in plasma, only rhein (M39) was the parent compound. The peak rhein concentration (Cmax) in plasma was 7.23 µg/ml. The peak concentration of

M19, a metabolite of emodin, reached 8.05 μg/ml at 2 h after i.g. administration of rhubarb decoction. The concentrations of the 16 compounds were shown in Table 2.

Time (h)	M7	M10	M14	M18	M19	M20	M23	M24	M25	M26	M29	M31	M33	M35	M36	M39
1	2.55	0.72	1.76	6.53	4.14	0.33	1.02	1.11	0	4.01	3.40	1.34	3.90	0.80	3.56	7.23
2	1.46	3.57	2.93	0	8.05	0.89	0.19	0.40	0.30	0	5.33	1.48	5.44	0	2.79	3.19
3	0	4.07	1.40	1.18	5.53	0.65	0.11	0	0.35	0	3.89	1.64	0	0	0.62	1.27

Table 2. The concentration of the 16 compounds detected in plasma (μg/ml)

3.10 Tissue distribution of rhubarb

Tissue distribution of the metabolites at 1.0, 2.0 and 3.0 h after a single intragastric administration of 10 g/kg rhubarb decoction to SD rats are also studied. Among the 24 metabolites found, M36 and M39 were distributed in most of the tissues, tissue concentrations of M36 and M39 are shown in Fig.7. At 1.0 h after intragastric dosing, tissue concentrations in most tissues were higher than the corresponding concentrations at 2.0 and 3.0 h. M7, M13, M18, M26, M29 and M33 reached the highest amount of concentration in kidney, M3, M8, M15, M16, M17, M27, M28, M30 and M37 reached the highest amount in stomach at 1.0 h after intragastric dosing. A total of nine compounds were detected in heart samples, seven in liver samples, four in lung samples, ten in kidney samples, thirteen in stomach samples, one in large intestine samples, three in small intestine samples and one in testis samples. The metabolites detected were shown in Table 1. The highest level of most of the metabolites was observed in the stomach, while none of the metabolites was found in spleen and brain.

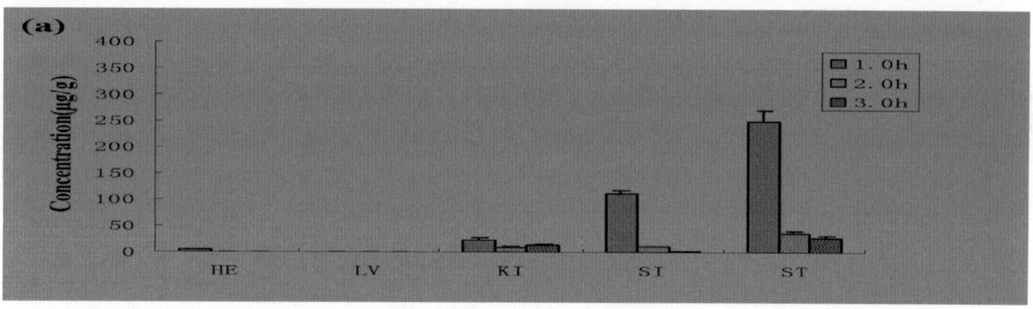

Fig. 7. Distribution of (a) M36, (b) M39 at 1.0h, 2.0h and 3.0h following intragastric administration of 10 g/kg rhubarb decoction to SD rats. Each value represents mean and SD of six animals.

4. Discussion

Many medicinal herbs have a long history of clinical use. However, the safety and efficacy of most of these herbs in relation to their pharmacological activities are poorly understood. Furthermore, knowledge of the pharmacokinetics of the main bioactive ingredients of these herbs is extremely limited. Dahuang is one of the most commonly prescribed Chinese medicinal herbs for the treatment of constipation. However, pharmacokinetics of the main bioactive ingredients in this herb is largely unknown.

In this paper, we developed a triple quadruple MS method for analysis and identification the main bioactive components and their possible metabolites in urine, plasma and tissues. Following a single intragastric administration of rhubarb decoction to rats, 21 constituents in urine samples and 16 compounds in plasma samples were identified. Some constituents of rhubarb were rapidly absorbed into blood and tissues, indicating that the compounds might be responsible for curative effects of rhubarb decoction. Ten compounds were detected in kidney samples, it may elucidate that rhubarb decoction has the effects of anti-diabetic and protecting chronic renal failure in rats. [9, 10].Their conjugations of glucosides, glucuronide and sulfates were also detected and two of the parent compound aloe-emodin and rhein. The developed method was simple, reliable and sensitive, which revealed that it will be appropriate for rapid analysis and identification the characterization of main bioactive components and their metabolites in biosamples. However, the present study still demonstrated the analytical potential of this approach for identification of metabolites. This identification and structure elucidation of these metabolites provided essential data for further pharmacological and clinical studies of rhubarb and related preparation.

5. Introduction

The root of *Scutellaria baicalensis*, called Huangqin in Chinese, is one of the most commonly used traditional Chinese medicines for the treatment of hepatitis, tumors, diarrhea, and inflammatory diseases [15]. It originated from Shennong Materia Medica, the earliest pharmacopoeia of China in Eastern Han (24-220 A.D.), and has been officially listed in the Chinese Pharmacopoeia for a long time. The major chemical constituents of Huangqin are flavonoids. Modern pharmacological studies have demonstrated that flavones have wide biological activities, such as anti-oxidants, anti-cancer, anti-inflammatory, *etc* [16,17,18]. Few data are available on the metabolism and metabolites of *S. baicalensis* extract *in vivo*. Therefore it is important to explicate the biotransformation of flavonoids *in vivo* so as to clarify the mechanism of pharmacological action and to promote its availability as well.

A simple and rapid high-performance liquid chromatographic-electrospray ionization (ESI) tandem mass spectrometric method has been developed for elucidation of the structures of the metabolites in rat plama, urine samples. LC-MS/MS is a more powerful analytical tool for the identification of durg metabolites in biological matrices by comparing changes in molecular masses (ΔM), retention-times, and spectral patterns of product ions with those of the parent drug [19,20].

6. Experimental

6.1 Chemicals and reagents

The roots of *Scutellaria baicalensis* Georgi were collected from Xi'an, ShanXi province, China, and authenticated by Professor Shen Jingui of Shanghai Institute of Materia Medica, Chinese Academy of Sciences. HPLC grade acetonitrile was purchased from Dikma Company (Dikma, USA). Water was deionized and double distilled. Other reagents used are of analytical grade.

6.2 Instrumentation

HPLC-MS experiments were performed with a Finnigan LCQ Advantage ion trap mass spectrometer (Thermo Finnigan, San Jose, CA) was connected to a Agilent 1100 HPLC instrument via an ESI source. The software Xcalibur version 1.2 (Finnigan) was applied for system operation and data collection. A high-speed desktop centrifuge (TGL-16C, Shanghai Anting Scientific Instrument Factory, Shanghai, China) was used to centrifuge urine, plasma sample. The urine, plasma sample were extracted on a C18 solid-phase extraction (SPE) cartridge (1ml/100mg, Supelco).

6.3 Chromatographic and mass spectrometric conditions

An Agilent series 1100 HPLC instrument (Agilent, Waldbronn, Germany) equipped with a quaternary pump, a UV detector, and a column compatment was used for analyses. The samples were separated on a Apollo C_{18} column (5μm, 4.6 × 250mm, Grace), including an EasyGuad Kit C_{18} (4 × 2mm) guard column. The column was maintained at 25°C. Detection wavelengths were set at 280nm. The flow rate was 0.8m/min. A gradient elution of 0.5% aqueous formic acid (A) and acetonitrile (B) was used as follows: 20% B in the first 10min, 20%~25% B at 10~11 min, then B held at 25% for 14min, linearly gradient to 35% B at 26 min and hold for 15min, 35%~55% B at 41~45 min, linearly gradient to 100%B at 50min and hold for 5min. The mass spectra were recorded in negative modes, drying gas flow rate 10L/min, drying gas temperature 35°C, nebulizer 35 psig., capillary voltage 4000V, fragmentor 100V, mass range 50-1500 m/z.

6.4 Administration

Male Sprague-Dawley (SD) rats (220 ± 10g body weigh, laboratory Animal Center of Shanghai University of Tradition Chinese Medicine) were divided into a blank group and drug group. Prior to oral administration, each rat was fasted for 24h in a metabolic cage with free access to water, and were then administered 1.2g/Kg the extract of *S. baicalensis* by i.g. Urine were collected separately at 2h, 4h, 6h, 8h, 10h and 24h. Samples were stored at -20°C until analysis. Blood samples were collected at 0.25, 0.5, 1, 3, 5, 7, and 24h after dosing from the caudal vein of the rats, then shaken and centrifuged at 4000rpm for 10min. The supernatant was decanted, and immediately frozen at -20°C until analysis.

6.5 Sample preparation

Solid phase extraction (SPE) with C18 cartridge (1ml/100mg, Supelclean™, Dikma) was used to purify the above supernatants of urine, plasma samples, for LC-MS/MS analysis. Before use, SPE columns were conditioned by 4ml methanol, 2ml deionized water. Then the selected supernatant sample was loaded, and the column was washed with 3ml deionized water to elute the impurity and 1ml methanol to elute the analytes in turn. The eluent was evaporated to dryness at 37°C in vacuum, and the residue dissolved in 100μl of 100% methanol. After centrifugation at 8000rpm. for 10min, 10μl of the supernatant was introduced into the HPLC system for HPLC-MS.

7. Results and discussion

7.1 Identification of metabolites

To elucidate the active constituents responsible for the pharmacological action, it is necessary to perceive the metabolic changes *in vivo* and chemical constituent profile in biological system. Therefore, the full-scan mass spectrum total-ion current chromatogram obtained from rat urine and plasma (Figs. 8(c), 9(b)) after *i.g.* of extract of *S. baicalensis* was compared with that from blank urine to find probable metabolites. The results show that the total peaks and corresponding peak areas in metabolic chromatograms were different when collected at different periods, and the most abundant metabolites were found at 4-6h in urine samples. These compounds were then analyzed by LC-MS/MS. Using negative ion electrospray tandem mass spectrometry, a total of 12 and 6 metabolites were detected in drug-containing urine and plasma samples in comparison with the extract of *S. baicalensis* and blank sample.

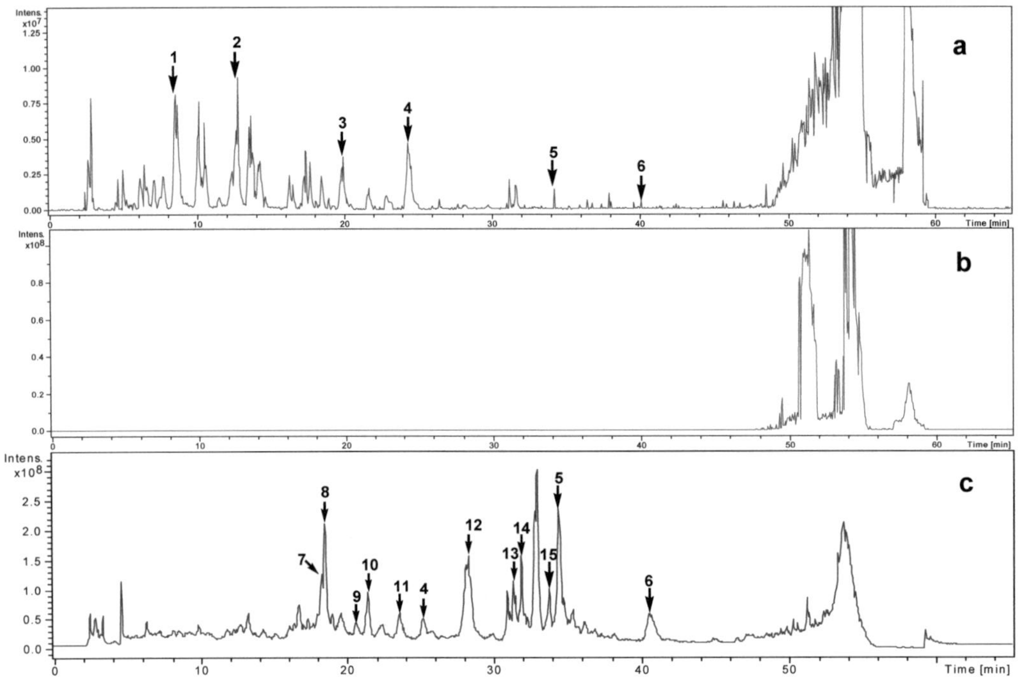

Fig. 8. HPLC-MS total ion current of the *S. baicalensis* decoction and its metabolites in negative mode. (a) The decoction of *S. baicalensis*; (b) Blank rat urine; (c) Urine sample after oral administration.

Peak 4 and 5 , 6 were confirmed as original components, baicalin (4) , wogonoside (5) and baicalein (6). The $[M-H]^-$ ion of baicalein at *m/z* 269 produced an ion at *m/z* 251, which should result from the loss of H_2O. The ion at *m/z* 241 was due to the loss of CO, and the *m/z* 223 ion was due to the successive loss of H_2O and CO.
Peak 6 showed $[M-H]^-$ m/z 445.3, with retention a Baicalin is an O-glucuronide. Upon CID, the glycosidic bond was easily cleaved to generate an ion at *m/z* 269, which resulted from the neutral loss of a glucuronic acid (Δm = 176u). In the MS^3 experiment, ion at *m/z* 269 produced the same ions as baicalein described above.
Wogonin is a methoxylated flavone. It exhibited a significant radical anion $[M-H-CH_3]^{-\bullet}$ as the base peak. In MS^3 spectra, we observed the significant ion at *m/z* 239 $[M-H-CH_3^{-\bullet}$ -$COH^\bullet]^-$, and the low signal intensity ions at *m/z* 163 ($^{0,2}A^-$), 212 $[M-H-CH_3^\bullet-2CO]^{-\bullet}$, 223 $[M-H-CH_3^\bullet-CO_2H^\bullet]^-$, 240 $[M-H-CH_3^\bullet-CO]^{-\bullet}$, which is identical with the previous report.
Peak 7 showed a $[M-H]^-$ m/z 607.4, with retention time at 18.3min on HPLC. Its MS^2 produced an ion at m/z 431 $[M-H-176]^-$, indicating the existence of a glucuronic acid.

Additionally, the successive yielded the ion at m/z 269 [M-H-176-162]-. Based on these data and by the knowledge on the flavones in *S. baicalensis*, compounds 1 were identified as Baicalein glucoside glucuronide conjugate.

Peak 8 gave a [M-H]- ion at *m/z* 621.4, with retention time at 18.5min on HPLC. CID of this compound produced an ion of [M-H-176]- at *m/z* 445, which resulted from the neutral loss of a glucuronic acid residue. In the MS^3 of *m/z* 445, fragments of *m/z* 430 and 269 indicated the presence of a H_2O and a glucuronic acid, respectively. Therefore, this compound was thus proposed as Baicalin glucuronide conjugate.

With a retention time at 19.6min on HPLC, peak 9 generated a [M-H]- at *m/z* 635.3 in MS spectrum and a [M-H]- at *m/z* 459 ([M-H]- -176, loss of a glucuronic acid) in MS^2. In the MS^3 experiment, ion at *m/z* 283 produced the same ions as wogonoside described above. Therefore, compound 9 was thus proposed as Wogonoside glucuronide conjugate.

Peak 10 displayed a [M-H]- ion at *m/z* 577.4, with retention time at 20.6min on HPLC. The MS^2 and MS^3 spectra gave ions at *m/z* 401 and 269, suggesting sequential losses of glucuronic acid (176 Da) and arabinose (132 Da) residues, respectively. This compound was thus identified as Baicalein xyloside glucuronide conjugate.

Peak 11 showed a $[M-H]^-$ ion at *m/z* 417.3, with retention time at 21.4min on HPLC. In the MS^2 speetrum of m/z 417.3, the fragment ion of 241 and 399 was generated by natural loss of a glucuronic acid and a H_2O, then the successive yielded the ion at m/z 199 [M-H-GlcA-$C_2H_2O]^-$ in MS^3. Therefore, it was tentatively identified as pinosylvin 2-hydroxymethyl glucuronide conjugate.

Peaks 12 and 15 are sulfation metabolites. Peak 12 with a retention at 23.6 min on HPLC, showed a $[M-H]^-$ m/z 539.4. In the MS^2 speetrum, the fragment ion of 363 and 459, indicating loss of a glucuronic acid and SO_3, respectively. Based on these data and by the knowledge on the flavones in *S. baicalensis*, this compound were identified as wongonoside sulfate conjugate. Peak 16 with a retention time at 33.7min on HPLC, yield MS fragments at m/z 363.2 and [M-H]- m/z 282.9 ([M-H]- - 80 Da, loss of a SO_3) in MS^2. Based on these data and by the knowledge on the flavones in *S. baicalensis*, this compound could be confirmed as wogonin sulfate conjugate.

Peak 13 gave a [M-H]- ion at *m/z* 447.3, with retention time at 31.3min on HPLC. CID of this compound produced an ion of [M-H-176]- at *m/z* 270.9, which resulted from the neutral loss of a glucuronic acid residue. Based on these data and by the knowledge on the flavones in *S. baicalensis*, this compound was thus proposed as baicalein glucuronide conjugate.

Peak 14, appearing at 31.8min on HPLC , had a [M-H]- at m/z 446 and yield a major ion at m/z 268.9 ([M-H]- - 176 Da, loss of a glucuronic acid unit) in MS^2 and a MS^3 fragment [M-H]- at m/z 251.0 ([M-H]- -176 Da–18 Da, loss of a glucuronic acid unit and one molecule of H_2O). Therefore it was presumed as apigenin glucuronide conjugate, which acts as one of the major apigenin metabolites in urine.

7.2 Plasma metabolites

The direct comparison of the TIC chromatograms of the blank rat plasma and the rat plasma samples collected at 0.5, 1, 2, 3, 4h after the oral administration of the extract of *S. baicalensis*. It showed that the information in the chromatogram at 1h post administration was more sufficient (Fig.9(b)). Including two original components, two metabolites, were tentatively elucidated as baicalin glucuronide conjugate (16), baicalin (4), norwogonoside glucuronide conjugate (17), wogonoside sulfate conjugate (18), wogonoside (5).

Peak 17 with retention time at 33.7min on HPLC, showed a $[M-H]^-$ ion of m/z 621.1. The MS^2 and MS^3 spectra gave ions at *m/z* 445 and 269, suggesting sequential losses of two glucuronic acid (2 ×176 Da) residues. In the MS^3 experiment, ion at *m/z* 225 produced $[M-2Glc\ A-CO-H]^-$. Base on these data, the structrue of 17 could be identified as norwogonoside glucuronide conjugate.

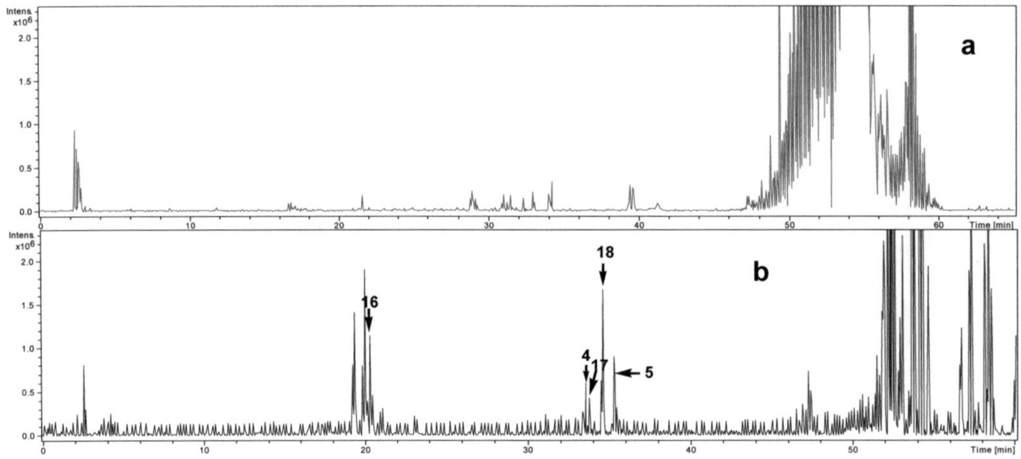

Fig. 9. HPLC-MS total ion current of the *S. baicalensis* decoction and its metabolites in negative mode. (a) Blank rat plasma; (b) Plasma sample after oral administration.

7.3 Identification of Baicalin metabolites in rat blood

Some reported that baicalin are the main active components of *S. baicalensis* [21]. In order to further study of baicalin metabolism *in vivo*. The metabolites of baicalin were studied further in rat plasma.

We identified three metabolites and the parent drug in rat plasma after administration of baicalin by healthy rats. Their protonated molecular ions ($[M-H]^-$) were at m/z 621, 643, and 564, respectively. MS^n spectra of motabolites, obtained by CID of their molecular ions, were used for more precise structural identification of metabolites. Among them, the retention time, the MS^2 and MS^3 spectra of the molecular ion at m/z 445 (M0) were the same as those of baicalin. Therefore, M0 is the unchanged parent drug.

M1 was observed at the retention time of 19.9 min and gave an deprotonated molecule $[M-H]^-$ at m/z 621. The ion at m/z 621 was increased by 176Da compared to that of unchanged baicalin and glucuronidation was a very common metabolic pathway of drug in vivo, indicating that M1 might be a conjugate of baicalin with glucuronic acid, which was confirmed by the characteristic fragment ions presented in the following MS^n spectrum. The $[M-H]^-$ ion at m/z 621 of M1 generated the base peak at m/z 445 in the MS/MS spectrum, attributed to the loss of 176 Da, suggesting the loss of a glucuronic acid. Then the product ion at m/z 445 was subjected to MS^3 analysis and produced an intense ion at m/z 268 by loss of a glucuronic acid group (176Da) again. Therefore, M1 was elucidated as baicalin glucuronide conjugate.

M2, eluted at 20.1 min, exhibited $[M-H]^-$ signal at m/z 643 which was 198 Da greater than that of parent compound, which indicated that M2 was a Na glucuronide metabolite of baicalin. The MS^2 spectrum of m/z 643 produced a significant radical ion at m/z 467 (Fig.10) via the loss of glucuronic acid (176Da). Then the ion at m/z 467 was successively subjected to MS[3] analysis and produced ion at m/z 269 by the loss of Na and glucuronic acid (198 Da). At the same time, the bask peak at m/z 241 was observed in the MS[4] spectrum by the loss of CO (28Da) from the ion at m/z 269. Therefore, M2 was tentatively proposed to be the baicalin Na glucuronide conjugate.

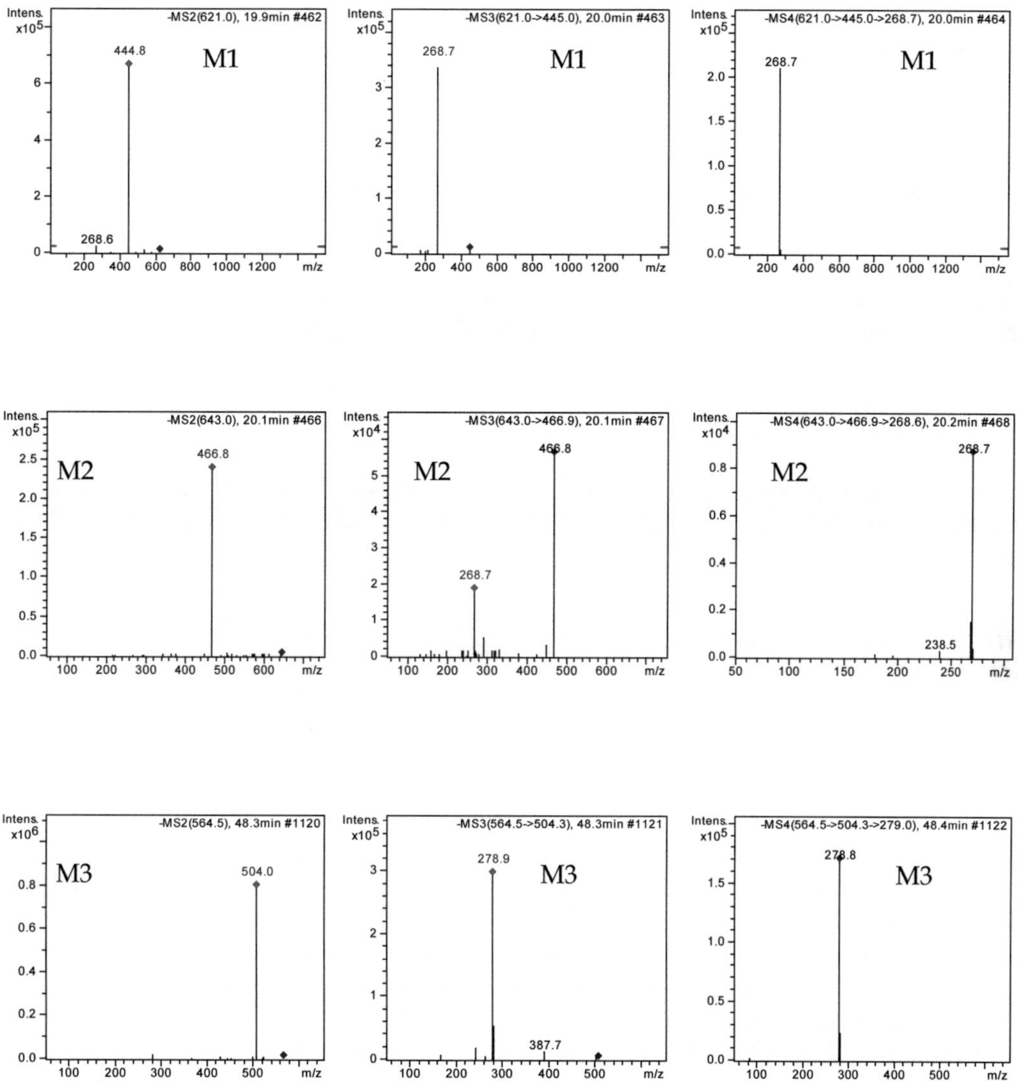

Fig. 10. Negative ion ESI-MS[n] spectra of baicalin metabolites in rat plasma

M3 was detected as a deprotonated molecule [M-H]- at m/z 564, with the retention time of 48.3 min. The molecular ion at m/z 564 was increased by 119 Da compared to that of the parent compound and there may be cysteine (119Da) reactions occurring at the baicalin skeleton. The molecular ion at m/z 564 by loss of the neutral fragment $C_2O_2H_3N$(60Da) produced the product ion at m/z 504 (Fig.10C) in the MS^2 spectrum. The obtained ion was subjected to MS^3 fragmentation, in which the base peak at m/z 389 was observed by the losing a glucuronic acid(176 Da). Based on the above results, M3 could be characterized as the baicalin cysteine conjugate.

8. Conclusion

In this paper, we discribe a strategy using liquid chromatogrphic-electrospray ionization (ESI) tandem ion trap mass spectrometric for fast analysis of the metabolic profile of *S. baicalensis* and baicalin. Using negative ion mode and applying the MS fragmentation rules of flavonoids reported before, 3 organic components, 9 metabolites in urine, 2 organic and 3 metabolites in plasma, were identified or tentatively identified in the extracts of *S. baicalensis.* 3 metabolites were identified in bacailin. However, several new analogues were identified in the present study, which proved that HPLC-MS is a powerful and rapid method to discover new constituents in Chinese medicinal herbs and its metabolites, help to lay the foundation of further study *in vivo.*

9. Acknowledgements

We thank the National Science & Technology Major Project "Key New Drug Creation and Manufacturing Program" (no. 2009ZX09301-001; 2009ZX09501-030; 2009ZX09308-005) and the National Natural Science Foundation of China (no. 20805054; 81030065) for financial support of this work.

10. References

[1] J. Wang, H. Zhao, W. Kong, C. Jin, Y. Zhao, Y. Qu, X. Xiao (2010). Microcalorimetric assay on the antimicrobial property of five hydroxyanthraquinone derivatives in rhubarb (*Rheum palmatum* L.) to *Bifidobacterium adolesentis*. *Phytomedicine*, 17: 684-689.

[2] K. Suresh Babu, P.V. Srinivas, B. Praveen, K. Hara Kishore, U. Suryanarayana Murty, J. Madhusudana Rao (2003). Antimicrobial constituents from the rhizomes of Rheum emodi. *Phytochemistry*, 62: 203-207.

[3] Mi Kyoung Moon, Dae Gill Kang, Jun Kyong Lee, Jin Sook Kim, Ho Sub Lee (2006). Vasodilatory and anti-inflammatory effects of the aqueous extract of rhubarb via a NO-cGMP pathway. *Life Sciences*, 78: 1550-1557.

[4] Sook-Kyoung He, Hyun-Jeong Yun, Eui-Kyu Noh, Sun-Dong Park (2010). Emodin and rhein inhibit LIGHT-induced monocytes migration by blocking of ROS production. *Vasc Pharmacol*, 53: 28-37.

[5] Hai-Rong Xiong, Jun Luo, Wei Hou, Hong Xiao, Zhan-Qiu Yang (2011). The effect of emodin, an anthraquinone derivative extracted from the roots of Rheum

tanguticum, against herpes simplex virus in vitro and in vivo. *J Ethnopharmacol*, 133: 718-23.

[6] Zhi-Heng He, Ming-Fang He, Shuang-Cheng Ma, Paul Pui-Hay But (2009). Anti-angiogenic effects of rhubarb and its anthraquinone derivatives. *J Ethnopharmacol*, 121: 313-317.

[7] Akira Iizuka, Osamu T. Iijima, Kazuo Kondo, Hiroshige Itakura, Fumihiko Yoshie, Hiroko Miyamoto, Masayoshi Kubo, Masami Higuchi, Hiroshi Takeda, Teruhiko Matsumiya (2004). Evaluation of Rhubarb using antioxidative activity as an index of pharmacological usefulness. *J Ethnopharmacol*, 91: 89–94.

[8] Li Liu, Shifang Yuan, Yin Long, Zhenjun Guo, Yang Sun, Yuhua Li, Yinbo Niu, Chen Li, Qibing Mei (2009). Immunomodulation of Rheum tanguticum polysaccharide (RTP) on the immunosuppressive effects of dexamethasone (DEX) on the treatment of colitis in rats induced by 2, 4, 6-trinitrobenzene sulfonic acid. *Int Immunopharmacol*, 9: 1568-1577.

[9] Jiabo Wang, Yanling Zhao, Xiaohe Xiao, Huifang Li, Haiping Zhao, Ping Zhang, Cheng Jin (2009). Assessment of the renal protection and hepatotoxicity of rhubarb extract in rats. *J Ethnopharmacol*, 124: 18-25.

[10] Jianfeng Xue, Wenjun Ding, Yan Liu (2010). Anti-diabetic effects of emodin involved in the activation of PPARγ on high-fat diet-fed and low dose of streptozotocin-induced diabetic mice. *Fitoterapia*, 81: 173–177.

[11] Chun-Hui Ma, Zhi-Xiong Li, Long-Xing Wang, Yi-Hong Tang, Hong-Bin Xiao, Cheng-Gang Huang (2009). Identification of Major Alkaloids in Rat Urine by HPLC/DAD/ESI-MS/MS Method Following Oral Administration of Cortex *Phellodendri* Decoction. *Helv Chim Acta*, 92: 379-397.

[12] Guan Ye, Hai-Yan Zhu, Zhi-Xiong Li, Chun-Hui Ma, Ming-Song Fan, Zhao-Lin Sun, Cheng-Gang Huang (2007). LC-MS characterization of efficacy substances in serum of experimental animals treated with *Sophora flavescens* extracts. *Biomed Chromatogr*, 21: 655-660.

[13] Rui Song, Lei Xu, Fengguo Xu, Zhe Li, Haijuan Dong, Yuan Tian, Zunjian Zhang (2010). *In vivo* metabolism study of rhubarb decoction in rat using high-performance liquid chromatography with UV photodiode-array and mass-spectrometric detection: A strategy for systematic analysis of metabolites from traditional Chinese medicines in biological samples. *Journal of Chromatography A*, 1217: 7144–7152.

[14] Susana González-Manzano, Ana González-Paramás, Celestino Santos-Buelga and Montserrat Dueñas (2009). Preparation and Characterization of Catechin Sulfates, Glucuronides, and Methylethers with Metabolic Interest. *J Agric Food Chem*, 57: 1231-1238.

[15] Pharmacopoeia of the People's Republic of China. Beijing: China Medical Technology Press. *National Commission of Chinese Pharmacopoeia*, 2010: 282.

[16] D.F. Birt, S. Hendrich, W.Q. Wang (2001). *Pharmacol Therapeut*, 90: 157.

[17] C.A. Williams, J.B. Harborne, H. Geiger, J. Robin, S. Hoult (1999). *Phytochemistry*, 51: 417

[18] A. Mantas, E. Detetey, F.H. Ferretti, M.R. Estrada, I.G. Csizmadia (2000). *J Mol Struct (Theochem)*, 504: 171.

[19] Y. Li, D. F. Zhong, S. W. Chen, I. Maeba (2005). *Acta Pharmacol Sin*, 26: 1519.
[20] A. Li, M. P. May, J. C. Bigelow (2006). *J Chromatogr B: Anal Technol Biomed Life Sci*, 836: 129.
[21] J. Han, M. Ye, M. Xu, J.H. Sun, B.R. Wang, D. Guo (2007). *J Chromatogr B*, 848: 355.

22

Traditional Chinese Medicine Active Ingredient-Metal Based Anticancer Agents

Zhen-Feng Chen, Hong Liang and Yan-Cheng Liu
Guangxi Normal University,
China

1. Introduction

Traditional Chinese medicine (TCM) possesses a rich and ancient history, tracing its roots back several thousand years. The practice of TCM, highly influenced by the development of Chinese culture, involves physical therapy using acupuncture, moxibustion (application of heat to the acupuncture point by burning a piece of the Chinese plant Artemisia moxa on the skin or the acupuncture needle), and chemical therapy. TCM natural products are isolated as decoctions of animal, mineral and herbal materials (Chan, 1995; Shibata, 1985;). The objective of the system of TCM is on the patient rather than disease, which fundamentally intention to promote health and enhance the quality of life, with therapeutic strategies for treatment of specific disease or symptoms in holistic fashion. TCM represents an old Chinese philosophical thinking, where the human is considered the centre of the universe and acts as an antenna between celestial and earthly elements of the world. The world is a single unit and its movement affords yin and yang, the two main antithetic aspects. Moreover, Chinese believe that yin and yang are not absolute but relative. Consistent with the modern view of homeostasis, yin and yang are interchanged to meet the view that yang decline and yin rises? Or yang is raised to produce a decline of yin? The four bodily humors (qi, blood, moitsture and essence) and internal organ systems (zang fu) play an important role in balancing the yin and yang in human body. Proper formation, maintenance and circulation of these energies are essential for health. When the two energies fall out of harmony, and the balance is broken, disease develops (Patwardhan et al., 2005). The physician takes into account this concept while treating patients. Drugs or herbs are used to correct this imbalance of yin-yang in the human body (Cheng, 2000; Gibert, 1998).

Different from TCM, western science and medicine are focused on the mechanism, which belongs to reductionism. Rather than addressing the overall well being of a patient, it is only the disease that is analyzed at the cellular, molecular, and pharmacological level. The history, philosophy, theory and practice of TCM can been seen in recent reviews (Liu, 1988), herein, we do not give unnecessary details.

Although medicinal herbs have played an important role in Western medicine from ancient to modern times, medicinal plants gradually lost their importance as synthetic pharmaceuticals advanced in Western countries during the 20th century. Currently, there is a revival of interest in bioactive natural products as chemical lead compounds for the generation of semi-synthetic derivatives, namely regression nature.

Traditional Chinese medicine (TCM) has held, and still holds, an important position in primary health care over vast rural areas of China and is appreciated in urban and well-developed areas because of its 5000-year-old tradition. Recently, the Chinese government has undertaken enormous efforts to modernize TCM by investing capital in scientific research, technology programs, and in the economic development of TCM therapies. In the Western world, interest in TCM is increasing due to the belief that it may lead to novel TCM-Western hybrid medicines and treatments.

Since the discovery of cisplatin (**1**, Fig. 1) in 1969, great progress has been made expanding the diversity of platinum anticancer drugs and the conditions they treat (Alt et al., 2007; Clark et al., 1999; Giandomenico, 1999; Jung & Lippard, 2007; Orvig & Abrams, 1999; Rosenberg et al., 1969; Wataru et al., 2008; Wong & Jamieson & Lippard, 1999; Zutphen & Reedijk, 2005). Cisplatin is currently used to treat bladder, non-small cell lung, head and neck, ovarian, cervical, and other cancers, being curative in nearly all cases of testicular cancers. Several similar platinum complexes with fewer toxic side effects, carboplatin (**2**, Fig.1) and oxaliplatin (**3**, Fig.1) were approved as a first-line treatment for colorectal cancer. Nedaplatin (**4**, Fig. 1) was approved for use in Japan, and lobaplatin (**5**, Fig.1) was approved for use in China (Lovejoy & Lippard, 2009). During the past three decades, medicinal chemists have investigated many approaches to enhance antitumor activity, reduce side effects, and overcome drug resistances. To data, thousands of platinum compounds have been synthesized, characterized, and their antitumor activity investigated; however, only 30 platinum compounds have entered clinical trials. Moreover, none have exceeded the anticancer activity of cisplatin. Obviously, current synthetic strategies for development of metal-based anticancer are inefficient (Kelland, 2007). Although non-platinum antitumor metal complexes exhibit different action mechanisms and structural characteristics compared to platinum drugs, the antitumor activity of these non-platinum compounds needs to be determined and their action mechanisms await further investigation. Recent research has shown that metal complexes based on TCMs afforded a novel approach to a potential (pro-) drugs (Chen et al., 2009; Ho et al., 2001; Liu et al., 2009).

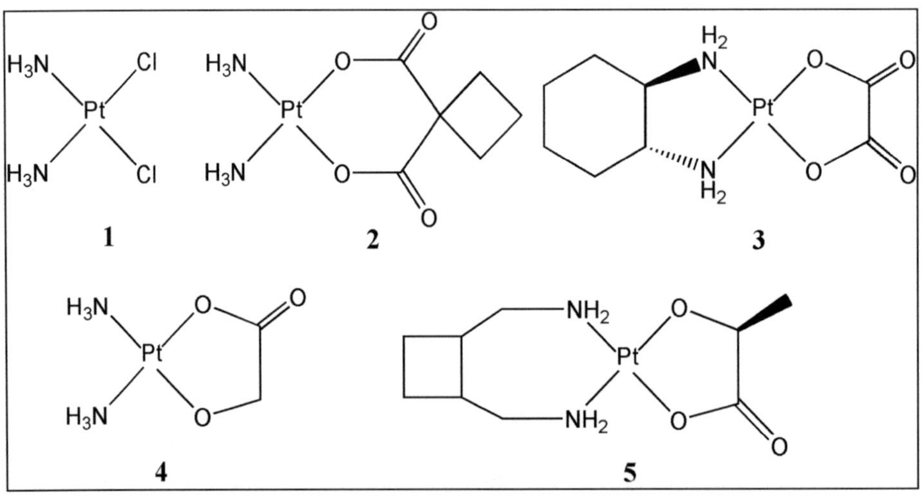

Fig. 1. Strucutres of platinum compounds currently in clinical use. 1: cisplatin, 2: carboplatin, 3: oxaliplatin, 4: nedaplatin, 5: lobaplatin.

2. The anticancer metal-based agents based on TCM active ingredients

Considering the low success rate of current metal-based anticancer synthetic strategies, some bioinorganic chemists have shifted focus to TCM derivatives. There are many successful examples of TCM-derived anticancer agents through organic modification of the active TCM constituents, which is considered a shortcut to discover new anticancer drugs, however, the TCM-metal based anticancer agents are still lack of enough attention, which represent another approach of modification. It is well known that metals and metal complexes can make significant contributions to drug development, but are not receiving the attention they merit. Metal complexes are relative easy to prepare, and the additional geometric possibilities resulting from the use of six-coordinate metal centres (compared to four-coordinate carbon) make this an attractive approach for the rapid development of new species, either as drugs or as probes of the geometric requirements of active sites (Hambley, 2007). Along with the TCM coordination chemistry theory springs up, it is convinced of that metal ion existence plays important role in TCM. Moreover, due to many active compounds containing hydroxyl, carboxylic acid, and amine groups, they are excellent donor atoms that may easily form coordination bonds. Developing TCM coordination complexes may lead to novel therapies that synergistically combine the functions of TCM and metals, generating a novel strategy that bridges traditional Chinese medicine to rational cancer therapy. This concept has attracted increased interest in TCM-metal based antitumor agents. Herein, we review the progress in TCM-metal based anticancer agents according to the TCM active gradient category.

2.1 Alkaloid-metal based anticancer agents

Alkaloids, which are generally defined as nitrogen-containing natural molecules independently of the basic character of the nitrogen, are abundant secondary metabolites in plants and represent one of the most widespread class of compounds endowed with multiple, varied pharmacological properties, including anticancer, antibacterial, anti-fungi, and even anti-virus activities. Up to now, the alkaloid-metal based anticancer agents mainly include oxoaporphine, matrine, β-carboline alkaloid-metal based anticancer agents.

2.1.1 Liriodenine-metal based anticancer agents

Among alkaloids, the aporphinoids constitute a broad subgroup of benzylisoquinoline compounds, with more than 500 alkaloids isolated up to now. They are widely distributed in a large number of plant families including *Annonaceae, Magnoliaceae, Monimiaceae, Menispermaceae, Hernandiaceae, Renunculaceae*. Our group has widely carried out a series of investigations on oxoaporphine-metal based anticancer agents. Liriodenine (**6**, Fig. 2), as an oxoaporphine alkaloid, was isolated for the first time form Liriodendron *tulipifera L.* and was subsequently found mainly in the family of *Annonaceae, Rutaceae, Magnoliaceae, Monimiaceae, Menispermaceae*, ect. (Bentley, 2001; Lan et al., 2003; Lin et al., 1994; Hsien et al., 2005; Nissanka et al., 2001; Woo et al., 1997; Wu et al., 1990). Liriodenine has a wide range of pharmacological activities, such as anti-bacterial, anti-fungi, antitumour and even anti-virus activities. Due to its planar aromatic structure, liriodenine can intercalate into the neighbouring base pairs of DNA double helix, to which its significant antitumor activity can be primarily attributed. Moreover, it also catalytically inhibits topoisomerase to block DNA synthesis and increase p53 and iNOS expression to induce cell cycle G1 arrest (Chang et al, 2004). Liriodenine has been isolated by our group from a classical Chinese herb richly yield in Guangxi Province of China, *Zanthoxylum nitidum* Var. *Fastuosum*, known for its significant anticancer properties. Based on the planar character of liriodenine and its N-7/O-8 donor sites, it can ligate metal ions (M^{n+}) to form metal-based bifunctional compounds with potential synergistic effects on antitumor activity.

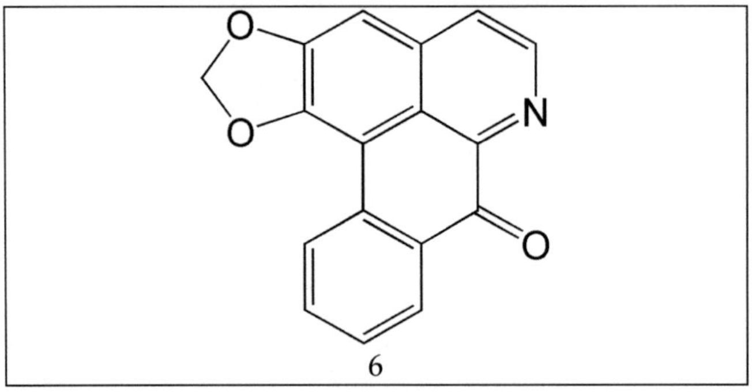

Fig. 2. Structure of liriodenine.

Reaction of liriodenine (L) with Pt(II), Ru(II), Mn(II), Fe(II), and Zn(II) as well as a series of lanthanides afforded a series of metal complexes. The crystal structures of *cis*-[Pt(L)(DMSO)Cl_2] (7), *cis*-[Ru(L)(DMSO)Cl_2]·1.5H_2O (**8**) (Chen et al., 2009); [MnCl_2(L)$_2$] (**9**), [FeCl_2(L)$_2$] (**10**), [Zn_2(L)$_2$(μ_2-Cl)$_2$$Cl_2$] (**11**) (Fig.3) (Liu et al., 2009); [Ce(L)$_2$(NO_3)$_3$] (12), [Pr(L)$_2$(NO_3)$_3$] (**13**), [Sm(L)$_2$(NO_3)$_3$] (**14**), [Eu(L)$_2$(NO_3)$_3$] (**15**) (Fig. 4) (Chen et al., 2011), were determined by single crystal X-ray diffraction methods. These complexes were fully characterized by elemental analysis, IR, ^{1}H and ^{13}C NMR spectroscopy, and ESI-MS spectrometry.

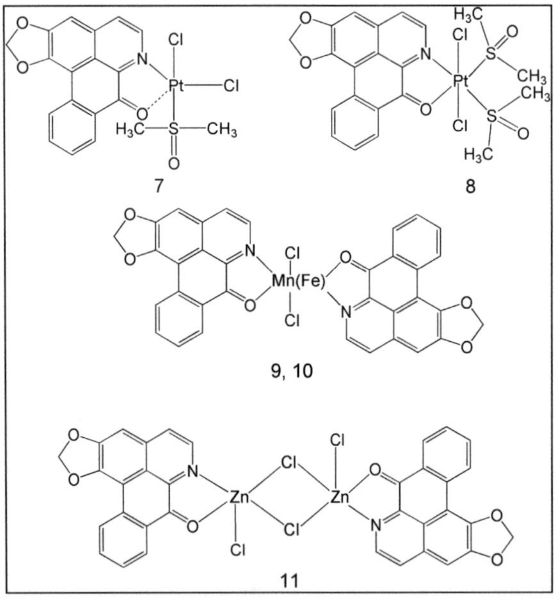

Fig. 3. Crystal structures of *cis*-[PtCl_2(L)(DMSO)] (7), *cis*-[RuCl_2(L)(DMSO)$_2$] (**8**), MnCl_2(L)$_2$] (**9**), [FeCl_2(L)$_2$] (**10**), and [Zn_2(L)$_2$(μ_2-Cl)$_2$$Cl_2$] (**11**).

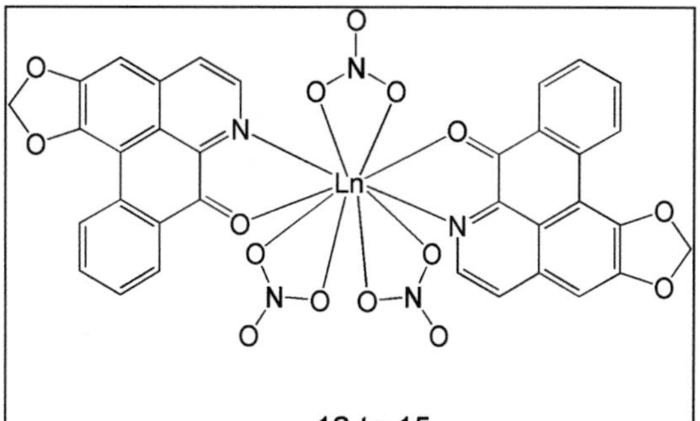

Fig. 4. Structures of four lanthanide complexes (**12** to **15**) with liriodenine.

The *in vitro* cytotoxicity of L and a series of its metal complexes against a panel of tumour cell lines have been evaluated by MTT method. The results show that these liriodenine metal-based compounds exhibit enhanced cytotoxicity *vs.* free L in most cases, and the IC_{50} values are in range of μM, suggesting that these compounds display synergic effect in the combination of metal ions and liriodenine. Although there is some evidence to suggest that other biological targets, including RNA or proteins, may be important in the cisplatin action mechanism, it is generally accepted that DNA is the primary target. Similarly, interactions between small molecules and DNA rank among the primary action mechanisms of anticancer activity. DNA replication in tumour cells will be blocked by the small molecule intercalation of the neighboring base pairs of DNA. On the other hand, topoisomerases are ubiquitous molecules that relieve the torsional stress in the DNA helix generated as a result of replication, transcription, and other nuclear processes; they are also specific targets for a number of anticancer agents (Baraldi et al., 2004), including the camptothecins, indolocarbazoles, and indenoisoquinolines. These compounds bind to a transient topoisomerase I (TOPO I)-DNA covalent complex and inhibit the resealing of a single-starnd nick that the enzyme creates to relieve superhelical tension in duplex DNA (Holfalnd et al, 2000; Staker et al., 2005). Therefore, in our researches, we investigated the interactions of these compounds with DNA and TOPO I. The interactions between ct-DNA and L or its Pt(II) and Ru(II) complexes through UV-Vis, fluorescence, EB competition binding, CD spectra, viscosity and agarose gel electrophoretic experiments reveal that these compounds mostly adopted a classical intercalation mode with DNA, but the metal complexes may bind covalently to DNA simultaneously because they easily hydrolyze to give coordinate active sites. Based on quantitative analysis of spectral titration experiments, it can conclude that the Pt(II) and Ru(II) complexes have higher binding ability than L itself does, suggesting that the metal complexes of planar L reinforce the binding ability. Although these results do not display a good coherence with what has been revealed in quantitative spectral analysis, however, it still confirms that DNA is an important target in cellular systems for these metal-based compounds derived from TCM. To introduce a TCM as a ligand to form bifunctional metal-based anticancer compounds (Herein, bifunction means TCM moiety intercalation and complex covalent binding to DNA, and differs from the meaning appearing in previous literature (Song et al., 2002; Wu et al., 2005) is a new effective strategy to achieve promising potential metal-based anticancer drug.

The *in vitro* cytotoxicity of three divalent transition metal (Mn(II), Fe(II), Zn(II)) complexes against 10 human tumor cell lines shows that most of these metal complexes exhibit higher cytotoxicity than L or cisplatin does, suggesting a probable synergistic effect upon liriodenine (L) coordinated to metal ions. The interactions between ct-DNA and L or its four divalent later transition metal complexes studied by UV-Vis, fluorescence, EB competition binding and CD spectra, as well as viscosity measurements and gel mobility shift assay experiments, reveal that these compounds mostly adopted an intercalation mode with DNA. Complexes **9**, **10** have higher binding affinity than L itself, suggesting that the metal complexes of planar L reinforce the binding ability. But it is lower than that of typical metallointercalator, which could be attributed to dichloride complex species (neutral) without chloride ligand exchange for water in short incubation period. In contrast, for biological assay on tumor cell lines, the long period incubation could allow (inside the cell) the conversion to diaqua species (dicationic) with a better interaction with NDA, and exhibit satisfied cytotoxicity. The electrostatic interactions between complex **11** and the polyanionic backbone of DNA helix should be considered simultaneously. Complex **11** tends to hydrolyze to form coordination unsaturated species, $[Zn(L)]^{2+}$, which can covalently bound to DNA. In addition, complexes **9–11** exhibit significant topoisomerase I inhibition ability at lower concentrations in contrast to L, implying topoisomerase I may be another molecular target. Although the exact molecular mechanism (including the real complex species in these metal complexes interacting with ct-DNA and tumour cell lines) needs further more detailed investigation, anyway, the three synthesized divalent later transition metal complexes of liriodenine exhibit significant enhanced cytotoxicity, offering a new effective strategy to achieve promising potential dual targeting cytotoxic agents by combining bioactive non-cytotoxic metal ions with cytotoxic active components from TCM.

The *in vitro* cytotoxicity of the lanthanide complexes **12–15** of liriodenine against four selected cell lines (7702, SK-OV-3, 7404, NCI-H460) were tested using MTT colorimetric method. The results indicate that the metal complexes exhibit enhanced cytotocicity against the four selected cell lines than that of liriodenine, which display the synergistic effects. All the complexes exhibit higher cytotoxicity to the tested tumor cells than ligand and cisplatin does. Remarkably, among these complexes, complexes **13** and **14** exhibit the highest cytotoxicity to tumour cells SK-OV-3, with IC_{50} values of 0.22±0.09 and 0.23±0.05 μM. The interactions between the liriodenine, its complexes and DNA were investigated by using various spectroscopic methods such as UV-Vis, fluorescence, CD, as well as viscosity and agarose gel electrophoresis experiments. The results indicate that liriodenine and its metal complexes interacted with DNA in an intercalation binding mode due to the liriodenine having good planarity and the π cyclic conjugated system. DNA has negative charge, there exist electrostatic interactions between liriodenine, its complexes. The interaction of complexes and DNA are stronger than that of liriodenine, it is agreed well with the results of antitumor activity tests. Overall, these liriodenine-metal complexes interact with DNA mainly by intercalation and electrostatic interaction, which blocks DNA synthesis and replication and induces cytotoxicity.

2.1.2 Oxoglaucine-metal based anticancer agents

Oxoglaucine (OG, **16**, Fig. 5) is an oxoaporphine alkaloid that has been isolated from overground parts of plants belonging to different families such as *Annonaceae* (Chang et al., 1998; Chen et al., 1996), *Lauraceae* (Chen et al., 1998), *Magnoliaceae* (Chen et al., 1976), *Fumariaceae* (Blanco et al., 1993; Tojo et al., 1991), *Menispermaceae* (Ohiri et al., 1982) and *Papveraceae* (Sari, 1999), which is also found widely exist in many traditional Chinese medicine, such as *aquilegia ecalcarata Maxim* (*Ranunculaceae*) mainly distributed in Sichuan and Yunnan Provinces of China and used for the treatment of necrotic boils, pustulosis and other infections (Wu et al., 1998). The primary screening results reveal that oxoglaucine possesses strong anticancer activity, such as against HCT-8 (ED_{50} = 1.00 μg/ml) and K_B (ED_{50} = 2.00 μg/ml) (Chang et al., 2002; Chen et al., 2002; Wu et al., 1989). In addition, oxoglaucine exhibits other important pharmacological activities including antiplatelet aggregation (Chang et al., 1998; Jantan et al., 2006), immunomodulatory activity (Ivanovska et al., 1997 and 2000), treatment of adjuvant arthritis (Ivanovska & Hristova, 2000), anti-inflammatory (Remichkova et al., 2009), antifungal activity (Clark et al., 1987).

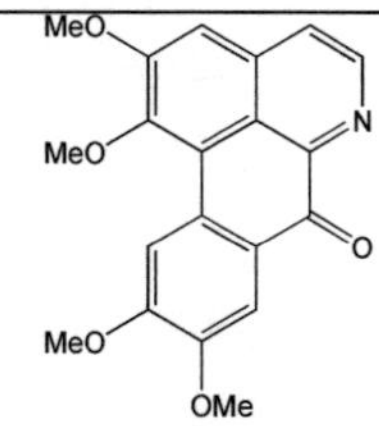

16

Fig. 5. Structure of oxoglaucine (**16**).

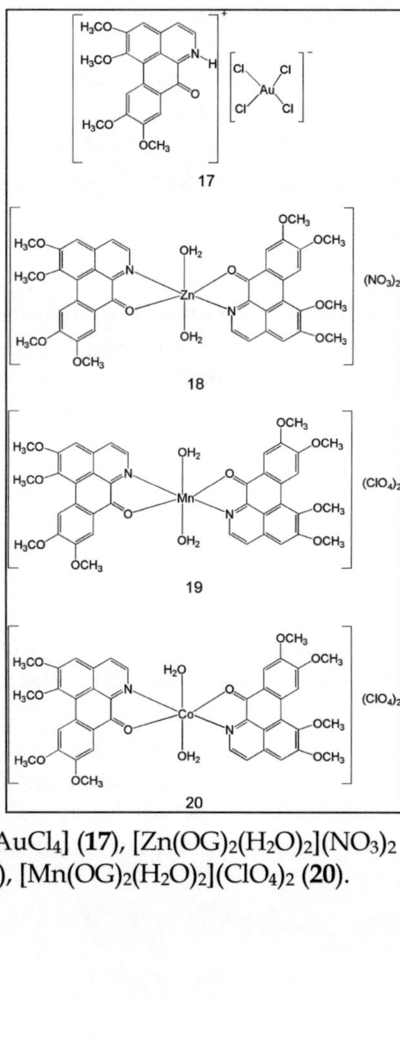

Fig. 6. Structures of $[OGH][AuCl_4]$ (**17**), $[Zn(OG)_2(H_2O)_2](NO_3)_2$ (**18**), $[Mn(OG)_2(H_2O)_2](ClO_4)_2$ (**19**), $[Mn(OG)_2(H_2O)_2](ClO_4)_2$ (**20**).

Oxoglaucine alkaloid (OG) was synthesized via a two-step reaction route. Using OG as ligand to react with corresponding transition metal salts gave rise to four metal-based compounds: $[OGH][AuCl_4]\cdot DMSO$ (**17**), $[Zn(OG)_2(H_2O)_2](NO_3)_2$ (**18**), $[Mn(OG)_2(H_2O)_2](ClO_4)_2$ (**19**), $[Co(OG)_2(H_2O)_2](ClO_4)_2$ (**20,** Fig. 6), whose structures were determined by X-ray single crystal diffraction analysis. The *in vitro* cytotoxicity of **17–20** against various tumour cell lines was assayed by MTT method. The results show that most of these metal-based compounds of oxoglaucine exhibit enhanced cytotoxicity *vs.* oxoglaucine and corresponding metal salts, with IC_{50} values ranging from 1.4 to 32.7 μM for sensitive cancer cells, implying a positive synergistic effect. Moreover, these complexes seem to be selectively active against certain cell lines. The interactions of oxoglaucine and its metal complexes with DNA and topoisomerase I were investigated by spectroscopic, viscosity and agarose gel electrophoresis measurements, which indicate that these OG metal–based compounds interact with DNA mainly *via* intercalation mode. Of special note, these metal-based compounds effectively inhibit Topoisomerase I even at low concentration, implying topoisomerase I may be another molecular target. However, the exact molecular mechanism requires further detailed investigation. Cell-cycle analysis revealed that these OG-metal complexes cause S-phase cell arrest.

2.1.3 Matrine-metal based anticancer agents

Matrine, a quinolizidine alkaloid matrine (MT), a main component found in roots of the Chinese herb *Sophora* including *Sophora flavescens* and *Sophora tonkinensis,* was selected as an active ligand. Matrine has been extensively used in China for the treatment of viral hepatitis and cardiac diseases (Liu et al., 2007). Matrine also exhibits inhibition activity toward many tumour cells (such as HeLa cell and gastric cancer MKN45 cell) (Galasso et al., 2006; Luo et al., 2007; Ruan et al., 2006; Zhang et al., 2001 & 2007).

Three TCM-metal compounds of Ga(III), Au(III), with Sn(IV) and matrine (MT), $[H\text{-}MT][GaCl_4]$ (**21**), $[H\text{-}MT][AuCl_4]$ (**22**) and $[SnCl_5(H\text{-}MT)]$ (**23,** Fig. 7), have been synthesized and characterized. The crystal structure analyses reveal that **21** and **22** are ionic compounds, while **23** is a coordination compound formed by monodentate MT *via* its carbonyl O (Fig.7). But the ESI-MS results show that they may exist with ionic species: $[H\text{-}MT]^+$, $[GaCl_4]^-$, $[AuCl_4]^-$ and $[SnCl_5]^-$ in water solution. The *in vitro* cytotoxicities of **21,** **22** and **23** against eight selected human tumour cell lines are different. In some case, they exhibit significant enhanced antitumour activity, such as **21** to SW480, **22** to HeLa, HepG2 and MCF-7, which exceed matrine and cisplatin, and display synergistic contribution of their components. However, in the case of **23**, such synergistic effect could not be observed due to the electronic structure alteration of lactam group of matrinium, thus **23** exhibits lower antitumour activity than that of compounds **21** and **22**. Although the spectroscopic and agarose gel electrophoresis assay show that these compounds bind to DNA inducing only small structural changes in the duplex, it could lead to a different cellular response. The cell cycle analyses show that compounds **21, 23** and MT exhibit cell cycle arrest at the G2/M phase. Their interactions with ct-DNA indicate that these metal-matrine compounds may be act mainly via intercalation mode of H-MT. In addition, **21** and **22** exhibit potent TOPO I inhibition ability, implying topoisomerase I may be another molecular target. However, the exact molecular mechanism requires further detailed investigation (Chen et al., 2011).

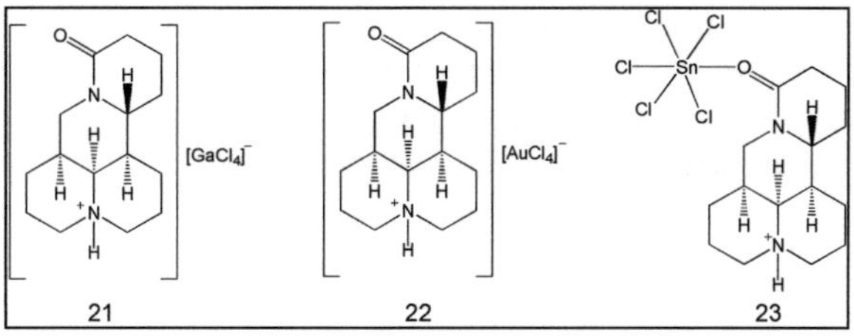

Fig. 7. Structures of [H-MT][$GaCl_4$] (**21**), [H-MT][$AuCl_4$] (**22**) and [$SnCl_5$(H-MT)] (**23**).

2.1.4 β-Carboline alkaloid-metal based anticancer agents

β-Carboline alkaloids, naturally occurring nitrogen-containing ligands, for example, harmaline (4,9-dihydro-7-methyl-3H-pyrido[3,4-b]indole), harmalol (4,9-dihydro-1-methyl-3H-pyrido[3,4-b] indole-7-ol), harmine (7-methoxy-1-methyl-9H-pyrido[3,4-b]indole), and harmane (1-methyl-9H-pyrido[3,4-b]indole), are extremely effective as antituberculosis, analgesic, and antimicrobial agents. Al-Allaf and co-worker reported the synthesis and cytotoxic evaluation of a series of novel biologically active platinum(II) (**24**, **26**, **28**, **30**) and palladium(II) (**25**, **27**, **29**, **31**, **32**, Fig. 8) complex of some β-carboline alkaloids (harmaline, harmine, and harmane). These complexes exhibited promising antitumour activity. The IC_{50} of the complexes varied from 0.2 to 2.0 μg/mL in the antiproliferative assays against three tumour cell lines, and the calculated therapeutic index varied again from 10 to 20 μg/mL (Al-Allaf et al., 1990; Al-Allaf & Rashan, 1998).

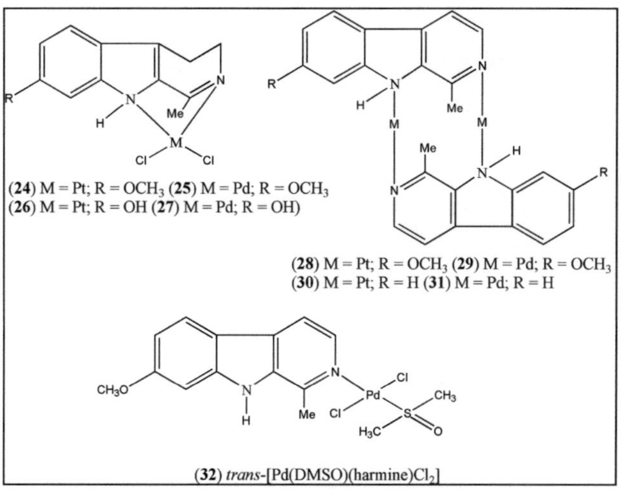

Fig. 8. Structures of β-carboline alkaloid-metal complexes (**24-32**).

2.2 Flavonoid-metal based anticancer agents

Flavonoids are found in many plants and belong to a group of natural substances occurring in TCM with variable phenolic structures. Their therapeutic effects were known long before they were isolated (Nijveldt et al., 2001). Flavonoids display many important biological effects including antitumour, antioxidative, anti-inflammatory (inhibition of cyclooxygenase and lipoxygenase), antiviral, antibacterial, and antifungal actions. They also were shown to be effective inhibitors of platelet aggregation (Narayana et al., 2001; Nijhoff et al., 1995).

2.2.1 Chrysin, morin-metal based anticancer agents

Chrysin (5, 7-di-OH-flavone) is one flavonoid occurring in TCM, a natural ligand for benzodiazepine receptors with anticonvulsant properties. Complexes with Co(II), Ni(II), Cu(II), Pb(II), Fe(III) and Y(III) etc., have been synthesized and characterized. [Ansari, 2008; Engelmann et al., 2005; Pusz et al., 1997, 2000] Recently, Tang et al. reported chrysin-La(III) complex, La(chrysin)$_2$(OAc)·7H_2O (**33**, Fig. 9), which exhibited high inhibition rate (*in vitro*) to A549 and P388 with 74.5% and 42.4 at 10μM, respectively; and higher too much than that of chrysin (4.9% and 16.7%). The intrinsic binding constants of La(III) complex and chrysin are 1.29×10^6 and $5.44 \times 10^5 M^{-1}$, respectively, which are considered both them bind to DNA by intercalation (Zeng et al., 2003).

Morin (2', 3, 4', 5, 7-pentahydroxyflavone) occurs in TCM and has antitumour activity (Alldrick et al., 1986). Wang et al. synthesized and characterized two complexes, Zn(morin)$_2$·3H_2O (**34**, Fig. 9) and Cu(morin)$_2$·2H_2O (**35**, Fig. 9) The two complexes exhibit higher *in vitro* antitumour activity to Hep-2, BBHK-2, BHK21 and HL-60 than morin alone, but the antitumour activity of the cobalt(II) complex (**36**, Fig. 9) is lower than morin (Zhang et al., 1996). Song and co-worker investigated the Zn(II) and Co(II) complexes of morin bound to ct-DNA by spectroscopic and voltammetric methods. The results indicate that they have different spectral characteristics and electrochemical behaviour, which suggests that the mode and affinity of Zn(II) and Co(II) complexes of morin bound to ct-DNA, may be responsible to their different antitumor activity (Song et al., 2003).

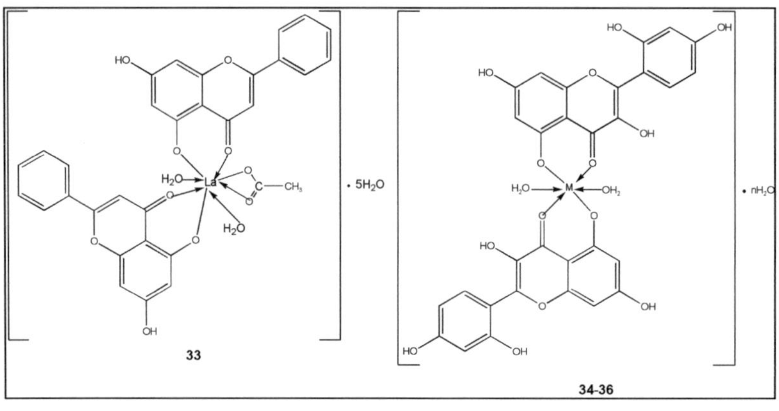

Fig. 9. Structure of La(chrysin)$_2$(OAc)·7H_2O (**33**) and the possible structure of the complexes. M = Zn(II) (**34**), Cu(II) (**35**), Co(II) (**36**), n = 0, or 1.

2.2.2 Hesperetin, naringenin, and apigenin-metal based anticancer agents

Hesperetin (5, 7, 3-trihydroxy-4-methoxy-flavanone), naringenin (4, 5, 7-trihydroxyflavanone) and apigenin (4, 5, 7-trihydroxyflavone), are biologically active flavonoids, commonly found in TCM (Tripoli et al., 2007). They have been reported to exhibit antitumour effects against breast cancer and hepatoma HepG2 cell lines (Korkina & Afanasev, 1997; Pereira et al., 2007). In addition, some metal complexes of hesperetin and naringenin have been found to exhibit antioxidant and anticancer activity (Chiang et al., 2006; So et al., 1996). The Naringenin Schiff base La(III) complex is more potent against the A-549 cell line than cisplatin under reasonable experimental concentrations (Li et al., 2008; Wang et al., 2006). Copper(II) complex of naringenin Schiff base possesses potent antioxidant activity, better than standard antioxidants like vitamin C and mannitol (Li et al., 2007). Our group reported three new copper(II) complexes of hesperetin, naringenin, and apigenin of general composition $[CuL_2(H_2O)_2]{\cdot}nH_2O$ (**37–39**, Fig. 10). The *in vitro* antitumor activity of the copper(II) complexes *vs* free ligand against human cancer cell lines HepG-2, SGC-7901, and HeLa have been assayed. Hesperetin-Cu(II) and apigenin-Cu(II) complexes were found to exhibit growth inhibition of SGC-7901 and HepG2 cell lines with respect to the free ligands; the inhibitory rate of hesperetin-Cu(II) complex is 43.2% and 43.8%, while apigenin-Cu(II) complex is 46% and 36%, respectively. Both hesperetin-Cu(II) complex and hesperetin were found to bind DNA in intercalation modes, and the binding affinity of the complex was stronger than that of free hesperetin (Tan et al., 2009).

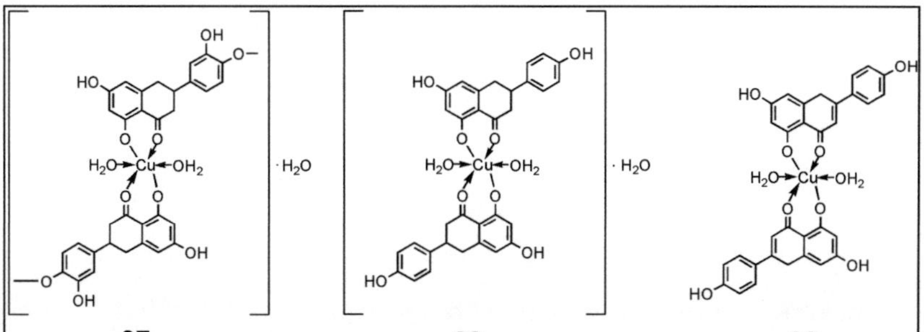

37 **38** **39**

Fig. 10. The possible structure of the hesperetin-Cu(II) (**37**), naringenin-Cu(II) (**38**) and apigenin-Cu(II) (**39**) complexes.

2.2.3 Quercetin-metal based anticancer agents

Quercetin (3, 5, 7, 3′, 4′-pentahydroxyflavone), a widely occurring compound in TCM, protects DNA from damage induced by reactive oxygen species (ROS) (Russo et al., 2000). Quercetin can chelate metal ions to form metal complexes that have better antioxidation and antitumour activity than quercetin alone (Zhou et al., 2001). Williams and co-worker reported the synthesis, characterization, antitumoural and osteogenic activities of quercetin vanadyl(IV) complexes. It was found that the free ligand quercetin might be a good candidate to be further evaluated in the treatment of bone tissue tumours because its effect has been more deleterious for tumoural osteoblasts that for the normal cells. However, the complexation of quercetin with vanadium center does not improve its potential anticarcinogenic properties. On the other hand, quercetin vanadyl(IV) complex seems to be a promising compound because it activates type I collagen production and shows a slight inhibitory effect on ALP specific activity, two markers of osteoblastic differentiation. It was believed that the activation of ERK pathways seems to be involved at least as one possible mechanism in the biological effects of quercetin vanadyl(IV) complex (Ferrer et al., 2006). Wang et al. investigated in detail the DNA binding, cytotoxicity, apoptotic inducing activity, and potential molecular mechanism of quercetin zinc(II) (46, Fig. 11) and copper(II) (47, Fig. 11) complexes. The quercetin znic(II) complex exhibits significant cytotoxicity against three tumour cell lines (HepG2, SMMC7721, and A549), which might be related to its intercalation into DNA (Tan et al., 2009). The quercetin zinc(II) complex displays strong DNA hydrolytic cleavage activity, which successfully promotes the cleavage of plasmid DNA, producing single and double DNA strand breaks, supported by evidence from free radical quenching, thiobarbituric acid-reactive substances (TBARS) assay, and T4 ligase ligation (Tan et al.,

2007). Tan et al. systematically investigated the mode of DNA binding, oxidative DNA cleavage activity, and apoptosis-inducing activity of the quercetin copper(II) complex. The results showed that the antitumour mechanism of the quercetin copper(II) complex involves not only its oxidative DNA damage with generation of ROS but also its specific interaction with DNA (Tan et al., 2009).

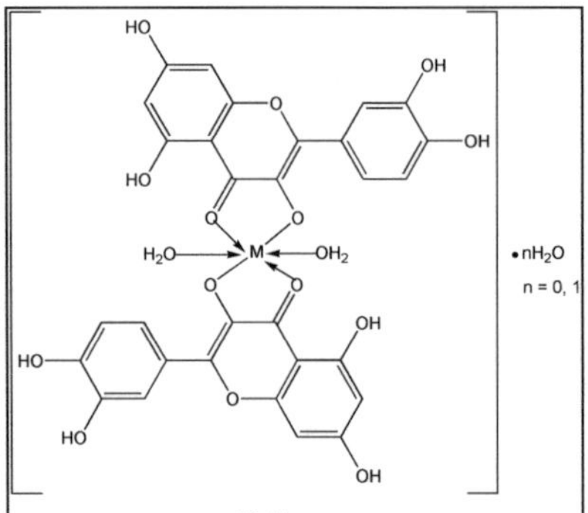

40-41

Fig. 11. The possible structures of quercetin metal complexes (M = Zn(II) (**40**), Cu(II)(**41**)).

In conclusion, flavonoids possess many potential pharmacological activity, represent a large type of TCM ligands, but because the flavonoids contain rich phenolic and carbonyl groups, chelate to metal ion, very easily to form polymeric structures, resulting in poor solubility, that limit the actual applications. Therefore, investigation of flavonoid metal-based antitumour agents, the excellent synthetic and characterized techniques is required, the good choice of flavonoids is very important.

2.3 Other TCM active ingredient-metal based anticancer agents

2.3.1 Coumarin-metal based anticancer agents

It is well documented that coumarin and a variety of coumarin derivatives have antitumour and antiproliferative activity. They have been shown to inhibit proliferation of particular human malignant cell lines *in vitro*, as well as affecting tumour activity against several in vitro tumour types (Kostova & Momekov, 2006). Kostova et al. synthesized a series of new zirconium(V) complexes with bis-coumarin ligands containing pyrazole or pyridine rings. The cytotoxic screening by MTT assay to HL-60 and the chronic myeloid leukemia LAMA-84 indicates that the zirconium(V) complexes of coumarins proved to be less potent than the corresponding free ligands (Kostova & Momekov, 2006). Egan and coworker investigated in vitro antitumour and cytoselective effects of coumarin-3-carboxylic acid and three of its hydroxylated derivatives, along with their silver-based complexes using human epithelial carcinoma cell lines (A-498 and Hep-G2). The *in vitro* antitumour assay results indicated that all of the ligands and their silver complexes induced a concentration-dependent cytotoxic effect. Hydroxylation of C-3-COOH and its subsequent complexation with silver led to the production of a series of compounds with dramatically enhanced cytotoxicity, with 6-OH-C-3-COO-Ag having the greatest activity, and all of the metal-based complexes were selectively cytotoxic to both carcinoma-derived cell lines, relative to normal renal and hepatic cells. The IC_{50} values obtained with Hep-G2 cells were between 2 and 5.5 times more cytotoxic than cisplatin. All of the coumarin-silver complexes inhibited the DNA synthesis, which did not appear to be mediated *via* intercalation. These findings suggest that both hydroxylation, particularly in the 6th position, and complexation with silver give rise to a cytotoxic-selective agent that significantly targets cancer cells, relative to normal cells (Thati et al., 2007). In addition, Kostova and co-worker investigated the cytotoxic activity of new lanthanum (III) and cerium (III) complexes of bis-coumarins. Their findings suggest that the coumarin-lanthanide complexes exhibited cytotoxic activity in micromolar contrations. Their *in vitro* effects are clearly expressed (Kostova et al., 2005, 2006). Recently, Creaven et al. reported the antibacterial and anticancer activities, coordination modes of copper(II) complexes of Schiff based-derived coumarin ligands (Creaven et al., 2010). Therefore, these coumarin-metal compounds have potential to develop as anticancer drugs, which provides hope for the pursuit of non-platinum anticancer drugs.

2.3.2 Cantharidin-metal based anticancer agents

Cantharidin is the active principle of Epicanta gorhami or Mylabris("blister beetles), which has long been applied as a TCM treatment for liver, lung, intestinal and digestive tract tumours (Wang, 1989). Cantharidin has severe side effects such as dysphagia, hematemesis, and dysuria (Wang, 1989). Cantharidin and its derivatives have been reported to have strong affinity and specificity for a protein phosphatase 2A (Li & Casida, 1992). Demethylcantharidin (norcantharidin, DMC) is a synthetic analogue of cantharidin and has potent antitumour activity but without the latter's adverse effects (Wang, 1989). Ho and coworker have carried out systematic, innovative research on the combination of demethylcantharidin with a platinum moiety to give a series of TCM-based platinum compounds $[Pt(C_8H_8O_5)(NH_2R)_2]$ (**42-46**, Fig. 12). These platinum complexes exhibit selective cytotoxicity toward SK-Hep-1 (human liver cell line), and circumvention of cross-resistance. They may possess a novel dual mechanism of antitumour action: inhibition of PP2A and platination of DNA (Ho et al., 2001 & 2003; To et al., 2004). Ho et al. determined the release of hydrolyzed demethylcantharidin from norcantharidin-Pt(II) compounds with anticancer activity by gas chromatography, in which the TCM component was slowly released from the norcantharidin-Pt(II) compounds over 24h, leading to PP2A inhibition. These complexes may prove to be new anticancer agents with novel mechanisms of cytotoxic action (To et al., 2002). The *in vitro* anti-proliferative activity of compounds **42-46** was investigated in human hepatocellular carcinoma (HCC) cell lines using MTT assay, which showed that compounds **42-46** were approximately 2-20 and 20-200 times more potent than cisplatin and carboplatin, respectively, in SK-Hep1 and HepG2 cells. The *in vivo* antitumour efficacies of **42-46** were evaluated in a s.c. inoculated SK-Hep1 xenograft model in nude mice. Compounds **42-46** exhibited definite *in vivo* activity without undue toxicity, contrasting the lack of activity of cisplatin and carboplatin. For *in vivo* cisplatin resistance model of human HCC, compounds **42-46** performed the same level of tumour growth suppression as in the control tumours, indicating the circumvention of cisplatin (To et al., 2005). Further studies indicated that compounds **42-46** were considerably less reactive to sulfur-containing nucleophiles than cisplatin, implying that they had reduced toxicity when compared with cisplatin, but the antitumour activity still remained (To et al., 2006). In order to determine the influence of the isomers on their anticancer activity, a series of platinum complexes integrating demethylcantharidin (CMC) with isomers of 1, 2-diaminocyhexane (DACH) have been synthesized. These compounds exhibit superior *in vitro* anticancer activity against colorectal and human hepatocellular cancer cell lines comparing with oxaliplatin, cisplatin, and carboplatin. The flow cytometric analysis results showed that the *trans*-DACH-Pt-DMC analogues presented similar behaviour to oxaplatin on affecting the cell cycle of the HCT116 colorectal cancer cells, but different from that of cisplatin or carboplatin. The DACH component obviously dictates the *trans*-DACH-Pt-DMC complexes to act similar to oxaliplatin, whereas the DMC ligand enhanced the compounds' overall anticancer activity. It was speculated these compounds accelerated the cell cycle from G1 to S-phase with subsequent onset of G2/M arrest and accompanying apoptosis (Yu et al., 2006). Ho's group also studied the pharmacokinetics and tissue distribution of these DMC-Pt anticancer agents in rats. Their findings suggested that the novel DMC-Pt compounds might afford higher clinical efficacy and reduced systemic side effects in contrast to cisplatin (Wang et al., 2007).

Moreover, the synergistic interaction between platinum-based antitumour agents and demethylcantharidin were investigated *in vitro* and *in vivo*, which demonstrated that synergistic effects occurred by combining demethylcantharidin with platinum-based antitumour agents. The demethylcantharidin might play a role in enhancing the efficacy of cisplatin in the treatment of various solid human tumours such as HCC, and overcoming cisplatin resistance. The demethylcantharidin has considerable promise as an adjuvant to chemotherapy (To et al., 2005).

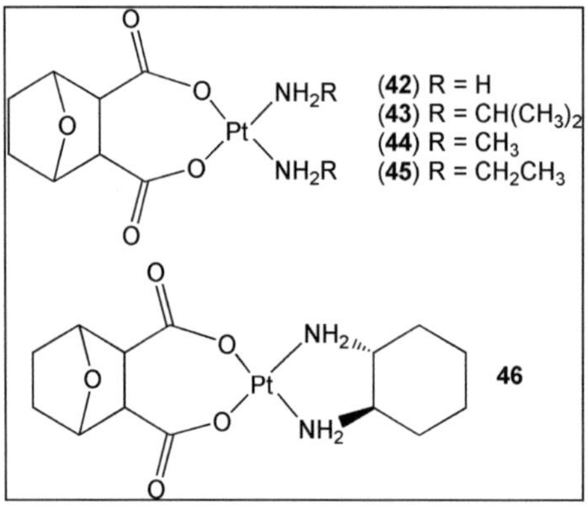

Fig. 12. Structures of $[Pt(C_8H_8O_5)(NH_2R)_2]$ (**42-46**) .

The systematic work carried out by Ho's group on cis-DMC-Pt anticancer agents provides a successful paradigm for future research of TCM metal-based anticancer agents by utilization of multi-targets and multi-mechanisms of TCM-metal based compounds. Their achievement make us to believe that innovative metal-based anticancer drugs enable to develop by integration of the multiple advantages of metals and metal complexes with TCM's multi-target and multi-mechanism features.

2.3.3 Plumbagin-metal based anticancer agents

Plumbagin (PLN) is a potent toxic natural product extracted from TCM *Plumbago Zeylanica* L. (*Plumbaginaceae*), which has been used in China as well as other Asian countries for the treatment of rheumatoid arthritis, dysmenorrhea, injury by bumping, and even cancer. The anticancer property of PLN against HeLa, P388 lymphocytic, leukemia, colon cancer and hepatoma has been reported (Aziz et al., 2008; Kuo et al., 2006; Lin et al., 2003; Olagunju et al., 1999; Srinivas et al., 2004). Our group carried out the studies on plumbagin metal-based antitumour agents. The anticancer TCM, plumbagin (PLN), was isolated from *Plumbago Zeylanica*. Reaction of plumbagin with Cu(II) salt, afforded $[Cu(PLN)_2]\cdot 2H_2O$ (47, Fig.13).

With 2,2′-bipyridine (bipy) as a co-ligand, PLN reacts with Cu(II) to give rise to $[Cu(PLN)(bipy)(H_2O)]_2(NO_3)_2{\cdot}4H_2O$ (48, Fig. 13). The two complexes were characterized by elemental analysis, IR, and ESI-MS. Their crystal structures were determined by single crystal X-ray diffraction methods (Fig. 13) And the *in vitro* cytotoxicity of PLN and the two copper complexes against seven human tumour cell lines was assayed. The metal-based compounds exhibit enhanced cytotoxicity vs. that of PLN, suggesting that these compounds display synergy in the combination of metal ions with PLN. The binding properties of PLN and the two copper complexes to DNA were investigated with UV-vis, fluorescence, CD spectroscopy, and gel mobility shift assay, which indicated that the two copper complexes of plumbagin were non-covalently binding and mainly intercalated in the neighboring base pairs of DNA. PLN and its copper complexes exhibit inhibition activity to topoisomerase I (TOPO I), but the metal complexes were more effective than PLN (Chen et al., 2009).

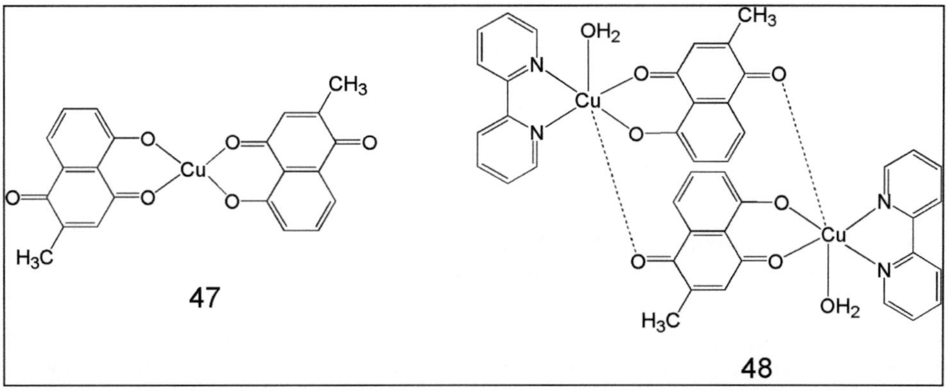

Fig. 13. Crystal structures of $[Cu(PLN)_2]$ (**47**) and $[Cu(PLN)(bpy)(H_2O)](NO_3)_2$ (**48**).

This work has recently been reviewed by Professor Roy Planalp. He thought that this work is very exciting with regards to the enhanced antitumour properties of a natural substance by complexation with a common biometal (Saxton, 2010).

In order to investigate the cytotoxicity of plumbaginate lanthanide complexes, five new lanthanide(III) complexes of deprotonated plumbagin: $[Y(PLN)_3(H_2O)_2]$ (**49**), $[La(PLN)_3(H_2O)_2]$ (**50**), $[Sm(PLN)_3(H_2O)_2]{\cdot}H_2O$ (**51**), $[Gd(PLN)_3(H_2O)_2]$ (**52**), and $[Dy(PLN)_3(H_2O)_2]$ (**53,** Fig. 14) were synthesized by the reaction of plumbagin with the corresponding lanthanide salts, in amounts equal to ligand/metal molar ration of 3:1. The PLN-lanthanide(III) complexes were characterized by different physicochemical methods: elemental analyses, UV-visible, IR and 1H NMR and ESI-MS as well as TGA. The plumbagin and its lanthanide(III) complexes **49–53**, were tested for their in vitro cytotoxicity against BEL7404 (liver cancer) cell lines by MTT assay. The five PLN-lanthanide (III) complexes **49–53** effectively inhibited BEL7404 cell lines growth with IC_{50} values of 11.0±3.5, 5.1±1.3, 6.1±1.1, 6.4±1.3, and 9.8±1.5μM, respectively, and exhibited a significantly enhanced cytotoxicity compared to plumbagin and the corresponding lanthanide salts, suggesting a synergistic effect upon plumbagin coordination to the Ln(III) ion. The lanthanide complexes under investigation also exerted dose- and time-dependent cytotoxic activity. $[La(PLN)_3(H_2O)_2]$ (**50**) and plumbagin interact with calf thymus DNA (ct-DNA) mainly via intercalation mode, but for $[La(PLN)_3(H_2O)_2]$ (**50**), the electrostatic interaction should not be excluded; the binding affinity of [La(PLN)$_3$(H$_2$O)$_2$] (**50**) to DNA is stronger than that of free plumbagin, which may correlate with the enhanced cytotoxicity of the PLN-lanthanide(III) complexes (Chen et al. 2011).

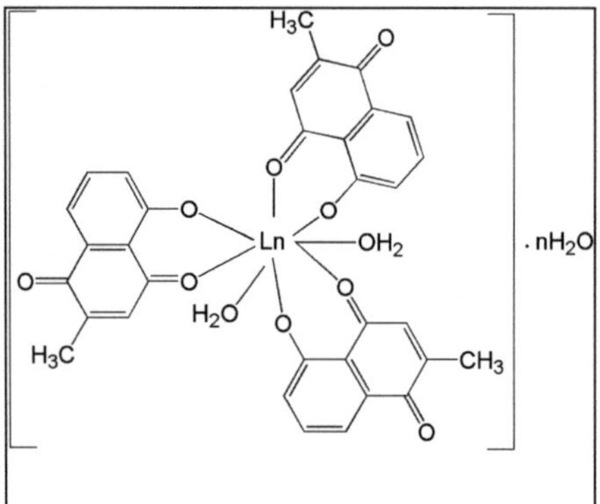

49 to 53

Fig. 14. The possible structure of complexes **49–53** (n=0, Ln = Y(III) (**49**), La(III) (**50**), Gd(III) (**52**), Dy(III) (**53**); n = 1, Ln = Sm(III) (**51**)).

2.3.4 Curcumin-metal based anticancer agents

Curcumin, an extract of turmeric, Curcuma longa L., has been used for centuries in variety of TCM pharmaceutical applications (Sharma, 1976), including treatment of arthritis (Deodhar et al., 1980), as an anti-inflammatory agent (Rao et al., 1982; Srimal & Dhawan, 1973) and as an orally available treatment for diabetes (Arun & Nalini, 2002). Thompson and co-worker synthesized a novel vanadyl curcumin complex (VO(cur)$_2$) (**54**, Fig. 15) and studied its anticancer potential in inhibiting mouse lymphoma cell growth. The complex was more effective than uncoordinated curcumin (Thompson et al., 2004).

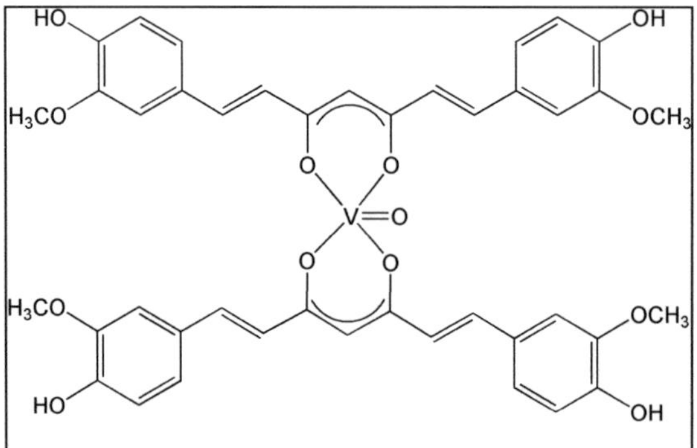

54

Fig. 15. Structure of vanadyl curcumin complex (VO(cur)$_2$ **54**).

2.3.5 Camphorato-metal based anticancer agents

Camphor has long been used as TCM to relieve pain, stop tickle, anti-inflammation, cure ulcers and sores, dental caries, and kill worms and acariasis as early as the Ming Dynasty. Camphoric acid can be obtained by the oxidation of camphor and is used in pharmaceuticals as exciting centre and respiration analeptic agent. Gou and coworker synthesized eight new camphorato platinum complexes (**55**, Fig. 16) and evaluated their in vitro cytotoxicity against HL-60, 2AO, BEL-7402 and A549 cells. The results show that most complexes exhibited good cytotoxic activity against the selected cell lines. One complex displayed not only higher *in vivo* antitumour activity, but also less toxicity than oxaliplatin when it was administered intravenously at a dose of 6 mg/Kg three times. Gou and coworkers research provides a new selection to find chiral leaving groups from TCM (Wang et al., 2005).

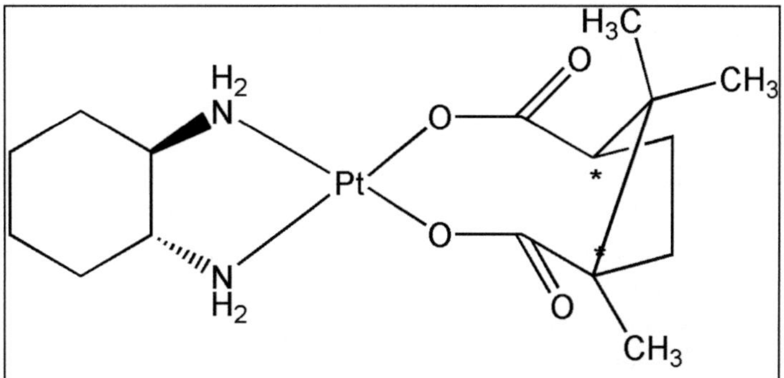

55

Fig. 16. *trans*-1R, 2R-Daiminocyclohexane camphorate-Pt complex (**55**).

3. Conclusion

TCM is a natural "combination chemical resources armoury", which has undergone several thousands years worth of clinical practice and screening. TCM possess multi-component, multi-target and co-regulatory features which meet the view points of multi-target drugs through the network approach (Csermely et al., 2005) and robustness-based approach to systems-oriented drug design (Kitano, 2007). TCM metal-based antitumor agents have at least two remarkable advantages: either TCM playing key role or metal complex making multiple contributions in development of drugs. In this review, the alkaloids, flavonoids, cantharidin, coumarins, plumbagin, curcumin and camphoric acid metal-based compounds with antitumor activity were summarized. Generally, TCM-metal based compounds formed *via* metal ions coordinating to TCM with O, N donors, exhibiting enhanced activity and synergistic effect with multi-targets and multi-mechanisms. With the Chinese government promotion of the modernization of TCM (Normile, 2003) and carrying out the *herbalome* (Stone, 2008), as well as the advancements of genome, proteome, metabolome, there is the possibility to design new TCM metal-based anticancer drugs and develop modern TCM, which will benefit to overcoming multidrug resistance (MDR). The promising trends have been supported by great potential of TCM metal-based antitumor agents mentioned above. We believe that innovative metal-based anticancer drugs enable to develop by integration of the multiple advantages of metals and metal complexes with TCM's multi-target and multi-mechanism features. But the action species and multi-target and multi-mechanism in cell and *in vivo* of the TCM metal-based antitumor agents still need to be widely and deeply investigated by adopting modern genome, proteome, metabolome technologies.

4. Acknowledgment

This work was supported National Basic Research Program of China (Nos. 2009CB526503, 2010CB534911), the National Natural Science Foundation of China (20861002), and Natural Science Foundation of Guangxi Province of China (Nos. 0991012Z, 0991003, and 2010GXNSFF013001).

5. References

Al-Allaf, T. A. K.; Ayoub, M. T.; Rashan, L. J. (1990). Synthesis and characterization of novel biologically active platinum(II) and palladium(II) complexes of some β-carboline alkaloids. *J. Inorg. Biochem.*, Vol.38, No.1, (January 1990), pp. 47-56, ISSN 0162-0134.

Al-Allaf, T. A. K.; Rashan, L. J. (1998). Synthesis and cytotoxic evaluation of the first trans-palladium(II) complex with naturally occurring alkaloid harmine. *Eur. J. Med. Chem.*, Vol.33, No.10, (October 1998), pp. 817-820, ISSN 0223-5234.

Alldrick, A. J.; Flynn J.; Rowland, I. R. (1986). Effects of plant-derived flavonoids and polyphenolic acids on the activity of mutagens from cooked food. *Mutat. Res.*, Vol.163, No.3, (December 1986), pp. 225-232, ISSN 0027-5107.

Alt, A.; Lammens, K.; Chiocchini,C.; Alfred Lammens, A.; Pieck, J. C.; Kuch, D.; Karl-Peter Hopfner, K.-P.; Carell, T. (2007). Bypass of DNA lesions generated during anticancer treatment with cisplatin by DNA polymerase eta. *Science*, Vol. 318, No.5852, (November, 2007), pp. 967-970, ISSN 0036-8075.

Ansari, A. A.(2008). ^{1}H NMR and spectroscopic studies of biologically active yttrium (III)-flavonoid complexes. *Main Group Chem.*, Vol.7, No.2, (February 2008), pp. 133-145, ISSN 1024-1221.

Arun, N.; Nalini, N. (2002). Efficacy of turmeric on blood sugar and polyol pathway in diabetic albino rats. *Plant Foods Hum. Nutr.*, Vol.57, No.1, (January 2002), pp. 41-52, ISSN 0921-9668.

Aziz, M. H.; Dreckschmidt, N. E.; Verma, A. K. (2008). Plumbagin, a medicinal plant-derived naphthoquinone, is a novel inhibitor of the growth and invasion of hormone-refractory prostate cancer. *Cancer Res.*, Vol.68, No.21, (November 2008), pp. 9024-9032, ISSN 0008-5472.

Baraldi, P. G.; Bovero, A.; Fruttarolo, F.; Preti, D.; Tabrizi, M. A.; Pavani, M. G.; Romagnoli, R. (2004). *Med. Res. Rev.*, Vol.24, No.4, (April 2004), pp. 475-496, ISSN 0198-6325.

Bentley, K. W. (2001). β-Phenylethylamines and the isoquinoline alkaloids. *Nat. Prod. Rep.*, Vol.18, No.2, (February 2001), pp. 148-170, ISSN 0265-0568.

Blanco, O. M.; Castedo, L.; Villaverde, M. C. (1993). *Phytochemistry*, Vol.32, No.4, (March 1993), pp. 1055–1057, ISSN 0031-9422.

Chan, K. (1995). Progresseses in traditional Chinese medicine. *Trends Pharmacol. Sci.*, Vol.16, No.6, (June 1995), pp. 182-187, ISSN 0165-6147.

Chang, F.-R.; Hsieh, T.-J.; Huang, T.-L.; Chen, C.-Y.; Kuo, R.-Y.; Chang, Y.-C.; Chiu, H.-F.; Wu, Y.-C. (2002). Cytotoxic constituents of the stem bark of neolitsea *acuminatissima*. *J. Nat. Prod.*, Vol.65, No.3, (March 2002), pp. 255–258, ISSN 0163-3864.

Chang, H. C.; Chang, F. R.; Wu, Y. C.; Lai, Y. H. (2004). Anti-cancer effect of liriodenine on human lung cancer cells. *Kaohsiung J. Med. Sci.*, Vol.20, No.8, (August 2004), pp. 365-371, ISSN 1607-551X.

Chen, C.-L.; Chang, H.-M.; Cowling, E. B.; Huang Hsu, C.-Y.; Gates, R. P. (1976). *Phytochemistry*, Vol.15, No.7, (July 1976), pp. 1161–1167, ISSN 0031-9422.

Chen, K.-S.; Chang, F.-R.; Chia, Y.-C.; Wu, T.-S.; Wu, Y.-C. (1998). Chemical constituents of Neolitsea parvigemma and Neolitsea konishii. J. Chin. Chem. Soc., Vol.45, No.1, (January 1998), pp. 103–110, ISSN 0009-4536.

Chen, S.-B.; Gao, G.-Y.; Yu, S.-C.; Xiao, P.-G. (2002). Cytotoxic Constituents from *Aquilegia ecalcarata. Planta Med.*, Vol.68, No.6, (June 2002), pp. 554–556, ISSN 0032-0943.

Chen, Z.-F.; Liu, Y.-C.; Liu, L.-M.; Wang, H.-S.; Qin, S.-H.; Wang, B.-L.; Bian, H.-D.; Yang, B.; Fun, H.-K.; Liu, H.-G.; Liang, H.; Orvig, C. (2009). Potential new inorganic antitumour agents from combining the anticancer traditional Chinese medicine (TCM) liriodenine with metal ions, and DNA binding studies. *Dalton Trans.*,Vol.38, No.2, (January 2009), pp. 262-272, ISSN 1477-9226.

Chen, Z.-F.; Mao, L.; Liu, L.-M.; Liu, Y.-C.; Peng, Y.; Hong, X.; Wang, H.-H.; Liu, H.-G.; Liang, H. (2011). Potential new inorganic antitumour agents from combining the anticancer traditional Chinese medicine (TCM) matrine with Ga(III), Au(III), Sn(IV) ions, and DNA binding studies. *J. Inorg. Biochem.*, Vol.105, No.2, (February 2011), pp.171-180, ISSN 0162-0134.

Chen, Z.-F.; Shi, Y.-F.; Liu, Y.-C.; Hong, X.; Geng, B.; Peng, Y.; Liang H. (2011). Unpublish results.

Chen, Z.-F.; Tan, M.-X.; Liu, L.-M.; Liu, Y.-C.; Wang, H.-S.; Yang, B.; Peng, Y.; Liu, H.-G.; Liang H. and Orvig, C. (2009). Cytotoxicity of the traditional Chinese medicine (TCM) plumbagin in its copper chemistry. *Dalton Trans.*, Vol.38, No.48, (December 2009), pp. 10824-10833, ISSN 1477-9226.

Chen, Z.-F.; Tan, M.-X.; Liu, Y.-C.; Peng, Y.; Wang, H.-H.; Liu, H.-G.; Liang, H. (2011). Synthesis, characterization and preliminary cytotoxicity evaluation of five lanthanide-plumbagin complexes. *J. Inorg. Biochem.*, Vol.105, No.2, (February 2011), pp. 308–316, ISSN0162-0134.

Chen, Z.-F.; Tao, L.; Liu, Y.-C.; Liang, H. (2011), unpulish results.

Cheng, J. T. (2000). Review: drug therapy in Chinese traditional medicine. *J. Clin. Pharmacol.*, Vol.40, No.5, (May, 2000), pp. 445-450, ISSN 0091-2700.

Chiang, L.-C.; Ng, L. T.; Lin, I.-C.; Kuo, P.-L.; Lin, C.-C. (2006). Anti-proliferative effect of apigenin and its apoptotic induction in human Hep G2 cells. *Cancer Lett.*, Vol.237, No.2, (June 2006), pp. 207–214, ISSN 0304-3835.

Clark, A. M.; Watson, E. S.; Ashfaq, M. K.; Hufford, C. D. (1987). *In vivo* efficacy of antifungal oxoaporphine alkaloids in experimental disseminated candidiasis. *Pharmaceutical Res.*, Vol.4, No.6, (December 1987), pp. 495–498, ISSN 0724-8741.

Clarke, M. J.; Zhu, F.; Frasca, D. R. (1999). Non-platinum chemotherapeutic metallopharmceuticals. *Chem. Rev.*, Vol.99, No.9, (August 1999), pp. 2511-2533, ISSN 0009-2665.

Creaven, B. S.; Czegledi, E.; Devereux, M.; Enyedy, E. A.; Kia, A. F.-A.; Karcz, D.; Kellett, A.; McClean, S.; Nagy, N. V.; Noble, A.; Rockenbauer, A.; Szabo-Planka, T.; Walsh, M. (2010). Biological activity and coordination modes of copper(II) complexes of Schiff based-derived coumarin ligands. *Dalton Trans.*, Vol.39, No.45, (December 2010), pp. 10854–10865, ISSN 1477-9226.

Csermely, P.; Ágoston, V.; Pongor, S. (2005). The efficiency of multi-target drugs: the network approach might help drug design. *Trends Pharmacol. Sci.*, Vol.26, No.4, (April2005), pp. 178-182, ISSN 0165-6147.

Deodhar, S. D.; Sethi, R.; Srimal, R.C. (1980). Preliminary study on antirheumatic activity of curcumin (diferuloyl methane). *Indian J. Med. Res.*, Vol.71, No.4, (April 1980), pp. 632-634, ISSN 0971-5916.

Engelmann, M. D.; Hutcheson, R.; Cheng, I. F. (2005). Stability of ferric complexes with 3-hydroxyflavone (flavonol), 5,7-dihydroxyflavone (chrysin), and 3′,4′-dihydroxyflavone. *J. Agric. Food Chem.*, Vol.53, No.8, (March 2005), pp. 2953-2960, ISSN 0021-8561.

Ferrer, E. G.; Salinas, M. V.; Correa, M. J.; Naso, L.; Barrio, D. A.; Etcheverry, S. B.; Lezama, L.; Rojo, T.; Williams, P. A. M. (2006). Synthesis, characterization, antitumoral and osteogenic activities of quercetin vanadyl(IV) complexes. *J. Biol. Inorg. Chem.*, Vol.11, No.6, (October 2006), pp. 791-801, ISSN 0949-8257.

Galasso, V.; Asaro, F.; Berti, F.; Pergolese, B.; Kovac, B.; Pichierri, F. (2006). On the molecular and electronic structure of matrine-type alkaloids. *Chem. Phys.*, Vol.330, No.3, (November 2006), pp. 457-468, ISSN 0301-0104.

Gibert, T. F. (1998). Thought on traditional Chinese medicine and its pharmacopeia. *Ann. Pharm. Fr.*, Vol.56, No.6, (November 1998), pp. 282-285, ISSN 0003-4509.

Hambley, T. W. (2007). Metal-based therapeutics. *Science*, Vol.318, No.5855, (November 2007), pp. 1392-1393, ISSN 0036-8075.

Hofland, K.; Petersen, B. O.; Falck, J.; Helin, K.; Jensen, P. B.; Sehested, M. (2000). Differential cytotoxic pathways of topoisomerase I and II anticancer agents after overexpression of the E2F-1/DP-1 transcription factor complex. *Clin. Cancer Res.*, Vol.6, No.4, (April 2000), pp. 1488-1498, ISSN 1078-0432.

Ho, Y.-P.; Au-Yeung, S. C. F.; To, K. K. W. (2003). Platinum-based anticancer agents: innovative design strategies and biological perspectives. *Med. Res. Rev.*, Vol.23, No.5, (September 2003), pp. 633-655, ISSN 0198-6325.

Ho, Y.-P.; To, K. K. W.; Au-Yeung, S. C. F.; Wang, X.; Lin, G.; Han, X. Potential new antitumor agents from an innovative combination of demethylcantharidin, a modified traditional Chinese medicine, with a platinum moiety. *J. Med. Chem.*, Vol.44, No.13, (June, 2001), pp. 2065-2068, ISSN 0022-2623.

Hsieh, T. J.; Liu, T. Z.; Chern, C. L.; Tsao, D. A.; Lu, F. J.; Syu, Y. H.; Hsien, P. Y.; Hu, H. S.; Chang, T. T.; Chen, C. H. (2005). Liriodenine inhibits the proliferation of human hepatoma cell lines by blocking cell cycle progressesesion and nitric oxide-mediated activation of p53 expression. *Food and Chem. Toxicol.*, Vol.43, No.7, (July 2005), pp. 1117-1126, ISSN 0278-6915.

Ivanovska, N.; Hristova, M.; Philipov, S. (2000). Immunosuppression and recovery of drug-impaired host resistance against Candida albicans infection by oxoglaucine. *Pharmacol. Res.*, Vol.41, No.1, (January 2000), pp. 101–107, ISSN 1043-6618.

Ivanovska, N.; Hristova, M. (2000). Treatment with oxoglaucine can enhance host resistance to Candida albicans infection of mice with adjuvant arthritis. *Diagnostic Microbiology and Infectious Disease*, Vol.38, No.1, (September 2000), pp. 17–20, ISSN 0732-8893.

Ivanovska, N.; Philipov, S.; Georgieva, P. (1997). *Pharmacol. Res.*, Vol.35, No.4, (April 1997), pp. 267–272, ISSN 1043-6618.

Jamieson, E. R.; Lippard, S. J. (1999). Structure, recognition, and processing of cisplatin-DNA adducts. *Chem. Rev.*, Vo.99, No.9, (August, 1999), pp. 2467-2498, ISSN 0009-2665.

Jantan, I.; Raweh, S. M.; Yasin, Y. H. M.; Murad, S. (2006). Antiplatelet activity of aporphine and phenanthrenoid alkaloids from Aromadendron elegans Blume. *Phytother. Res.*, Vol.20, No.6, (June 2006), pp. 493–496, ISSN 0951-418X.

Jung, Y.; Lippard, S. J. (2007). Direct cellular responses to platinum-induced DNA damage. *Chem. Rev.*, Vol.107, No. 5, (May, 2007), pp. 1387-1407, ISSN 0009-2665.

Kelland, L. (2007). The resurgence of platinum-based cancer chemotherapy. *Nature Rev.*, Vol.7, No.8, (August 2007), pp. 573-584, ISSN 1474-175X.

Kitano, H. (2007). A robustness-based approach to systems-oriented drug design. *Nature Rev. Drug Discovery*, Vol.6, No. 3, (March 2007), pp. 202-210, ISSN 1474-1776.

Korkina, L. G. & Afanasev, I. B. (1997). Antioxidant and chelating properties of flavonoids. *Adv. Pharmacol.*, Vol.38, No.2, (February 1997), pp. 151–163, ISSN 1054-3589.

Kostova, I.; Manolov, I.; Momekov, G.; Tzanova, T.; Konstantinov, S.; Karaivanova, M. (2005). Cytotoxic activity of new cerium (III) complexes of bis-coumarins. *Eur. J. Med. Chem.*, Vol.40, No.12, (December 2005), pp. 1246-1254, ISSN 0223-5234.

Kostova, I.; Momekov, G. (2006). New zirconium (IV) complexes of coumarin with cytotoxic activity. *Eur. J. Med. Chem.*, Vol.41, No.6, (June 2006), pp. 717-726, ISSN 0223-5234.

Kostova, I.; Momekov, G.; Zaharieva, M.; Karaivanova, M. (2005). Cytotoxic activity of new lanthanum (III) complexes of bis-coumarins. *Eur. J. Med. Chem.*, Vol.40, No.6, (June 2005). pp. 542-551, ISSN 0223-5234.

Kostova, I.; Momekov, G.; Tzanova, T.; Karaivanova, M. (2006). Sythesis, characterization, and cytotoxic activity of new lanthanum (III) complexes of bis-coumarins. *Bioinorg. Chem. Appl.*, Doi 10.1155/BCA?2006/25651, ISSN 1687-479X.

Kuo, P.-L.; Hsu, Y.-L.; Cho, C.-Y. (2006). Plumbagin induces G2-M arrest and autophagy by inhibiting the AKT/mammalian target of rapamycin pathway in breast cancer cells. *Mol. Cancer Ther.*, Vol.5, No.12, (December 2006), pp. 3209-3221, ISSN 1535-7163.

Lan, Y. H.; Chang, F. R.; Yu, J. H.; Yang, Y. L.; Chang, Lee, Y. L.; S. J.; Wu, Y. C. (2003). Cytotoxic styrylpyrones from Goniothalamus amuyon. *J. Nat. Prod.*, Vol.66, No.4, (April 2003), pp.487-490, ISSN 0163-3864.

Li, T.-R.; Yang, Z.-Y.; Wang, B.-D. (2007). Synthesis, characterization and antioxidant activity of naringenin Schiff base and its Cu(II), Ni(II), Zn(II) complexes. *Chem. Pharm. Bull.*, Vol.55, No.1, (January 2007), pp. 26-28, ISSN 0009-2363.

Li, T.-R.; Yang, Z.-Y.; Wang, B.-D. Qin, D.-D. (2008). Synthesis, characterization, antioxidant activity and DNA-binding studies of two rare earth(III) complexes with naringenin-2-hydroxy benzoyl hydrazone ligand. *Eur. J. Med. Chem.*, Vol.43, No.8, (August 2008), pp. 1688–1695, ISSN 0223-5234.

Li, Y. M.; Casida, J. E. (1992). Cantharidin-binding protein: identification as protein phosphatase 2A. *Proc. Natl. Acad. Sci. USA*, Vol.89, No.24, (December 1992), pp. 11867-11870, ISSN 1091-6490.

Lin, C. H.; Chang, G. J.; Su, M. J.; Wu, Y. C.; Teng, C. M.; Ko, F. N. (1994). Pharmacological characteristics of liriodenine, isolated from Fissistigma glaucescens, a novel muscarinic receptor antagonist in guinea-pigs. *Br. J. Pharmacol.*, Vol.113, No.1, (September 1994), pp. 275-281, ISSN 0007-1188.

Lin, L. C.; Yang L. L. and Chou C. J. (2003). Cytotoxic naphthoquinones and plumbagic acid glucosides from Plumbago zeylanica. *Phytochemistry*, Vol.62, No.4, (February 2003), pp. 619-622, ISSN 0031-9422.

Liu, Y.-C.; Chen, Z.-F.; Liu, L.-M.; Peng, Y.; Hong, X.; Yang, B.; Liu, H.-G.; Liang, H. and Orvig, C. (2009). Divalent later transition metal complexes of the traditional chinese medicine (TCM) liriodenine: coordination chemistry, cytotoxicity and DNA binding studies. *Dalton Trans.*, Vol.38, No.48, (December 2009), pp. 10813-10823, ISSN 1477-9226.

Liu, J. Y.; Hu, J. H.; Zhu, Q. G.; Li, F. Q.; Wang, J.; Sun, H. J. (2007). Effect of matrine on the expression of substance P receptor and inflammatory cytokines production in human skin keratinocytes and fibroblasts. *International Immunopharmacol.*, Vol.7, No.6, (June 2007), pp. 816-823, ISSN 1567-5769.

Liu, Y. C. (1988). *The essential book of traditional Chinese medicine: theory, clinical practice*, Columbia University Press.

Lovejoy, K. S. and Lippard, S. J. (2009). Non-traditional platinum compounds for improved accumulation, oral bioavailability, and tumor targeting. *Dalton Trans.*, Vol.38, No.48, (December 2009), pp. 10651-10659, ISSN 1477-9226.

Luo, C.; Zhu, Y. L.; Jiang, T. J.; Lu, X. Y.; Huang, J. (2007). Matrine induced gastric cancer MKN45 cells apoptosis via increasing pro-apoptotic molecules of Bcl-2 family. *Toxicology*, Vol.229, No.3, (January 2007), pp. 245-252, ISSN 0300-483X.

Narayana, K. R.; Reddy, M. S.; Chaluvadi, M. R.; Krishna, D. R. (2001). Bioflavonoids classification, pharmacological, biochemical effects and therapeutic potential. *Indian J. Pharmacol.*, Vo.33, No.1, (February 2001), pp. 2-16, ISSN 0253-7613.

Nijveldt, R. J.; van Nood, E.; Hoorn, D. E. C.; Norren, K.; Leeuwen, P. A. M. (2001). Flavonoids: a review of probable mechanisms of action and potential applications. *Am. J. Clin. Nutr.*, Vol.74, No.4, (October 2001), pp. 418-425, ISSN 0002-9165.

Nijhoff, W. A.; Bosboom, M. A.; Smidt, M. H.; Peters, W. H. M. (1995). Enhancement of rat hepatic and gastrointestinal glutathione and glutathione S-transferases by alpha-angelicalactone and flavone. *Carcinogenesis*, Vol.16, No.3, (March 1995), pp. 607-612, ISSN 0143-3334.

Nissanka, A. P. K.; Karunaratne, V.; Bandara, B. M. R.; Kumar, V.; Nakanishi, T.; Nishi, M.; Inada, A.; Tillekeratne, L. M. V.; Wijesundara, D. S. A.; Gunatilaka, A. A. L. (2001). Antimicrobial alkaloids from Zanthoxylum tetraspermum. and caudatum.. *Phytochemistry*, Vol.56, No.8, (April 2001), pp. 857-861, ISSN 0031-9422.

Normile, D. (2003). The new face of traditional Chinese medicine. *Science*, Vol.299, No.5604, (October 2003), pp. 188-190, ISSN 0036-8075.

Ohiri, F. C.; Verpoorte, R.; Baerheim Svendsen, A. (1982). Alkaloids from Chasmanthera dependens. *Planta Med.* Vol.46, No.12, (December 1982), pp. 228–230, ISSN 0032-0943.

Olagunju, J. A.; Jobi, A. A.; Oyedapo, O. O. (1999). An investigation into the biochemical basis of the observed hyperglycaemia in rats treated with ethanol root extract of plumbago zeylanica. *Phytother. Res.*, Vol.13, No.4, (June 1999), pp. 346-348, ISSN 0951-418X.

Orvig, C.; Abrams, M. J. (1999). Medicinal inorganic chemistry: introduction. *Chem. Rev.*, Vol.99, No.9, (August 1999), pp. 2201-2203, ISSN 0009-2665.

Patwardhan, B.; Warude, D.; Pushpangadan, P. and Bhatt, N. (2005). Ayurveda and traditional Chinese medicine: a comparative overview. *Evid. Based Complement. Altern. Med.*, Vol.2, No.4, (December 2005), pp. 465-473, ISSN 1741-427X.

Pereira, R. M. S.; Andrades, N. E. D.; Paulino, N. Sawaya, A.C. H.; Eberlin, M. N.; Marcucci, M. C.; Favero, G. M.; Novak., E. M.; Bydlowski, S. P. (2007). Synthesis and characterization of a metal complex containing naringin and Cu, and its antioxidant, antimicrobial, antiinflammatory and tumor cell cytotoxicity. *Molecules*, Vol.12, No.7, (July 2007), pp. 1352–1366, ISSN 1420-3049.

Pusz, J.; Nitka, B. (1997). Synthesis and physicochemical properties of the complexes of Co(II), Ni(II), and Cu(II) with chrysin. Microchem. J., Vol.56, No.3, (July 1997), pp. 373-381, ISSN 0026-256x.

Pusz, J.; Nitka, B.; Zieliska, A.; Wawer, I. (2000). Synthesis and physicochemical properties of the Al(III), Ga(III) and In(III) complexes with chrysin. Microchem. J., Vol.65, No.3, (October 2000), pp. 245-253, ISSN 0026-265X.

Rao, T. S.; Basu, N.; Siddiqui, H. H. (1982). Anti-inflammatory activity of curcumin analogues. *Indian J. Med. Res.*, Vol.75, No.2, (April 1982), pp. 574-578, ISSN 0971-5916.

Remichkova, M.; Dimitrova, P.; Philipov, S.; Ivanovska, N. (2009). Toll-like receptor-mediated anti-inflammatory action of glaucine and oxoglaucine Fitoterapia, Vol.80, No.7, (July 2009), pp. 411–414, ISSN 0367-326X.

Rosenberg, B.; VanCamp, L. V.; Trosko, J. E.; Mansour, V. H. (1969). Platinum compounds: a new class of potent antitumour agents. *Nature*, Vol.222, No.5191, (April 1969), pp. 385-386, ISSN 0028-0836.

Ruan, L.-P.; Chen, S.; Yu, B.-Y.; Zhu, D.-N.; Cordell, G. A.; Qiu, S. X. (2006). Prediction of human absorption of natural compounds by the non-everted rat intestinal sac model. *Eur. J. Med. Chem.*, Vol.41, No.5, (May 2006), pp. 605-610, ISSN 0223-5234.

Russo, A.; Acquaviva, R.; Campisi, A.; Sorrenti, V.; Di Giacomo, C.; Virgata, G.; Barcellona, M. L.; Vanella, A. (2000). Bioflavonoids as antiradicals, antioxidants and DNA cleavage protectors. *Cell Biol. Toxicol.*, Vol.16, No.2, (April 2000), pp. 91-98, ISSN 0742-2091.

Sakai, W.; Swisher, E. M.; Karlan, B. Y.; Agarwal, M. K.; Higgins, J.; Friedman, C.; Villegas, E.; Jacquemont, C.; Farrugia, D. J.; Couch, F. J.; Nicole Urban, N.; Taniguchi, T. (2008). Secondary mutations as a mechanism of cisplatin resistance in BRCA2-mutated cancers. *Nature*, Vol.451, No.7182, (February 2008), pp. 1116-1120, ISSN 1476-4687.

Sari, A. (1999). Alkaloids from *Glaucium leiocarpum*. *Planta Med.*, Vol.65, No.5, (June 1999), pp. 492, ISSN 0032-0943.

Saxton, C. (2010). Natural remedy shows anticancer activity. *Highlights in Chemical Science*, 01.

Sharma, O. P. (1976). Antioxidant activity of curcumin and related compounds. *Biochem. Pharmacol.*, Vol.25, No.5, (August 1976), pp. 1811-1812, ISSN 0006-2952.

Shibata, S. (1985). In *Advances in Chinese Medicinal Materials Research* (Chang, H. M.; Yeung, H. W.; Tso, W. W. and Koo, A.; eds), pp3-16, World Scientific Publishing.

So, F. V.; Guthrie, N.; Chambers, A. F.; Moussa, M. and Carroll, K. K. (1996). Inhibition of human breast cancer cell proliferation and delay of mammary tumorigenesis by flavonoids and citrus juices. *Nutr. Cancer*, Vol.26, No.2, (August 1996), pp. 167–181, ISSN 0163-5581.

Song, Y.; Kang, J.; Wang, Z.; Lu, X.; Gao, J.; Wang, L. (2002). Study on the interactions between CuL2 and Morin with DNA. *J. Inorg. Biochem.*, Vol.91, No.3, (August 2002), pp. 470-474, ISSN 0162-0134.

Song, Y.; Yang, P.; Yang, M.; Kang, J.; Qin, S.; Lü, B. (2003). Spectroscopic and vlotammetric studies of the cobalt(II) complex of morin bound to calf thymus DNA. *Transition Met. Chem.*, Vol.28, No.6, (June 2003), pp. 712-716, ISSN 0340-4285.

Srimal, R. C.; Dhawan, B.N. (1973). Pharmacology of diferuloyl methane (curcumin) a non-steroidal anti-inflammatory agent. *J. Pharm. Pharmacol.*, Vol.25, No.6, (June 1973), pp. 447-452, ISSN 0022-3573.

Srinivas, P.; Gopinath, G.; Banerji, A.; Dinakar, A.; Srinivas, G. (2004). Plumbagin induces reactive oxygen species, which mediate apoptosis in human cervical cancer cells. *Mol. Carcinogen.*, Vol.40, No.4, (August 2004), pp. 201-211, ISSN 1098-2744.

Staker, B. L.; Feese, M. D.; Cushman, M.; Pommier, Y.; Zembower, D.; Stewart, L.; Burgin, A. B. (2005). Structures of three classes of anticancer agents bound to the human topoisomerase I−DNA covalent complex. *J. Med. Chem.*, Vol.48, No.7, (February, 2005), pp. 2336-2346, ISSN 0022-2623.

Stone, R. (2008). Lifting the veil on traditional Chinese medicine. *Science*, Vol.319, No.5864, (February 2008), pp. 709-710, ISSN 0036-8075.

Tan, M.-X.; Zhu, J.-C.; Pan, Y.M.; Chen, Z.-F.; Liang, H.; Liu, H.-G.; Wang, H.-S. (2009). Synthesis, cytotoxic activity, and DNA binding properties of copper (II) complexes with hesperetin, naringenin and apigenin. *Bioinorg. Chem. Appl.*, doi:10.115/2009/347872, ISSN 1687-479X.

Tan, J.; Wang, B. C.; Zhu, L. C. (2007). Hydrolytic cleavage of DNA by quercetin zinc(II) complex. *Bioorg. Med. Chem. Lett.*, Vol.17, No.5, (March 2007), pp. 1197-1199, ISSN 0960-894X.

Tan, J.; Wang, B. C.; Zhu, L. C. (2009). DNA binding and oxidative DNA damage induced by a quercetin copper(II) complex: potential mechanism of its antitumor properties. *J. Biol. Inorg. Chem.*, Vol.14, No.5, (June 2009), pp. 727-739, ISSN 0949-8257.

Tan, J.; Wang, B. C.; Zhu, L. C. (2009). DNA binding, cytotoxicity, apoptotic inducing activity, and molecular modeling study of quercetin zinc(II) complex. *Bioorg. Med. Chem.*, Vol.17, No.2, (January 2009), pp. 614–620, ISSN 0968-0896.

Thati, B.; Noble, A.; Creaven, B. S.; Walsh, M.; McCann, M.; Kavanagh, K.; Devereux, M.; Egan, D. A. (2007). In vitro anti-tumour and cyto-selective effects of courmarin-3-carboxylic acid and three of its hydroxylated derivatives, along with their silver-based complexes, using human epithelial carcinoma cell lines. *Cancer Lett.*, Vol.248, No.2, (April 2007), pp. 321-331, ISSN.

Thompson, K. H.; Böhmerle, K.; Polishchuk, E.; Martins, C.; Toleikis, P.; Tse, J.; Yuen, V.; McNeill, J. H.; Orvig, C. (2004). Complementary inhibition of synoviocyte, smooth muscle cell or mouse lymphoma cell proliferation by a vanadyl curcumin complex compared to curcumin alone. *J. Inorg. Biochem.*, Vol.98, No.12, (December 2004), pp. 2063-2070, ISSN 0162-0134.

To, K. K. W.; Wang, X.; Yu, C.-W.; Ho, Y.-P.; Au-Yeung, S. C. F. (2004). Protein phosphatase 2A inhibition and circumvention of cisplatin cross-resistance by novel TCM-platinum anticancer agents containing demethylcantharidin. *Bioorg. Med. Chem.*, Vol.12, No.17, (September 2004), pp. 4565-4573, ISSN 0968-0896.

To, K. K. W.; Ho, Y.-P.; Au-Yeung, S. C. F. (2002). Determination of the release of hydrolyzed demethylcantharidin from novel traditional Chinese medicine-platinum compounds with anticancer activity by gas chromatography. *J. Chromatogr. A*, Vol.947, No.2, (February 2002), pp. 319-326, ISSN 0021-9673.

To, K. K. W.; Ho, Y.-P.; Au-Yeung, S. C. F. (2005). *In vitro* and *in vivo* suppression of growth of hepatocelular carcinoma cells by novel traditional Chinese medicine-platinum anti-cancer agents. *Anti-cancer Drugs*, Vol.16, No.8, (September 2005), pp. 825-835, ISSN 0959-4973.

To, K. K. W.; Au-Yeung, S. C. F.; Ho, Y.-P. (2006). Differential nephrotoxicity of cis-platin and a novel series of traditional Chinese medicine-platinum anticancer agents correlates with their chemical reactivity towards sulfur-containing nucleophiles. *Anti-cancer Drugs*, Vol.17, No.6, (July 2006), pp. 673-683, ISSN 0959-4973.

To, K. K. W.; Ho, Y.-P.; Au-Yeung, S. C. F. (2005). Synergistic interaction between platinum-based antitumor agents and demethylcantharidin. *Cancer Lett.*, Vol.223, No.2, (June 2005), pp. 227-237, ISSN 0304-3835.

Tojo, E.; Dominguez, D.; Castedo, L. (1991). *Phytochemisrry*, Vol.30, No.3, (March 1991), pp. 1005–1010, ISSN 0031-9422.

Tripoli, E.; Guardia, M. L.; Giammanco, S.; Majo, D. D. and Giammanco, M. (2007). Citrus flavonoids: Molecular structure, biological activity and nutritional properties: A review. *Food Chem.*, Vol.104, No.2, (September 2007), pp. 466–479, ISSN 0308-8146.

Wang, B.-D.; Yang, Z.-Y.; Wang, Q.; Cai, T.-K.; Crewdson, P. (2006). Synthesis, characterization, cytotoxic activities, and DNA-binding properties of the La(III) complex with naringenin Schiff-base. *Bioorg. Med. Chem.*, Vol.14, No.6, (March 2006), pp. 1880–1888, ISSN 0968-0896.

Wang, G. S. (1989). Medical uses of mylabris in ancient China and recent studies. *J. Ethnopharm.*, Vol.26, No.2, (September 1989), pp. 147-162, ISSN0378-8741.

Wang, L.; Gou, S.; Chen, Y., Liu, Y. (2005). Potential new antitumour agents from an innovative cmbination of camphorato, a ramification of traditional Chinese medicine, with a platinum moiety. *Bioorg. Med. Chem. Lett.*, Vol.15, No.14, (July 2005), pp. 3417-3422, ISSN 0960-894X.

Wang, X.; Au-Yeung, S. C. F.; Ho, Y.-P. (2007). Pharmacokinetics and tissue distribution of novel traditional Chinese medicine-platinum anticancer agents in rats. *J. Inorg. Biochem.*, Vol.101, No.6, (June 2007), pp. 909-917, ISSN 0162-0134.

Wong, E.; Giandomenico, C. M. (1999). Current status of platinum-based antitumor drugs. *Chem. Rev.*, Vol.99, No. 9, (August 1999), pp. 2451-2466, ISSN 0009-2665.

Woo, S. H.; Reynolds, M. C.; Sun, N. J.; Cassady, J. M.; Snapka, R. M. (1997). Inhibition of topoisomerase II by liriodenine. *Biochem. Pharmacol.*, Vol.54, No.4, (August 1997), pp. 467-473, ISSN 0006-2952.

Wu, J.-Z.; Yuan, L.; Wu, J.-F. (2005). Synthesis and DNA binding of □-[2,9-bis(2-imidazo[4,5-f][1,10]phenanthroline)-1,10-phenanthroline]bis[1,10-phenanthroline-copper(II)]. *J. Inorg. Biochem.*, Vol.99, No.11, (November 2005), pp. 2211-2216, ISSN 0162-0134.

Wu, Y. C.; Duh, C. Y.; Wang, S. K.; Chen, K. S.; Yang, T. H. (1990). Two new natural azafluorene alkaloids and a cytotoxic aporphine alkaloid from Polyalthia longifolia. *J. Nat. Prod.*, Vol.53, No.5, (September 1990), pp. 1327-1331, ISSN 0163-3864.

Wu, Y.-C.; Liou, Y.-F.; Lu, S.-T.; Chen, C.-H.; Chang, J.-J.; Lee, K.-H. (1989). *Planta Med.*, Vol.55, No.2, (April 1989), pp. 163–165, ISSN 0032-0943.

Wu, Z. Y.; Zhou, T. Y.; Xiao, P. G. (1998). *Xin Hua Compendium of Materia Medica (I)*, Sahnghai: Shanghai Science & Technology Press, 1998: pp. 113–117.

Yu, C.-W.; Li, K. K. W.; Pang, S.-K. ; Au-Yeung, S. C. F.; Ho, Y.-P. (2006). Anticancer activity of a series of platinum complexes integrating demethylcantharidin with isomers of 1, 2-diaminocyclohexane. *Bioorg. Med. Chem. Lett.*, Vol.16, No.6, (March 2006), pp 1686-1691, ISSN 0960-894X.

Zeng, Y.-B.; Yang, N.; Liu, W.-S.; Tang, N. (2003). Synthesis, characterization and DNA-binding properties of La(III) complex of chrysin. *J. Inorg. Biochem.*, Vol.97, No.3, (November 2003), pp. 258-264, ISSN 0162-0134

Zhang, Q.; Wang, L.; Liu X. (1996). Synthesis, characterization and antitumour properties of metal(II) solid complexes with morin. *Transition Met. Chem.*, Vol.21, No.1, (January 1996), pp. 23-27, ISSN 0340-4285.

Zhang, L. J.; Wang, T. T.; Wen, X. M.; Wei, Y.; Peng, X. C.; Li, H.; Wei, L. (2007). Effect of matrine on HeLa cell adhesion and migration. *Eur. J. Pharmacol.*, Vol.563, No.1-3, (June 2007), pp. 69-76, ISSN 0014-4285.

Zhang, L. P.; Jiang, J. K.; Tam, J. W. O.; Zhang, Y.; Liu, X. S.; Xu, X. R.; Liu, B. Z.; He, Y. J. (2001). Effects of Matrine on proliferation and differentiation in K-562 cells. *Leuk. Res.*, Vol.25, No.9, (Septmber 2001), pp. 793-800, ISSN 0145-2126.

Zhou, J.; Wang, L.; Wang, J.; Tang, N. (2001). Antioxidative and anti-tumour activities of solid quercetin metal(II) complexes. *Transition Met. Chem.*, Vol.26, No.1-2, (January 2001), pp. 57-63, ISSN 0340-4285.

Zutphen, S.; Reedijk, J. (2005). Targeting platinum anti-tumour drugs: Overview of strategies employed to reduce systemic toxicity. *Coord. Chem. Rev.*, Vol.249, No.24, (December 2005), pp. 2845-2853, ISSN 0010-8545.

23

The Producing Area of Chinese Medicine and Famous Region Drug Research – Magnolia Officinalis

Guo Li
Jiangxi University of Traditional Chinese Medicine, Nanchang, Jiangxi, PRC

1. Introduction

1.1 Producing area

Under the guidance of the theory of the Traditional Chinese Medicine, many plants, animals and minerals in China can be medicines to treat the human diseases. Synchronously, the capacious land, sea and rich mineral deposits supply resources for them. Before they become medicines, they need grow and be gathered in some areas. But in these areas the weather, geographic features and biologic distributions are very different such as the different natural zones. Therefore these comprehensive factors endow Chinese medicines with different biological features and effects. After long time use, the medical practitioners gradually found the quantity or quality of some Chinese medicines which were produced in different areas were also different. An appellation came into being, which was called famous region drug.

1.2 Famous region drug

This appellation means those medicines which have good breeds and higher quality grow in some characteristic regions and feasible growing environments. They are cultivated and processed reasonably and output is great.

One thousand and five hundred years ago, in (Annotated Shen Nong's Herbal), Jinghong Tao had discussed the producing areas of Chinese Medicine. But at Yuan dynasty, famous region drug were first written in (Peony Pavilion) Xianzu Tang wrote. Until Tang dynasty, the government divided the country into ten areas according natural form. So Simiao Sun recorded famous region drugs producing in these areas in(a supplement to the essential prescriptions worth a thousand gold). (commentaries on the illustrations)written by Song Su and (Compendium of Materia Medica)written by Shizhen Li both recorded the regions and quality of Chinese Medicine. Now some places in China are famous regions of Chinese Medicines, such as Sichuan province, Guangdong province, Shandong province where respectively produced Rhizoma Chuanxiong, Fructus Amomi, Equus asinus L.

1.3 Magnolia officinalis

Magnolia officinalis are from the barks of Magnolia officinalis Reha. et Wils. and Magnolia officinalis Reha. et Wils.var. biloba. Reha. et Wils which belong to Magnoliaceae [1]. Its producing areas mainly include Sichuan, Hubei and Jiangxi province [2]. The characters of its medicinal materials usually showed single or double drum, grey outer surface with vertical wrinkles, purple brown inter surface with wiped oil mark and section with fine crystallization. Microstructure of its medicinal materials usually showed stone and oil cells or starch grains. The modern research also showed that its main effective component is magnolol and honokiol.

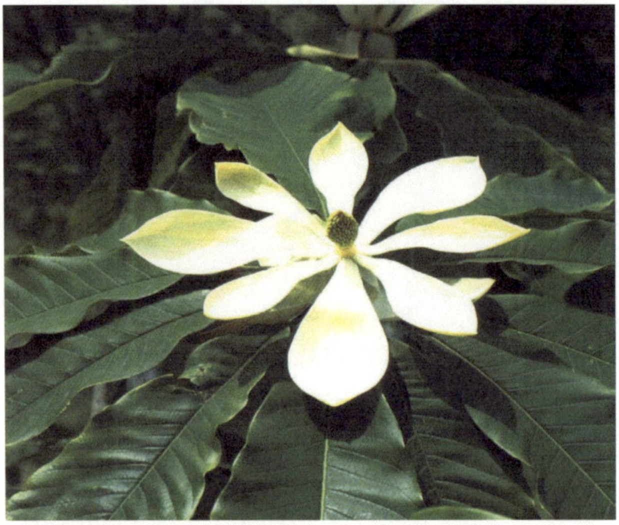

Fig. 1. Medicinal plant of Magnolia officinalis

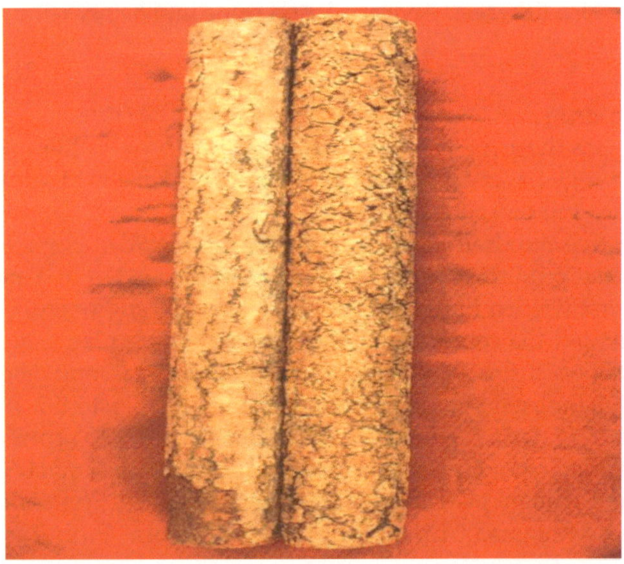

Fig. 2. Medicinal materials of Magnolia officinalis

It is wide used in clinic due to the effect of eliminating dampness and phlegm, promoting qi and removing distention. But the resource of Magnolia officinalis is decreasing and the imbalance between supply and demand is outstanding in recent years. It has been involved in natural protected Chinese medicine. Its variety research seems very urgent for looking for its substitute.

2. Purpose

To explore the exact substitute and the quality evaluation, optimization methods of Magnolia officinalis, the comprehensive varieties researches based on its adulterants and substitutes and quality evaluation methods were reviewed.

3. Methods

The appearance characters, microstructure, physical and chemical(including Thin-Layer Chromatography and high performance liquid chromatography) and randomly amplified polymorphic DNA(RAPD) identification, 1H Nuclear magnetic resonance spectroscopy, powder X-ray diffraction fourier fingerprint, polyamide chromatography of different adulterants and substitutes were applied according to the records. And they were reviewed. The results showed that they totally contained ten families and forty - three varieties. The influence factors on the quality of Magnolia officinalis and the other quality evaluation methods were also reviewed.

4. Result and conclusion

4.1 Families and varieties of plants identified with Magnolia officinalis and identified methods

The difference between Magnolia officinalis and these adulterants and substitutes were significant through the research. Firstly the morphological and(or) histological characters of some varieties were different from Magnolia officinalis, such as sikimmi, aleurites montana, Magnolia rostrata w w smith, Manglietia szechuanica Hu., Neolitsea levinei Merr., phyllanthi fructus, White yulan Magnolia, bigleaf magnolia bark, Wudang yulan magnolia, Magnolia wilsonii, camphortree bark , M.szechuanica Hu, M.insignis(Wal1.)Bl, Manglietia chingii Dandy, Manglietia yuyuanensis Law, sprenger magnolia bark, sargent magnolia bark, Magnolia wilsonii , Magnolia campbellii Hook.f.et Thoms., Mountain yulan Magnolia, M.szechuanica Hu, Manglietia chingii Dandy [3-14]. Secondly some physical and chemical identification showed significant results between Magnolia officinalis, Wudang magnolia bark, Magnolia campbellii Hook.f.et Thoms., albiziae , thinleaf machilus and Ormosia balansae. [15-17].The thin-Layer Chromatography analyzing also showed Magnolia officinalis were very different from the following adulterants and substitutes: (1)Wudang magnolia bark, Xikang magnolia bark and sargent magnolia bark were identified with cyclohexane-chloroform-ethanol (7:3:1) as developer and 5% vanillin sulfuric acid solution as coloration using silica gel G and observed at 254 nm using ultraviolet lamp [18]. (2)White yulan Magnolia, biond magnolia flower, shikimmi, red nanmu, aleurites montana, schima root-bark, Albizziakal Kora(Roxb).Prain., arbutus were identified with benzene-methanol (27:1) as developer and vanillin sulfuric acid solution as coloration using silica gel G and observed at 365 nm using ultraviolet lamp [19]. (3)Magnolia campbellii Hook.f.et Thoms.was identified with benzene-methanol (9:1) as developer and 1% vanillin sulfuric acid solution as coloration using silica gel G [20]. (4) Guangxi Manglietia was identified with benzene-methanol (8:2) as developer and 5% vanillin sulfuric acid solution as coloration

families	varieties numbers	varieties
Magnoliaceae	26	sprenger magnolia bark、sargent magnolia bark、Magnolia campbellii Hook.f.et Thoms.、Xikang magnolia bark 、Wudang yulan magnolia、white yulanMagnolia、Mountain yulan Magnolia、Magnolia wilsonii、Tianmu mountain magnolia immature flower、bigleaf magnolia bark、Magnolia rostrata w. w. smith、purple yulan Magnolia、magnolia bioudii、Mt. Huang magnolia bark、M.szechuanica Hu、M.insignis(Wall.)Bl、Manglietia chingii Dandy、Manglietia yuyuanensis Law、 Guangxi Manglietia、liriodendron 、biond magnolia flower、 shikimmi 、Michelia maudiae、Qinshi Manglietia、Magnolietia patungensis、Michelia champaca L..
Euphorbiaceae	2	phyllanthi fructus、 aleurites montana
lauraceae	4	red nanmu、 thinleaf machilus 、 camphortree bark 、 Neolitsea levinei Merr.
Juglandaceae	3	Engelhardia roxburghiana Wall 、 wild walnut 、 Juglans mandshurica Maxim.
myricaceae	1	arbutus
araliaceae	1	Manglietia szechuanica Hu.
Scrophulariaceae	1	Paulownia tomentosa (Thunb.) Steud.
Theaceae	1	schima root-bark
Leguminosae	3	Albizziakal Kora(Roxb).Prain.、 Ormosia balansae 、 albiziae
Oleaceae	1	Fraxinus rhynchophylla Hance

Table 1. Families and varieties of plants identified with Magnolia officinalis

using silica gel G [21]. (5) Juglans mandshurica Maxim.,Wild walnut, Paulownia tomentosa (Thunb.) Steud.and Mountain yulanMagnolia were identified with benzene-methanol (27:1) as developer and 1% vanillin sulfuric acid solution as coloration using silica gel G [22-25]. (6) Tianmu mountain magnolia immature flower was identified with benzene-ethyl acetate-methanol (27:1) as developer using silica gel G [26]. (7)Mt. Huang magnolia bar k, Manglietia yuyuanensis Law, Michelia maudiae were identified with benzene-methanol (27:1) as developer and 5% vanillin sulfuric acid solution as coloration using silica gel G [27]. (8) Qinshi Manglietia was identified with chloroform-methanol as developer and 5% vanillin sulfuric acid solution as coloration using silica gel G [28]. (9)Engelhardia roxburghiana Wall was identified with benzene-methanol (9:1) as developer and 1% vanillin sulfuric acid solution as coloration using silica gel G [29]. High performance liquid chromatography(HPLC) detection showed the total amount of magnolol and honokiol in Magnolia wilsonii, sprenger magnolia bark, and sargent magnolia bark were corresponding with PRC codex 2005 which was on Permaphase ODS, under the condition of mobile phase of benzene:phosphate(70:30) with the flow rate of 1.0ml/min. The calibration curves showed linear regression $r > 0.9989$. The recoveries ranged from 99.04% to 105.45%. [30]. But there was no magnolol and honokiol in white yulan Magnolia, purple yulan Magnolia, magnolia bioudii and Wudang yulan magnolia on Permaphase ODS, under the condition of mobile phase of benzene:water (74.5:25.5) with the flow rate of 1.0ml/min. Most of manglietia and Mountain yulan Magnolia contain small amounts of magnolol and honokiol [31]. The randomly amplified polymorphic DNA was also used to identify the certified products and the adulterants and substitutes of Magnolia officinalis like yulan magnolia, magnolia bioudii, Wudang yulan magnolia, purple yulan Magnolia, Mountain yulan Magnolia, Manglietia chingii Dandy, M.insignis(Wal1.)Bl and liriodendron.The result showed that the DNA Fingerprinting of Magnolia officinalis was very different from that of these adulterants and substitutes [32]. 15 samples of cortex Magnolia officinalis from different origin, 1 standard sample of Magnolia officinalis and 1 Wudang yulan magnolia were identified by 1H Nuclear magnetic resonance spectroscopy. The fingerprint showed that 1H-NMR could be an accurate and feasible method for the quality control of Magnolia officinalis [33]. Powder X-ray diffraction fourier fingerprint pattern was developed to identify and analyze Magnolia officinalis. Experiments and analysis were carried out on 3 samples of cortex Magnoliae officinals, 3 samples of cortex Magnolia bilobae, 14 samples of substitute and one counterfeit of cortex Magnolia officinals. It was found that this method can be used for identification on Chinese medicinal material Cortex Magnolia officinals [34].The characteristic chromatogram for cortex Magnolia officinalis was established by using polyamide chromatography (PC) to identify the cortex Magnolia officinalis from different origin and its substitute and false products. The result showed that this method could be used for the identification and quality evaluation for cortex Magnolia officinalis [35].

4.2 Influence factors and determinative methods of quality of Magnolia officinalis

The content of magnolol and honokiol of Magnolia officinalis collected from 7 provinces, 11 counties and Jingning provenance testing forest of Zhejiang province were detected as quality standards by using HPLC. And the correlation analysis between the factors which would affect the quality of Magnolia officinalis and the content of magnolol and honokiol was applied. The result showed that many factors would affect the quality of Magnolia officinalis significantly, such as provenance, producing area, blade profile, DBH, tree height, crown width, tree age, bar thickness, powder color, oiliness, grindability, bark type and position of sampling, etc. Among them, provenance, blade profile, powder color, bark thickness, DBH and position of sampling were more significant factors, especially the variety [36]. However some other researches showed tree age and length of storage period would be two factors which affected the quality of Magnolia officinalis [37-38]. After analysis, geographical position and Climate, blade profile and variety firstly maybe would affect the quality of Magnolia officinalis, especially the provenances with a sharpened leaf tip from Hubei Province has a highest content of phenols, and that with a concave leaf tip from the Lushan Mountain has a lowest content of phenols [39-40]. Secondly, there was positive correlation between the growth factors of Magnolia officinalis including tree age, DBH, tree height, crown width and content of phenols of Magnolia officinalis, especially the DBH [41]. Thirdly, appearance characters including bark thickness, powder color, grindability and bark roughness were regarded as the main traditional basis for the quality evaluation of Magnolia officinalis, which accorded with the research [42]. Position of sampling was also a basis for the quality evaluation of Magnolia officinalis which included dry hide, root bark, shoot cortex, etc. Content of phenols of root bark from Magnolia officinalis was 3-5 times higher than that of shoot cortex from Magnolia officinalis [41].

Besides the TLC and HPLC, amplified fragment length polymorphism analysis was applied as a method for further study with molecular markers in the field of genetic diversity, for breeding new cultivars, and for genetic relationships with Magnolia officinalis [43]. First derivative of UV spectrophotometry was also used to analyze compositions of Magnolia officinalis. The result showed that this method could eliminate interference of other impurity and make all samples exhibit maximum absorbance at 300nm [44]. A gas chromatography/mass spectrography was developed to identify the compositions of Magnolia officinalis, including magnolol, honokiol, δ-selinene and β-eudeomol, etc. And the content of magnolol and honokiol were determined [45]. The second order derivative synchronous fluorescence spectra of magnolol, honokiol and their mixture in 0.08%-0.16% methanol solution were studied. The experiment results indicated that their second order derivative synchronous fluorescence spectra were separated absolutely, which eliminated the disturbance between them [46]. To detect the contents of six trace elements (Fe ,Cu ,Zn ,Mn ,Ca ,Mg) in cortex Magnolia officinalis by flame atomic absorption spectroscopy, the contents of six trace elements (Fe ,Cu ,Zn , Mn ,Ca and Mg) were determined by calibration curve method. The result showed that the Cortex Magnolia officinalis is rich in trace elements which are necessary for people [47]. Quantitative Measurement of magnolol and honokiol was tested by using excitation–emission Matrix Fluorescence coupled with second–order calibration algorithm. It showed that the second-order calibration methods could quantify the analysis of interest from overlapped chromatographic profiles and give the accurate predicted results by utilizing mathematical-separation instead of physics-separation [48]. Fluorescent determination of magnolol has been effected employing the sensitivity- and stability-enhancing action of the non-ionic surface active emulsifier OP. As a result, the accuracy of determination was raised by 2 orders of magnitude as compared to that of ultraviolet spectrophotometry [49]. A highly sensitive and selective method was developed for the determination of honokiol and magnolol by HPLC-electrochemical detection, using a microbore column. The result showed that this method could be proposed for the determination of honokiol and magnolol in traditional Chinese medicines and human plasma sample [50].

All above-mentioned researches showed there were four kinds of factors mainly affecting the quality of Magnolia officinalis. And many methods had been used to determinate the content or compositions of Magnolia officinalis for the identification or quality control. Making and following the comprehensive and well-considered plans to develop famous region drugs would benefit protecting the environment, rare Chinese Medicine and highlighting characteristic of Chinese Medicines significantly.

5. References

[1] Chinese Pharmacopoeia Commission, *Pharmacopoeia of the People's Republic of China*, vol. 1, 2005,176.

[2] Z.L.Zheng, Y.S.Zheng, *Journal of Fujian Forestry Science and Technology*, 2010, 37, 103

[3] W.B.Duan,*Chinese Journal of Misdiagnostics*, 2002, 2, 797.

[4] Q.J.Shen,*Base Journal of Chinese Materia Medica*, 1997, 11, 14.

[5] M.Xu,*Journal of Modern Applied Pharmacy*, 1995,12,22.

[6] L.Wei,*Base Journal of Chinese Materia Medica*,2000,14,32.
[7] S.L.Yu,M.R.Zhu,Z.P,Li, Shandong Journal of Traditional Chinese Medicine,1998, 17, 227.
[8] S.H.,Yang,*Strait Pharmaceutical Journal*,1994,6 ,67.
[9] H.P.Zhu,*Shandong Journal of Traditional Chinese Medicine*.2008,27,629..
[10] C.Q.Xu,L.W.Cao,F.J.Xiang, Jorunal of Chinese Medicinal Materials, 1994, 17, 16.
[11] C.Q.Xu,L.W.Cao,F.J.Xiang,China Journal of Chinese Meteria Medica,1994,19,579
[12] Q.H.Wang,*Journal of Practical Traditional Chinese Internal Medicine*,2007,21,94.
[13] S.X.Peng,Modern Journal of Integrated Traditional Chinese and Western Medicine,2008,17,5642
[14] Y.Liu,Z.L.Yang, *Nonwood Forest Research*,2002,20,45.
[15] H.L.Zhang,*Chinese Journal of Modern Applied Pharmacy*,2000,17,108.
[16] X.Yu,Y.C.Zhuang,J.X.Yi,*Lishizhen Medicine and Materia Medica Research*,2008,19,2023.
[17] H.Chen,*Yunnan Journal of Traditional Chinese Medicine and Materia Medica*,1999, 20,40.
[18] W.G.Song,Strait Pharmaceutical Journal, 2003, 15, 57.
[19] J.G.Ye,Y.L.Wang, Heilongjiang Journal of Traditional ChineseMedicine, 2000, (6), 57.
[20] Z.M.Bai,X.X.Su, Research and Practice on Chinese Medicines, 2007, 21, 28.
[21] Y.Cao,Research and Practice on Chinese Medicines, 2004,18,33.
[22] A.W.Sun,*Chinese Licensed Pharmacist*,2007,(6),30.
[23] Q.Peng,*Journal of Chinese Medicinal Materials*,1992,15,20.
[24] Q.Peng,Journal of Chinese Medicinal Materials,1993, 16, 15.
[25] S.H.Wang,B.H.Li,M.Liu,Journal of Chinese Medicinal Materials,1999, 22,397.
[26] Q.Q.Yang,*Lishizhen Medicine and Materia Medica Research*, 2005,16,42.
[27] S.F.Li,F.Zhu,J.H.Wang, Journal of Chinese Medicinal Materials,1992, 15,16.
[28] H.D.Fu,J.M.Zheng, *China Pharmaceuticals*, 2008,17,67.
[29] R.L.Lin,*Strait Pharmaceutical Journal*, 2004, 16, 79.
[30] Y.P.Zhou,X.M.Fu,*Medical Journal of the Chinese People' s Armed Police Forces*,2002,13,618.
[31] .W.Su,C.Q.Xu,C.H.Sui,R.Q.Sun,Y.J.Wang,H.L.Liu,X.H.Shen, *Journal of She-nyang Pharmaceutical University*,1992,9 ,185.
[32] B.L.Guo, M.Wu, J.P.S, J.S.Li, *Journal of pharmaceutical practice*, 2000, 18, 314
[33] Y.Nie, W.F.Yao, W.B.Shen. Jiangsu Journal of Traditional Chinese Medicine, 2008, 40, 91
[34] L.Wu, L.Ma, Q.T.Zheng, W.Z.Song, Y.Lv. *Chinese Traditio nal Patent Medicine*, 2004,26, 861
[35] H.M.Jiang, D.H.Sun, J.Q.Lu, F.Huang, Y.Cao. *China Hospital pharmacy Journal*, 2004, 24, 221
[36] J.P.Si, Z.K.Tong, Y.R.Zeng. China Journal of Chinese Materia Medica, 2000, 25, 466
[37] Y.R.Zeng, Z.K.Tong, Y.Q.Zhu, J.P.Si, X.P.Pan. Journal of Chinese Materia Medica, 1999, 22, 379
[38] X.Y.Jiang, J.P.Si, Y.R.Zeng, Y.Q.Zhu. Journal of Zhejiang University of Traditional Chinese Medicin, 2003, 27, 82
[39]] Z.Li, M.Zhang, X.Lin, Y.M.Hou. *China Journal of Chinese Materia Medica*, 1989, 14, 15
[40] J.P.Si. Journal of Chinese Materia Medica, 2000, 23, 373
[41] J.P.Si, X.P.Pan, M.Y.Pan, R.Liu, X.L.Mei. *Journal of Zhejiang Forestry Science and Technology*, 1994,14,21
[42] Y.Q.Zhu, Y.R.Zeng, X.P.Pan, J.P.Si, Z.L.Wang. *Journal of Zhejiang Forestry College*, 1999, 16, 387
[43] Y.F.Jiang, J.P.Si, H.H.Huang, L.J.Cheng. *Journal of Zhejiang Forestry College*, 2010, 27, 304

[44] X.M.Wang, T.M.Ding, C.Chen. China Journal of Chinese Materia Medica, 1992, 17, 169
[45] Y.Wang. Strait Pharmaceutical Journal, 1998, 10, 45
[46] J.Yang, D.S.Yu, S.P.Liu, G.F.Tian, B.B.M.*Chinese Journal of Analytical Chemistry*, 2009, 37, 107
[47] J.L.Li, S.Z.Wu, Y.B.Li, L.Yu, Q.S.Li. *China Pharmacy*, 2008, 19, 2843
[48] L.Q.Hu, C.L.Ying, Y.Yang, L.W.Chui. *Journa l of Pingdingshan University*, 2010, 25, 53
[49] W.J.Liu, B.Q.Wang, Z.G.Pang, H.Cheng. *China Journal of Chinese Materia Medica*, 1991, 16, 101
[50] D.L.Wang, Q.S.Wang, D.R. Jin. *Chinese Journal of Pharmaceutical Analysis*, 2007, 11, 1820

24

Separation and Quantification of Component Monosaccharides of Cold Water-Soluble Polysaccharides from *Ephedra sinica* by MECC with Photodiode Array Detector

Haixue Kuang, Yong-Gang Xia and Bing-You Yang
Key Laboratory of Chinese Materia Medica,
(Heilongjiang University of Chinese Medicine), Ministry of Education, Harbin,
China

1. Introduction

The *Ephedra* plant, or "Mahuang" of traditional Chinese medicine, is one of the oldest medicinal plants known to mankind. More than 45 species of *Ephedra* plants exist and are indigenous to regions of Asia, North, Central and South America and Europe. Mahuang contains ephedrine alkaloids as their principal components, which are primarily localized in the aerial parts of the plant [1]. In recent years, many herbs used in popular medicine have been reported to contain polysaccharides with a great variety of biological activities and the polysaccharides are also demonstrated to be one of the main bioactive constituents of *Ephedra* plant except for a series of ephedrine alkaloids [2-4]. For these reasons, great interest arose on the reliable analytical methods of the Mahuang polysaccharides, which can be used for exploring the new functional products with polysaccharides due to its pharmacological importance and application in the pharmaceutical industry. Immunosuppressive effects of acidic polysaccharides from the stems of *E. sinica* have been demonstrated by carbon clearance test, delayed type hypersensitivity reaction and humoral immune response *in vivo* [2].

The commonly used separation techniques for carbohydrate analysis are gas chromatography (GC), high-performance liquid chromatography (HPLC), and capillary electrophoresis (CE) [5-7]. GC is a very classical method to analyze monosaccharide compositions of polysaccharides. Neutral monosaccharides are derivatized by silylation or acetylation before analysis, whereas acidic monosaccharides such as glucuronic acid and galacturonic acid can not be derivatized at all [8]. The uronic acid contents can be calculated by the difference between before and after carboxyl reduction of polysaccharides [9, 10]. So it is very laborious to calculate the uronic acid contents by GC method. Most of the HPLC and CE techniques are often used labeling with either fluorescence or UV tags for enhanced detection because these native carbohydrates are lack of chromophores or fluorophores in the structure. The reagent 1-phenyl-3-methyl-5-pyrazolone (PMP) is one of the popular labels that react with the reducing carbohydrate under mild conditions, requiring no acid catalyst and causing no desialylation and isomerization [11-16]. CE seems to possess several advantages over HPLC by offering higher separation efficiencies, yielding shorter analysis time, requiring small sample amounts, and consuming lower amounts of expensive reagents and solvents. It has the potential to become an important analytical separation tool for carbohydrate determination. Capillary zone electrophoresis (CZE) has been developed and successfully applied to analyze and quantify the aldoses and uronic acids [11-16]. However, few reports were proposed using MECC for the separation of the aldoses and uronic acids. The present paper is specifically concerned with the simultaneous separation of the 8 monosaccharides (aldoses and uronic acids) possibly found in natural herbs using pre-column PMP derivatization MECC and UV detection at 254 nm. Furthermore, the developed MECC method was applied to the quantitative analysis of component monosaccharides in the cold water-soluble polysaccharides from *E. sinica*.

2. Materials and methods

2.1 Rragents and standards

D-mannose (Man), L-rhamnose (Rha), D-glucose (Glc), D-galactose (Gal), L-arabinose (Ara), D-xylose (Xyl), D-glucuronic acid (GlcUA), D-galacturonic acid (GalUA) and sulfuric acid (H_2SO_4) were purchased from Sigma (St. Louis, USA). Trifluoroacetic acid (TFA) was obtained from Merck (Darmstadt, Germany). 1-Phenyl-3-methyl-5-pyrazolone (PMP), purchased from Beijing Reagent Plant (Beijing, China), was recrystallized twice from chromatographic grade methanol before use. Throughout the study deionised water was used, prepared by a Milli-Q water system (Millipore, MA, USA). The pH value of the electrolyte solution was measured with a Sartorius PB-20 pH meter with Sartorius pH/ATC electrode (Sartorius, CO, Germany) calibrated with commercial buffers of pH 7.00, 10.00, and 12.0 (Titrisol, Merck kGaA, Germany). All other chemicals were of the highest grade available.

2.2 Plant material

The dry stems of *E. sinica* were collected in March 2007 from Datong of Shanxi Province, China and identified by Prof. Zhenyue Wang of Heilongjiang University of Chinese Medicine. The voucher specimen (20070016) was deposited at Herbarium of Heilongjiang University of Chinese Medicine, Harbin, P. R. China.

2.3 Extraction of polysaccharides from *E. sinica*

The dry stems of *E. sinica* were ground to powders, and submitted to extractions as follows: dry powders (1.0 kg) were extracted 3 times with 10 vol of 95% EtOH under reflux for 3 h each time to remove lipids. The residue was dried in air and then extracted 3 times with 10 vol of distilled water for 24 h (each time) at 4 °C. The combined aqueous extracts were filtered, concentrated 10-fold, and 95% EtOH added to final concentration of 80%. The precipitate was dissolved in 600 mL of water and deproteinated 15 times with 200 mL of 5:1 chloroform -*n*-butanol as described by Staub (1965). The resulting aqueous fraction was extensively dialyzed (cut-off M_w 3500 Da) against tap water for 48 h and distilled water for 48 h and precipitated again by adding a 5 fold volume of ethanol. After centrifugation, the precipitate was washed with anhydrous ethanol and then dissolved in water and lyophilised to yield the cold water soluble polysaccharide (8.5 g) was collected by centrifugation (3000 rpm, 10 min, 20 °C).

2.4 MECC equipment and conditions

The analysis of PMP-labeled monosaccharides was carried out on a P/ACE MDQ capillary electrophoresis instrument (Beckman Coulter, Fullerton, CA, USA). An integrated P/ACE 32 Karat Station (software version 4.0) was used to perform the data collection and to control the operational variables of the system. Separation was carried out in an unmodified fused silica capillary (48.5 cm × 50 μm i.d., effective length 40 cm). Both the capillary and samples were thermostatted to 25 °C. The samples were injected with a pressure of 0.5 psi for 5 s. The separation voltage was raised linearly within 0.2 min from 0 to 20 kV. Detection was done with direct UV monitoring using a photodiode array detector at wavelength 254 nm.

A new capillary from Yongnian Optical Fiber Factory (Hebei Province, China) was activated by washing consecutively with each of 0.1 M phosphoric acid (15 min), water (10 min), 0.1M sodium hydroxide (15 min), and water (10 min). At the beginning of each working day, the capillary was prewashed with 0.1 M phosphoric acid (2 min), water (2 min), 0.1 M sodium hydroxide (2 min), water (2 min) and running buffer (2 min), respectively. Between analyses the capillaries were consecutively rinsed with 0.1 M sodium hydroxide (1 min), water (1 min) and running buffer (1 min).

2.5 Complete acid hydrolysis

20 mg of polysaccharide sample was dissolved in 2 ml of 2 M TFA in an ampoule (5 ml). The ampoule was sealed under a nitrogen atmosphere and kept in boiling water bath to hydrolyze the polysaccharide into component monosaccharides for 10 h. After being cooled to room temperature, the reaction mixture was centrifugated at 1000 rpm for 5 min. The supernatant was collected and dried under a reduced pressure. The hydrolyzed and dried sample solutions are added with 1 ml distilled water and then ready for the following experiments.

2.6 Derivatization procedure

PMP derivatization of monosaccharides was carried out as described previously with proper modification [11-17]. 200 μl of individual standard monosaccharide, or mix standard monosaccharide solutions, or the hydrolyzed polysaccharide samples were placed in the 2.0 ml centrifuge tubes, respectively, then 0.5 M methanol solution (100 μl) of PMP and 0.3 M aqueous NaOH (100 μl) were added to each. Each mixture was allowed to react for 30 min at 70 °C water bath, then cooled to room temperature and neutralized with 100 μl of 0.3 M HCl. The resulting solution was performed on liquid-liquid extraction with same volume of isoamyl acetate (two times) and chloroform (one time), respectively. After being shaken vigorously and centrifuged, the organic phase was carefully discarded to remove the excess reagents. Then the aqueous layer was filtered through a 0.45 μm membrane and diluted with water before MECC analysis.

2.7 Method validation

The regression equations were calculated in the form of $y = a\,x + b$, where y was the peak areas and x was the concentration of analytes. The signal-to-noise of 3:1 and 10:1 were used to establish LOD and LOQ, respectively. The measurement of intra- and inter-day variability was utilized to determine the precision of this newly developed method. The intraday variation was determined by analyzing the same mixed standard water solution for five times within 1 day. While for inter-day variability test, the solution was examined in triplicate for consecutive 3 days. Stability of sample solution was tested at 0, 4, 8, 12, 24 and 48 h within 2 days. All solutions were kept at 4 °C before analysis. The analytes showed stable in water solution (RSD<3.45%) at 4 °C during the tested period.

3. Results and discussion

3.1 Method development

We can only label carbohydrates according to Fig. 1 [16], usually yields neutral sugar derivatives which become negatively charged in aqueous basic solutions due to the partial dissociation of the enolic hydroxyl group of the PMP tag. In this study, the method development was achieved by optimizing background electrolyte pH, SDS and borax concentration of the buffer, applied voltage and capillary temperature.

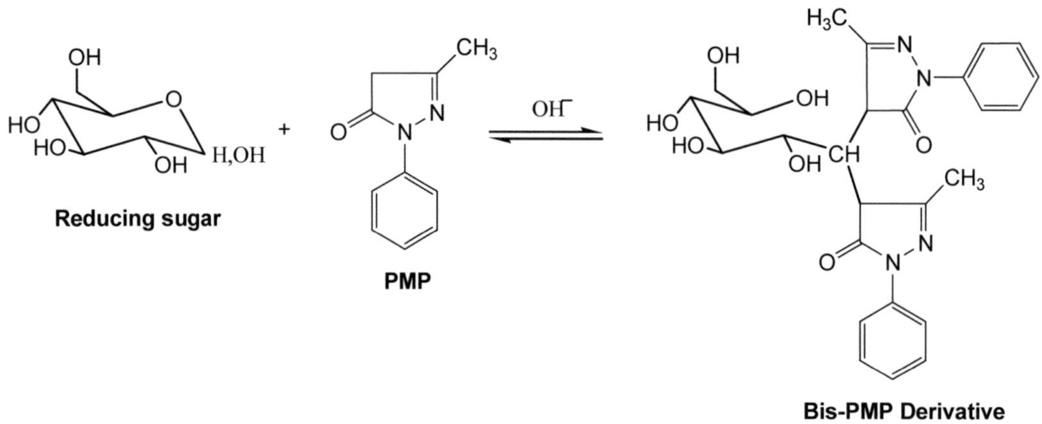

Fig. 1. Illustration of condensation reaction with PMP

3.1.1 Effect of pH

The effect of pH on the separation was also investigated in the pH range from 9.7 to 10.75 using borate buffer solutions as background electrolytes. Fig. 2 is comparison of four pH electrolytes in the analysis of 8 carbohydrates, from which the separation conditions are revealed more clearly. The result reveals that the pH of buffer had great influence on the resolutions and the migration time. Supposing an appropriate pH (9.70) chosen, ara and glc have been co-eluted as one peak. Only man, gal, glcUA and galUA have the high resolutions. If a higher pH (10.0 or 10.23) is adopted, there are poor resolutions between ara and glc. And if we use pH 10.75, good symmetry and the resolution for each analyte was achieved. Thus pH 10.75 was chosen as the optimal running buffer condition.

3.1.2 Effect of buffer and SDS concentration

The separation of PMP-labeled carbohydrates was very sensitive to borate buffer concentrations and SDS concentration in MECC. In this study, borate concentration in the range of 20–33 mM was evaluated (Fig. 3). The results indicated that the migration time of PMP-labeled carbohydrates generally increased with a gradual increasing of buffer concentrations. Taking the shorter run-time and good resolution into consideration, 25 mM borate buffer solution was selected and the maximum resolution was obtained.

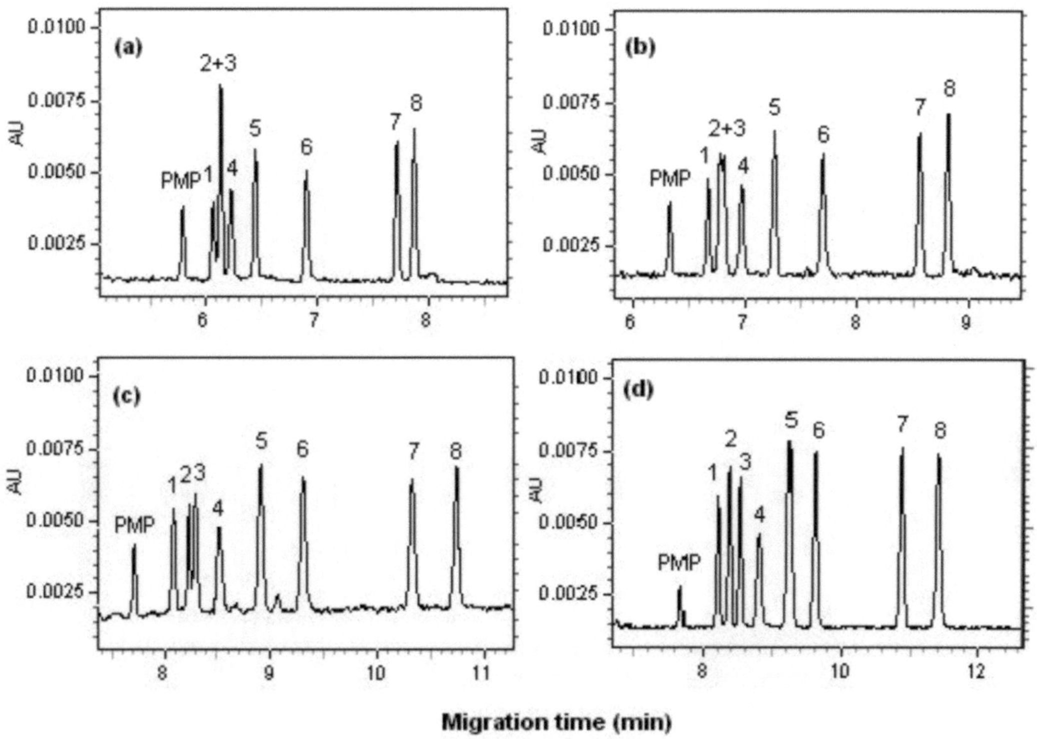

Fig. 2. Comparison of electropherograms of PMP derivatives of 8 standard monosaccharides with 25 mM borate buffer and 30 mM SDS at four pH electrolytes, 1 mM each. Peak identities: 1, xyl; 2, ara; 3 glc; 4 rha; 5, man; 6, gal; 7, glcUA; 8, galUA. Separation conditions: applied voltage, +20 kV; Separation conditions: +25 kV; detection, 254 nm direct mode; injection pressure, 0.5 psi for 5 s; capillary, fused-silica 40.0/48.5 cm (*L*det/*L*tot); separation temperature, 25 °C. The pH of borate buffer: (a) pH 9.70; (b) pH 10.00; (c) pH 10.23; (d) pH 10.75

Different concentrations of SDS (25, 30 and 35 mM) at pH 10.75 and 25 mM borate buffer on the separation of analytes were studied (Fig. 4). It was found that Xyl and Ara were not well separated at 20 mM SDS with poor resolution, but best resolution and highest theory plates were achieved at 30 mM SDS. Increasing SDS concentration, however, remarkably increased the migration time of all analytes. Therefore, 30 mM SDS was chosen as the optimal SDS concentration thus it was chosen for the further experiments.

3.1.3 Effect of capillary temperature and voltage

The temperature of the analysis may sometimes be important in MECC, as fluctuations in the temperature may affect the viscosity of the running buffer, leading to higher analyte electrophoretic mobilities and shorter analysis time. The temperature changes can also affect the pH of the buffer. In this case, 25 °C is most optimal. In addition, the effects of three voltage values (10-28 kV) on separation of the analytes also were studied. The results showed that the good resolution and acceptable migration time were achieved at 25 kV.

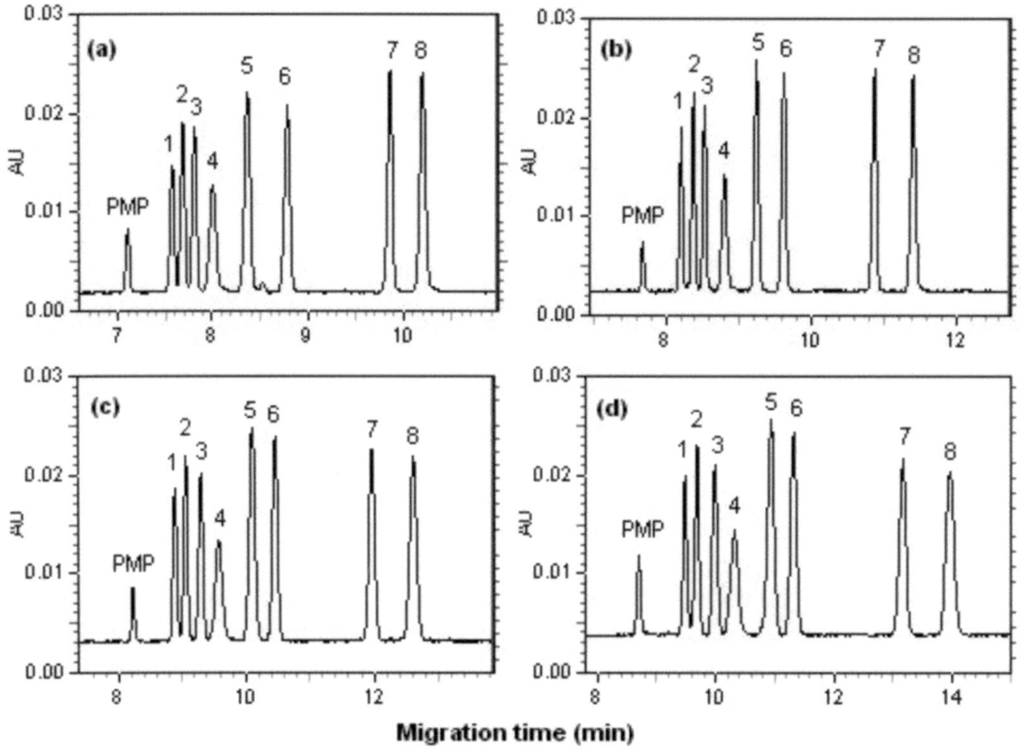

Fig. 3. Comparison of electropherograms of PMP derivatives of 8 standard monosaccharides at four buffer concentration electrolytes, 1 mM each. Borate concentration: (a) 20 mM; (b) 25 mM; (c) 27 mM; (c) 30 mM. Peak identities and other analytical conditions were in Fig. 2.

To achieve optimal separation, the operation at 20 mM of borax and 30 mM SDS at pH 10.75, capillary temperature 25 °C and applied voltage 20 kV, a complete baseline resolution for carbohydrate derivatives can be achieved within the shortest time. Under the proposed conditions, the separation of nine PMP-labeled carbohydrates is achieved within 12 min. The separation of standard mixture consisting of 8 PMP-labeled carbohydrates is shown in Fig. 5A.

3.2 Validation of the method developed

The MECC method was validated in terms of linearity, reproducibility, limit of detection (LOD) and precision. The linearity was verified by the analysis of six points in the range of 37.5 - 600.00 µM, and the linear regression parameters of the calibration curves were shown in Table 1. As a consequence, the good linearity (correlation coefficient $R^2 > 0.9993$) between y (peak area ratio of the analytes with internal standard) and x (concentration of the standards) was achieved in the tested range. Furthermore, LOD of each tested analyte was obtained by injecting 0.5 psi for 5 s of gradational dilutions of a standard mixture

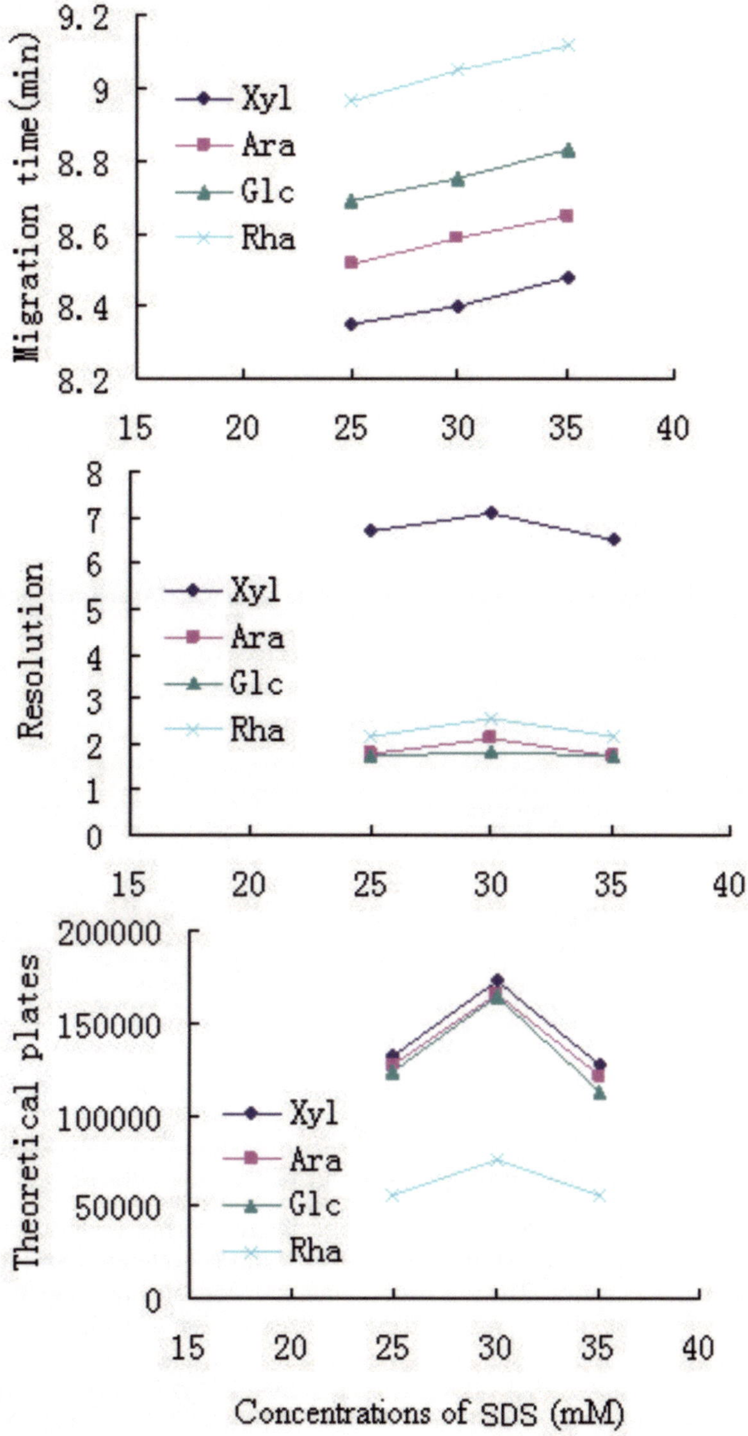

Fig. 4. Effects of SDS on the migration time, resolution and theory plates.

derivatized as mentioned above in the derivatization procedure, followed by the comparison of peak height with baseline noise level and a signal-to-noise ratio (S/N) of 3 assigned the detection limit. The results showed that the LOD of the monosaccharides was in the range from 10.5 to 11.7 μM (Table 1), indicating that the sensitivity of the method was satisfactory.

Carbohydrats[a]	Regression equation (y = a + b x)[b]		correlation coefficient	LOD[c] (μM)	LOQ[d] (μM)
	a	b			
Xyl	-0.2106	0.0134	0.9998	10.5	33.6
Ara	-0.2681	0.0172	0.9994	11.2	35.8
Glc	-0.1576	0.0078	0.9993	11.4	36.4
Rha	-0.1196	0.0086	0.9997	11.7	37.5
Man	-0.1049	0.0203	0.9995	10.9	34.8
Gal	-0.26	0.0225	0.9995	11.3	36.0
GalUA	-0.4612	0.0232	0.9992	10.8	34.6

[a] Quantitated with a calibration curve at = 254 nm

[b] The y and x are peak area ratio of the analytes to internal standard (GlcUA) and concentration of the analytes (37.5-600μM), respectively

[c] LOD corresponds to concentrations giving a signal-to-noise ratio of 3.

[d] LOQ corresponds to concentrations giving a signal-to-noise ratio of 10.

Table 1. Linearity of CE method of different carbohydrate

Carbohydrats	Intra-day precision (RSD%, n = 5)		Inter-day precision (RSD%, n = 3)	
	Retention time	Peak area	Retention time	Peak area
Xyl	1.25	2.38	1.36	3.21
Ara	2.03	2.97	1.58	3.56
Glc	1.69	1.97	2.21	4.03
Rha	2.31	2.46	1.99	3.69
Man	2.09	2.36	2.16	2.79
Gal	1.95	2.57	1.94	2.88
GlcUA	1.85	2.77	2.37	4.35
GalUA	1.38	2.89	1.96	4.27

Table 2. Precision of the retention time and peak area of analytes in the present method

Moreover, method precision was also determined by measuring repeatability (intra-day variability) and intermediate precision (inter-day variability) of retention time and peak area for each tested monosaccharide. The precision of method was calculated as the coefficient of variation (RSD) for five successive injections of each tested monosaccharide at the concentration of 1 mM and the results were summarized in Table 3. The results showed that the intra-day reproducibility (RSD values) were less than 2.31% for the migration time and 2.97% for the peak areas, and the interday RSD values were less than 2.37% for the migration time and 4.35% for the peak areas, indicating that the method precision was satisfactory.

Component	added amount (μM)	found amount (μM)	recovery(%)[a] means ± SD	RSD (%)[b]
Ara	270	270.2	100.15 ± 4.03	4.02
Glc	62	61.7	99.51 ± 3.63	3.65
Rha	35	35.4	105.13 ± 2.79	2.76
Man	25	24.6	98.45 ± 2.86	2.91
Gal	53	53.5	103.97 ± 3.51	3.48
GalUA	30	29.7	97.28 ± 3.73	3.83

a Recovery (%) = [(mean of measured concentration−spiked concentration)/spiked concentration]×100.
b RSD (%) = (SD/mean)×100

Table 3. Recoveries of six monosaccharides in sample analysis (n= 6)

3.3 Analysis of the cold water-soluble polysaccharide extract from E. sinica

This experiment was designed to develop a rapid, repeatable and accurate MECC method for the quantification of the component carbohydrates in the cold water-soluble polysaccharide extract from *E. sinica*. In order to evaluate the applicability of the proposed method, the polysaccharide was hydrolyzed with 2M TFA, and PMP-labeled as described in the experimental section and finally, the released monosaccharide derivatives were analyzed by the described MECC method under the optimized conditions using GlcUA as internal standard. Fig. 5B shows a typical chromatogram of the cold water-soluble polysaccharide sample. As can be seen, the PMP derivatives of the component monosaccharides released from the Mahuang polysaccharide sample could be still baseline separated and the component monosaccharides could be identified by comparing with the chromatogram of the mixture of standard monosaccharides (Fig. 5A). The results showed that the cold water-soluble polysaccharide extract from *E. sinica* was a typical heteropolysaccharide and was composed of arabinose, glucose, rhamnose, mannose, galactose and galacturonic acid in the molar rate of 4.36:1.43:1.00:0.55:0.41:0.85:0.45, and their corresponding mole percentages were 57.24%, 13.12%, 7.16%, 5.40%, 11.17%, and 5.87% (mol%), respectively. It was clear that the predominantly composition monosaccharides in the cold water-soluble polysaccharide extract from *E. sinica* were arabinose up to 57.24% (mol%) of total carbohydrates, and only 5.87% of total carbohydrates was galacturonic acid.

Furthermore, recovery experiments were performed in order to investigate the accuracy of the method. Known amounts of each monosaccharide solute were added to the sample detected, and the resulting spiked sample was subjected to the entire analytical sequence. Each solute was spiked at a close concentration with the sample and recoveries were calculated based on the difference between the total amount determined in the spiked samples and the amount observed in the non-spiked samples. All analyses were carried out in triplicate. The results showed that the recoveries of all the monosaccharides ranged between 97.28% and 105.13% and the RSD values were within 2.76–4.02% (Table 3). Such results further demonstrated that this method is precise and practical for the analysis of polysaccharide samples from *E. sinica*.

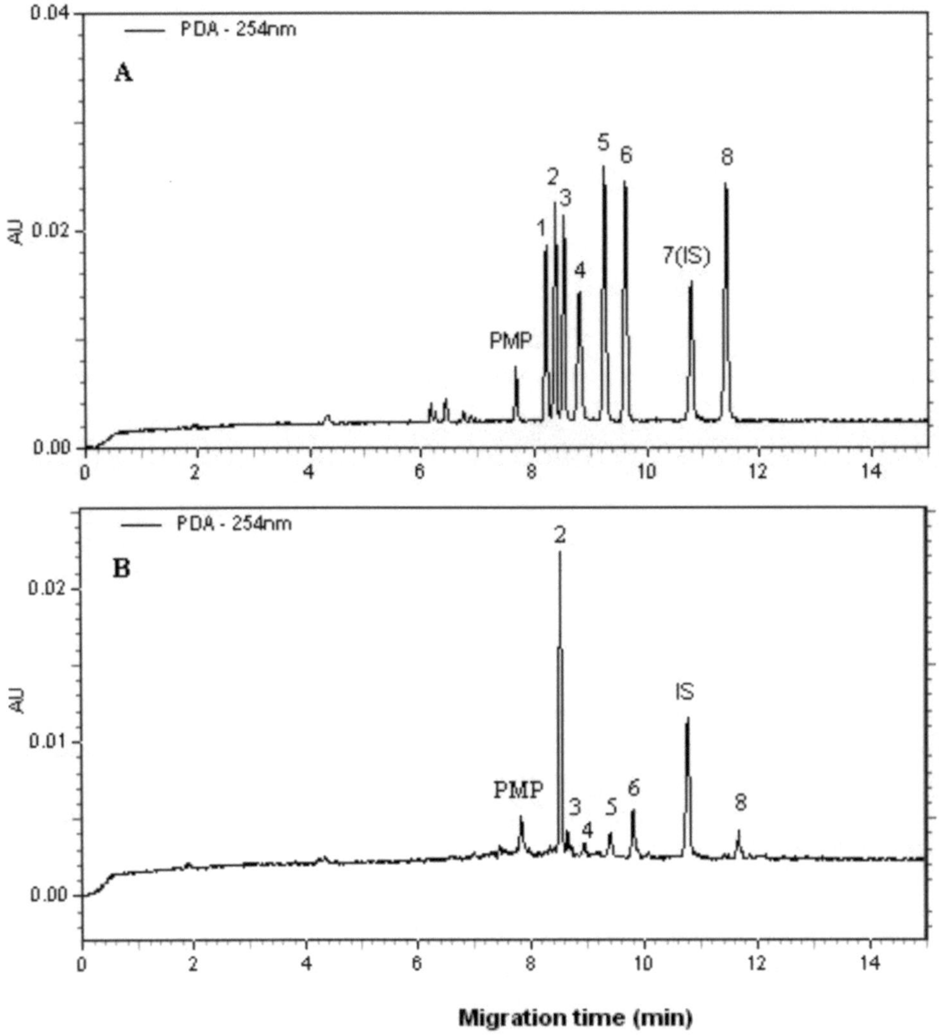

Fig. 5. Electropherograms of PMP derivatives of standard monosaccharides (A) and the sample (B). Peak identities and other analytical conditions were in Fig. 2.

4. Conclusions

In recent years, the monosaccharides PMP derivatives mentioned above were successfully separated by CZE and HPLC although the analysis was accomplished for a long time [11-16]. However, in this study, as shown in Fig. 5A, various PMP derivatives of monosaccharides were shown to separate quite nicely in MECC within 12 min and seven composition monosaccharides were successfully identified and the assay results were satisfactory. The separation is based on the differential distribution of the PMP derivatives between the aqueous mobile phase and the micellar phase. The applicability of the SDS micellar system was extended to the identification and quantitation of monosaccharides obtained from carbohydrate hydrolyzates from polysaccharide. The shape of the peaks was very sharp and it was clear that a substantial improvement in the separation of neutral sugar and uronic acid derivatives was obtained by MECC method, and thus, the analytical cost is lower and is also eco-friendly for its non-consumption of organic solvents as compared with other analytical techniques.

5. Acknowledgements

The authors wish to thank financial support for this study by the Major State Basic Research Development Program of China (973 Program 2006CB504708), State Key Creative New Drug Project of 12th Five-year Plan of China (2011ZX09102-006-01), National Natural Science Foundation of China (30973870), China Postdoctoral Science Foundation project (20110490111), Heilongjiang Postdoctoral Science Foundation project (LBH-Z10019) and Heilongjiang University of Chinese Medicine Doctor Innovative Foundation project (B201002).

6. References

[1] Jiangsu New Medical College (1986). *Dictionary of Chinese Materia Medica*. Shanghai: Shanghai people's press; p. 2221-2224.

[2] Kuang, H. X., Xia, Y. G., Yang, B.Y., Wang, Q. H., and Wang, Y. H. Screening and comparison of the immunosuppressive activities of polysaccharides from the stems of *Ephedra sinica* Stapf. *Carbohydrate Polymers*, 2010, 83 (2), 787-795.

[3] Cheng, R. M., Zhu, G. X., and Xu, Z. Y. (2001). Effect of different extracts from Ephedra on cell immunity. *Journal of Nanjing TCM University, 17*, 234–236.

[4] Meng, D. L., Yan, S. H., and Xu, Z. Y. (2007). Effect of ephedran on erythrocytolysin formation of mouse caused by sheep erythrocyte. *Journal of Jiangsu University, 17*, 379–381.

[5] Guo, L., Xie, M. Y., Yan, A. P., and Wan, Y. Q. (2006). Simultaneous determination of five synthetic antioxidants in edible vegetable oil by GC-MS. *Analytical and Bioanalytical Chemistry, 386*, 1881-1887.

[6] Daotian, F., and Roger, A. (1995). Monosaccharide composition analysis of oligosaccharides and glycoproteins by high-performance liquid chromatography. *Analytical Biochemistry, 227*, 377-384.

[7] Lv, Y., Yang, X. B., Zhao, Y., Ruan, Y., Yang, Y., and Wang, Z. Z. (2009). Separation and quantification of component monosaccharides of the tea polysaccharides from *Gynostemma pentaphyllum* by HPLC with indirect UV detection. *Food Chemestry, 112*, 742-746.

[8] Chen, Y., Xie, M. Y., Wang, Y. X., Nie, S. P., and Chang, L. (2009). Analysis of the monosaccharide composition of purified polysaccharides in *Ganoderma atrum* by capillary gas chromatography. *Phytochemical Analysis, 20*, 503-510.

[9] Perry, M. B., MacLean, L. L., Patrauchan, M. A., and Vinogradov, E. (2007). The structure of the exocellular polysaccharide produced by *Rhodococcus sp.* RHA1. *Carbohydrate Research, 342*, 2223-2229.

[10] Xia, Y. G., Liang, J., Yang, B. Y., Wang, Q. H., and Kuang, H. X. A new method for quantitative determination of two uronic acids by CZE with direct UV detection. *Biomedical chromagraphy*, doi:10.1002/bmc.1564.

[11] Andersen, K. E., Bjergegaard, C., Mller, P., Srensen, J. C., and Srensen, H. (2003). High performance capillary electrophoresis with indirect UV detection for determination of α-galactosides in leguminose and brassicaceae. *Journal of Agricultural and Food Chemistry, 51,* 6391-6397.

[12] Daotian, F. and Roger, A. (1995). Monosaccharide composition analysis of oligosaccharides and glycoproteins by high-performance liquid chromatography. *Analytical Biochemistry, 227,* 377-384.

[13] Honda, S., Akao, E., Suzuki, S., Okuda, M., Kakehi, K., and Nakamura, J. (1989). High performance liquid chromatography of reducing carbohydrates as strongly ultraviolet-absorbing and electrochemically sensitive 1-phenyl-3-methyl-5-pyrazolone derivatives. *Analytical Chemistry, 180,* 351-357.

[14] Honda, S., Suzuki, S., and Taga, A. (2003). Analysis of carbohydrates as 1-phenyl-3-methyl-5 -pyrazolone derivatives by capillary/microchip electrophoresis and capillary electrochro -matography. *Journal of Pharmaceutical and Biomedical Analysis, 30,* 1689-1714.

[15] Wang, Q. J. and Fang, Y. Z. (2004). Analysis of sugars in traditional Chinese drugs. *Journal of Chromatography B, 812,* 309-324.

[16] Xia, Y. G., Wang, Q. H., Liang, J., Yang, B. Y., Li, G. Y., and Kuang, H. X. Development and application of a rapid and efficient CZE method coupled with correction factors for determination of monosaccharide composition of acidic hetero-polysaccharides from *Ephedra sinica. Phytochemical Analysis*, 2011, 22, 103-111.

[17] Zhang, L. Y., Xu, J., Zhang, L. H., Zhang, W. B., and Zhang, Y. K. (2003). Determination of 1-phenyl-3-methyl-5-pyrazolone-labeled carbohydrates by liquid chromatography and micellar electrokinetic chromatography. *Journal of Chromatography B, 793,* 159-165.

25

Phytochemicals as Antidepressants: The Involvement of Serotonin Receptor Function, Stress Resistance and Neurogenesis

Rui Wang[1] and Ying Xu[2]
[1]*Program of Pharmacology, Weill Graduate School of Medical Science, Cornell University, New York, NY,*
[2]*Department of Behavioral Medicine and Psychiatry, West Virginia University Health Science Center, Morgantown, WV, USA*

1. Introduction

Mood disorders are among the most prevalent forms of mental illness and a major cause of morbidity worldwide. Depression is one of the top ten causes of morbidity and mortality worldwide based on a survey by the World Health Organization (Berton and Nestler, 2006). Depression (major depressive disorder, major depression, unipolar depression, clinical depression) is a chronic, recurring and potentially life-threatening mood disorder that has been estimated to affect 21% of the world population (Schechter et al., 2005). It is estimated that 40% of the risk for depression is genetic, though the specific genes involved in the risk is still limited understanding. The other 60% non-genetic risk remains poorly defined, with suggestions as diverse as acute or chronic stress, childhood trauma, viral infections and even random processes during brain development might be involved (Akiskal, 2000; Berton and Nestler, 2006).

Stress occurs in every day life. Among psychiatric disorders, depression is probably the most common stress-related diseases. The theoretical premise is that depression is the outcome of an eventual inability to cope with a stream of dissimilar unpleasant stimuli imposed by the environment (Ferretti et al., 1995). The link between genetic predisposition and life stressors in the etiology of depression remains unclear because the mode of transmission of mood disorders is likely to be complex. However, interactions between a genetic predisposition and some environmental stressors are probably necessary to induce depression (Caspi and Moffitt, 2006). In addition, not only the hypothalamic-pituitary-adrenal (HPA) axis, but also brain neuronal systems, including the monoaminergic systems and in particular the serotonin (5-HT) containing neuronal one, play critical roles in stress-related disorders (Lanfumey et al., 2008; Xu et al., 2006). The structural alterations of neurons in stress-induced depression, such as a progressive decrease in the volume of the frontal cortex and hippocampus, have also been found to be related to dysfunctions of HPA axis, abnormalities in 5-HT and its receptors (Drevets, 2000; Reinés et al., 2008; Tsuji et al., 2001). But, so far, no clear consensus has evolved in pathological mechanism of inter-neuronal communication and post-receptor signal transduction of depression.

Early theories of depression focused on imbalance of neurotransmitter system, especially depletion of the serotonin (5-HT), norepinephrine (NE) and/or dopamine in depression and related mood disorders, since the efficacy of tricyclic antidepressants and monoamine oxidase inhibitors (MAOIs) in the treatment of these disorders. Current theoretical and experimental developments in serotonin and noradrenaline research extend the previous studies, the robust therapeutic effects of newer antidepressants are discovered, such as selective serotonin reuptake inhibitors (SSRIs), noradrenaline reuptake inhibitors (NRIs) and serotonin and noradrenaline reuptake inhibitors (SNRIs). However, the current therapeutic options of depression are far from ideal: most of the pharmacological interventions are not effective in more than 50% cases, and are often associated with a range of serious side effects and drug-drug/drug-food interactions (Baker et al., 2003; Meijer et al., 2004).
Polyphenolic nutraceuticals (phytochemicals) present in vegetables and fruits are believed to reduce the risk of several major diseases including cardiovascular, autoimmune and neurodegenerative disorders. Six such polyphenols are curcumin, low molecular proanthocyanidin, resveratrol, fisetin, piceatannol and ferulic acid, which have been used throughout Asia as traditional herbal medicines. They show strong antioxidant and anti-inflammatory properties. The wide ranging activity of these compounds and the repeated demonstration that they can decrease the stress response, oxidative damage, inflammation, neuronal damage and act as neuroprotectants, strongly suggest these compounds might have a significant impact on stress-induced depression and other affective disorders.
In this review, we integrate our current knowledge to define the present state of depression and assessment of the position of serotoninergic function in the pathophysiology of depression. We also summarize the status of a few novel approaches and compounds that are under investigation for the treatment of major depression. We attempt to provide a progress report on the pharmacological profile of multiple polyphenolic phytochemicals as promising herbal antidepressants.

2. Biological correlates of stress-induced depression and neurogenesis: Evidence for serotoninergic function

2.1 Stress, corticosterone and depression

Glucocorticoid release is regulated by the HPA axis in physical conditions. Corticotropin-relaesing hormone (CRH) released by the paraventricular nucleus of the hypothalamus stimulates the release of corticotropin (ACTH) from the anterior pituitary, which, in turn, stimulates glucocorticoid secretion from the adrenal cortex. HPA axis is an essential component of an individual's capacity to cope with stress (Berton and Nestler, 2006). Stress may be described as any environmental change, either internal or external, that disturbs the maintenance on homeostasis (Leonard, 2005). The stress response is to maintain homeostasis, which includes a series of physiological reactions such as endocrine activation (especially of the HPA axis) and cardiovascular changes (Sapolsky, 2003). The symptomatology, such as irritability, anxiety and a feeling of being unable to cope with, may ultimately result in depression when exposure to a prolonged and sustained stress (Lanfumey et al., 2008). Chronic stress often acts as a trigger to the onset of major depression and is associated with a decreased sensitivity to HPA axis feedback inhibition by cortisol in primates or corticosterone in rodents. Excessive stimulation of the axis further increases the secretion of glucocorticoids, which affects many aspects of peripheral and neuronal function, including immune, epithelial cell growth and energy mebabolism, neuronal connections, and synaptic transmission (McEwen and Stellar, 1993).

It is a common finding that around 50% of depressed patients (80% if severely depressed) show hyperactivity of the HPA axis (Young et al., 1991). Interestingly, similar changes in the hyperactivity of the HPA axis have been reported in animals subjected to chronic stress (Leonard, 2005). Elevated corticosterone level is a hallmark of HPA axis feedback inhibition evidenced by animal studies (Centeno and Volosin, 1997). This feedback is mediated by two types of corticosteroid receptors in the brain, the mineralocorticoid receptor (MR) and the GR (McEwen, 2000). The MR is a high-affinity receptor which binds corticosterone at low concentration (Kd ~0.5nM). MR is almost completely occupied (90%) by basal corticosterone levels and this contributes to maintaining homeostasis. When normal secretion of glucocorticoids is altered during stress, leading to increased levels of corticosterone, GR becomes substantially occupied by the hormone ligand. GR has a widespread distribution in limbic regions such as the hippocampus, paraventricular nucleus (PVN), the locus coeruleus and the dorsal raphe nucleus (DRN) (Harfstrand et al., 1986; Reul and de Kloet, 1986). Glucocorticoids diffuse passively through cellular membranes and bind to intracellular glucocorticoid receptors (GR), causing their translocation into the nucleus (Gillespie and Nemeroff, 2005). In the nucleus, these ligand-activated transcription factors bind to specific DNA response elements and alter gene expression. In the brain, glucocorticoid-regulated gene changes mediate a variety of effects on neuronal excitability, neurochemistry and structural plasticity (McEwen, 2000).

2.2 Serotonin and its receptors in depression

5-HT was discovered in 1948 and is a phylogenetically conserved neurotransmitter (Rapport et al., 1948; Barnes and Sharp, 1999). It is synthesized from L-tryptophan both in the peripheral nervous system and the CNS, via tryptophan hydroxylase 1 and 2, respectively (Walther et al., 2003). In the CNS, 5-HT neurons are localized in the raphe nuclei and project, via ascending and descending pathways, to a wide range of brain regions (Dahlström and Fuxe, 1964). These receptors affect a wide range of physiological and psychopathological processes such as mood disturbances, sleep, temperature control appetite, sexual behavior, movement, pain perception, and gastrointestinal motility. It is well established that the 5-HT is a phylogenetically conserved monoaminergic neurotransmitter which is crucial for a number of physiological processes and is dysregulated in several disease states including depression, anxiety and schizophrenia. As an important neurotransmitter, serotonin exerts its functions through 14 5-HT subtypes receptors. Exposure of experimental animals to various stressors, such as restraint stress and electroshock, has been shown to increase the turnover of serotonin and its receptors in the frontal cortex, hippocampus, amygdala and other brain regions (Inoue et al., 1994).

Fourteen different 5-HT receptors have been cloned and pharmacologically characterized (Barnes and Sharp, 1999; Dahlstrom and Fuxe, 1964; Walther et al., 2003; Millan et al., 2008). The human 5-HT receptors are divided into 7 distinct families (5-HT_{1-7}) (Davis et al., 2002). With the exception of the 5-HT_3 receptor as a ligand-gated ion channel, all other serotonin receptors (5-HT_{1A-E}, 5-HT_{2A-C}, 5-HT_4, 5-HT_5, 5-HT_6, 5-HT_7) are G protein-coupled receptors that activate an intracellular second messenger cascade to produce an excitatory or inhibitory response. Activation of the specific G-protein can affect enzymes (5-HT_1- and 5-HT_5-class receptors decrease cAMP formation; 5-HT_2-class receptors increase inositol triphosphate and diacylglycerol formation; and 5-HT_4, 5-HT_6 and 5-HT_7 receptors increase cAMP formation) and the function of cation channels especially K^+ and Ca^{2+} (Kushwaha and Albert, 2005).

5-HT, as an important neurotransmitter, has long been reported to exert an important mitogenic action in the central neural system (CNS) during development (Lauder et al., 1981; Whitaker-Azmitia,1991). In the adult CNS, serotonin is involved in neuronal and synaptic plasticity, and its action on the serotonin 5-HT_{1A} receptor is particularly significant in this regard (Azmitia and Whitaker-Azmitia, 1997). It was also found that the powerful mitogenic effect of fenfluramine (a releaser of serotonin throughout the CNS) on the granule cell layer of the adult rat dentate gyrus (DG) could be completely blocked by pretreatment with a specific 5-HT_{1A} antagonist (Jacobs, 2002).

The 5-HT_{1A} and 5-HT_{2A} receptors are the most studied receptors in relation to affective disorders. It has been shown, in both human and animal studies, that 5-HT_{1A} (Blier et al., 1993; Nishi et al., 2009), 5-HT_{1B} (Benjamin et al., 1990; Clark et al., 2002; Kaiyala et al., 2003; O'Connor et al., 1994; Saudou et al.,1994; Sari, 2004), 5-HT_{2A} (Bhagwagar et al., 2006), and a 5-HT transporter (5-HTT) (Bhagwagar et al., 2007) play important roles in affective disorders as well as the action of antidepressants. Evidence is accumulating that dysfunction in the brain serotonergic system relates to mood and behavior disorders (Soares and Mann, 1997). The 5-HT_{1A} receptor is not only a presynaptic autoreceptor (as described earlier) but also a postsynaptic receptor, which is similar to the 5-HT_{2A} receptor and highly distributed in limbic areas and hypothalamus. In rodents, 60% of the neurons in the prefrontal cortex are expressing 5-HT_{1A} and/or 5-HT_{2A} receptors (Amargós-Bosch et al., 2004). Both of these receptors are expressed in different cell types including pyramidal cells and GABAergic inter neurons in both frontal cortex and hippocampus. The 5-HT neurons in the dorsal raphe are regulated by somatodendritic presynaptic 5-HT_{1A} receptors and distal feedback via postsynaptic 5-HT receptors which regulate the glutamatergic neurons in the prefrontal cortex (Celada et al., 2001; Martín-Ruiz et al., 2001; Puig et al., 2003).

The potential role of 5-HT_{1A} receptors in the function and structure (e.g. DG neurogenesis) of hippocampus-related depressive disorders has been reported earlier (Gould, 1999; Radley and Jacobs, 2002), and the 5-HT_{1A} receptor is present at a particularly high concentration in the hippocampus, especially in the DG. The consistent neuroendocrine evidence in depression has already demonstrated a reduction in 5-HT_{1A} receptor function and number (Porter et al., 2004; Riedel et al., 2002; Drevets et al., 1999). The clinical reports have pointed out that the low level of 5-HT_{1A} receptors represents a risk factor in mood disorders (O'Neill and Conway, 2001; Cryan et al., 2005). Animal studies also suggest that the increase in the neurotransmission at postsynaptic 5-HT_{1A} receptors may mediate the therapeutic effects of some antidepressants (Welner et al., 1989). In addition, many studies suggest that increases in adult neurogenesis after the SSRI administration require the activation of 5-HT_{1A} receptors (Santarelli et al., 2003), which is consistent with the results that 5-HT_{1A} receptor antagonists or knockout mice decrease or lack cell proliferation in the dentate gyrus, respectively (Radley and Jacobs, 2002; Santarelli et al., 2003). Furthermore, it has been reported that the antidepressant effect of SSRIs are mediated by 5-HT_{1A} receptors (Tatarczynska et al., 2002; Hirano et al., 2002) by changing the receptor-medicated G-protein-coupled inwardly rectifying potassium (GIRK) currents (Cornelisse et al., 2007). Therefore, 5-HT_{1A} is definitely involved in depression as well as the action of antidepressants.

Recent studies have also pointed out an important role for 5-HT_2 receptors in the pathology of depression as well as the action of many antidepressants (Cryan and Leonard, 2000; Cryan and Lucki, 2000; Boothman et al., 2006). Treatment of some established antidepressants results in a reduction of 5-HT_2 receptor density in rat frontal cortex (Klimek et al., 1994; Subhash et al., 1997). Indeed, most antidepressants can primarily down-regulate $5\text{-}HT_{2A}$ receptors, which indicates the therapeutical potential of this receptor (Toth and Shenk, 1994). In addition, some $5\text{-}HT_{2A/2C}$ receptor antagonists are found to enhance the antidepressant-like effects of SSRIs when given jointly (Redrobe and Bourin, 1997; Redrobe and Bourin, 1998), which suggests that the antagonism of these receptors may be implicated in the action of such antidepressants. Moreover, it has been reported that mRNA levels of $5\text{-}HT_{1A}$ and $5\text{-}HT_2$ remained unchanged after the treatment of imipromine or citalopram, implying that the antidepressant outcome may involve the changes of the 5-HT receptor density as well as the functional effects of 5-HT receptors (Butler et al., 1993; Burnet et al., 1994; Spurlock et al., 1994).

2.3 Neurotrophic mechanisms in depression

Animal studies have already shown that acute or chronic stress can activate HPA axis and inhibit the cell proliferation in adult hippocampus (Warner-Schmidt and Duman, 2006; Paizanis et al., 2007). It has been shown that the psychosocial and physical stressors can inhibit the neurogenesis in various animal models and thus lead to decreased cell proliferation and survival (Joëls et al., 2007). In the chronic stressed model, both neurogenesis and proliferation were reduced in all rats (Joëls et al., 2007, Li et al., 2006). Moreover, treatment with diverse antidepressants, such as lithium, will reverse these changes (Knijff et al., 2007).

It is widely accepted that both stress and corticosteroid can decrease the levels of some neurotrophic factors in hippocampus while many classes of antidepressant as well as electroconvulsive shock treatment can reverse the decrease and prevent the action of stress, which is the base of the neurotrophic mechanism of depression (Duman and Monteggia, 2006). Neurotrophic factors, such as BDNF, NGF, neurotrophin-3 (NT-3), NT-4, NT-5 and NT-6, have been shown to enhance the cell proliferation and neurogenesis in the subgranular layer of the dentate gyrus (Banasr et al., 2004). These neurotrophic factors are critical to the viability and function of the neurons. Local infusion of BDNF into the midbrain or hippocampus regions has antidepressant-like effects in behavioral animal models of depression (Siuciak et al., 1994; Duman and Monteggia, 2006). For human studies, reduced levels of BDNF were detected in postmortem brain tissues of the depressed patients while antidepressant treatment can reverse it (Chen et al., 2001). All these data suggest that the action of antidepressants might be mediated via activating BDNF signaling in the hippocampus.

Increasing evidence has shown that the neuroprotective effects of the neurotrophic factors are mainly mediated by inhibiting the cell death/apoptosis pathways (Du et al., 2003). BDNF, as a major neurotrophic factor, can initiate various signaling pathways, such as MAPK/ERK and PI-3K/Akt pathways, through binding to its tyrosine kinase TrkB receptor and thus activate the downstream molecules which can promote neurogenesis and cell survival. The phosphor-ERK and PI-3K/Akt can further phosphorylate and activate cyclic adenosine monophosphate (cAMP) response element binding (CREB) (Banasr et al., 2004; Chen and Manji, 2006). For instance, BDNF and CREB levels are decreased in cerebral cortex of depressive patients, while the treatment of antidepressants can enhance the BDNF levels in patients (Karege et al., 2002). In the CREB knockout mice, BDNF up-regulation is abolished after the antidepressant treatment (Conti et al., 2002). Moreover, a variety of antidepressants, regardless of their mechanisms, up-regulate the BDNF expression in rodent hippocampus, while the non-antidepressant drugs are not effective (Duman and Monteggia,

2006). In addition, the phosphorylation of CREB will consequently activate the transcription of many survival-promoting genes, such as B-cell lymphoma 2 (bcl-2) and BDNF.
Bcl-2, a critical anti-apoptotic protein, has been shown to be upregulated by mood stabilizers in multiple animal studies (Chen et al., 1999; Manji et al., 2000; Chang et al., 2009). Reduced level of bcl-2 was also observed after stress: bcl-2 mRNA level was decreased by 70% when exposed to aggressive social stress after ischemia. Moreover, overexpression of bcl-2 will attenuate the infracts caused by high level of corticosterone (DeVries et al., 2001). Actually, the survival-promoting effect of CREB might be attributed to its induction of bcl-2 transcription (Finkbeiner, 2000). There is accumulating evidence that CREB is a common target for different classes of antidepressants. Various kinds of antidepressants significantly increase the Phospho-CREB level as well as CREB binding activity in rat hippocampus (Nibuya et al., 1996; Koch et al., 2003). Moreover, the activation of CREB will in turn promote the transcription and synthesis of more BDNF (Riccio et al., 1999).
As discussed above, the serotonergic system is intensely involved in the pathology and treatment of depression (Mattson et al., 2004). It is also widely accepted that 5-HT receptor activation is important for the pharmacotherapeutic effects of antidepressants (Ivy et al., 2003). Actually, there exist interactions between BDNF and serotonin systems (Martinowich and Lu, 2008). A critical pathway following 5-HT stimulation is cAMP/PKA signaling transduction which results in the phosphorylation of CREB (Nestler et al., 2002). Moreover, the CREB activation can induce BDNF transcription and then increase cell proliferation (Tao et al., 1997). Indeed, there is crosstalk between the two pathways: the activation of 5-HT receptors coupled to cAMP production and CREB activation can induce transcription of BDNF gene; on the other hand, increased BDNF synthesis will promote the growth and sprouting of 5-HT neuron axons which can increase the neuronal plasticity and survival (Mamourias et al., 1995). For example, BDNF can promote the neurogenesis of 5-HT neurons (Mamounas et al., 1995) and change the 5-HT receptor expression (Lyons et al., 1999). Moreover, the activation of 5-HT receptors will lead to the phosphorylation of the transcription factor cAMP responsive element binding protein (CREB), which will start the transcription of BDNF (Mattson et al., 2004). All these observations indicate the downregulation of neurotrophic factors might mediate, at least in part, the decreased neurogenesis and structural damage in the stressed brain. Under the "neurogenesis hypothesis", neurtotrophic factors might also serve as promising targets for the treatment of depression.

3. Phytochemicals as antidepressants

3.1 Phytochemicals and serotonergic system

Health benefits associated with Mediterranean diets are due to the large intake of functional plant foods and beverages, i.e., fruits, vegetables, cereals, legumes, nuts, wine, beer, and olive oil, containing a great array of bioactive phytochemicals or nutraceutical compounds. Therefore, the low risk of chronic diseases, such as coronary hearth disease and certain cancers, observed in some population groups, results from a diverse eating style, either in term of foods or food components. The paradigm of the relationship between the chemical diversity of a particular food and the array of its biological activities may be symbolized by grape. Despite the extensive knowledge about phenylpropanoids, principally polyphenols (stilbenes and anthocyanins) and condensed tannins (proanthocyanidins), in grape and wine, little it is known about the other compounds, such as tetrahydro-b-carbolines.

Recently, it has been attached importance to the dietary indoleamines, melatonin, and serotonin, in different plant foods, including grape, thus further supporting the hypothesis that health benefits, associated with Mediterranean dietary style, are due to plant food chemical diversity. Besides, because of plant sessile status, synthesis of phytochemicals represents a major strategy for counteracting unfavorable conditions, in terms of natural selection, biological evolution, and biodiversity.

Plant natural products can be roughly ascribed to three main classes of compounds, phenylpropanoids, isoprenoids, and alkaloids, widely distributed in plant foods and medicinal herbs (Facchini, 2001; Holstein and Hohl, 2004; Iriti and Faoro, 2004). Polyphenolic phytochemicals, which are active components found in many medicinal plants and regulate a variety of enzymes as well as cell receptors, are a group of plant secondary metabolites characterized by the presence of more than one phenolic unit which is linked directly to the aromatic rings (Bravo, 1998). These compounds are categorized by the number of phenol rings as well as the structural elements linked between the rings. The major classes include phenolic acids, flavonoids, stilbenes and lignans (Manach et al., 2004). A growing number of researchers have shown interests in polyphenolic phytochemicals. The major reasons include their antioxidative effects and potentials in preventing oxidative stress-induced diseases, such as neurodegenerative diseases and cancer (Scalbert et al., 2005).

Curcuma longa, one of the most extensively studied phytochemicals, is a major constituent of many traditional Chinese medicines, such as Xiaoyao-san, and has been used widely in Asian countries to manage mental disorders effectively. Curcumin is a major active component of C. longa and its antidepressant-like effect has been previously demonstrated in animal models of depression such as the forced swimming test (Xu et al., 2005) and chronic unpredictable mild stress modle (Li et a., 2009). Moreover, the antidepressant effect of curcumin can be potentiated by various kinds of antidepressants when given jointly, such as fluoxetine, venlafaxine, and bupropion. Enhanced serotonin level has also been found in mice after curcumin administration (Kulkarni et al., 2008). The concomitant administration of curcumin and piperine, a bioavailability enhancer, showed a significantly enhanced level of serotonin (Bhutani et al., 2009). Wang et al., also demonstrated that the antidepressant effect of curcumin in the forced swimming test may involve 5-HT receptors, especially 5-HT1A/1B and 5-HT_{2C} subtypes (Wang et al., 2008). The recent study also showed that curcumin attenuated the stress-induced decrease in 5-HT_{1A} mRNA level in rat hippocampus (Xu et al., 2007).

Resveratrol is a key antioxidant that present in grapes and red wine. The trans-resveratrol, as the active component of *Polygonum cuspidatum* which is traditionally used to treat neropsychiatric disorders in Asia countries, has been studied for anti-inflammation, amelioration of learning and memory impairment, and neuroprotection (Tredici et al., 1999; Chen et al., 2007; Kumar et al., 2007; Ranney and Petro, 2009). The recent studies have already shown the inhibitory effects of resveratrol on noradrenaline and 5-HT uptake activity in rats (Yáñez et al., 2006). Moreover, significantly decreased immobility time in mouse model of despair tests as well as the enhanced levels of serotonin and noradrenaline in brain regions have been demonstrated after trans-resveratrol application (Xu et al., 2010). The reduced activity of MAO, which catalyze the oxidative deamination of dietary amines and monoamine neurotransmitters, such as 5-HT, have been shown in both in vivo and in vitro experiments (Mazzio et al., 1998; Xu et al., 2010). All these data indicate the antidepressive effect of Resveratrol.

Proanthocyanidins, known as oligonols (catechin-type monomers, dimmers and trimmers) and oligomeric proanthocyanidins (oligomers), exists commonly in plants, such as grape seeds (DalBó et al., 2006). People have shown that proanthocyanidins have a wide range of pharmacological activities, including antioxidant effect, antinociceptive and cardioprotective properties (Preuss et al., 2000; Uchida et al., 2008; Sato et al., 2001). Recently, Xu et al. have shown that proanthocyanidin can reduce the duration of immobility in both tail suspension and forced swimming test. Moreover, significantly enhanced 5-HT concentrations were found in frontal cortex, hippocampus and hypothalamus of mice after the proanthocyanidin administration (Xu et al., 2010). However, the mechanisms underlying the antidepressant effect of proanthocyanidin is still not clear.

3.2 Phytochemicals and neurotrophic mechanisms

The emerging neurotrophic hypothesis of antidepressant actions suggests that the stress-induced BDNF reduction could, at least in part, induce the structural damage as well as the reduced neurogenesis, and most antidepressant treatment share the effect of increasing BDNF and neurogenesis, which might be via downstream mechanisms (Duman et al., 1997; Duman, 2004). Through cAMP-PKA and IP3-Ca^{2+} dependent protein kinase secondary messenger systems, CREB can be regulated by 5-HT receptors (Duman, 1998; Rajkumar and Mahesh, 2008). The activation of CREB will start the BDNF transcription, which leads to the activation of downstream cascades including Ras-Raf-ERK and PI-3K/AKT via the TrkB receptor (Berton and Nestler, 2006). Accordingly, the chronic treatment of antidepressants increases cell proliferation and neurogenesis, accompanied with enhanced phosphorylated CREB (Sasaki et al. 2007; Li et al., 2009).

A number of researches have suggested that phytochemicals are neuroprotective. In the transient middle cerebral artery occlusion animal model, Cyanidin-3-O-beta-D-glucopyranoside extracted from mulberry extract showed a neuroprotective effect against the brain injury (Kang et al., 2006). Low concentration of (–)-epigallocatechin-3-gallate from green tea can reduce the neuronal cell death in serum-starved cells, and promote the neurite outgrowth (Reznichenko et al, 2005). Low dose of curcumin has been shown to activate the ERK signaling and enhance the neurogenesis in adult hippocampus, which indicates its capability to enhance neural plasticity and repair (Kim et al., 2008b). The oral administration of 10 and 20 mg/kg curcumin to mice can prevent the stress-induced decrease of BDNF level in hippampus and enhance the hippocampal neurogenesis, which suggests that curcumin might protect hippocampal neurons from further damage in response to chronic stress via up-regulating BDNF in hippocampus (Xu et al., 2007). Curcumin application also prevents the cultured rodent cortex cells against glutamate excitotoxicity (Wang et al., 2008). Recently, it has been demonstrated in the chronic unpredictable mild stress (CUMS) rats, curcumin was also able to improve the CREB activity (Li et al., 2009). More importantly, studies have also shown that curcumin exerts the neuroprotective effects via BDNF/TrkB-mediated PI-3K/Akt and MAPK/Erk cascades, and thus stimulating the transcription factor CREB (Wang et al., 2008; Wang et al., 2010).

It has been reported that resveratrol and its methylated derivertives exhibit neuroprotective effects in SH-SY5Y cells against parkinsonian mimetic 6-hydroxydopamine (6-OHDA)-induced neurotoxicity (Chao et al., 2010). Pretreatment of resveratrol has been shown to provide neuroprotection in animal models of cerebral ischemia (Della-Morte et al., 2009), which might be mediated through NMDA and estrogen receptor (Saleh et al., 2010). Moreover, Piceatannol (3,4,3',5'-tetrahydroxy-*trans*-stilbene) isolated from the seeds of

Euphorbia lagascae, is a metabolite of resveratrol existing in grapes and red wine (Ferrigni et al., 1984; Larrosa et al., 2004). Previous studies have shown that piceatannol exhibited protective effect against Aβ-induced neuronal cell death in cultured PC-12 cells (Kim et al., 2008). The following studies further demonstrated that the neuroprotective effect against oxidative stress is likely due to the inhibition on JNK (Kim et al., 2008) or c-Jun N-terminal kinase activity (Jang et al., 2009). Although the mechanisms of the neuroprotective effects of resveratrol and piceatannol are still unclear, their diverse pharmacological properties have already attracted wide attention.

Fisetin (3,3′,4′7′-tetrahydroxylflavone) is a flavonoid which exists in many plants and foods, such as strawberries (Arai et al., 2000). Recently, people have demonstrated that fisetin can protect neuronal cells from oxidative stress induced cell death, and demonstrate neurotrophic effect of improving the differentiation of PC-12 cells (Ishige et al., 2001), which might depend on the activation of ERK signaling pathway (Sagara et al., 2004). Moreover, the recent studies found that fisetin can facilitate long-term memory in rats, which is mediated via ERK signaling and the CREB phosphorylation (Maher et al., 2006). All these data indicate that fisetin has neurotrophic effect and can promote cell proliferation, and therefore it may be useful in treating mental disorders, including depression.

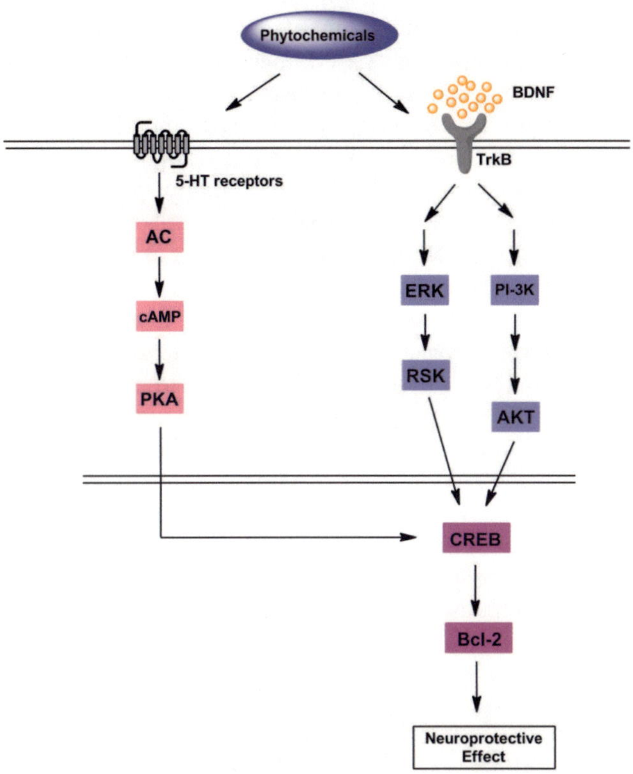

Fig. 1. Neuroprotective pathways targeted by phytochemicals. The activated BDNF receptor TrkB will initiate ERK and PI-3K signaling pathways. 5-HT receptors, which are usually coupled to G proteins, will activate the AC/PKA cascade. Phytochemicals can stimulate both 5-HT and BDNF signaling cascades which interweave and result in activation of CREB, and thus exert their neuroprotective effects.

Ferulic acid (4-hydroxy-3-methoxycinnamic acid; FA) is an ample phenolic phytochemical found in plant components (Srinivasan et al., 2007). Ferulic acid has been reported to have a number of pharmacological activities including antioxidative, anti-inflammatory, anti-cancer, anti-diabetic, anti-atherogenic and neuroprotective effects (Mukhopadhyay et al., 1982; Kawabata et al., 2000; Balasubashini et al., 2004; Kim and Kim, 2000; Yogeeta et al., 2006). Ferulic acid can prevent neurons from Aβ-induced cell death, which is associated with its antioxidative activity (Sultana et al., 2005; Picone et al., 2007). The recent studies found that oral administration of ferulic acid can attenuate the stress-induced behavior in the depression-like model mice. Moreover, treatment of ferulic acid can increase the CREB phophorylation. Accordingly, BDNF mRNA level in the hippocampus is also enhanced (Yabe et al., 2010). Although the molecular mechanisms of the antidepressant effect of ferulic acid still needs to be clarified, the current result indicated its therapeutic potential in the treatment of depressive disorder.

4. Future directions

It is widely accepted that phytochemicals are neuroprotective. The actions of the antidepressive effects of phytochemicals appear to involve many mechanisms, including monoamine neurotransmitters-based mechanism, HPA axis-based mechamism, and neurotrophic factors, or neurogenesis, based mechanisms. All these effects seem to be associated with the activation of the signaling cascades in brain, which can trigger a number of responses, such as promoting the neuronal survival and differentiation and inhibiting neuronal apoptosis. Despite the great advances in our understanding of depression, little is known about the antidepressant mechanisms of many phytochemicals because their antidepressant effects always involve multiple complex mechanisms. Therefore, it is very important to identify the bio-molecules and signaling network that can be specifically regulated by individual phytochemical.

There are many advantages of phytochemicals in regard to application to development of antidepressants. For instance, phytochemicals are natural products, or even isolated from some herbal medicines, so they can be readily moved to the clinical trials on humans. Moreover, chemical analogues of the druggable phytochemcals can be developed for better bioavailability and lower toxicity. However, although the consensus is developing that phytochemcals are potential antidepressant candidates, our understanding and knowledge of the active phytochemicals as well as their mechanisms of actions are limited. It is therefore of critical need to develop high-throughput assays to identify antidepressive phytochemicals. Further *in vivo* and *in vitro* studies are required to reveal in more details about the antidepressive mechanisms of phytochemcals.

5. References

Akiskal HS. Mood disorders: introduction and overview. In: Comprehensive Textbook of Psychiatry. B.J. Sadock and V.A. Sadock, (eds). Lippincott, Williams & Wilkins, 2000. 1284-1298.

Amargós-Bosch M, Bortolozzi A, Puig MV, Serrats J, Adell A, Celada P, Toth M, Mengod G, Artigas F. Co-expression and in vivo interaction of serotonin1A and serotonin2A receptors in pyramidal neurons of prefrontal cortex, Cereb. Cortex 2004; 14, 281–299.

Arai Y, Watanabe S, Kimira M, Shimoi K, Mochizuki R, Kinae N. Dietary intakes of flavonols, flavones and isoflavones by Japanese women and the inverse correlation between quercetin intake and plasma LDL cholesterol concentration. J Nutr. 2000;130(9):2243-2250.

Azmitia BC, Whitaker-Azmitia PM. Development and adult plasticity of serotoninergic nevirons and their target cells. In: Baumgarten HG, Gothert M, editors. Handbook of experimental pharmacology. Berlin: Springer; 1997; 1-39.

Baker CB., Johnsrud MT., Crismon ML, Rosenheck RA, Woods SW. Quantitative analysis of sponsorship bias in economic studies of antidepressants. Br. J. Psychiatry. 2003; 183, 498-506.

Balasubashini MS, Rukkumani R, Viswanathan P, Menon VP. Ferulic acid alleviates lipid peroxidation in diabetic rats. Phytother Res. 2004;18(4):310-314.

Bambico FR, Nguyen NT, Gobbi G. Decline in serotonergic firing activity and desensitization of 5-HT1A autoreceptors after chronic unpredictable stress. Eur Neuropsychopharmacol. 2009;19(3):215-228.

Banasr M, Hery M, Printemps R, Daszuta A. Serotonin-induced increases in adult cell proliferation and neurogenesis are mediated through different and common 5-HT receptor subtypes in the dentate gryus and the subventricular zone. Neuropsychopharmacology. 2004;29(3):450-460.

Barden N. Regulation of corticosteroid receptor gene expression in depression and antidepressant action. J. Psychiatry Neurosci. 1999; 24, 25-39.

Barnes NM, Sharp T. A review of central 5-HT receptors and their function, Neuropharmacology 1999; 38: 1083–1152.

Benjamin D, Lal H, Meyerson LR. The effects of 5-HT1B characterizing agents in the mouse elevated plus-maze. Life Sci. 1990; 47 (3), 195–203.

Berton O, Nestler EJ. New approaches to antidepressant drug discovery: beyond monoamines. Nat. Rev. Neurosci. 2006;7(2):137-151.

Bhagwagar Z, Hinz R, Taylor M, Fancy S, Cowen P, Grasby P.Increased 5-HT(2A) receptor binding in euthymic, medication-free patients recovered from depression: a positron emission study with [(11)C]MDL 100, 907. Am J Psychiatry. 2006;163(9):1580-1587.

Bhagwagar Z, Murthy N, Selvaraj S, Hinz R, Taylor M, Fancy S, Grasby P, Cowen P. 5-HTT binding in recovered depressed patients and healthy volunteers: a positron emission tomography study with [11C] DASB. Am J Psychiatry. 2007;164(12):1858-1865.

Bhutani MK, Bishnoi M, Kulkarni SK. Anti-depressant like effect of curcumin and its combination with piperine in unpredictable chronic stress-induced behavioral, biochemical and neurochemical changes. Pharmacol Biochem Behav. 2009;92(1):39-43.

Blier, P., Lista, A., De Montigny, C., Differential properties of pre- and postsynaptic 5-hydroxytryptamine1A receptors in the dorsal raphe and hippocampus: II. Effect of pertussis and cholera toxins. J. Pharmacol. Exp. Ther. 1993; 265, 16–23.

Boothman LJ, Mitchell SN, Sharp T. Investigation of the SSRI augmentation properties of 5-HT2 receptor antagonists using in vivo microdialysis. Neuropharmacology 2006; 50, 726–732.

Bravo L. Polyphenols: chemistry, dietary sources, metabolism, and nutritional significance. Nutr Rev. 1998;56(11):317-33.

Butler MO, Morinobu S, Duman RS. Chronic electroconvulsive seizures increase the expression of serotonin2 receptor mRNA in rat frontal cortex. J Neurochem 1993; 61:1270-1276.

Burnet PW, Michelson D, Smith MA, Gold PW, Sternberg EM. The effect of chronic imipramine administration on the densities of 5-HT_{1A} and 5-HT_2 receptors and the abundances of 5-HT receptor and transporter mRNA in the cortex, hippocampus and dorsal raphe of three strains of rat. Brain Res 1994; 638: 311-324.

Caspi A, Moffitt TE. Gene-environment interactions in psychiatry: joining forces with neuroscience. Nat. Rev. Neurosci. 2006; 7, 583-590.

Celada P, Puig MV, Casanovas JM, Guillazo G, Artigas F. Control of dorsal raphe serotonergic neurons by the medial prefrontal cortex: Involvement of serotonin-1A, GABA(A), and glutamate receptors. J Neurosci. 2001;21(24):9917-9929.

Centeno VA, Volosin M. Chronic treatment with desipramine: effect on endocrine and behavioral responses induced by inescapable stress. Physiol. Behav. 1997; 62, 939-944.

Chang YC, Rapoport SI, Rao JS. Chronic administration of mood stabilizers upregulates BDNF and bcl-2 expression levels in rat frontal cortex. Neurochem Res. 2009;34(3):536-541

Chao J, Li H, Cheng KW, Yu MS, Chang RC, Wang M. Protective effects of pinostilbene, a resveratrol methylated derivative, against 6-hydroxydopamine-induced neurotoxicity in SH-SY5Y cells. J Nutr Biochem.2010;21(6):482-489.

Chen B, Dowlatshahi D, MacQueen GM, Wang JF, Young LT. Increased hippocampal BDNF immunoreactivity in subjects treated with antidepressant medication. Biol Psychiatry. 2001;50(4):260-265.

Chen G, Huang LD, Jiang YM, Manji HK. The mood-stabilizing agent valproate inhibits the activity of glycogen synthase kinase-3. J Neurochem. 1999;72(3):1327-1330.

Chen G, Manji HK. The extracellular signal-regulated kinase pathway: an emerging promising target for mood stabilizers. Curr Opin Psychiatry. 2006;19(3):313-323.

Chen LW, Wang YQ, Wei LC, Shi M, Chan YS. Chinese herbs and herbal extracts for neuroprotection of dopaminergic neurons and potential therapeutic treatment of Parkinson's disease. CNS Neurol Disord Drug Targets. 2007;6(4):273-281.

Chen MJ, Nguyen TV, Pike CJ, Russo-Neustadt AA. Norepinephrine induces BDNF and activates the PI-3K and MAPK cascades in embryonic hippocampal neurons. Cell Signal. 2007;19(1):114-128.

Clark MS, Sexton TJ, McClain M, Root D, Kohen R, Neumaier JF. Overexpression of 5-HT1B receptor in dorsal raphe nucleus using Herpes Simplex Virus gene transfer increases anxiety. J Neurosci. 2002; 22(11):4550-4562.

Cornelisse LN, Van der Harst JE, Lodder JC, Baarendse PJ, Timmerman AJ, Mansvelder HD, Spruijt BM, Brussaard AB. Reduced 5-HT1A and GABAB receptor function in dorsal raphe neurons upon chronic fluoxetine treatment of socially stressed rats. J. Neurophysiol., 2007; 98, 196-204.

Conti AC, Cryan JF, Dalvi A, Lucki I, Blendy JA. cAMP response element-binding protein is essential for the upregulation of brain-derived neurotrophic factor transcription, but not the behavioral or endocrine responses to antidepressant drugs. J Neurosci. 2002;22(8):3262-3268.

Cryan JF, Leonard BE. 5-HT1A and beyond: the role of serotonin and its receptors in depression and the antidepressant response. Hum. Psychopharmacol. 2000; 15, 113–135.

Cryan JF, Lucki I. Antidepressant-like behavior effects mediated by 5-hydroxytryptamine (2C) receptors. J. Pharmacol. Exp. Ther. 2000; 295, 1120–1126.

Cryan JF, Valentino RJ, Lucki I. Assessing substrates underlying the behavioral effects of antidepressants using the modified rat forced swimming test. Neurosci. Biobehav. Rev. 2005; 29, 547–569.

Dahlström A, Fuxe K, Localization of monoamines in the lower brain stem, Experientia. 1964; 20: 398–399.

DalBó S, Jürgensen S, Horst H, Soethe DN, Santos AR, Pizzolatti MG, Ribeiro-do-Valle RM. Analysis of the antinociceptive effect of the proanthocyanidin-rich fraction obtained from Croton celtidifolius barks: evidence for a role of the dopaminergic system. Pharmacol Biochem Behav 2006;85:317–323.

Davis KL, Charney D, Coyle JT, Nemeroff CB. (Eds.), Neuropsychopharmacology: The Fifth Generation of Progress, 5th ed., Lippinkott Williams & Wilkins, Nashville, 2002.

Della-Morte D, Dave KR, DeFazio RA, Bao YC, Raval AP, Perez-Pinzon MA. Resveratrol pretreatment protects rat brain from cerebral ischemic damage via a sirtuin 1-uncoupling protein 2 pathway. Neuroscience. 2009;159(3):993-1002.

DeVries AC, Joh HD, Bernard O, Hattori K, Hurn PD, Traystman RJ, Alkayed NJ. Social stress exacerbates stroke outcome by suppressing Bcl-2 expression. Proc Natl Acad Sci. 2001; 98(20):11824-11828.

Drevets WC, Frank E, Price JC, Kupfer DJ, Holt D, Greer PJ, Huang Y, Gautier C, Mathis C. PET imaging of serotonin 1A receptor binding in depression. Biol. Psychiatry 1999; 54, 597-606.

Drevets WC. Neuroimaging studies of mood disorders. Biol. Psychiatry 2000; 48, 813-829.

Du J, Gould TD, Manji HK: Neurotrophic signaling in mood disorders; in Finkel T, Gutkind JS (eds): Signal Transduction and Human Disease. Hoboken, Wiley, 2003: 411–446.

Duman RS, Heninger GR & Nestler EJ. A molecular and cellular hypothesis of depression. Arch. Gen. Psychiatry 1997; 54, 597–606.

Duman RS. Novel therapeutic approaches beyond the serotonin receptor. Biol. Psychiary 1998; 44, 324-335.

Duman RS. Structural alterations in depression: cellular mechanism underlying pathology and treatment of mood disorders. CNS Spectr. 2002, 7, 140-142, 144-147.

Duman RS. Role of neurotrophic factors in the etiology and treatment of mood disorders. Neuromolecular Med. 2004; 5, 11–25.

Duman RS, Monteggia LM. A neurotrophic model for stress-related mood disorders. Biol. Psychiatry 2006, 59, 1116–1127.

Facchini PJ. Alkaloid biosynthesis in plants: biochemistry, cell biology, molecular regulation and metabolic engineering. Annu Rev Plant Physiol Plant Mol Biol. 2001; 52:29-66.

Ferretti C, Marinella B, Gamalero SR, Ghi, P. Biochemical and behaviour changes induced by acute stress in a chronic variate stress model of depression: the effect of amitripltyline. Eur. J. Pharmacol. 1995; 280, 19-26.

Ferrigni NR, McLaughlin JL, Powell RG, Smith CR. Use of potato disc and brine shrimp bioassays to detect activity and isolate piceatannol as the antileukemic principle from the seeds of Euphorbia lagascae. J Nat Prod 1984;47:347–352.

Finkbeiner S. CREB couples neurotrophin signals to survival messages. Neuron. 2000; 25(1):11-14.

Gillespie CR, Nemeroff CB. Hypercortisolemia and depression. Psychosom. Med. 2005; 67, S26-S28.

Gould E. Serotonin and hippocampal neurogenesis. Neuropsychopharmacology 1999; 21:46S–51S.

Harfstrand A, Fuxe K, Cintra A, Agnati LF, Zini I, Wikstrom AC, Okret S, Yu ZY, Goldstein M, Steinbusch H, Verhofstad A, Gustafsson JA. Glucocorticoid receptor immunoreactivity in monoaminergic neurons of rat brain. Proc. Natl. Acad. Sci. 1986; 83, 9779-9783.

Hirano K, Yamada S, Kimura R. Effects of fluvoxamine and fluoxetine on 5-HT_{1A} and 5-HT_{2A} receptors in mouse brain. Pharmacol. Rev. Commun. 2002; 12, 215-221.

Holstein SA, Hohl RJ. Isoprenoids: remarkable diversity of form and function. Lipids 2004; 34:293–309.

Inoue T, Tsuchiya K, Koyama T. Regional changes in dopamine and 5-hydroxytryptamine activation with various intensity of physical and psychological stress in rat brain. Pharmacol. Biochem. Behav. 1994, 49, 911-920.

Iriti M, Faoro F. Plant defense and human nutrition: the phenylpropanoids on the menu. Curr. Top. Nutr. Res. 2004; 2:47–65.

Ishige K, Schubert D, Sagara Y. Flavonoids protect neuronal cells from oxidative stress by three distinct mechanisms. Free Radic Biol Med. 2001;30(4):433-446.

Ivy AS, Rodriguez FG, Garcia C, Chen MJ, Russo-Neustadt AA. Noradrenergic and serotonergic blockade inhibits BDNF mRNA activation following exercise and antidepressant. Pharmacol. Biochem. Behav. 2003; 75: 81-88.

Jacobs BL. Adult brain neurogenesis and depression. Brain Behav. Immun. 2002;16:602–609.

Jang YJ, Kim JE, Kang NJ, Lee KW, Lee HJ. Piceatannol attenuates 4-hydroxynonenal-induced apoptosis of PC12 cells by blocking activation of c-Jun N-terminal kinase. Ann N Y Acad Sci. 2009;1171:176-182.

Joëls M, Karst H, Krugers HJ, Lucassen PJ. Chronic stress: implications for neuronal morphology, function and neurogenesis. Front Neuroendocrinol. 2007;28(2-3):72-96.

Kaiyala KJ, Vincow ES, Sexton TJ, Neumaier JF. 5-HT_{1B} receptor mRNA levels in dorsal raphe nucleus: inverse association with anxiety behavior in the elevated plus maze. Pharmacol. Biochem. Behav. 2003, 75 (4), 769–776.

Kang TH, Hur JY, Kim HB, Ryu JH, Kim SY. Neuroprotective effects of the cyanidin-3-O-beta-Dglucopyranoside isolated from mulberry fruit against cerebral ischemia. Neurosci Lett. 2006;391(3):122-126.

Karege F, Perret G, Bondolfi G, Schwald M, Bertschy G, Aubry JM. Decreased serum brain-derived neurotrophic factor levels in major depressed patients. Psychiatry Res. 2002; 109(2):143-148.

Kawabata K, Yamamoto T, Hara A, Shimizu M, Yamada Y, Matsunaga K, Tanaka T, Mori H. Modifying effects of ferulic acid on azoxymethane-induced colon carcinogenesis in F344 rats. Cancer Lett. 2000;157(1):15-21.

Kim HJ, Lee KW, Lee HJ. Protective effects of piceatannol against beta-amyloid-induced neuronal cell death. Ann N Y Acad Sci. 2007;1095:473-82.

Kim HJ, Lee KW, Kim MS, Lee HJ. Piceatannol attenuates hydrogen-peroxide- and peroxynitrite-induced apoptosis of PC12 cells by blocking down-regulation of Bcl-XL and activation of JNK. J Nutr Biochem. 2008a;19(7):459-466.

Kim SJ, Son TG, Park HR, Park M, Kim MS, Kim HS, Chung HY, Mattson MP, Lee J. Curcumin stimulates proliferation of embryonic neural progenitor cells and neurogenesis in the adult hippocampus. J. Biol. Chem. 2008b;283(21):14497-14505.

Kim SR, Kim YC. Neuroprotective phenylpropanoid esters of rhamnose isolated from roots of Scrophularia buergeriana. Phytochemistry. 2000;54(5):503-509.

Klimek V, Zak-Knapik J, Mackowiak M. Effects of repeated treatment with fluoxetine and citalopram, 5-HT uptake inhibitors, on 5-HT1A and 5-HT2 receptors in the rat brain. J. Psychiatry Neurosci. 1994; 19, 63-67.

Knijff EM, Breunis MN, Kupka RW, de Wit HJ, Ruwhof C, Akkerhuis GW, Nolen WA, Drexhage HA. An imbalance in the production of IL-1beta and IL-6 by monocytes of bipolar patients: restoration by lithium treatment. Bipolar Disord. 2007;9(7):743-753.

Koch JM, Kell S, Aldenhoff JB. Differential effects of fluoxetine and imipramine on the phosphorylation of the transcription factor CREB and cell-viability. J. Psychiatr. Res. 2003; 37: 53-59.

Kushwaha N, Albert PR. Coupling of 5-HT1A autoreceptors to inhibition of mitogen-activated protein kinase activation via G beta gamma subunit signaling. Eur. J. Neurosci. 2005; 21, 721-732.

Kulkarni SK, Bhutani MK, Bishnoi M. Antidepressant activity of curcumin: involvement of serotonin and dopamine system. Psychopharmacology (Berl) 2008;201:435-442

Kumar A, Naidu PS, Seghal N, Padi SS. Neuroprotective effects of resveratrol against intracerebroventricular colchicine-induced cognitive impairment and oxidative stress in rats. Pharmacology. 2007;79(1):17-26.

Ishige K, Schubert D, Sagara Y. Flavonoids protect neuronal cells from oxidative stress by three distinct mechanisms. Free Radic Biol Med. 2001;30(4):433-446.

Lanfumey L, Mongeau R, Cohen-Salmon C, Hamon M. Corticosteroid-serotonin interactions in the neurobiological mechanisms of stress-related disorders. Neurosci Biobehav Rev. 2008;32(6):1174-1184.

Larrosa M, Tomas-Barberan FA, Espin JC. The grape and wine polyphenol piceatannol is a potent inducer of apoptosis in human SKMel-28 melanoma cells. Eur J Nutr 2004;43:275–84.

Lauder JM, Wallace JA, Krebs H. Roles for serotonin in neuroembryogenesis. Adv. Exp. Med. Biol. 1981;133:477–506.

Leonard BE, 2005. The HPA and immune axes in stress: the involvement of the serotonergic system. Eur. Psychiatry. 20, S302-306.

Lesch KP, Mayer S, Disselkamp-Tietze J., Hon A., Wiesmann M., Osterheider M., Schulte H.M., 1990. 5-HT1A receptor responsivity in unipolar depression. Evaluation of ipsapirone-induced ACTH and cortisol secretion in patients and controls. Biol. Psychiatry. 1990; 28, 620-628.

Li YC, Wang FM, Pan Y, Qiang LQ, Cheng G, Zhang WY, Kong LD. Antidepressant-like effects of curcumin on serotonergic receptor-coupled AC-cAMP pathway in chronic unpredictable mild stress of rats. Prog Neuropsychopharmacol Biol Psychiatry. 2009;33(3):435-449.

Li YF, Chen HX, Liu Y, Zhang YZ, Liu YQ, Li J. Agmatine increases proliferation of cultured hippocampal progenitor cells and hippocampal neurogenesis in chronically stressed mice. Acta Pharmacol Sin. 2006;27(11):1395-1400

Li YF, Huang Y, Amsdell SL, Xiao L, O'Donnell JM, Zhang HT. Antidepressant- and anxiolytic-like effects of the phosphodiesterase-4 inhibitor rolipram on behavior depend on cyclic AMP response element binding protein-mediated neurogenesis in the hippocampus. Neuropsychopharmacology. 2009;34(11):2404-19.

Lyons WE, Mamounas LA, Ricaurte GA, Coppola V, Reid SW, Bora SH, Wihler C, Koliatsos VE, Tessarollo L. Brain-derived neurotrophic factor-deficient mice develop aggressiveness and hyperphagia in conjunction with brain serotonergic abnormalities. Proc. Natl. Acad. Sci. 1999; 96, 15239-15244.

Maher P, Akaishi T, Abe K. Flavonoid fisetin promotes ERK-dependent longterm potentiation and enhances memory. Proc Natl Acad Sci. 2006;103(44):16568-73.

Mamounas LA, Altar CA, Blue ME, Kaplan DR, Tessarollo L, Lyons WE. BDNF promotes the survival and sprouting of serotonergic axons in the rat brain. J. Neurosci., 1995; 15, 7929-7939.

Manji HK, Lenox RH. The nature of bipolar disorder. J Clin Psychiatry. 2000;61 Supp 13:42-57.

Manach C, Scalbert A, Morand C, Rémésy C, Jiménez L. Polyphenols: food sources and bioavailability. Am J Clin Nutr.2004; 79(5):727-47.

Martín-Ruiz R, Puig MV, Celada P, Shapiro DA, Roth BL, Mengod G, Artigas F. Control of serotonergic function in medial prefrontal cortex by serotonin-2A receptors through a glutamate-dependent mechanism. J Neurosci. 2001; 21(24):9856-9866.

Martinowich K, Lu B. Interaction between BDNF and serotonin: role in mood disorders. Neuropsychopharmacology 2008; 33: 73-83.

Mattson MP, Maudsley S, Martin B. BDNF and 5-HT: a dynamic duo in age-related neuronal plasticity and neurodegenerative disorders. Trends Neurosci. 2004; 27(10):589-594.

Mazzio EA, Harris N, Soliman KF. Food constituents attenuate monoamine oxidase activity and peroxide levels in C6 astrocyte cells. Planta Med. 1998;64(7):603-606.

McEwen BS, Stellar E. Stress and the individual. Mechanisms leading to disease. Arch. Intern. Med. 1993; 153, 2093-2101.

McEwen BS. The neurobiology of stress: from serendipity to clinical relevance. Brain Res. 2000; 886, 172–189.

Meijer WE, Heerdink ER, Nolen WA, Herings RM, Leufkens HG, Egberts AC. Association of risk of abnormal bleeding with degree of serotonin reuptake inhibition by antidepressants. Arch. Intern. Med. 2004; 164, 2367-2370.

Millan MJ, Marin P, Bockaert J, Mannoury la Cour C. Signaling at G-protein-coupled serotonin receptors: recent advances and future research directions. Trends Pharmacol Sci. 2008;29(9):454-464.

Mukhopadhyay A, Basu N, Ghatak N, Gujral PK. Anti-inflammatory and irritant activities of curcumin analogues in rats. Agents Actions. 1982;12(4):508-515.

Nestler EJ, Barrot M, DiLeone RJ, Eisch AJ, Gold SJ, Monteggia LM. Neurobiology of depression. Neuron 2002; 34, 13-15.

Nishi K, Kanemaru K, Diksic M. A genetic rat model of depression, Flinders sensitive line has a lower density of 5-HT_{1A} receptors, but a higher density of 5-HT1B receptors, compared to control rats. Neurochem. Int. 2009; 54 (5–6), 299–307.

Nibuya M, Nestler EJ, Duman RS. Chronic antidepressant administration increases the expression of cAMP response element binding protein (CREB) in rat hippocampus. J Neurosci. 1996;16(7):2365-72.

Nibuya M, Morinobu S, Duman RS. Regulation of BDNF and trkB mRNA in rat brain by chronic electroconvulsive seizure and antidepressant drug treatments. J Neurosci 1995; 15: 7539 -7547.

O'Connor JJ, Rowan MJ, Anwyl R. Long-lasting enhancement of NMDA receptor-mediated synaptic transmission by metabotropic glutamate receptor activation. Nature 1994; 367 (6463): 557–559.

O'Neill MF, Conway MW. Role of 5-HT1A and 5-HT1B receptors in the mediation of behavior in the forced swim test in mice. Neuropsy- chopharmacology 2001; 24, 391–398.

Paizanis E, Kelaï S, Renoir T, Hamon M, Lanfumey L. Life-long hippocampal neurogenesis: environmental, pharmacological and neurochemical modulations. Neurochem. Res. 2007; 32, 1762–1771.

Picone P, Bondi ML, Montana G, Bruno A, Pitarresi G, Giammona G, Di Carlo M. Ferulic acid inhibits oxidative stress and cell death induced by Ab oligomers: improved delivery by solid lipid nanoparticles. Free Radic Res. 2009; 43(11):1133-1145.

Preuss HG, Wallerstedt D, Talpur N, Tutuncuoglu SO, Echard B, Myers A, et al. Effects of niacin-bound chromium and grape seed proanthocyanidin extract on the lipid profile of hypercholesterolemic subjects: a pilot study. J Med 2000; 31:227–246.

Porter RJ, Gallagher P, Watson S, Young AH. 2004. Corticosteroid-serotonin interactions in depression: a review of the human evidence. Psychopharmacology (Berl). 2004;173(1-2):1-17

Puig MV, Celada P, Díaz-Mataix L, Artigas F. In vivo modulation of the activity of pyramidal neurons in the rat medial prefrontal cortex by 5-HT2A receptors: relationship to thalamocortical afferents. Cereb Cortex. 2003;13(8):870-882.

Radley JJ, Jacobs BL. 5-HT1A receptor antagonist administration decreases cell proliferation in the dentate gyrus. Brain Res 2002;955:264–267.

Rajkumar R, Mahesh R. Assessing the neuronal serotonergic target-based antidepressant stratagem: impact of in vivo interaction studies and knockout models. Curr Neuropharmacol. 2008;6(3):215-234.

Ranney A, Petro MS. Petro, Resveratrol protects spatial learning in middle-aged C57BL/6 mice from effects of ethanol. Behav Pharmacol. 2009;20(4):330-336.

Rapport MM, Green AA, Page IH., Crystalline Serotonin. Science. 1948; 108(2804):329-330.

Reznichenko, L., Amit, T., Youdim, M. B. and Mandel, S. Green tea polyphenol (-)-epigallocatechin-3-gallate induces neurorescue of long-term serum-deprived PC12 cells and promotes neurite outgrowth. J. Neurochem. 2005; 93, 1157–1167.

Redrobe JP, Bourin M. Partial role of 5-HT2 and 5-HT3 receptors in the activity of antidepressants in the mouse forced swimming test. Eur. J. Pharmacol. 1997; 325, 129–135.

Redrobe JP, Bourin M. Clonidine potentiates the effects of 5-HT1A, 5-HT1B and 5-HT2A/2C receptor antagonists and 8-OH-DPAT in the mouse forced swimming test. Eur. Neuropsychopharm. 1998; 8, 169–173.

Reul JM, de Kloet ER. Anatomical resolution of two types of corticosterone receptor sites in rat brain with in vitro autoradiography and computerized image analysis. J. Steroid Biochem. 1986; 24, 269-272.

Riedel W, Klaassen T, Griez E, Honig A, Menheere P, Van Praag HM, 2002. Dissociable hormonal, cognitive and mood responses to neuroendocrine challenge: evidence for receptor-specific serotonergic dysregulation in depressed mood. Neuropsychopharmacology. 26, 358-367.

Reinés A, Cereseto M, Ferrero A, Sifonios L, Podestá MF, Wikinski S. Maintenance treatment with fluoxetine is necessary to sustain normal levels of synaptic markers in an experimental model of depression: correlation with behavioral response. Neuropsychopharmacology 2008; 33, 1896-1908.

Riccio A, Ahn S, Davenport CM, Blendy JA, Ginty DD (1999). Mediation by a CREB family transcription factor of NGF-dependent survival of sympathetic neurons. Science 286: 2358–2361.

Sagara Y, Vanhnasy J, Maher P. Maher, Induction of PC12 cell differentiation by flavonoids is dependent upon extracellular signal-regulated kinase activation. J Neurochem. 2004;90(5):1144-1155.

Saleh MC, Connell BJ, Saleh TM. Resveratrol preconditioning induces cellular stress proteins and is mediated via NMDA and estrogen receptors. Neuroscience. 2010; 166(2):445-454.

Santarelli L, Saxe M, Gross C, Surget A, Battaglia C, Dulawa S, et al. Requirement of hippocampal neurogenesis for the behavioral effects of antidepressants. Eur J Pharmacol 2003; 301:805–809.

Sari Y. Serotonin1B receptors: from protein to physiological function and behavior. Neurosci. Biobehav. Rev. 2004; 28 (6), 565–582.

Sapolsky RM. Taming stress. Sci. Am. 2003; 289: 86-95.

Sasaki T, Kitagawa K, Omura-Matsuoka E, Todo K, Terasaki Y, Sugiura S, Hatazawa J, Yagita Y, Hori M. The phosphodiesterase inhibitor rolipram promotes survival of newborn hippocampal neurons after ischemia. Stroke 2007; 38:1597–1605.

Sato M, Bagchi D, Tosaki A, Das DK. Grape seed proanthocyanidin reduces cardiomyocyte apoptosis by inhibiting ischemia/reperfusion-induced activation of JNK-1 and C-JUN. Free Radic Biol Med 2001;31:729–737.

Saudou F, Amara DA, Dierich A, LeMeur M, Ramboz S, Segu L, Buhot MC, Hen R. Enhanced aggressive behavior in mice lacking 5-HT1B receptor. Science 1994; 265 (5180), 1875–1878.

Scalbert A, Manach C, Morand C, Rémésy C, Jiménez L. Dietary polyphenols and the prevention of diseases. Crit Rev Food Sci Nutr. 2005;45(4):287-306.

Schechter LE, Ring RH, Beyer CE, Hughes ZA, Khawaja X, Malberg JE, Rosenzweig-Lipson S. Innovative approaches for the development of antidepressant drugs: current and future strategies. J. Am. Soc. Exp. Neurother. 2005; 2, 590-611.

Siuciak JA, Altar CA, Wiegand SJ, Lindsay RM. Antinociceptive effect of brain-derived neurotrophic factor and neurotrophin-3. Brain Res. 1994;633(1-2):326-30.

Spurlock G, Buckland P, O'Donovan M, McGuffin P. Lack of the effect of antidepressant drugs on the levels of mRNAs encoding serotonergic receptors, synthetic enzymes and 5-HT transporter. Neuropharmacology 1994; 33:433-440.

Srinivasan M, Sudheer AR, Menon VP. Ferulic Acid: therapeutic potential through its antioxidant property. J Clin Biochem Nutr. 2007;40(2):92-100.

Soares JC, Mann JJ. The functional neuroanatomy of mood disorders. J. Psychiatr. Res. 1997; 31, 393–432.

Subhash MN, Jagadeesh S. Imipramine-induced changes in 5-HT2 receptor sites and inositoltrisphosphate levels in rat brain., 1997. Neurochem Res. 22, 1095-1099.

Sultana R, Ravagna A, Mohmmad-Abdul H, Calabrese V, Butterfield DA. Ferulic acid ethyl ester protects neurons against amyloid beta- peptide(1-42)-induced oxidative stress and neurotoxicity: relationship to antioxidant activity. J Neurochem. 2005 Feb;92(4):749-758.

Tao X, Finkbeiner S, Arnold DB, Shaywitz AJ, Greenberg ME. Calcium influx regulates BDNF transcription by a CREB family transcription factor-dependent mechanism. Neuron 1997; 20: 709–726.

Tatarczynska, E., Klodzinska, A., Chojnacka-Wojcik, E. Effects of combined administration of 5-HT1A and/or 5-HT1B receptor antagonists and paroxetine or fluoxetine in the forced swimming test in rats. Pol. J. Pharmacol. 2002; 54, 615-623.

Toth M, Shenk T. Antagonist-mediated down-regulation of 5-hydroxytryptamine type 2 receptor gene expression: modulation of transcription. Mol. Pharmacol., 1994; 45, 1095-1100.

Tredici G, Miloso M, Nicolini G, Galbiati S, Cavaletti G, Bertelli A. Resveratrol, map kinases and neuronal cells: might wine be a neuroprotectant? Drugs Exp Clin Res. 1999; 25(2-3):99-103.

Tsuji M, Takeda H, Matsumiya T. Protective effects of 5-HT1A receptor agonists against emotional changes produced by stress stimuli are related to their neuroendocrine effects. Br. J. Pharmacol. 2001; 134, 585-595.

Uchida S, Hirai K, Hatanaka J, Hanato J, Umegaki K, Yamada S. Antinociceptive effects of St. John's wort, Harpagophytum procumbens extract and grape seed proanthocyanidins extract in mice. Biol Pharm Bull 2008;31:240–245.

Walther DJ, Peter JU, Bashammakh S, Hörtnagl H, Voits M, Fink H, Bader M. Synthesis of serotonin by a second tryptophan hydroxylase isoform. Science. 2003;299(5603):76

Warner-Schmidt JL, Duman RS. Hippocampal neurogenesis: opposing effects of stress and antidepressant treatment. Hippocampus 2006; 16, 239–249.

Wang R, Xu Y, Wu HL, Li YB, Li YH, Guo JB, Li XJ. The antidepressant effects of curcumin in the forced swimming test involve 5-HT1 and 5-HT2 receptors. Eur J Pharmacol. 2008; 578(1):43-50

Wang R, Li YB, Li YH, Xu Y, Wu HL, Li XJ. Curcumin protects against glutamate excitotoxicity in rat cerebral cortical neurons by increasing brain-derived neurotrophic factor level and activating TrkB. Brain Res. 2008;1210:84-91.

Wang R, Li YH, Xu Y, Li YB, Wu HL, Guo H, Zhang JZ, Zhang JJ, Pan XY, Li XJ. Curcumin produces neuroprotective effects via activating brain-derived neurotrophic factor/TrkB-dependent MAPK and PI-3K cascades in rodent cortical neurons. Prog Neuropsychopharmacol Biol Psychiatry. 2010;34(1):147-153.

Welner SA, De Montigny C, Desroches J, Desjardins P, Suranyi-Cadotte BE. Autoradiographic quantification of serotonin 1A receptors in rat brain following antidepressant drug treatment. Synapse 1989; 4:347–352.

Whitaker-Azmitia PM. Role of serotonin and other neurotransmitter receptors in brain development: basis for developmental pharmacology. Pharmacol Rev. 1991; 43(4):553-561.

Xu Y, Ku BS, Yao HY, Lin YH, Ma X, Zhang YH, Li XJ. Antidepressant effects of curcumin in the forced swim test and olfactory bulbectomy models of depression in rats. Pharmacol Biochem Behav. 2005;82(1):200-206.

Xu Y, Ku B, Cui L, Li X, Barish PA, Foster TC, Ogle WO. Curcumin reverses impaired hippocampal neurogenesis and increases serotonin receptor 1A mRNA and brain-derived neurotrophic factor expression in chronically stressed rats. Brain Res. 2007;1162:9-18.

Xu Y, Ku B, Tie L, Yao H, Jiang W, Ma X, Li X. Curcumin reverses the effects of chronic stress on behavior, the HPA axis, BDNF expression and phospphorylation of CREB. Brain Res. 2006; 1122: 56-64.

Xu Y, Li S, Chen R, Li G, Barish PA, You W, Chen L, Lin M, Ku B, Pan J, Ogle WO. Antidepressant-like effect of low molecular proanthocyanidin in mice: involvement of monoaminergic system. Pharmacol Biochem Behav. 2010; 94(3):447-53.

Xu Y, Wang Z, You W, Zhang X, Li S, Barish PA, Vernon MM, Du X, Li G, Pan J, Ogle WO. Antidepressant-like effect of trans-resveratrol: Involvement of serotonin and noradrenaline system. Eur Neuropsychopharmacol. 2010; 20(6):405-13.

Yabe T, Hirahara H, Harada N, Ito N, Nagai T, Sanagi T, Yamada H. Ferulic acid induces neural progenitor cell proliferation in vitro and in vivo. Neuroscience. 2010; 165(2):515-24.

Yáñez M, Fraiz N, Cano E, Orallo F. Inhibitory effects of cis- and trans-resveratrol on noradrenaline and 5-hydroxytryptamine uptake and on monoamine oxidase activity. Biochem Biophys Res Commun. 2006; 344(2):688-95.

Yogeeta SK, Gnanapragasam A, Kumar SS, Subhashini R, Sathivel A, Devaki T. Synergistic interactions of ferulic acid with ascorbic acid: its cardioprotective role during isoproterenol induced myocardial infarction in rats. Mol Cell Biochem. 2006;283(1-2):139-146.

Young EA, Haskett RF, Murphy-Weihberg V, Watson SJ, Akil H. Loss of glucocorticoid fast feed back in depression. Arch. Gen. Psychiatry. 1991; 48, 693-699.